YOUR
MONEY
&
YOUR
HEALTH

JORDAN BRAVERMAN, MPH

YOUR MONEY & YOUR HEALTH

How to Find Affordable, High-Quality Healthcare

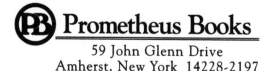

Prometheus Books

59 John Glenn Drive
Amherst, New York 14228-2197

Published 2006 by Prometheus Books

Inquiries should be addressed to
Prometheus Books
59 John Glenn Drive
Amherst, New York 14228–2197
VOICE: 716–691–0133, ext. 207
FAX: 716–564–2711
WWW.PROMETHEUSBOOKS.COM

10 09 08 07 06   5 4 3 2 1

Library of Congress Cataloging-in-Publication Data

Braverman, Jordan.
    Your money and your health : how to find affordable, high-quality healthcare / by Jordan Braverman.
        p. cm.
    Includes bibliographical references and index.
    ISBN 1–59102–393–9 (pbk. : alk. paper)
    ISBN 978–1–59102–393–7
    1. Medical care, Cost of—United States. 2. Medical care—United States.
3. Consumer education—United States. 4. Patient education—United States. I. Title.

RA410.53.B734 2006
338.4'33621—dc22

                                                                                            2005035127

Printed in the United States of America on acid-free paper

To my parents, Morris and Molly Braverman,
who taught my brother, Irwin, and me
that good health is the true wealth of life

The Most Precious Gift

It is the most valuable possession we have.
It is with us every moment of our lives.
We enact laws to protect it;
We seek to protect it from laws.
We cannot buy it. We cannot sell it,
But we can inherit and pass it on.
We spend billions to keep it,
Billions to improve it,
Billions to find it when it is lost.

It is valued and accepted;
It is ignored and abused.
As a science it is glamorized;
As an art it is criticized;
As an issue it is politicized.
It affects the private purse of each of us;
It affects the public purse of an entire nation.
Some enrich themselves from it;
Some are impoverished by it.
It is the core of our soul, our essence,
Our well-being—it is our health.

CONTENTS

CHAPTER FOUR—MANAGED CARE 184

CHAPTER FIVE—MEDICAID AND MEDICARE   **232**

CHAPTER NINE—HOME HEALTHCARE AND HOSPICE CARE   437

PREFACE

As American healthcare enters the twenty-first century, consumer-patients are confronted with a bewildering array of institutions, organizations, and programs—public and private—that are constantly evolving as they seek to find quality medical care at reasonable costs. As examples, these diverse groups include hospitals, nursing homes, ambulatory care centers, home healthcare and hospice programs, insurance and pharmaceutical companies, health maintenance organizations, preferred provider plans, and a host of public and private programs like Medicare and Medicaid.

In addition, consumer-patients must become conversant and knowledgeable about a new lexicon of terminology, concepts, and acronyms that have arisen as they to try to wend their way through the healthcare maze, including managed care, point-of-service plans, Medigap, COBRA, gatekeepers, coordinated care, MRIs, MACs, CATs, and others. Insurance companies are now called carriers, or third-party payors; doctors are referred to as providers; medical suppliers are called vendors; hospitals are now medical centers, which are part of multicenter healthcare systems as a result of mergers or acquisitions and have SICUs (surgical intensive care units) or MICUs (medical intensive care units); and primary care physicians are called "gatekeepers" who in managed care decide whether patients can see specialists or do something else that is costly.

As another century is upon us, American society must resolve many complex issues in regard to the kind of healthcare it will receive in the ensuing decades and the costs such services will entail. The aging of the baby boomer generation of the late 1940s and beyond represents a demographic time bomb. Until the twentieth century, few people lived into old age. Less than 1 percent of the world's population was sixty-five or older in 1900. In 1996, 6 percent were that old; 12 percent in the United States. By 2050 as many as a quarter of Americans will be in this age group. In the decade beginning in 2010, while the population as a whole is expected to increase by 2 percent, the number of retirees will grow by 30 percent, fifteen times as fast. Whereas in 1996 there were about four workers helping to pay the medical care of each senior citizen, according to the US General Accountability Office, as the twenty-first century progresses, the number of workers by 2030 financially supporting each of the elderly through Social Security has been projected to shrink even further to about three working-age persons. This overall decline of the retiree-to-worker ratio will be due to both the increase in retirees brought about by the aging baby boomer generation and falling fertility rates, which translates into relatively fewer workers in the future. How will the financial support of the elderly be accomplished? What impact will government reform of the welfare system have upon those who use Medicaid to purchase medical care, especially our children? How many more jurisdictions, like Oregon and its health plan of 1994, will begin to ration public medical care? At what financial and emotional cost to our citizens? These are but a few of the issues that American society must resolve in the twenty-first century.

Toward this end, I have written this book so that consumer-patients will be able to master and understand the American healthcare system so that they can find the kind of quality services they need for their own well-being at prices that are reasonable for consumers to afford. Whether it be deciding upon joining a health maintenance organization (HMO), or a preferred provider plan, or using traditional fee-for-service health insurance; finding and judging the quality of doctors or dentists, or a nursing home or home health program; understanding the complexities and obligations of Medicare; understanding the use of prescription drugs and saving money on such expenditures; lowering a hospital bill as well as understanding the operation of such institutions to make a stay easier; or knowing when and how to obtain a second surgical opinion and asking the right questions—this book will provide you, the consumer-patient, with answers to these and many other healthcare questions. Regardless of your personal health status, whether you are single or married, male or female, working or unemployed, an individual or an organization, this book will allow you to make the most effective use of today's and tomorrow's healthcare system. In this fashion, you can become adept in obtaining and using the kind of healthcare services you desire both for yourself and those for whom you are responsible.

With my wish that you are all able to live life as fully and as healthfully as possible, remember the words of ancient Greek, Roman, and Middle Eastern cultures that are as relevant today as when they were first expressed millennia ago. First, those of Hippocrates, a physician of ancient Greece who is often called the "father of medicine": "A wise man should consider that health is the greatest of human blessings, and learn how by his own thought to derive benefits from his illness," for, as both an epigram from 66 CE, the era of the Roman Empire, and a Middle Eastern proverb note, "life is not merely being alive, but being well" because "he who has health has hope; and he who has hope has everything."

Finally, to those whose labors in the healthcare field are represented in this book, be they licensed professionals or not, and to all others outside the field whose efforts directly or indirectly contribute to it and thus help improve the health condition of humankind, Marcus Tullius Cicero, Roman lawyer, politician, and philosopher, once characterized your station in life as follows. In successfully defending a

Roman soldier, Quintus Ligarius, charged with treason, before Julius Caesar (*Pro Ligario* [XII]), Cicero, in part, said in Latin: "Homines enim ad deos nulla re propius accedunt quam salutem hominibus dando," which means, "In nothing do men approach so nearly to the gods, as in giving health to men."

Jordan Braverman
Washington, DC

ACKNOWLEDGMENTS

Beginning with the very first word of this book and until I wrote the very last, I did not realize the years it would take to bring together in one volume a lifetime of experience in the healthcare field. Drawing upon my other books, papers, columns, and research, published and unpublished, stretching as far back as the 1960s up until today, as well as the works and writings of many others both within and outside the healthcare field, I tried to write this book as a faithful portrait of consumer healthcare in the twenty-first century—its progress, its problems, its questions, and its answers. Whatever shortcomings the book has are solely my responsibility.

Healthcare today is as modern as a handheld computer and telemedicine and as old as the basic questions of centuries ago: What's wrong with me? Will I get well? This book traces and discusses it all: healthcare at its most fundamental level of asking questions that will never change regardless of a century's number and healthcare on the cutting edge of new technologies and programs that speed our healing. I have tried to bring it all together in this one volume.

But my manuscript would not exist as a book at all if it were not for the efforts of several individuals who I wish to acknowledge and thank. First, Mr. Steven L. Mitchell, editor in chief of Prometheus Books, whose very great interest and vision of the value of this manuscript brought it into publication. Second, Ms. Nancy Rosenfeld, my literary agent, whose many hours of hard work and enthusiasm for the book was indispensable for bringing the manuscript as a project to a successful conclusion. Third, Ms. Peggy Deemer, my editor, whose editorial interest, meticulousness, and very arduous efforts were invaluable in bringing into the public arena an original manuscript of nearly nine hundred pages and of varying conceptual complexities in terms of its subject matter. I also want to acknowledge and thank the following advisory board members for taking time from their own very busy schedules to review and read the drafts of my manuscript and offer me their insightful comments, critiques, and suggestions. These are:

Professor Sherry Glied, chair, Department of Health Policy and Management,

Mailman School of Public Health, Columbia University, whose very constructive comments led me to rethink and revise my health insurance chapter. Professor Glied has served as senior economist for healthcare and labor market policy to the President's Council on Economic Advisors under both President George H. W. Bush and President William J. Clinton and is the author of *Chronic Condition*, a book on healthcare reform.

Dr. Elizabeth Morgan, a Los Angeles plastic surgeon, whose years of experience as both an author and in the practice of medicine and surgery at Harvard University, Yale University Medical School, and as an Oxford University fellow, raised many provocative questions about the definition of some surgical concepts that are headlined in the public arena today and which I hope will stir debate as to the true status of surgical practice in this country. In addition to other books, Dr. Morgan is the author *The Complete Book of Cosmetic Surgery: A Candid Guide for Men, Women, and Teens* and *The Making of a Woman Surgeon.*

Dr. Michael J. Tabacco, prosthodontist and clinical assistant professor, Department of Restorative Dentistry, Baltimore College of Dental Surgery, Dental School, University of Maryland, not only is teaching and training future dental specialists but also conducts his own practice in such a manner that the patients are informed to their benefit on dental procedures as if the patients are taking a course in dentistry themselves. The reader is the beneficiary of his comments on my writings about dental care.

Professor Albert Wertheimer, Temple University School of Pharmacy and director of the Center of Pharmaceutical Health Services Research, whose knowledge of managed care and the pharmaceutical industry were of incalculable value to me in his commentary on my writings. Dr. Wertheimer is an international authority in pharmaeconomics and outcomes research, editor of the *Journal of Pharmaceutical Finance, Economics, and Policy*, and the author of *Managed Care Pharmacy: Principles and Practice, US Healthcare System and Pharmacy* as well as other books.

Dr. Mervin H. Zimmerman, who, as a clinical professor of ophthalmology at George Washington University, took time out from his busy schedule of training hospital residents to review my draft about eyecare and eyewear and whose very helpful suggestions improved the draft immensely. In addition to serving as Consulting Ophthalmologist, US Department of State, Dr. Zimmerman, among other activities, has been president of the Washington, DC, Ophthalmological Society and the Pan American Medical Society and has served on the executive committee of George Washington University Hospital.

Again, to all my deepest appreciation for your interest in my book.

ADVISORY BOARD MEMBERS

Sherry Glied, MA, PhD
Professor and Chair
Department of Health Policy and Management
Mailman School of Public Health
Columbia University

Elizabeth Morgan, MD, PhD, FACS
Plastic Surgeon
Author of *The Complete Book of Cosmetic Surgery: A Candid Guide for Men,
Women, and Teens*
Fellow, American College of Surgeons
Fellow, American Society of Plastic Surgeons
Fellow, American Society of Aesthetic Plastic Surgeons

Michael J. Tabacco, MS, DDS, FACP, FICD
Clinical Assistant Professor
Department of Restorative Dentistry
Baltimore College of Dental Surgery, Dental School, University of Maryland
Fellow, American College of Prosthodontists
Fellow, International College of Dentists

Albert Wertheimer, MBA, PhD
Professor of Pharmacy Administration
Director, Center for Pharmaceutical Health Services Research
School of Pharmacy
Temple University

Mervin H. Zimmerman, MD, FACS
Clinical Professor of Ophthalmology
George Washington University
Fellow, American College of Surgeons
Fellow, American Academy of Ophthalmology

INTRODUCTION

If any word captures the revolution that American healthcare has been undergoing with the advent of the twenty-first century, it is the word *reform*. New organizations, new concepts, new payment mechanisms, and alterations of existing delivery and payments systems continue to evolve as the healthcare system seeks to resolve the increasing costs of healthcare and at the same time meet the quality care needs of an aging but growing American population.

Many questions continue to concern American consumers today. How does managed care affect the kind of medical care I am receiving? What are health maintenance organizations (HMOs), preferred-provider organization (PPOs), and exclusive provider organization (EPOs) plans? What are Medicare HMOs and how does my joining affect my purchasing Medigap insurance? What do I need to know about COBRA and the health insurance law of 1996 that allows my health insurance to become portable if I lose or change jobs? What should I tell my physician about the state of my health if I am a woman? How I can save money purchasing prescription drugs yet receive quality drugs to meet my medical needs? What should I know about purchasing long-term care insurance? What are my rights as a nursing home, hospice care, or hospital patient and how can I control the costs of my personal care in such institutions and programs and judge the quality of care I wish to receive? What should I know about homecare benefits, services, and programs? What kind of questions should I ask before undergoing surgery?

This book not only answers these questions but many others in comprehensive chapters that address physician care, dental care, private health insurance, managed care, Medicare and Medicaid, surgery and second surgical opinion programs, hospitals, nursing homes, hospice and homecare, and prescription drugs. In addition, the book contains a directory of organizations and Web sites that you may contact for additional information about those medical problems that concern you as well as a glossary of health-related terminology to help you understand today's healthcare system.

As noted, this book provides many questions about how to obtain information, what information to get, and how to obtain financing for health services and pay for them as economically as possible so as to lower your medical bills. While these questions can be very many for one person who may not receive an answer to each and every one, that is not their intent. All this information and these questions have been brought together in one volume and in varying degrees in each chapter so that you, the reader, do not have to go to many different sources to find out the same information or what questions you should ask to elicit the information you are seeking. Thus, as a reader, you can use as many or as few or possibly none of the questions at all to obtain the answers that you may need on any subject and on any occasion. The questions and information are there for you to use whether it be today or sometime in the future.

It is the author's belief that the worst question in healthcare is the one you never asked and wish you had or the one you were not even aware of to ask, whether it be in regard to deciding on a medical procedure, finding a nursing home, buying health insurance, choosing a physician, or any other issue for which you require information in order to maintain your own health or that of a loved one in as best a state as possible.

It is very important that you become knowledgeable about today's healthcare system. As more and more of the decision-making process about the care you receive falls under the aegis of organizations other than your own personal physician, it becomes increasingly important that you have as much if not more understanding of the system as those who deliver and finance such services so that you receive and your provider delivers the medical care you require. Toward this end, this book has been written and will allow you to become a more prudent purchaser and user of healthcare services. It is my belief that what this book states will help you achieve this goal.

CHAPTER ONE

PHYSICIAN CARE

INTRODUCTION

American medicine has entered the twenty-first century. It is Internet Web sites, electronic mail, electronic medical records, handheld computers transmitting medical information, and telemedicine where patients in one country are treated by physicians in another. It is laparoscopic surgical procedures whereby telescopic devices within the human body guide the surgeon's hands. It is the use of lasers to improve our eyesight and other parts of the body, in addition to many other technological advances.

Yet American medicine is still in the twentieth century as well as those that preceded it. For the consumer-patient, it is house calls, not knowing how to reduce a medical bill, nor knowing the kind of questions to ask, nor always understanding the answers being given to ensure as quick and as healthful a recovery as possible or the maintenance of one's health.

For the consumer-patient and those who deliver medical care, American medicine today is a mixture of the old and the new. It has always been and will always be. It is care that is quite affordable and care that is beyond an individual's means. It is as primitive an emotion as the fear of a diagnosis yet the hope of its treatment. American medicine was, is, and will always be an art of uncertainty and a science of precision where the possibilities are beyond human imagination.

Those who practice the healing arts, be they physicians, dentists, nurses, or others, and the consumer-patient who is receiving their care are confronted with a bewildering array of choices in a system that at times changes as slow as a snail's pace; and other times as fast as a bullet's velocity. At the center of the swirling vortex of the health system's nursing homes, hospitals, homecare agencies, hospice programs, HMOs, PPOs, Medicare/Medicaid programs, health insurance plans, and other entities stands the consumer-patient and the physician whose interaction with each other sets off a chain of activities throughout the system whose dimensions are difficult to measure and whose reverberations are never ending.

It is the purpose of this chapter and this book to help the consumer-patient enter, travel through, and understand the American health system and its dizzying array of changes and choices so that the consumer-patient hopefully will no longer find our healthcare system "a riddle wrapped in mystery inside an enigma," as Winston Churchill once described the former Soviet Union. Rather, the consumer-patient will become knowledgeable about a system whose dimensions, components, and choices will be easier to discern, enabling the consumer-patient to make the kind of decisions that will allow him to live in as healthful a state as possible. More specifically, it is the purpose of this book to inform consumer-patients how to find various health services, judge their quality, and pay for them as economically as possible so as to lower their medical bills. So now let us enter and travel through America's healthcare system, beginning with the provider who stands at its very core—the physician.

As of 1999, the United States had 29.1 active physicians (doctors of medicine and doctors of osteopathy) for each 10,000 of its population. According to the American Medical Association, as of 2000 there were an estimated 813,770 physicians in the United States. Of this number there were about 473,431 in office-based patient care and 157,032 in hospital-based patient care. Almost one-third practiced as either primary care generalists (33.7 percent) or a much smaller number as primary care specialists (6.4 percent).[1]

The largest number practiced in internal medicine, followed by family practice.[2] Yet millions of Americans live in communities that lack a doctor. In fact, as of 2005 one-fifth of the US population—about 60 million people—lived in rural areas spread over 80 percent of the country. In counties with a population of less than 10,000, there were far fewer doctors per capita than in urban and suburban areas.[3] According to the National Health Service Corps, the shortage of doctors in rural America has led the federal government to designate such areas as health professional shortage areas, and, according to the US Office of Rural Health Policy, 10 percent of doctors live in rural areas.[4] Given this situation, a very basic question arises for the prospective patient: Does a person's geographic area lack or have a surplus of adequate medical services and practitioners? Whichever the case may be, further questions arise: *How can I find a doctor who will meet my needs? How can I judge a physician's ability to provide quality care?*

By tradition, the physician is the centerpiece of the healthcare system. He has the principal role in the delivery of medical care, whether it is provided in the hospital or in an office or a community-based setting. The physician has the ultimate responsibility for the accurate diagnosis and treatment of diseases. When a patient visits a physician, it is the doctor who decides when the patient returns, what other medical services or medical specialists he requires, what drugs he needs, and whether hospitalization or another kind of institutionalization is necessary and for how long. In addition, the physician often supervises other healthcare personnel, frequently is the focus of reimbursement under health insurance plans, and contributes to the formulation of our national health policies.

The components of primary care include general and family practice, internal medicine, and pediatrics. Primary care physicians are distinguished by the fact that they are the first contact for the patient. They make the initial health assessment and attempt to solve as many of the patient's health problems as possible. Moreover, they are responsible for coordinating the remainder of the healthcare team who serve the patient (including consultants, when necessary) and provide continued contact with the patient in acting as an adviser, confidant, and advocate.

However, despite the large number of physicians in this country, be they primary care physicians or other specialists, access to medical care services, which varies among different segments of our population, remains a basic problem. The reasons for this situation include the shortage of physicians in primary care despite their large numbers, the distances patients must sometimes travel to receive medical services, and the lengthy time patients must occasionally wait before receiving a medical appointment.

In addition, many patients have little or no access to the more specialized medical services they require because accurate diagnoses and timely referrals do not always occur readily or soon enough at the primary care levels.[5]

Look what happened to Jack. He was in a real dilemma. He had just moved from New York to Washington, DC, because he had accepted a high appointment in the federal government and knew he had to have a physician in Washington to care for his rare chronic illness. The only thought on Jack's mind was, "Where am I going to find such a physician? I can't go to the Yellow Pages *like I'm buying an automobile. I don't have any friends to ask yet. I don't know my new colleagues at work well enough to judge their suggestions. I can't ask my relatives; I don't have any in Washington."*

Then Jack had a great idea. He called up his former specialist in New York to ask him if he knew of any doctors in Washington who might treat him. Well, his doctor didn't, but he did know the chairman of the department of the Albert Einstein Medical School in New York City that treated patients that had Jack's illness. Because departmental chairmen network with other chairmen involved in the same field throughout the country, that chairman contacted the chairman of the department at George Washington University Medical School. The chairman in Washington sent back his recommendations to New York, and these recommendations were then transmitted to Jack. Jack then interviewed several of the physicians on the list and made his choice. Well, obviously not everyone can be like Jack, but there are other steps you can take to find a physician best suited to your needs. The following suggestions will help you do this.

SELECTING A PHYSICIAN

Medical doctors (MDs) and osteopathic doctors (DOs) are the only providers who are legally called physicians. Both are total physicians, meaning that they have received the same basic medical training and are licensed to treat the whole body, perform surgery, and prescribe drugs. The difference between them is that osteo-pathic physicians receive additional training in palpation and manipulative proce-dures (a form of manual pressure applied to joints, bones, and muscles), which they use along with the other more traditional forms of diagnosis and treatment. How-ever, some MDs are also beginning to use manipulation in their practice, but they call it biomechanics. Whether you wish to use the services of an MD or a DO, the best time to look for and select a physician is when you are still healthy. A physician who already is familiar with your medical history and your normal state of health will provide the best care for you when you become ill. Therefore, as a patient, you should take the following steps when seeking a physician.

Keep in Mind Your General Needs for Medical Care

An internist or a general family practitioner should be responsible for your overall medical care and that of your family. These primary physicians are specifically trained for general medical care. Unlike general practitioners, family physicians complete a full three-year residency in family practice, making them eligible to take a board-certifying examination. This length of residency training follows four years of medical school and is the same length of time required to become an internist or a pediatrician.

Family physicians differ from pediatricians and internists in that they take care of both adults and children. However, they are also more likely to deal with prob-lems in the fields of dermatology, minor surgery, office orthopedics, and office gyne-cology. But like general internists and pediatricians, family physicians perform gen-eral physical examinations and diagnose and treat acute medical problems like ear infection, pneumonia, sprains, and vaginal infection. They also care for people with chronic medical problems like hypertension, diabetes, cancer, and heart disease. Family practitioners and internists will be able to lead you and your family through the maze of the modern healthcare delivery system, as needed, to appropriate med-ical specialists, hospitals, and other medical services.

Interview several doctors or groups before making your decision. Not everyone is comfortable doing this. Many doctors will want to give you an initial examination and charge for it. Some are willing to offer a ten-minute initial interview without charge. Telephone and ask about this. When you settle on a primary care doctor, realize that, to do his or her job well, he or she should see you at regular intervals, not just when you are ill, to get to know you and your family.

Compile a Roster of Prospective Physicians

You can put together a list of prospective physicians from friends, coworkers, com-munity hospitals, medical schools, or your local county medical society. Do not, however, make your choice only on the basis of a local county medical society. Membership in these organizations only tells you that a physician is licensed to prac-tice medicine and has paid his dues to the society. One important positive sign of a physician's ability will be his membership on the medical staff of a good hospital, especially a hospital that maintains an affiliation with a medical school.

Try telephoning the chief of staff, chief of medicine, or chief resident at any major hospital or medical center or its public relations officer to find or check upon the quality of a physician. If you are moving, your present doctor or pharmacist may be able to refer you to a good physician in your new community. One of the newest and most popular sources of finding and choosing a physician for medical treatment is the online directories on the Web. Directories can be searched by city, state, zip code, medical specialty, and doctors' names.

Plan members also can request a list of doctors within a specified number of miles from their city or zip code. In addition, the directories may contain other information concerning a physician's qualifications and medical practice. But a word of caution: these online directories are subject to errors. Many doctors don't always tell their insurers when they move or retire.

Also, the publication of a doctor's office fees can present a problem. If the physician raises his office fees after the directory is published, he may receive many complaints from his patients about the price of his services. Price information may be inaccurate if the physician directory is not continually updated. Therefore, notice the directory's publication date and ask your physician whether the fees listed in the directory are correct or whether they have changed and, if so, to what price level.

The database of providers can list hundreds of thousands of providers, so it is difficult to keep the changes up-to-date on a timely basis, though some states, like Maryland, have a law that requires insurers to update their online directories every fifteen days, and they can be fined if the information is not correct. Other insurers have notices on their Web sites telling customers that they should double-check the accuracy of the listings and list a "legal notice" in which they inform the customers that they assume complete responsibility for using the information on that site.

Thus, these listings can include wrong telephone numbers and addresses, doctors who are deceased, those who closed their practice more than two years ago, or those whose licenses have even been suspended. So be very careful in using such directories.

Medicare Physicians

If you are a Medicare beneficiary and need to find a physician, you can go to a Medicare Web site that will tell you about the medical backgrounds of thousands of physicians who participate in the Medicare program. The directory is available at http://www.medicare.gov. Medicare's National Participating Physician Directory includes information about physicians as to their medical school and year of graduation, any board certification in a medical specialty, and the hospitals at which an individual physician has admitting privileges. The directory, which is updated monthly, includes each participating physician's office telephone number and any foreign language abilities. In the future, the directory will contain information on whether the doctor is accepting new Medicare patients.

Make Use of Physician Referrals

Many doctors may have such full schedules that they cannot add new patients to their practices; often, however, they are willing to recommend other physicians. A referral by a respected physician is especially valuable.

Consider a Geriatrician

As America's aging population increases in number, elderly patients may wish to use the services of a geriatrician, a physician who specializes in geriatric medicine. If you are such a patient, remember that few physicians have formal training in this field. According to the American Geriatrics Society, as of 2001 there were about 7,600 certified geriatricians in the United States and by 2030 the country will need 36,000 trained geriatricians as the number of adults age sixty-five years and older is projected to double to seventy million. Most geriatricans are either internists or family practitioners who were certified since 1988 under a grandfather clause that allowed practicing physicians with experience in geriatrics to take a qualifying exam. Those who passed the boards, offered by the American Board of Internal Medicine and the American Board of Family Medicine, through 1994 earned a certificate of added qualifications in geriatric medicine. In addition, since 1991, the American Board of Psychiatry and Neurology has offered board certification in geriatrics. If you need to find a geriatric psychiatrist, the American Association for Geriatric Psychiatry (AAGP) can provide you with contact information for two or three board-certified geriatric psychiatrists in your geographic area—or the geographic area of someone about whom you care. You may also ask your family doctor to refer you to a geriatric psychiatrist.

To access the AAGP's online referral service, go to http://www.aagponline.org and click on "Need a Referral?" You may also write to the AAGP, Suite 1050, 7910 Woodmont Avenue, Bethesda, MD 20814-3004.

Geriatric psychiatrists complete four years of medical school, four years of postgraduate residency psychiatric training, and then a one- to two-year intensive fellowship in geriatric psychiatry. They must also pass a certification exam in geriatric psychiatry as well as one in general psychiatry. The geriatric psychiatrist can help spot the earliest signs of Alzheimer's disease and differentiate them from other forms of dementia or drug interventions, can see warning signs of substance abuse, can spot hidden suicidal tendencies among the elderly that elude other doctors, and can specialize in dealing with family members as well as with the patient. Basically, the ongoing changes that accompany the aging process and often lead to acute loneliness, anxiety, depression, confusion, or other mental disorders among the elderly are the kind of conditions geriatric psychiatrists are trained to recognize and treat. Beginning in 1996, only physicians who have completed formal advanced training in geriatric medicine or a fellowship in geriatrics will be eligible to take the certification examination offered by the American Board of Internal Medicine and the American Board of Family Medicine.

Not everyone over sixty-five years of age must see a geriatrician, but many older patients who suffer from several medical problems and have difficulty managing multiple drug therapies may want to consider a doctor who is trained in geriatrics. Also, older patients who are concerned about a diagnosis or treatment, or who just feel their doctor doesn't spend enough time with them to understand the whole picture, may want to consider a geriatric assessment. Geriatric care has many benefits. These include diminished disability; less time as an inpatient in a hospital or nursing home; improved social functioning; lower rates of depression; more access to social support services; the preservation of physical function or the slowing of decline; and an increased patient and family satisfaction.

An interdisciplinary approach to medicine forms the basis of geriatric medicine. During a geriatric assessment, a physician evaluates the patient's physical and mental condition and often calls on and works with other professionals as a team— possibly a social worker, a pharmacist, a nurse practitioner, a physician's assistant, a physical and/or occupational therapist, a nutritionist, or a geriatric psychiatrist— to help identify factors that may be affecting the patient's quality of life. These factors may include the lack of a caregiver, no access to community services, poor diet, or depression caused by isolation. Make sure your physician doesn't frequently attribute your problems to "old age."

Geriatricians specialize in managing chronic medical conditions rather than curing them. For example, one of the keys to taking care of elderly patients is a thorough knowledge of drugs. Many older people take medicines prescribed by different doctors, so geriatricians generally look for possibilities of what they can do with less medication rather than constantly adding more. Sometimes the best solution to a problem is no medicine at all. Most geriatric clinics affiliated with hospital centers accept Medicare payments, while some geriatricians in private practice do not.

According to some geriatricians, since Medicare does not have a reimbursement code for geriatric assessments, most payments to doctors represent a portion of their costs. Basically, what this means is that, unlike many services Medicare covers, the program does not have a specific amount of money that it will pay a physician who provides a geriatric assessment of a patient. Therefore, the payment the physician receives from Medicare may not cover the costs the physician bears in providing this service. If the payment is less than the physician's expenses for such a service, a physician conceivably could decide not to provide it anymore, to the detriment of a patient's health.

To find a geriatrician, you can call local hospitals or medical schools to see if they have a geriatrician on staff or ask your own doctor for a referral. Some geriatricians are listed in the *Yellow Pages*.

Also, the American Geriatrics Society in New York maintains a national directory of geriatricians. For information call 1-212-308-1414 or toll free 1-800-563-4916. For additional information about geriatrics, you may visit the organization's Web site at http://www.americangeriatrics.org.[6] In addition, to gain more health information about the elderly and their medical conditions such as arthritis, stroke,

Alzheimer's disease, osteoporosis, and others, you can go to http://www.nihsenior health.gov, a Web site that has been established by the National Institutes on Aging and the National Library of Medicine, both part of the National Institutes of Health.

Make Sure You Are Satisfied with Your Physician

Choose a doctor you respect and with whom you feel comfortable—then stay with him. Make sure your doctor will not abandon you, no matter how difficult your problems become. A relationship established over the years of consultation and treatment means the best healthcare for you and your family. Your physician will maintain a permanent record of your medical history and, by knowing your background, will be more knowledgeable to detect any illness and treat you as promptly and effectively as possible. Also, do not assume that because everyone in the community is acquainted with a physician, that familiarity is a reflection of his medical ability. Do your own investigating and decision making.

Remember, if you join a health maintenance organization (HMO), it usually means that you have to leave your own doctor of many years. So at least make sure you have several doctors to choose from in the HMO and insist on meeting them before you make any kind of commitment. Also, be careful of selecting any physician who regularly diagnoses and prescribes medications for you just over the telephone. Hopefully, the physician will be a person who is someone you can talk with and someone who communicates with you the options that are available to you in regard to your health alternatives.

Your physician should be someone who asks precise questions—what, where, when, and why—shows curiosity about you and intellectual curiosity about medicine, is a partner who presents explanations and alternatives and helps you decide what should be done, not just what might be done, and then teaches you how to manage your care. In addition, he/she should keep abreast of the latest medical advances and information; allow you to take an active role in your own care; and follow up after days, weeks, or months to find out how a treatment worked. Your physician should not be offended if you ask questions about your care and should admit what he occasionally doesn't know; find time to research answers when he must, and regularly confer with colleagues to check and sharpen his knowledge, or teach or act as an "attending" or volunteer staff member at a university or other teaching hospital. Physicians who teach also learn by teaching, and the fact that they are allowed to teach is an indication of their medical competence.

If for any reason you are not happy with your physician later, tell your doctor how and why he or she is failing you. The doctor cannot be held accountable without the opportunity to respond. Both the positive and the negative issues that occur between doctor and patient need to be discussed, not avoided.

Observe How the Physician's Office Functions

The first line of observation is the people who answer the office phones. To avoid I-can't-be-bothered lines at your life-and-death moments, check out the physician's office staff. Observe and use your instincts. Judge their telephone rapport. When you call, are you put on hold for long periods of time? Are your messages taken accurately? Are your questions for the doctor relayed in an effective manner or are you told just to come in? If your potential doctor has more than one office, what happens when you call at one location when the physician is at another? Despite your physical ailments, are you ordered to call the following day when the doctor can check your charts in another office, or are your messages and records relayed carefully? Remember, the manner in which the office operates comes from the physician in charge. Also, find out about vacation coverage. Make sure someone will be responsible when your doctor is not in town.

Find out who covers for your doctor in emergencies and at other times. Who has access to your charts in an emergency? Who takes responsibility? Remember, doctors have their own lives as well, and no physician will always be there. How a physician covers his office is extremely important to your health.

Find Out Whether Your Physician Is Board Certified

Today, there are 24 medical specialty boards and 110 subspecialties including pediatric surgery, aerospace medicine, and forensic psychiatry, all members of the American Board of Medical Specialties (ABMS). The following are the 24 boards that the ABMS recognizes: Allergy & Immunology; Anesthesiology; Colon and Rectal Surgery; Dermatology; Emergency Medicine; Family Practice; Internal Medicine; Medical Genetics; Neurological Surgery; Obstetrics & Gynecology; Ophthalmology; Otolaryngology; Orthopedic Surgery; Pathology; Pediatrics; Physical Medicine and Rehabilitation; Plastic Surgery; Preventive Medicine; Psychiatry and Neurology; Radiology; Surgery; Thoracic Surgery; and Urology. To determine whether a subspecialty is officially recognized or whether a doctor is board certified, you can call the American Board of Medical Specialties at 1-866-275-2267 (toll free) or 1-847-491-9091. Its mailing address is American Board of Medical Specialties, 1007 Church St. Suite 404, Evanston, IL 60201-5913 and its Web site is http://www.abms.org.

Each of the previous boards is responsible for the formulation of training requirements and other qualifications as well as the administration of certifying examinations in a particular medical specialty. To be eligible to take the official specialty board examination, a doctor must have successfully completed one of the accredited American residency training programs. Graduates of foreign medical schools are eligible if they complete a US residency program; doctors who successfully finished a residency in Canada or England may be exempt from this requirement. Residencies vary in length. Most are three years, although some surgery residencies can last seven years.[7] A physician who passes the American Board exam-

Figure 1-1

DEFINITION OF PHYSICIAN SPECIALTIES

Allergist—Diagnoses and treats allergies.

Anesthesiologist—Specializes in the application of medications to ensure that the patient is unconscious during surgery.

Bariatrician—Specializes in the prevention of obesity and its treatment.

Cardiologist—Diagnoses and treats heart problems.

Emergency medicine specialist—Expert at treating patients suffering from such traumas as shootings, automobile accidents, and other life-threatening emergencies.

Endocrinologist—Diagnoses and treats glandular diseases, including diseases of the male and female sex glands.

Family practitioner—Today's counterpart of the former general practitioner.

Forensic pathologist—Specializes in determining the cause of death in criminal cases.

Gastroenterologist—Diagnoses and treats disorders of both the stomach and the intestines such as Crohn's disease (Ileitis).

Gynecologist—Diagnoses and treats diseases of the female reproductive organs.

Hematologist—Diagnoses and treats diseases of the blood.

Immunologist—Works on problems involving the body's immune system.

Neonatologist—Specializes in the care of any newborn infants with health problems.

Nephrologist—Diagnoses and treats disorders of the kidneys.

Neurologist—Diagnoses and treats disorders of the nervous system as well as patients who suffer from epilepsy, strokes, meningitis, encephalitis, and multiple sclerosis.

Obstetrician—Cares for women through their pregnancies.

Oncologist—Diagnoses tumors and treats cancer patients.

Ophthalmologist—Diagnoses and treats eye disease.

Orthopedist—Specializes in disorders of the bones, joints, ligaments, tendons, ligaments, and muscles.

Otolaryngologist—Diagnoses and treats illness of the ear, nose, and throat.

Pathologist—Supervises technicians in the analysis of blood and tissue specimens.

Pediatrician—Diagnoses and treats children's diseases.

Physical medicine and rehabilitation specialist—Treats disabled patients and instructs them on how to successfully cope with their handicaps.

Perinatologist—Specializes in diagnosing and treating disorders and diseases in infants while they are still in the womb and immediately after birth.

Proctologist—Diagnoses and treats patients with disorders of the colon, rectum, and anus.

Pulmonary diseases specialist—Treats diseases of the lungs and pulmonary arteries.

Radiologist—Uses x-rays and other forms of radiation to diagnose and treat certain diseases.

Rheumatologist—Diagnoses and treats arthritis and other diseases of the joints and connective tissues.

Urologist—Diagnoses and treats disorders of the urinary tract of both sexes and the genital tract of men only.

ination within a specialty area becomes *board certified* and is known as a *diplomate* of that board. Many physicians who are *board eligible* by virtue of their medical training have not taken the qualifying examinations. In many of the board specialties, a doctor may also be a member of a "college," an honorary body whose principal concern is continuing medical education within the specialty.

Once certain qualifications have been met, the physician may be elected a fellow of the college. Thus, certain initials may follow your doctor's name, such as FACP (Fellow of the American College of Physicians) or FACS (Fellow of the American College of Surgeons). Ask your physician what the initials after his name mean, for they show that your doctor is a fellow of a particular college and, very probably, a *diplomate* in that medical specialty. The lack of board certification does not necessarily reflect on a doctor's medical competence.

A comprehensive listing of all diplomates of the various specialty boards is published in the *Directory of Medical Specialists*, which is available in some libraries. For your own informational needs, ask your local public library or an institutional library, perhaps in your community hospital or medical school, whether it has such a directory. As a prospective patient, you should know that any physician can legally practice surgical or medical specialties without the specialized training that the board certification reflects. Therefore, the initials after your physician's name offer added reassurance that your doctor is qualified to practice his specialty. While it is unlikely that a reputable hospital would allow an unqualified practitioner to apply complex medical or surgical techniques to his patients, this situation may not be universally true.

Find Out about the Various Sources of Medical Assistance in Your Community

Should an emergency arise and no physician is immediately available, one of the most convenient sources of assistance in any urban or suburban community is the local fire or police department. Your community may even maintain a volunteer ambulance corps that provides emergency transportation to a hospital. Remember, hospitals also maintain emergency room facilities that are staffed twenty-four hours a day.

If you must go to a hospital emergency room, be ready to look out for yourself or try to have someone go along with you. The following suggestions may help you obtain good service:

- When you contact your physician, ask if he or she can meet you, or at least telephone you, at the hospital.
- Tell the emergency room staff your doctor's name.
- Before treatment begins, tell the staff you want your own doctor to get your medical records.
- If you don't have a doctor, telephone the emergency department yourself to ask if they can take care of you. This may help the staff to get ready for you. Ask whether the doctor treating you is a hospital resident (a medical graduate

in internship or specialty training). Some residents have two or three years of additional experience and great expertise; some are just out of school. If a resident is treating you, ask to have the staff physician check on the treatment. (In asking, be tactful. "I'm sure you are a competent doctor, but I would feel more comfortable if a supervisor looked at me, too.")
- Be polite. It helps lower the hospital staff's tension and also allows you to tell them your medical needs more effectively.[8]

Remember, it is a real emergency if you are risking death or permanent damage if you don't receive care in thirty minutes or less. If you just think this may be the case, telephone 911 or an ambulance first, stay as calm as possible, give clear directions, ask to have your address repeated, and if no one shows up in ten minutes, telephone again, and keep calling. Immediately after calling 911 or an ambulance, or if you have decided to drive to an emergency room in a less drastic situation, call your doctor, too, if you have one, and say what's happening. In its publication *Seconds Save Lives in Medical Emergencies*, the American College of Emergency Medicine recommends that you get help fast when the following warning signs appear:

- coughing or vomiting blood
- uncontrolled bleeding
- sudden or severe pain; chest pain lasting two minutes or more
- difficulty breathing; shortness of breath
- sudden dizziness, weakness, or change in vision
- severe or persistent vomiting or diarrhea
- change in mental status (e.g., confusion, difficulty arousing)

In addition to the previous list, according to the American College of Emergency Medicine, the following are also warning signs of a medical emergency:

- fainting or loss of consciousness
- suicidal or homicidal feelings
- upper abdominal pain or pressure
- head or spinal injury
- sudden, severe pain anywhere in the body
- ingestion of a poisonous substance
- sudden injury like a motor vehicle accident, burns or smoke inhalation, near drowning, deep or large wound, or other similar traumas[9]

If the problem is not urgent such as a sore throat or a bruise, go to your regular doctor, a hospital's outpatient department, or a community clinic and try to find a doctor who is able and willing to be there for follow-up or the next time you need care. In nonurgent cases, the emergency department may not be the best place to seek help because you may have to wait a very long time while they treat cases that are more serious than your own.[10] Also, you are likely to get a higher medical bill than if you went to some other treatment facility, such as a freestanding emergicenter. These alternative facilities are not designed to treat "life—or limb—threatening" cases but rather to treat episodic primary care like upper and lower respiratory tract infections, sprains, lacerations, and urinary tract infections.

Despite their speed and convenience, remember that facilities which are independent of hospitals may also be independent of medical regulations, licensing, and monitoring. Ask your doctor how emergicenters or even surgical or dental centers compare with your community's hospital facilities and visit such centers before you decide to use them. Also, find out whether your insurance policy covers procedures performed in such centers.

If you are worried about a symptom that hasn't become a life-threatening emergency as yet, that's the time to call your doctor's office and tell the assistant that your situation is urgent. (Symptoms in this category might include a fever of 102 degrees or over.) You should either be connected with a doctor on the spot or hear from the physician within an hour.[11]

Remember, use the hospital emergency room wisely. A hospital's emergency room is designed to handle illnesses and accidents that can't wait for an office visit before treatment. Emergency room services are costly and should be used only for illnesses requiring immediate medical care.

Look for a Doctor Exhibiting Good Qualities of Medical Practice

A good physician will be compassionate and interested in you as a patient, ask for a detailed medical history, and give you enough time to discuss your problems. After an examination, he will make sure you understand his diagnosis and the treatment he orders. When necessary, he will willingly refer you to specialists; he will also be conservative about recommending surgery. Once he has made a referral or recommended surgery, he will not desert you once such treatment has begun.

How to Avoid a Bad Doctor

Here are some questions to ask that may help you avoid choosing a bad doctor:

- Has the doctor been disciplined or formally charged with misconduct? You can find out by calling or writing the state medical board that licenses physicians in your state. Call the Federation of State Medical Boards (1-817-868-4000) for the telephone number to call in your area or visit its Web site at http://www.fsmb.org.
- Has your doctor lost hospital privileges? Ask the doctor.
- Is the doctor board certified? Check with the American Board of Medical Specialties. Call 1-866-275-2267 (toll free) or 1-847-491-9091. (Note: Lack of board certification does not necessarily reflect on the quality of a doctor. A

good doctor may not be board certified, while a bad doctor may have such certification.)

- Has your doctor's malpractice insurance ever been canceled? Why? Some state medical boards will tell you when a doctor has had insurance canceled. (But most doctors can get insurance no matter how bad their record.)
- What does the American Medical Association (AMA) have on file about your doctor? *The American Medical Directory*, published by the AMA, lists the affiliations of its members. It should be available at your public library. The AMA, for a charge, will also provide biographical information on physicians. Write: AMA, Department of Physician Data Services, Dept. P, 515 N. State St., Chicago, IL 60610.[12]

The federal government does have a very restricted file with the names of thousands of physicians who were involved in malpractice suits, were disciplined by state medical boards, or had adverse reviews regarding membership in professional medical societies. It is the National Practitioner Data Bank (NPDB). Only hospital medical boards and similar health providers can check the information in the data bank. While doctors can check on themselves, they cannot check on other doctors.

In August 1996 Massachusetts became the first state to establish a law that requires the release of information about physician malpractice payouts, disciplinary actions against doctors, and physician's criminal records. Anyone who wants information on a doctor's history—good or bad—can call the Massachusetts State Board of Registration in Medicine's toll-free hotline for residents of Massachusetts (1-800-377-0550) or those outside of the state can call 1-617-654-9800 or visit its Web site, http://www.massmedboard.org, and receive up to ten profiles faxed or mailed to them free. The profiles can also show a doctor's credentials. People can learn where a doctor went to medical school, whether he is board certified in a specialty, what honors he has received, and where he has published research. The listings also offer practical information, including whether doctors are accepting new patients, hospitals where they can practice, and insurance plans they accept. Other states are considering similar laws. Find out from your state medical society or state medical licensing board whether such a law has been passed in your state or whether it publishes any directories detailing such information about physicians. If your state does not publish such directories, ask whether there are any consumer-oriented organizations in your area that do so. You can check the training and history of a physician at http://www.healthgrades.com.

There are other signs that a physician may not be the proper doctor for you or other members of your family, including the following:

- The doctor doesn't display any respect for your modesty or makes improper remarks while conducting a pelvic or breast examination.
- The doctor fails to tell you of the potential risks, benefits, and side effects of prescription medicines or suggested procedures and tests. (Also, be wary of a

doctor who prescribes a drug to which you are allergic and you mentioned as being so.)

- The doctor does not like it if you say you would like to obtain a second opinion regarding your diagnosis or gives the impression that he or she knows everything and is adamant that his or her method of treatment is the only correct one.
- The doctor seems to have memory difficulties, or is hostile or has the smell of alcohol on his or her breath.
- What is the doctor's educational background? Where did the doctor go to medical school? If she or he has graduated from any foreign school outside western Europe, check for American, Canadian, or western European internship and residency.
- Is the doctor willing to make house calls? Under what conditions, if any?
- Does the physician have hospital privileges? If none, try someone else. You need a personal doctor with one or more appointments at respected hospitals.
- Does the doctor do any teaching? As already noted, doctors with "clinical" (part-time volunteer) teaching appointments not only instruct others but also learn from their experience as well.
- Is the physician's office accessible to the handicapped?
- Does the doctor practice alone or with others? There are fewer and fewer "solo" practitioners today, and many who practice alone make adequate arrangements for readily available backup when they're away. But some do not. Doctors who normally work together tend to consult and add to each other's strengths.

Physician Office Booklets

If your community does not have a physician's directory, then it is possible that your physician may have developed his own office booklet. The American Medical Association has encouraged physicians to create these publications. Such booklets improve patient relations in general, save the physician and his staff a great amount of time in explaining their office policies to patients, and represent a printed record of medical policy that is available to both the office staff and patients in case of any misunderstandings.

The American Medical Association, in a pamphlet titled *Preparing a Patient Information Booklet*, suggests that the following information be provided, most of which could also appear in a community's physicians' directory:

- physician's medical specialty and type of practice
- policy on appointments, cancellations, and missed appointments
- office hours and physician's schedule
- telephone calls—what can and cannot be accomplished by telephone
- policy on billing and collection of office fees
- policy on preparing insurance and legal forms[13]

Such printed information assures better comprehension of the physician's office procedures and policies than may be conveyed in personal patient-physician conversations.

Local County Medical Societies

In addition to community physician directories and individual physician office booklets, your county medical society may be another source of assistance for finding and judging the quality of physician services in your community. One excellent illustration of how medical societies may assist individuals in finding the doctor of their choice is the Montgomery County Medical Society of Maryland. This society established a program called the Patient Advocacy Referral Service, which has become a model in the nation for other societies to examine and, hopefully, adopt. You should ask whether your county medical society has a similar program.

The Montgomery County Medical Society program concerns itself with many kinds of patient problems, such as matching persons who have difficulty speaking English with physicians who speak the same language, informing patients where to find transportation to reach a doctor, or helping people who do not know how to find a doctor. The service has a register of doctors, all of whom are members of the county medical society. The concept of the service is to match the doctor to the individual's needs and offer a person a choice of several physicians. The Montgomery County Medical Society may do much as a model to resolve one of this nation's most vexing healthcare problems—how to find a qualified physician when you need help and do not know where to look.

CHOOSING YOUR CHILD'S DOCTOR

Aside from seeking a physician for your own needs, what about for other members of your family such as your children? Your relationship with your child's pediatrician or family physician can last from infancy to adulthood. They may even provide care to your grandchildren. It is wise to choose your child's doctor before your child is born. Take time to find someone with whom you feel comfortable and can communicate.

Mary, for example, had a problem with her four-year-old son. Playing with some tissue paper, he playfully stuffed it up his nose, and when he tried to get it out, he couldn't. Some of the tissue paper was still stuck in his nose and Mary panicked. She went to a family practitioner in her neighborhood who told Mary that the boy would have to be operated on to get the paper out. Mary became frightened at the doctor's suggestion. She didn't know what to do. She didn't want her boy's face scarred, perhaps for the rest of his life. She called a relative about the situation, and the relative recommended an ear, nose, and throat (ENT) specialist whom Mary called. Being an emergency, the ENT physician saw Mary as quickly as possible. The

ENT specialist told Mary that she should never to go to a doctor for treatment who does not have the experience in someone else's specialty. Medicine is too complex today to know everyone else's field. Just as a psychiatrist should not operate on a person's heart, so a family physician in general practice should not be providing the specialty treatments practiced by ENTs. The specialist told Mary that there were other ways besides an operation to remove the tissue from her son's nose. Mary followed the doctor's advice, and the ENT specialist successfully removed the tissue from her son's nose, and the boy is now well.

Thus, to begin your search:

- Ask your obstetrician, other health professionals, your family, your local medical society, friends, and hospitals for referrals. If using friends or relatives, remember that you must a visit a physician to find out whether the qualities your friends and family like in the physician also meet your personal requirements. Reputable hospitals, including children's hospitals, usually have a referral service that can give you the names of staff doctors who meet certain criteria that you may be looking for, such as their specialty, gender, and office location. For example, is the physician's office convenient to your own home, your workplace, the child's school, or his/her daycare center? But, remember a hospital's referral service is only providing you with a list of names. The service cannot assure you of the quality of care a physician provides. If you are a member of a managed care plan, find out what pediatricians are associated with it and whether the plan can provide you with any information about them. You may also contact the American Academy of Pediatrics, a professional organization that can tell you which of its member doctors practice in your community. Just send a self-addressed envelope and a note indicating the city and state where you are looking to the American Academy of Pediatrics, Department C-Pediatrician Referral, 141 Northwest Point Blvd., Elk Grove Village, IL 60007-1098. Its Web address is www.aap.org, and its telephone number is 1-847-434-4000.
- Interview several doctors before deciding. Ask whether the physician will bill you for the interview visit. Some won't; others may. Take a list of questions with you such as:
  - ▼ When are your office hours and do you have call-in times? If I have a question that may not be of an emergent nature, when is the best time to call your office? Be cautious of any doctor who does not telephone patients. Do you have specific hours when a patient can walk into your office for a visit without making an appointment?
  - ▼ Do you see patients after hours and on weekends in emergencies? When you are not available, who covers for you and what is their background? Do you have any information about these doctors that is available to the public which tells you about their education and other information pertaining to their professional background?

▼ With what hospitals are you affiliated? You need a personal physician who has one or more appointments at respected hospitals. If the physician does not have any, look for another doctor. Ask about his or her residency training. Where did he train? Pediatricians complete a three-year residency in pediatrics. Find out whether he/she is board certified in pediatrics and whether the doctor has a subspecialty. How much importance does the doctor place on a child's proper nutrition? Will the doctor send out reminders about your child's immunizations? Does the physician maintain any testing or diagnostic facilities where he practices? If not, to whom does his office usually refer?

▼ If the doctor is in a group practice, can you schedule appointments with the doctor of your choice?

▼ How does the doctor's office deal with billing? Must you pay immediately at the time of your visit? Will the physician accept your health insurance plan and submit your claims to the third-party payer? If not, how are insurance claims handled?

▼ What is the length of time that you must you wait for your first appointment? What about an emergency appointment? Has the doctor established different appointment times for well and sick children? Some doctors set up well-baby appointments for the morning hours and non-emergency illnesses in the afternoon to try and prevent the spread of diseases among those sitting in the waiting room. Some doctors even maintain separate waiting rooms at their office.

Remember that you and your doctor are a team, working together for the health of your child. If your child is not a newborn, bring the doctor a summary of your child's medical history, including childhood diseases, chronic illnesses, hospitalizations, and medications. If you are changing doctors, you can request such information from your former doctor. Also, don't forget to tell your doctor about your own family's health history since it directly affects your child's health risk factors. Remember, in addition to pediatricians, general and family practitioners can also provide medical care to your whole family from newborns to seniors. In either situation, whether selecting a pediatrician or a general and family practitioner in regard to your child's health, you should try to choose a physician while you are pregnant. In this manner, the physician can keep up-to-date on any health problems that occur during your pregnancy and which might affect the child and be there right after birth to give your baby a checkup. Regular visits to your doctor are good measures of preventive healthcare. When you take your child to your doctor for a checkup, the doctor should thoroughly examine your child to make sure that he or she is well nourished and that your child's immunizations are up-to-date. The physician should also follow your child's growth and development, and look for any physical problems before they become serious. You can prepare your child for the visit ahead of time. Tell your child what to expect. Library books about visiting the doctor can ease your child's fears.

During visits, notice the following:

- Does the doctor address your child directly or talk only to you?
- Does the doctor explain what's being done and why—in such a way that you understand? For example, does the physician explain why he is taking your child's blood pressure? On May 19, 2004, the Associated Press reported that the federal government's National High Blood Pressure Education Program of the National Heart, Lung, and Blood Institute recommends that doctors begin checking children for high blood pressure at age three to determine possible heart and blood vessel damage if they have high blood pressure, a danger that is increasing among children as Americans gain more and more weight.
- Does the doctor take time to answer all questions, including your child's?
- Is the doctor a good listener?
- Does the doctor show a caring attitude toward your child?
- Are the receptionist and nurses cheerful and approachable?
- Does the waiting area have washable toys and a play space?

The most important test for your pediatrician or family practitioner is how she or he cares for your child and responds to your concerns. If you cannot speak easily with your physician, think about finding another doctor, especially if your doctor is unwilling to explain a diagnosis or treatment thoroughly; makes you feel like you are bothering him/her by asking for details about an illness or telephoning him/her about a medical concern, wanting to obtain a second opinion; doesn't take enough time to treat the child by rushing through the child's checkup; or overtreats the child, ignores your concerns and observations, or if your child's fear of the doctor is way out of proportion, for example, to receiving a simple injection.

As a parent, you can ease your child's doctor's visit by taking the following steps:

- Explain to your child why the visit to the doctor is necessary.
- Listen to your child's questions and concerns.
- Be honest when answering your child's questions.
- Reassure your child that the visit to the doctor is not a punishment for something he or she did wrong.
- If a procedure at the doctor's is going to hurt, tell your child that it's okay to cry or yell "ouch." Don't expect your child to be big and brave. Children are little and uncertain, and that is to be expected.[14]

REDUCING YOUR MEDICAL BILL

Once you have found and selected the kind of physician you seek, there are a number of steps that you can take as a patient to control the costs of your physician's services.

Phil was very concerned about this. Even though he had health insurance coverage from his job, he found that his employer was asking him to contribute more and more for his own insurance coverage. Phil remembered a time when his employer used to pay 100 percent of the premium, but not anymore. Health insurance was getting too expensive not only for Phil but also for his employer, who didn't want to lay off Phil and others to save money on health insurance and who did not want to go out of business because health insurance costs were eating into his profits upon which his business expansion relied.

Phil said, "My insurance coverage now has so many gaps in it. I know I'm going to have to pay for these gaps out of my own pocket in addition to what is being deducted from my salary at work. I only take home so much money each week. How can I minimize the size of my medical bills not just for me but for my family members as well?" Phil's employer may have provided Phil with health insurance coverage at work to help pay for Phil's medical bills, but it was up to Phil to decide what kind of doctors he wanted to visit for treatment. These, too, have an impact on reducing the costs of your medical bills. So the following points are what you want to look into to control the cost of your medical bills.

Consider Different Doctors

Physician fees differ, even in the same community. Ask the doctor if you could see a fee schedule or have sample prices quoted over the telephone before making your first appointment.

Look at old and young physicians. Doctors who have been in practice long enough to remember when fees were very low for any office visit may not be disposed to raise their fees as fast as younger physicians. A semiretired physician usually can spend more time with patients. While he may not keep up-to-date on all the latest tests and drugs, he could be the doctor you are seeking if you are looking for a personal touch. Physicians who are just starting their medical practices often establish fees low enough to attract patients; once established, however, they can raise them quickly.

Beware of False Savings

Solo practitioners often charge less per visit than medical group practices. However, a medical group may charge less for the services of staff specialists (e.g., technicians) than you would pay if you were referred to the group by a solo general practitioner. Also, physicians in medical groups often routinely discuss selected cases among themselves, the equivalent of a free consultation for you. Medical groups sometimes employ paraprofessionals to perform routine procedures at less cost to you and many have their own laboratories where tests can be processed, saving you time and money. Know what the insurer considers emergency care, and don't use the emergency room as a doctor's office.

Discuss Fees and Payment Plans

Fees are flexible, and physicians will often arrange their payments to meet your economic circumstances such as establishing installment payments if you need treatment and paying promptly will be a problem. But make sure you talk about the physician's fee schedule at your first meeting and not after the doctor sends you the bill. Also, ask your doctor about the cost of a procedure that your insurer does not cover and that you must pay yourself and whether or not your treatment requires such a procedure. You cannot let doctor bills go unpaid for months anymore. Many doctors expect immediate payment for your first visit; a few won't bill patients ever. Some doctors have even started cash-only practices where there are no insurance cards whatsoever. Medical groups with computerized billing may add finance charges to past-due bills and may turn over months-old bills to collection agencies. Find out whether the physician accepts the type of insurance you use or whether the physician takes Medicare or Medicaid patients. Does he accept Medicare fees as full payment? If not, how much might you have to pay?

How are payments handled—immediately by cash, check, or charge card, or will the physician wait for insurance reimbursement? More and more physicians accept credit cards, which can be a way for you to juggle medical bills. Does the physician require payment at each visit or immediately thereafter of new patients? Will the doctor's office handle your insurance forms? Many will (or you may want a doctor at a health plan where there are no insurance forms, only a regular monthly or other kind of time payment). These are important questions you need to ask for your own financial well-being.

If you believe a fee is not reasonable after the medical service is provided, then you should try to negotiate the fee with your physician. Be especially careful to discuss fees initially with a specialist, who may be very expensive but who also may reduce and stretch out the payments for his charges to meet your budget.

Ask your doctor whether he lowers his fee if you pay for the medical services quickly so that you do not have to be billed. There is always the possibility that you will have to pay less for a service at the time you receive it than when you receive the physician's bill at a later date. The reason for this circumstance is that some services do not have a "routine" charge. Also, if you have to visit the doctor regularly for continuing treatment, such as once a week, ask him if the cost might be less if he bills you for the total service rather than for each visit. Remember, only the doctor can reduce his fees. Therefore, discuss your bill with the physician—not with his nurse or his waiting room secretary, who do not have the power to negotiate. If the doctor refuses to reduce the fee and you are still bothered by the bill, ask your county medical association to review the matter. Also, keep good records to avoid overlooking a missed reimbursement. If your claim for reimbursement is denied and you feel that this rejection is unfair, appeal the decision. Any health plan for which you sign up should provide an impartial appeal mechanism to hear such complaints when you know the rejection is arbitrary. Such panels are required by law in more than forty states and Washington, DC.

Take Advantage of Your Doctor's Schedule

If you must discuss something with your doctor that may take a long time, ask for the last appointment of the day. Not pressured by the next patient, your doctor may be easing off his day's schedule and be happy for a chance to sit and talk. On the other hand, if you need a diagnosis, try to make an appointment for as early in the day as possible when your physician may not be tired.

Ask If Telephone Calls or E-mails Are Okay

Some physicians prefer to renew prescriptions and give routine advice on the telephone, at no charge, rather than have you take up precious office time. Physicians sometimes set aside telephone hours for taking calls or returning them. If a physician charges for a patient's call, it would probably be at a fraction of the original fee.

Some physicians prefer e-mail contact with their patients. More e-mail contacts means fewer office visits, which means more time can be spent with patients who really do have to come in. Other doctors are concerned about e-mails because they lack face-to-face contact with the patient and also because insurers do not reimburse for e-mail time. But whether your physician prefers e-mail contact or not, remember that your physician can always tell you to visit his office if he has any doubts about your condition.

However, do not seek phone advice when you ought to be making an appointment. Don't call at night or on weekends about nonurgent matters. But if you think it's an emergency or if you are in pain, say so. Also, be aware that some physicians are caught between rising costs and lower revenues and are beginning to charge patients not only for telephone time but also for paperwork and other services. Among the new billable items, aside from talking on the telephone with or e-mailing patients and their relatives, are providing copies of medical records or sending files to another doctor; calling a pharmacy with a prescription refill; and completing forms for school, disability, medical leave, life insurance, or summer camp. Some practices are even charging patients for missed appointments or those cancelled without at least twenty-four hours' notice. While it is difficult to know how widespread this trend may be, medical experts say the trends are more likely to be found among the three primary care specialties that are the least lucrative and most patient intensive: internal medicine, pediatrics, and family practice.

Transfer Medical Records

If you move or change doctors, have your old medical records transferred. You may not have to repeat recent tests and incur more medical bills. When seeing a medical specialist for the first time, volunteer accurate information about diagnostic tests you have had recently.

Think about Homecare

Uncomplicated long-term illness and recovery can often be taken care of at home instead of in expensive hospital rooms. Insurers like this idea more and more. Public agencies and private companies provide homecare nursing.

How Physician's Assistants Can Help

Today, many physicians employ a paraprofessional called the *physician's assistant* (PA), and the PAs may help reduce your medical bill. The physician's assistant works under the supervision of a doctor who approves and ultimately is responsible for the PA's work.

The responsibilities of the PA may vary depending upon the setting in which he works, but the basic idea is that PAs help physicians in some of the routine medical tasks for which they receive special academic training. They are employed in such medical settings as physicians' offices, hospitals, health maintenance organizations (HMOs), nursing homes, clinics, and other medical sites. Typically, following two years of training in an accredited program, PAs receive certification after passing an examination. They also take courses in continuing education and a recertifying exam every six years, just like many of their physician colleagues.

Some of the medical procedures PAs perform include the taking of medical histories, doing physical examinations, ordering certain laboratory tests, and advising patients about their diagnosis and treatment. Studies demonstrate that PAs are cost effective, meaning that, within the range of their abilities, they can provide competent medical services at less expense than physicians. In addition, PAs often spend more time with patients than physicians do, providing important patient education instruction.

In addition, your doctor may also employ a nurse practitioner who performs duties similar to the physician's assistant. All have an RN and some have a BS degree. All nurse practitioners have had at least an additional twelve months of training in order to practice as a nurse practitioner and, like the PAs, know when to bring in the MD for problems they cannot handle.[15]

Treating Minor Ailments

Do not forget that a doctor's time is constrained and expensive. You and your physician are a partnership and together can do much to prevent medical bills from increasing. Dr. William A. Nolen, the distinguished surgeon/author, has stated that he believes that one-half of patient visits could be avoided and the patients' yearly medical expenses reduced by at least one-half if patients knew how to treat minor cuts and bruises, headaches, colds or flu, sprains and strains, backaches, and minor puncture wounds. Your physician can advise you on such treatments. In addition, you can buy and use one of the many do-it-yourself medical books that tells you how to treat minor problems and how to recognize which symptoms require a physician's consultation and which ones do not. Ask your physician if he/she could recommend any.

Also, keep a first aid kit in your home, resupplying it as you use the following items: different-sized Band-aids, adhesive tape, sterile gauze pads, antiseptic ointment/wipes, sterile eye wash, hydrocortisone cream, triangular bandages, rubber gloves, an instant ice pack, petroleum jelly, hydrogen peroxide, over-the-counter pain relievers, sterile cotton, a thermometer, a tweezers, a small flashlight, safety pins, and scissors.

If you have an ailment for which you need, or think you need, to see a doctor, make an appointment during his regular office hours. If you insist on seeing him on a Sunday, for example, for an illness you have had for a week, the visit may cost you a lot more than it would have for a routine scheduled office visit. Some doctors feel they should be paid more for their services if they are asked to work odd hours. This advice, however, does not apply to emergency service—only to routine care that can be treated in a routine office visit.

Purchasing Prescription Drugs

Do not pay more for a medication than you must. Ask your doctor to prescribe the drug by its generic name. For example, penicillin tablets sold under the generic name (penicillin) will probably cost much less, depending upon the pharmacist's markup, as an equivalent product sold under a brand name. Most drugs dispensed under their generic names are as reliable as and almost always cheaper than their brand-name equivalents. Also, if you cannot afford to purchase a prescription drug, ask your physician whether he can match you up with a pharmaceutical company aid programs. In addition, don't forget, if you qualify for Medicare, the program now covers out-of-hospital prescription drugs.

Preventive Self-Care

Some health plans still refuse to reimburse you for doctor's visits when you are well. Make sure that your plan does reimburse for such preventive healthcare because, as examples, routine screening can detect a susceptibility to heart disease and many cancers can be cured if found early enough. Before taking a screening test, find out if there is good evidence that the test works, that the person performing it has the qualifications to do so, and, as in the case of cancer, that the test helps prevents deaths rather than just finding the illness. Federal guidelines are a good place to perform your own research. To read the guidelines on various illnesses, go to the US Agency for Healthcare Research and Quality on the Web at http://www.ahrq.gov/clinic and click on "Interactive Preventive Services Selector." On various cancer screening tests themselves, information is also available on the Web from the National Cancer Institute at http://www.cancer.gov/cancertopics/screening. Meanwhile, there are preventive healthcare steps that you can take to ensure your own physical well-being.

- Keep your weight at normal levels. Overweight people are much more susceptible to illnesses such as diabetes, heart disease, and high blood pressure than are people of normal weight.
- Get sufficient rest and relaxation.
- Drive carefully and watch out for accident and fire hazards in the home.
- Maintain a wise, low-fat, low-cholesterol diet, light on meat and heavy on fruits and vegetables.
- Do not smoke. The problems cigarettes cause—bronchitis, emphysema, heart disease, lung cancer—are well publicized.
- If you drink alcohol, do so in moderation. Excessive drinking can lead to alcoholism and cirrhosis.
- Get regular, vigorous exercise. Regular means at least three times a week, and vigorous means an activity that will raise your normal pulse rate about 50 percent and keep it there at least twelve minutes. You should check with your physician before beginning any exercise regimen so that he can make sure that you are fit to begin and give you advice as to what regimen to follow. If you follow his instructions, the price of that one visit will save you lots of money in the future by helping you to stay healthy.

Seeking Physical Examinations

Some physicians now question whether patients must have annual physical examinations—unless, of course, they have medical problems that require repeated checkups, in which case the examinations would not be classified as "routine." Complete checkups are becoming very expensive. Despite the cost, many patients still insist on an annual physical examination, and many corporations demand that their officers have them.

In 1983, the American Medical Association revised and offered the following guidelines for medical examinations:

- If you are pregnant, you should visit your physician every 4 weeks for the first 28 weeks, every 2 to 3 weeks for the next 8 weeks, and then each week until delivery.
- Newborn infants should be seen by a physician 2 to 4 weeks after birth, 5 or 6 times within the first year of life, and thereafter every 1 to 2 years up through age 21.
- Between ages 2 and 20, you should have a physical every year or two.
- Between ages 21 and 39, you should have a physical every 5 years.
- Between ages 40 and 65, you should have a physical examination every 1 to 3 years.

Your physician may give you a complete and thorough physical examination, including a proctoscopy, chest x-rays, and an electrocardiogram (stress and regular).

Blood tests can detect anemia, infection, diabetes, kidney trouble, abnormal blood fats such as cholesterol that predispose one to heart attacks, cancer, and hepatitis. Other disorders or more exotic diseases such as Lyme disease or AIDS conditions can be found through targeted blood tests. Because of this extensive testing, your bill will probably be expensive.

After age sixty, according to Dr. Nolen, you are very fortunate if you do not have any problems that require regular office visits to a physician. For example, Pap smears (a test for cervical cancer) are no longer annually recommended for women of all ages even though the American College of Obstetricians and Gynecologists (ACOG) recommends annual Pap smears for women up to the age of thirty, with the first screen beginning three years after the first sexual intercourse or by age twenty-one, whichever comes first. Previously, the ACOG called for the first Pap smear by the onset of sexual activity or age eighteen, whichever came first. In 2003 the ACOG revised its guidelines and if you are a woman over thirty recommends Pap smears at least once every two to three years, especially if you are taking birth control pills and if you have a recent history of three or more consecutive normal Pap smears. Cervical cancer screening is generally not recommended for women over sixty-five or seventy or for women who had hysterectomies. But in a survey of women aged forty and over after the recommendations were published, 75 percent of women wanted annual Pap smears despite the recommendations for the two- to three-year interval. In addition, according to the American Cancer Society, women in their twenties and thirties should have clinical breast examinations about every three years, and after the age of forty, women should have a screening mammogram every year to detect breast cancer as well as a yearly clinical breast examination (CBE) by a health professional.[16]

If you need a mammogram, make sure the facility is approved by the Food and Drug Administration. You can find out by checking the certificate in the facility. Or call 1-800-422-6337 to find out the names of certified facilities near you.

Dr. Nolen believes that getting rid of the concept that most people need a complete annual checkup would probably reduce our national health budget by millions of dollars.[17] But, of course, the frequency of physical examinations is an individual and personal decision, and these guidelines are noted here in terms of present medical opinions.

Listen to Your Doctor's Advice

Don't ask for unnecessary prescriptions, office visits, shots, diagnostic tests, or x-rays. They will not only add to your medical bills but also your physician will tell you whether they are necessary for your recovery.

Your Physician's Role in Reducing Your Medical Bill

Not only must you exercise prudence in controlling your personal medical expenses, but your physician also has a role in this regard. Individual physicians can contribute significantly to the containment of medical costs, in part, through your patient care treatment plan. The American Medical Association, in suggesting ways your doctor can help reduce your medical expenses, asks physicians:

- When referring patients to another physician, do you send along all reports (lab tests, x-rays, etc.) that may be required in order to avoid costly duplication?
- Do you receive previous reports and lab results when a patient is referred to you?
- Do you stand up to patient pressure to prescribe tests, treatments, or medications that you feel are harmless but unnecessary?
- Do you know the cost of the diagnostic tests and x-rays you order?
- Are you familiar with the cost of the medications you prescribe? Are you aware of competitive brands that may offer your patient the same clinical effectiveness but at a lower cost?
- Do you emphasize to your patients that the emergency room is only for emergencies; that they should call you first if they are not certain that they require emergency room services?
- Do you avoid referring patients with nonemergency problems to the emergency room?
- Do you have an arrangement to provide physician coverage when you are unavailable so that patients who cannot locate you will not have to turn to the emergency room for minor problems?
- Do you explain medical procedures to your patients so they will know what aftereffects are to be expected and what aftereffects may require a follow-up phone call or visit?
- Have you considered employing other healthcare professionals in your office for patient education and routine procedures so that you may use your time more effectively?
- Do you schedule diagnostic tests or procedures on an outpatient basis whenever feasible?
- Do you or a qualified member of your staff provide your patients with information on prevention and self-care? Do you explain the importance of adhering to the treatment regimens, diets, and so on that you prescribe?
- Have you considered using patient education booklets or other patient information materials to explain procedures that you perform frequently or diets and other treatment regimens which are common in your practice?[18]

Although some of these questions were discussed earlier from the patient's viewpoint, they are applicable to the physician as well. By becoming more aware of the economic implications of their medical decisions, physicians can do much to alleviate rising medical costs while continuing to deliver high-quality medical services.

But there is also another trend, however small, that is emerging in American medicine for those patients who can afford it. This trend is called "boutique" medicine, as some doctors abandon large group plans for a small select clientele. For an annual fee that may amount to thousands of dollars, the medical industry will offer you round-the-clock phone service, appointments on demand, valet parking, interpreters in your native language, someone to accompany you to a specialist and to hospitals when required, in some cases someone to make house calls, coordinated care among specialists, and treatments such as a full body scan, emphasizing personal attention, prevention, nutrition counseling, exercise programs, and new technologies. Beyond that, patients must pay—in cash or through their insurance plans—for any medical services provided. While some concierge doctors accept private insurance and Medicare, most insurers and Medicare will not reimburse for a patient's annual fees or services the plans do not normally cover. Other doctors don't accept private insurance or participate in Medicare because they don't want to deal with the paperwork or constraints insurers require. Patients need to check about payment arrangements if they are considering the receipt of boutique care. A slight variation of this form of medical practice is VIP medicine, which, for an initiation charge and an annual fee, links the patient to elite specialists, promises twenty-four-hour access, and, in some instances, home visits.

EYECARE AND EYEWEAR

Another area where you may reduce your medical bill relates to the purchase of eyeglasses and contact lenses.

Frank was talking to his wife one day about his work situation, complaining that he seemed to be getting passed over for promotions at work because his physical appearance made him look older than his colleagues who were competing for the same position. He didn't know if he would look younger if he changed his eyewear to a more fashionable kind of style or whether wearing contact lenses would improve his chances for a promotion. In addition, he said jokingly to his wife, "You know, I think all the print magazines and newspapers are conspiring against me for some unknown reason, because they seem to be making the size of their words smaller and smaller the older I become. What's worse, I don't even know who I should go to for advice about my eyewear? Should I visit an ophthalmologist, an optometrist, or an optician? What is the difference among them?"

Frank would like to have a better understanding of what these different eyewear specialists do. He has heard that some even sell their own eyeglasses after an examination. Frank wants the best for his money and does not want to be forced to buy eyeglasses or contacts from the person examining him. Well, Frank does not have to worry. In the spring of 1978, the Federal Trade Commission ruled that ophthalmologists and optometrists must release a written prescription for eyeglasses to a patient who requests it. The rule also prohibits physicians and optometrists from charging patients extra for releasing the prescription and from requiring patients to buy eyewear that the examiner may sell. Some states also require the release of contact lens prescriptions. Check with your optometrist or ophthalmologist as to whether your state mandates such a prescription release.

Some physicians are concerned that when they write a prescription for contact lenses, they could be held responsible for any medical problem that could arise if you, the patient, fill the prescription elsewhere. When you are armed with this prescription and the information sellers of eyewear provide through advertisements, the Federal Trade Commission hopes you will be able to find the best combination of price and quality. Thus, you now have the opportunity to compare prices among different opticians who are responsible for making the glasses. Opticians are technicians who not only make and fit eyeglasses but also, in some places, dispense contact lenses. However, they cannot write a prescription for corrective lenses or diagnose eye diseases. Also, find out if your state requires formal licensing for opticians.

In 1993 only about half the states required formal licensing for opticians; in the others, just about anyone could open up a practice. But be aware that a state license or certification by the American Board of Opticianry may only be an indicator (but not a guarantee) of appropriate training. In addition to opticians, others who sell eyewear can include private optometrists, ophthalmologists, pharmacies, discount stores, and mail-order firms. When you compare prices, mail-order firms are not always the least expensive. Even when they match others' low prices, you still pay a shipping fee, while discount houses include no shipping fee and tend to be competitive. Make sure you compare the prices and quality of service among the various sellers of eyewear. They can vary greatly for the same lenses owing to the cost of doing business and the amount and quality of eyecare the wearer will receive.

More complicated prescriptions may also cost more at some optical offices because the offices don't do a high volume in specialized prescriptions. It is more trouble for them than it may be for a discount firm. And a doctor with a small practice who provides thorough aftercare for you, the patient, likely will charge more than a mail-order firm that deals in high volume and offers you no personal care. So select what's best for you.

When you visit a dispenser of eyewear, make sure the fitting is done carefully and exactly, with the center of the glass lined up at the visual axis of the eye. The dispenser should measure the distance between your eyes. Both you and the dispenser should make sure that the frame you select is not too large or too small. If the frame does not sit well on your face, your glasses might slip off your nose, creating distorted vision and a general feeling of discomfort. Also, large lenses can create a distortion at the edges. In selecting frames, be aware that higher prices may be due more to fashion and ornateness than quality. Remember, if you purchase corrective lenses from an optometrist, he is not a physician but a doctor of optometry (DO), who has received a minimum of six years of academic study, professional training, and clinical experience to examine eyes for vision problems, diagnose eye diseases, and prescribe glasses and contact lenses. Various states permit DOs to prescribe certain drugs to treat eye diseases.

The American Medical Association has noted that in the case of eyeglasses, an ophthalmologist (a physician specializing in eyecare) may want you to return for a visit after the prescription is filled so that he may verify the accuracy and wearing comfort of the eyeglasses. The ophthalmologist has completed several years of residency study diagnosing and treating eye diseases. Unlike optometrists, ophthalmologists can perform surgery. More and more, private ophthalmologists are checking eyes and selling eyeglasses and contact lenses. An ophthalmologist will determine whether the glasses themselves are centered and the pupil distance—the optical center of near and far vision—has been correctly measured. He will see to it that the base of the curvature of the lens has been accurately ground. With respect to contact lenses, an ophthalmologist will usually want to examine you after the initial fitting to make certain that the lenses are not causing any injury to your eyes. In some cases, such as patients who have had cataract surgery, lens modification may be necessary from time to time, thereby requiring changes in the patient's prescription. If you wear contact lenses, there are five basic types:

- *Soft contact lenses*, also known as daily-wear contacts, are the most commonly worn lenses in the United States. They are made with a soft, pliable plastic that allows oxygen to pass through the lenses. Traditional soft lenses are removed nightly, cleaned and disinfected, then worn again the next morning.
- *Extended-wear soft contact lenses* are plastic lenses that can be worn for up to seven days at a time before they must be removed for cleaning and disinfecting prior to being worn again. Because of increased infections, most ophthalmologists do not recommend sleeping in contact lenses.
- *Disposable soft contact lenses* look the same as standard soft contact lenses or extended-wear lenses. Their advantage is that they can be made cheaply enough to be discarded after seven days of use, thus eliminating cleaning and disinfecting. Some people double the life span of disposables by cleaning and disinfecting them just as they would standard soft contacts.
- *Rigid gas-permeable contact lenses* are made of a firmer plastic that has a longer life span than soft contacts. They must be removed daily for cleaning and disinfecting.
- *Traditional hard lenses* are made of a tough, inflexible plastic, which does not allow oxygen to pass through the lenses. Of all contacts, they last the longest but must be removed daily for cleaning and disinfecting. Few patients tolerate these lenses.

When purchasing contact lenses, ask the doctor about the pros and cons of each kind of lens in regard to your vision problems. For example, in 1989 a study published in the *New England Journal of Medicine* (September 21,1989) found that extended-wear contact users had a ten to fifteen times higher risk of developing ulcerative keratitis than contact wearers who removed and cleaned their lenses every day. Then, a study performed by John Hopkins Medical School between 1990 and1992 showed that patients who wore disposables had the greatest risk of eye infection. They were fourteen times more likely to develop ulcerative keratitis than people who wore standard soft lenses and seven times more likely to develop the problem than those who used nondisposable extended-wear contacts. These findings seem to indicate that disposable contact lenses worn overnight are associated with greater risk of corneal infection. If caught early enough, corneal infection can be cured with antibiotics. If not caught early, severe impairment of sight or, occasionally, blindness can result.

The cornea is the transparent covering of the iris and pupil on which the contact lens rests. A corneal ulcer is a raw, sore spot or eruption on the front surface of the eye that is caused by various infections.

Eye Infections

Pain in the eye is the main symptom of a corneal ulcer and *Acanthamoeba keratitis*, a rare and difficult-to-treat eye infection, which has been increasing in people wearing all types of contacts. Another infection is *Pseudomonas keratitis*, caused by the *Pseudomonas* bacteria, which has the tendency to stick to the surface of the contact lens and leads to pain, itchiness, redness, and irritation. Although the infection is more responsive to medication than is the *Acanthamoeba*, if it is not caught early enough, like the *Acanthamoeba*, it could cause enough corneal damage to cause permanent visual loss.

Another eye condition that is treatable is called presbyopia, which is related to aging and universally occurs after age forty. The eye loses its ability to focus at near distance and requires a separate lens correction, either as a bifocal or a separate reading glass. A procedure that is used today to correct vision is LASIK surgery, which improves vision by reshaping the cornea for people who have trouble seeing distant objects.

If you wear contacts and develop eye pain, see your eye doctor right away. Eye infections or minor trauma—such as wearing improperly cleaned contacts or keeping contacts in too long—can cause an ulcer to develop. So ask your doctor which contacts are the best for preventing the occurrence of ulcerative keratitis and about the various other risks that different kinds of contact lenses might pose for your eyesight. Other contact lens–related corneal problems include irritation, swelling, and scratching, which tend to be transient and not as severe. The milder conditions usually can be traced to an ill-fitting lens, a piece of dirt trapped under the lens, or a lens that itself is scratched or torn. The eyes itch, burn, and redden, and the best treatment is to take out the lens for a few days. If the lens is damaged or poorly fit, it needs to be replaced. Most doctors today advise patients to wear lenses for no more than six days, and if they are to be used again, they should be cleaned and disinfected. All contact lens wearers also need to have regular checkups, at least twice a year for regular contacts and four times a year for those who wear any type of extended-wear contact lenses. Should any redness, discomfort, light sensitivity, or excess tears occur, the contact should be removed immediately. And if it doesn't get better in an hour or two, call the ophthalmologist.[19]

To help reduce the risk of trouble with contact lenses, eye doctors recommend the following steps:

- Keep overnight use of contact lenses—even extended-wear lenses—to a minimum. The less they are worn while sleeping, the smaller the chance of having ulcers and infections develop.
- Never wear daily contact lenses overnight.
- Always wash your hands thoroughly with soap and water before handling contacts.
- Remove contact lenses before swimming or using a hot tub. Even chlorinated water will not kill all the pool bacteria, which can stick to the surfaces of contact lenses.
- Never put contact lenses in your mouth and then place them in your eye. The mouth is a rich source of bacteria.
- Use only sterilized cleaning or heat-processing sterilization to clean contacts. Avoid the use of salt tablets, distilled water, or homemade saline, which can't sterilize the lenses.
- Disinfect as well as clean all contact lenses by one of three methods: heat sterilization, hydrogen peroxide, or another chemical disinfectant.
- Remove, rinse, and clean contacts at the first sign of eye redness or irritation. Other warning signs: blurry vision, swollen lids, discharge, pain, or the sensation of a foreign object in the eye. Seek immediate medical attention if any of these symptoms persist.
- Allow lens cases to air-dry after each use. Wash them weekly. One study found that nearly half of the lens cases were contaminated with bacteria and fungi—even though the wearers had no signs of eye problems.
- Have eyes and lenses checked regularly by a medical professional. Extended-wear contact lenses that are not recommended for sleeping in should be double-checked every three to six months; soft wear daily-use lenses and hard lenses every six to twelve months.[20]

The American Medical Association encourages patients to see their ophthalmologist to foster good eyecare, although prescriptions for any drugs or devices may be filled anywhere. The ophthalmologist can suggest an appropriate interval between examinations depending upon your needs. For example, if a child is tested at age three, you will usually know if he has an astigmatism if he is farsighted or nearsighted. If he is not abnormally farsighted or nearsighted at three and is tested every year or two at school, the school authorities should be able to pick up any significant change. If you wear glasses by age twenty, your eyes usually change little at thirty up to forty.

Therefore, your ophthalmologist may suggest that your eyes be checked every two years after the age of forty. One reason for the more frequent examinations is that an eye examination can detect the onset of glaucoma, macular degeneration, diabetic retinopathy, or other illnesses. According to Dr. Susan Taub, a Northwestern University ophthalmologist, protecting your eyes from the sun, not smoking since smoking also damages eyes, and eating lots of vitamin-packed dark leafy vegetables may help prevent these diseases from ever forming.[21] Age-related macular degeneration, or AMD, steals vision from the center of the eye outward because the macula, a sensitive area in the retina responsible for central and detail vision, is damaged, again often causing loss of central vision. Glaucoma usually steals vision from the outside in, with gradual damage to the optic nerve that first destroys peripheral vision. Diabetic retinopathy is a diabetes complication in which retinal blood vessels break, leak, or become blocked, causing spotty vision. Like glaucoma, cataracts are another condition that interferes with clear vision and can be a natural part of the aging process. Many people over age sixty may have both conditions. Otherwise, the two are not related. With the exception of glaucoma owing to secondary causes such as trauma or steroids, glaucoma does not cause cataracts and cataracts do not result in glaucoma. Glaucoma is most often a problem with drainage—that is, the correct amount of fluid cannot drain out of the eye when the eye's drainage canals become clogged—causing the inner eye pressure (also called intraocular pressure, or IOP) to rise. Glaucoma is a group of diseases that steal eyesight without warning and without symptoms. The most common form is called Primary Open Angle Glaucoma and responds well to medication, especially if caught early and treated. The less common forms of glaucoma that you should ask your physician about are Angle Closure Glaucoma, Secondary Glaucoma, Normal Tension Glaucoma (NTG), and Pigmentary Glaucoma.

On the other hand, a cataract is the clouding of the eye's natural lens, the part of the eye responsible for focusing light and producing clear, sharp images, thus allowing less light to pass through. Cataracts do not form on the eye, but rather within the eye. The eye's lens is contained in a sealed bag or capsule. As old cells die, they become trapped within the capsule. Over time, the cells accumulate, causing the lens to cloud and making images look blurred or fuzzy. Eye injuries, certain medications, and diseases such as diabetes and alcoholism have also been known to cause cataracts. The commonality between glaucoma and cataracts is that both are serious conditions that can cause you to lose vision. However, loss of vision as a result of cataracts can be reversed with surgery. As yet, the loss of vision from glaucoma is not reversible.

If you want more information about these diseases, you can contact Prevent Blindness America at 1-800-331-2020 or visit its Web site at http://www.prevent blindness.org. By detecting any disease in its early stages, you may prevent more expensive treatments at a later date.

A thorough eye examination should include:

- *History.* The examiner should take a record of past and current eye problems, systemic disease, and family history. Diabetes and high blood pressure, in particular, can damage blood vessels in the retina, causing serious vision problems or blindness. The examiner should ask about any particular visual requirements in your job or hobbies and any medications you take.

- *Eye coordination.* The test tracks how well your eyes work together.
- *Visual acuity.* The doctor uses the familiar eye chart to judge far and near vision, with and without glasses.
- *Eye structure.* A "slit lamp" or biomicroscope plays light across the eye, permitting the examiner to check the lids, cornea, iris, pupil, and front of the lens. An "ophthalmoscope" is a lighted device that allows the doctor to see the retina and the optic nerve.
- *Refraction.* A "phoroptor," an instrument you look through with dial-in lenses for all possible prescriptions, allows the doctor to determine the amount of refraction—bending of light rays—that is required to correct your vision to normal.
- *Intraocular pressure.* Some doctors use an air-puff machine to measure pressure in the eye; high pressure is the cause of glaucoma. More precise measurement requires the use of drops to anesthetize the eye and an instrument that gently presses against the eyeball.
- *Field testing (peripheral vision).* Measuring peripheral vision can reveal retinal damage, other eye diseases, or neurological problems, including certain brain tumors.[22]

The American Optometric Association recommends a yearly exam for everyone from preschool to age twenty-five, exams every two years between ages twenty-five and thirty-five, and annual exams again for those thirty-five years and older. According to the US Public Health Service, diabetics should undergo an eye exam for possible retina damage every year. And persons at high risk for glaucoma— African Americans over the age forty and all people over sixty—should similarly be examined at least once every two years.[23]

DEVELOPING GOOD PATIENT-PHYSICIAN COMMUNICATIONS

In order to develop the best treatment program for you, your physician needs your assistance. Communication is the key here.

"But that's the problem," Janet told her husband. "Every time I go to my doctor, I become nervous. That white coat makes my doctor seem like such an authority or powerful figure. I am afraid to ask questions because I'm afraid he will think I am questioning his judgment, that he'll become angry and ask me to stop being his patient. I really don't want to lose him. Besides, doctors seem to treat men differently than women. Some are so friendly and take their time to listen to you like Marcus Welby on that old television program, while others seem to be in such a rush, are indifferent to your problems, and don't give you any time to ask them questions."

Janet complains that sometimes she feels like she's a number in the waiting room and on an assembly line. "There are times," Janet continues, "that if I see a doctor for five minutes, it seems like it's a lot of time. I spend more time with the nurses and assistants in my doctor's office than with my own doctor. I know he is very busy, but I would like to have a better relationship with him and be able to communicate with him better. But I don't even know where to begin or what kind of questions I should ask him or what kind of questions he may be asking me."

There are times Janet feels embarrassed to tell a doctor, even a woman doctor, very personal things about her medical or emotional condition, thinking he or she might think ill of her. "I only wish I knew how to prepare myself better when I visit the doctor so that no matter how much time he spends with me I will feel that I am getting the most of out my visit. I just wish I knew what kind of questions I should be asking him and what to expect when he is treating me. I think I would feel much better and less afraid when I visit my doctor if I only knew how to communicate with him without being afraid."

What to Ask and Tell the Physician

There are seven elements to a successful doctor-patient communications:

1. Be ready to make decisions when you visit your doctor.
2. Have your questions prepared in advance before visiting his office.
3. Ask about and know the advantages and disadvantages of whatever treatments your doctor may prescribe, and ask your doctor why he favors one form of treatment over another—for example, surgery versus drugs.
4. Discuss with your doctor any conflicts in the methods of treatment he prescribes—for example, if a drug makes you uncomfortable, ask for another drug. The doctor may feel the drug may not be as effective but at least the patient will take it. Unfortunately, some patients fail to give their physician all the information he or she may require. They may fail to mention drugs they are taking, drinking habits, sexual problems; and—not realizing how emotional disturbances can trigger or exacerbate physical illness—they neglect to discuss their depressed or anxious feelings and crises at work or at home.
5. Therefore, be honest about your lifestyle and habits such as not sticking to a recommended diet if a diabetic or not taking all the medications that have been prescribed for your condition(s). For your own physical and emotional well-being, you should be prepared to tell your physician everything you can about your problem, as succinctly as possible, including other treatments you have tried.
6. Before a visit, take your temperature. Fever is a common sign of infection, so your physician will want to know your temperature. Make a list of your symptoms—recall when they began, the order in which they appeared, whether they are they getting better or worse, what makes them better or

worse and how they changed, how long they lasted, whether they are affecting eating, sleeping, or other activities and, if so, how—and remember all the medications you are taking, including prescription, over-the-counter, as well as any natural remedies and their dosage. If you are aware of emotional discomfort, let the physician know. Don't self-diagnose. Don't hold back information or questions about symptoms or feelings or fears out of shyness or embarrassment. Many patients do. Don't assume that some symptoms are caused by aging or stress or the weather. Let your doctor decide. It is best to give information without applying your judgment to the problem. Do not leave your doctor's office feeling your questions have not been answered. That doesn't mean, however, that you shouldn't mention unusual aspects of the illness—just don't present them as its cause.

7. If you are talking to a specialist, have specialized information ready. For example, if your doctor is a gynecologist, you should have ready any information about changes relating to your gynecological health such as whether you've changed your contraceptive methods. There are certain problems that many women hesitate to raise with their doctor. A lot of women are afraid to report any symptom they think may indicate cancer. Because of this, the disease could be untreatable by the time they finally report it. Therefore, when visiting your gynecologist, especially when filling out your medical history, be prepared to tell your gynecologist the following information because of its medical implications for your personal health. This information includes the length of your period, your cycle regularity, any pain or heavy bleeding of cycles, any premenstrual symptoms (length and severity), the number of pregnancies you have had (number of deliveries, C-sections, miscarriages, or terminations), any history of infertility, your methods of contraception (if any), absent or reduced sexual desire or pleasure, any sexually transmitted diseases, and any symptoms if menopausal.

Another issue is sex-related health problems that are often not mentioned—even when they might be the primary complaint. If something is really bothering you, no matter how trivial you may consider it to be, be sure to ask your doctor about it. That is why your physician is there. It is possible that the question you do not ask could be the one that saves your life. Also, make sure you report anything unusual to your physician, especially any changes you may have noticed about your body. From age thirty-five on, the annual gynecological exam should be coupled with a comprehensive medical checkup that includes a cancer screening, a check for heart disease, and a check for osteoporosis, which is a condition that results in fragile bones.

Remember that drugs and illnesses differ between women and men. To obtain more information about women's health, men's health, and treatments for various medical conditions, you can go to the online magazine of Health Pages at http://www.thehealthpages.com.

In women drugs such as aspirin, acetaminophen, and Valium remain in the body longer. Women also tend to have higher incidences of migraines, eating disorders, osteoporosis, and heart-valve problems than men, and depression because their brain has less depression-fighting serotonin than men. As other examples, female diabetics are at much greater risk of heart diseases than male diabetics, while sexually transmitted diseases progress more quickly in women. This is why it is very important, as already noted, to discuss with your doctor all the issues that may be of concern, no matter how unimportant they may seem at the time. When your doctor recommends a prescription medicine or a procedure, find out whether its effect has been studied in women and not just in men. Medications, tested only in men, for example, but prescribed far more frequently for women, such as diet and psychiatric drugs, have caused serious side effects in women.

Therefore, make sure you are prepared before you visit your physician for the first time. Find out as much as you can about your family's medical history. If you wish to create a family history, visit the Mayo Clinic Web site at http://www.mayo clinic.com and search for family history. You may also visit the federal government's Centers for Disease Control and Prevention (CDC) Web site and its Family History Initiative, which provides information on this subject. Go to http://www.cdc.gov. If your physician requires that you answer a detailed patient history questionnaire, have it sent to you ahead of time so that you can find the answers. You should be able to provide the following information to your doctor:

- The name and strengths of all your medications and why, when, and how often you take them: Hourly? Twice a day? Before or after meals? (Sometimes patients forget why medicines were prescribed yet take them anyway. If you do this, be sure to tell your doctor. Wrong medication combinations can be deadly.)
- Vaccinations you have had.
- Illnesses that occur in your family.
- Any previous medical evaluations or diagnosed health problems, such as high blood pressure. Do you control it? With diet? Exercise? Medication?
- Men: Give your doctor the dates and results of your last prostate-specific antigen (PSA) blood test.
- Women: List the dates of your last Pap smear and mammogram. The American Cancer Society recommends a yearly mammogram for women beginning at age forty.
- Men and women: Ask your doctor how to submit stool tests for colon evaluation.
- If you are over fifty and have never had a colonoscopy, ask your doctor about getting one as soon as possible.
- Work with your doctor to find ways to make any prescribed lifestyle changes needed to improve your health. If quitting a habit like drinking doesn't cure a terminal illness, it might slow down or lessen your chances of getting one.

• Never fail to obtain a regular physical examination, even if you're feeling fine. Ask your doctor how often you should get a checkup. The tests your doctor performs and at what intervals depend upon your age, occupation, sex, family history, and other factors. Standard procedures include blood tests, an electrocardiogram, a mammogram, a colonoscopy (important at age fifty and every five years thereafter or more often if you have had any change in your bowel habits, blood in the stool, polyps removed, or a family history of colon cancer), a bone density test, PSA levels (for prostate disorders), as well as frequent monitoring of any abnormalities that may have been detected previously. According to Dr. Isadore Rosenfeld, Distinguished Professor of Clinical Medicine at the New York Hospital–Cornell Medical Center, if you are told the examination will take less than thirty minutes, that is not enough time. It takes forty-five minutes to an hour to have all the tests you require exclusive of any special procedures that may be performed such as electrocardiographic stress testing.[24]

To be fair, there are good reasons why patients may communicate poorly with their physicians. Their physicians may tell them things they do not understand and they neglect to ask what they mean. Some do not want to appear unintelligent; some, aware that other patients are waiting, do not wish to take up the physician's time; some may fear that they are questioning the physician's judgment. As a result, they go home bewildered—and often needlessly worried and anxious. Therefore, if you believe it will help, don't go to the doctor alone, especially if you have a language impairment problem from a stroke or other condition. Take along a friend or relative to help you ask questions. A second person can help you later remember more of what was said in the doctor's office and may be more insistent in getting firm answers than you are. Tell your doctor beforehand that you want to know all you can about your condition and let him know if you have a hearing or visual impairment. Thus, when your doctor makes a diagnosis, have him explain it clearly to you. Take notes if necessary. If your physician uses medical terms you do not understand, ask him to explain, and don't go on to the next question until you are positive you understand the explanation. If the doctor answers you with clichés or patronizing answers or avoids giving you a direct response, insist that he elaborate. Also, always look the doctor in the eye and speak forcefully. Otherwise, the doctor may think he doesn't have to be straightforward or complete with you. And when a physician prescribes a treatment, you have a right to know what it can reasonably be expected to do, in how long a time, any risks that may be involved, and any possible alternatives. Double-check your understanding of what you may have been told. In your own words, repeat to the physician what you understand to be the nature of your problem and your treatment.

Know whether your insurance policy covers or does not cover the costs of that treatment and whether the policy states that the procedure must have a prior written authorization so that your insurer will not reject your claim for that procedure. If you feel rushed by your doctor or he or she seems vague, impatient, or unwilling to answer your questions, ask him if there would be a more convenient time for you to question him at greater length. And if your physician repeatedly rushes you, will not listen, and avoids communicating effectively with you, then you probably should change doctors. It's important, before you find yourself in an emergency situation, to have a doctor with whom you can communicate. For the sake of your own personal health, you must understand the treatment your physician wishes you to follow; for your emotional well-being, you need to know why it is being prescribed. Such an understanding will contribute greatly to your recovery.[25]

Doctors should welcome the following interchange of questions when you visit:

- What is wrong with me, doctor?
- What caused it?
- What should be done about it?
- What will it cost?
- What tests should be performed?
- Why?
- What will you do next?
- Is it necessary?
- Do I, the patient, have alternatives?
- Is it dangerous?

When you visit your physician for the first time, expect him to take your medical history and give you a complete physical examination. The way a doctor examines you may tell you more about the doctor than any question. A thorough exam should include questions about you and your family, job, finances, or other problems that might affect your emotional as well as your physical health. The doctor will take a history of the present illness, asking such questions as when, where, and how did the problem begin? What makes it better or worse or doesn't affect it? Is it something that has occurred to you before or someone else in your family? Any recent foreign travels where you may have been exposed to new parasites, viruses, and bacteria? What about your energy levels and sleeping patterns? The doctor will also ask questions about your past medical history to put your current problem into perspective with your previously known medical problems such as previous surgeries, past blood transfusions, allergies, bad reactions to medicines, or alcohol, drug, and tobacco use.

Sometimes your social history—such as your occupation, the number of members of your household, your educational status, or recent events in your life—is as important as your family history. Asking you about your family's history can be useful in identifying a genetic risk for certain conditions. In some cases, the doctor will touch upon all these issues, and at other times the problem is so obvious that these details are not necessary. As already noted, most doctors agree that no doctor can take an initial history and do a thorough physical in less than thirty minutes, and that is fast. Many take an hour. If you said you wanted a thorough physical or you have a serious problem and your doctor does not have you take off all your clothes and examine you from head to foot, you have not had a thorough physical. If you have the feeling that you have not really been examined—you were not examined in significant places or you didn't have a chance to say something significant—you were probably slighted. If your doctor diagnoses your condition and prescribes treatment without examining you at all, you may have reason to suspect that you are receiving less than optimal care. If your physician fails to examine you in areas you wish him to look at, ask him to do so. Most doctors will readily comply.

It is not always possible that the diagnosis is clear or established after the history and the physical examination are completed. Instead, your physician may be left with a number of possible causes of the problem, the differential diagnosis. After considering the patient's history and exam, and matching it with the diseases in the differential diagnosis, the physician then puts all the pieces together to form an impression. This is a statement in which the possible causes of the chief complaint are discussed, usually in the order of decreasing likelihood. After formulating an impression, a plan is made. This is a statement about what the doctor wants to do next. It may include treatment, further diagnostic testing, watchful waiting, or referral to a specialist. The plan is usually known as "Doctor's orders."[26]

The following information should enable you to help your physician treat you and allow you to understand the reasons for his undertaking various medical procedures. Remember, there are no foolish questions. The only foolish question is the one you did not ask even though you wanted to.

Diagnostic Tests

If your physician orders diagnostic tests, try to have your doctor not use a scatter-shot approach—that is, doing every conceivable test and taking every possible x-ray because something is certain to be revealed. If your physician's treatment involves invasive, new, costly, or experimental testing, the following questions may help you. What do I have to do to prepare for the test? What are the chances the test will help? How is the test done? Does it cause any pain, discomfort, or complications? Has the test's value been established by good research? Has there been an adequate clinical trial in a large number of patients? What were the results? Ask what the physician hopes to learn from the test, and why that information is important in your case. If there are any risks involved, your physician should tell you what they are—and why he or she feels the benefits of the tests outweigh the risks.

If you take the tests the physician is ordering now, can the results possibly help you? Will they affect your treatment one way or the other? If the test turns out positive, will your doctor do anything to you that he/she would not do anyway? If not, why do the test? How accurate is it? If neither you nor your doctor would do anything differently regardless of how the test came out, then the test is medically unnecessary and you are ill advised to undergo the risks, expense, and inconvenience the test involves. For tests your doctor sends to a laboratory, ask which he or she uses and why. You may want to know that the physician chooses a particular laboratory because he has business ties to it or the health plan may require that the test go there. Find out if the laboratory is accredited by a group such as the College of American Pathologists (1-800-323-4040 or http://www.cap.org) or the Joint Commission on the Accreditation of Hospitals (1-630-792-5800 or http://www.jcaho.org). Ask how long it will take to get the results of the test and how you will get them.

What are the alternatives? What will happen to you if you don't do it? Is that a risk?

Is this something your physician does a lot? If there are risks, would he/she recommend using someone who performs this test more frequently? What would your physician do if he/she were in your situation and who would he/she go to? Are there any self-diagnostic tests that can be performed at home at less cost, such as checking your own blood pressure rather than going to the clinic every two or three weeks to do so?

What will the test cost? Remember, it is still your decision to take the tests and you have the right to refuse. Find out how long it will take to get a report of the results. If your doctor orders x- rays, ask what the dosage will be. Keep track of how many x-rays (including dental x-rays) you have received, and ask your doctor if your cumulative exposure is within a safe range.

When the test results are known, ask for the exact values, and get your doctor to tell you what the normal range is. If you are pregnant or think you are, be sure to tell your doctor before submitting to any x-rays. According to the American College of Radiology guidelines (1983), chest x-rays given automatically to persons who are asymptomatic in prenatal examinations and during preemployment physicals (except on a selective basis, dependent on people's jobs and medical history), tuberculosis screening, and hospital admissions are not necessary.

If a biopsy is performed, ask for the results of the pathologist's report. If any of the tests are abnormal, expect your doctor to find out why or to follow your progress until the results return to normal.

Understanding the Diagnosis

Once your physician finishes his diagnostic workup, you have the right to know what your doctor thinks is wrong and your outlook for the future. Find out what the diagnosis is in medical terms; knowing your "official" medical diagnosis is helpful when checking reference works or consulting other doctors. Ask your physician what findings were used to arrive at the final diagnosis. What do your test results mean? What body systems are involved? What is the disease process at work? What has caused the illness? Is it contagious or will it spread? Is there a chance that someone in my family might get the same condition? How could I have prevented the condition? What can I do to prevent it from occurring again? What can I do to help myself with my problem and to keep healthy? What changes, if any, will I have to make in my daily life? What will the course of the illness be? When can I expect to become better? What signs of worsening should I watch for? Will I need help at home for my condition? If so, what kind of help? You may wish to ask your physician to go over your medical chart with you to educate you about your illness. Also, ask your doctor if he feels qualified to treat you if this illness is outside of his specialty or expertise.

Also, you can telephone the medical director of the hospital to which you would be admitted to have your treatment performed and ask the medical director how frequently its doctors treat your condition. If you find that the closest qualified hospital is many miles away, ask your doctor if he can consult with the specialists there.

Support Groups

If, after receiving the diagnosis, you feel you need support in dealing with your condition, there are self-help groups that offer support to persons with disabilities, cancer, and many other health problems. The groups are made up of those who have already been there in a similar situation and who share their information and experiences. Contact the American Self-Help Clearinghouse for information on national groups (1-973-326-6789). The clearinghouse can also refer you to any state or local self-help clearinghouse. If you wish to begin your own self-help group, the clearinghouse has information to assist you at its Web site, http://www.selfhelpgroups.org.

Treatment of Illness

After your doctor explains his diagnosis to you, ask what forms of treatment are available. What are the risks and benefits of each? Which does your doctor recommend and why? What are the chances or odds that your doctor's recommended treatment will work? That is, ask how many patients with your condition are helped by this treatment? If helped, when will you see expected results? Are there any side effects to the treatment? What can be done about them? If the treatment is painful, can the pain be controlled? If the cause of your problem is unknown, why can this treatment be expected to help? What are the pros and cons of the treatment alternatives in the opinion of the experts? What will happen to you if you do nothing? How much does the treatment cost and find out if your health plan will pay for it. Since differences of opinion can exist as to what is appropriate therapy for your problem, try to obtain as much information as possible before making any decisions regarding the course of treatment. To understand the treatment guidelines for your condition, you can find them on the National Guideline Clearinghouse's Web site at http://www.guideline.gov. Although the material may be technical, showing it to your doctor may assist him or her to prescribe the appropriate treatment.

Ask your doctor if he could suggest someone for a second opinion. (You do not necessarily have to see the person who is recommended, but you lose nothing by asking.) Do not ask for a second opinion from another physician in your own doctor's practice. They may not wish to contradict each other. A doctor who works with a different hospital, preferably outside of your insurer's network, is usually the most unbiased (many insurance plans will pay part of the cost of consulting a specialist outside of your network).

If necessary, seek a third opinion if there is major disagreement between the first two. Some insurers will pay for a third opinion. Check with your insurer to see if it will do so. Also, ask your physician (or his nurse) where you can find reading material on your problem. He or she should be able to provide some references. Do not hesitate to seek information on your own. Check with a reference librarian at a health library if possible.

You may also wish to use the Internet to learn and do research on your condition. But a word of caution: While the Internet may be helpful, it can also be a source of misinformation, so use Web sites that are backed by known organizations. For example, a prominent one is MedlinePlus (located at http://www.medlineplus.gov), a site jointly operated by the US National Library of Medicine and the National Institutes of Health. Also, the site http://www.healthfinder.gov has links to more than eighteen hundred health-related organizations. A third example is the Stanford University Medical Center's Health Library, which offers free research help to anyone seeking information on an illness or treatment. To reach the Stanford University Medical Center's Health Library you can telephone toll-free 1-800-295-5177 or go to the site at http://healthlibrary.stanford.edu. Fourth, information about women's health, men's health, and treatments for arthritis, diabetes, and other conditions is available from Health Pages's online magazine at http://www.thehealthpages.com.

Also, seek to reduce the stress caused by the illness or problem. Stress is normal, expected, and usually not permanent. However, support mechanisms may be needed—support groups or seeing a therapist whose specialty is stress or illness counseling. Hobbies, vacations, exercise, and social interaction—finding other people with whom to share feelings—can help make the problems less overwhelming. Do not rush into any decision about your illness. If possible, take a few days or even a couple of weeks to ponder all your treatment options, including the ones your physician may not know about. Deciding on a treatment too quickly may cause you regret later on.

Be aware that in an effort to reduce healthcare costs, insurers and employers have hired thousands of nurses to coach patients and doctors to follow the standard protocols for each disease. This process is called *disease management*. This concept received a boost in 2003 when a Medicare reform bill called for trying out disease management on approximately four million senior citizens. The disease management companies employ sophisticated computer programs that alert nurses (and the physicians who want to check on their patients) exactly what the standard of care is for each disease and how each disease patient's care compares. Therefore, you as a patient or your doctor may be contacted by a nurse in regard to the latest standards in the treatment of a particular illness and whether you or your doctor are following these standards in your care. Not all doctors like the frequent monitoring of physician care by nurses, claiming that it interferes with their own judgment as to the best way to treat a patient's particular illness. Other doctors welcome such oversight, noting that nurses were catching patient problems earlier than their twice-yearly medical checkups as well as keeping their patients updated about the latest treatment standards through personal patient contact. Regardless of the pros and cons of disease management, many employers and almost every major private insurer offer this program.

Again, to help yourself with the treatment, ask the doctor about anything you don't understand. If you have problems following the doctor's direction, the sooner you tell the doctor the better it will be for you. If you have made any changes to the doctor's treatment plan, make sure you tell the doctor, and if you feel worse, develop new symptoms, or have side effects from the treatment, call your doctor.

Drug Therapy

If your physician prescribes drugs, you should be sure to obtain detailed information about each drug. What is the name of the drug? Why is it indicated for your diagnosis? What is the drug supposed to do? How does it work in the body? Ask about possible side effects or adverse reactions, and be sure to inform your doctor immediately if you notice any unexpected reactions or changes. Are any alternative drugs available? Is there an alternative to drug therapy? Ask your doctor whether the drug is on your insurer's formulary—the list of preferred drugs for which the insurer will make full reimbursement. Ask if it is safe to split pills. Consider using your insurer's mail-order service, which may provide you with a three-month supply of drugs for just one copayment. Don't hesitate to ask your doctor for samples as well as to shop around at different pharmacies, since drug prices can vary among pharmacies. These steps will not only allow you to obtain the proper prescriptions for your illness but also save you money on drugs as well.

If you decide to take the drug, make sure you know the dosage (how much should be taken and when), how to administer the drug to yourself, and how long you should take the drug. Find out what to do if you miss taking a pill at the right time. Can you take it at another time? Are there any other instructions to follow: Ask whether you should avoid any foods, activities, or other medications while taking the drug. And, as already noted, ask the doctor to prescribe the drug by its generic name, if possible, rather than the brand name, to save you money. If you are to take a medication for seven days or thirty days, take all the medication even if you feel better or the problem may return. Also, do not overdo medications. Taking more than a recommended dose may cause some harmful effect. If you have any unexpected adverse symptom while taking a drug, call and tell your doctor immediately. Also, make sure that your doctor is not too reliant on and too quick to prescribe drugs without dealing with the real causes of your medical problems. If you want to know more about a drug, ask your physician if there is any written information available about the drug.

Diet Advice

How important is this diet? What will happen if I don't follow it? Can I occasionally eat something not on it?

Taking Care of Yourself at Home

If a drug is the only treatment your physician recommends, you might want to ask if there are other things besides the prescription that will enable you to become well. For any treatment at home, ask about restrictions on activity, what precautions to take, and how long the treatment should be carried out. Ask what aftereffects to expect. And if your doctor recommends a course of action that you think will not work for you, do not hesitate to tell him so that alternatives can be examined. If the treatment plan will not fit into your schedule, you and your doctor may be able to work out something more realistic.

An Approach to Treatment

If married or otherwise with a companion, approach the illness as a couple problem. The fact that one person may be identified as having a problem does not cancel the effect on both. A workup, evaluation, and treatment are much better dealt with when the spouse or companion participates in at least some visits and has a good understanding of the problem. The more involved a couple is, the better able they are to support each other and make decisions on treatment options.

Before leaving your physician's office, find out whether and when you should report back or return. You may also want to ask whether you should telephone in for laboratory reports and what you should do if your condition worsens or if you experience an adverse reaction to a new medication. You may find it helpful to write a summary of your visit when you return home. If anything was not satisfactory, be sure to talk about it on your next visit or ask about the best time to telephone if more questions should occur to you after you leave the office.

Through these procedures and questions, you can help develop a partnership with your physician in treating the problem that brought you into his office. By educating yourself and having your physician educate you through your questions, you will obtain the most out of your visits with your physician and will do very much to overcome your illness.

In summary, therefore, to obtain the best personal care from your physician, complete a family history and ask your doctor to file a copy in your medical record. Then, develop a personalized health plan with your physician that sets specific goals and includes recommendations based on your family history, age, sex, weight, fitness, and lifestyle. Analyze your health risks and discuss with your physician the steps you can take to avoid, delay, or detect them early. Then, research the drugs prescribed for you. Ask if the drug has been studied in individuals similar to yourself—

for example, women, blacks, Asians, the elderly, or diabetics. Ask if there is anything in your personal or medical history that suggests a greater risk of side effects or the probability that one drug will work better for you than another.

If you are using the Internet for medical advice, note the creator of the Web site. Web sites ending in ".gov" (for government) or ".edu" (for an educational institution) are the most reliable. Look at the health or medical credentials of the Web site's author or medical advisory board to make sure they are appropriate. Also, check the Web documents for references in regard to any data and advice that they note. Look at the dates of these documents to make sure their information is up-to-date. Finally, be wary of bias since many "health" Web sites are simply disguised advertisements. Read their headings carefully to distinguish between facts and promotion. If you follow these guidelines, you will do a great deal to ensure that you are receiving the best treatment available to alleviate your medical condition and promote your personal health.

THE DO'S AND DON'TS OF HOUSE CALLS

If you are unable to visit your physician's office for treatment, you should ask whether he will make house calls.

"Those were the good old days," Bob was telling his neighbor. "I remember the time when all my parents had to do was to call Dr. Garber's office and he'd come to my home, and in his little black bag were all the weapons to fight illness. No crowded waiting rooms, no long waiting time even when you arrive on time for your appointment, no long insurance forms to fill out—just you and your doctor in the comfort of your home. I understand that medicine has become more technological and more complex than when I was a boy, and it's easier with all this technology for a doctor to treat you in his office than at home, but many times I wish those days were here again. Do you think there any doctors who still make house calls?"

Under emergency conditions, many physicians still do, but, in general, the house call is a vanishing form of treatment in American medicine today. Yet, despite this situation, the first nationwide online listing of house-call doctors who are currently accepting new patients is posted on the American Academy of Home Care Physicians Web site (http://www.aahcp.org). Another Web site, sponsored by the National Association for Home Care (http://www.nahc.org), includes a special consumer section about choosing a homecare provider plus other helpful house-call doctor resources.

The reasons for the decline of house calls are technological and economical. Due to the explosion of medical knowledge and technology, doctors' offices today contain a great deal—including technologically advanced equipment and medical records—that could never be squeezed into a black bag; consequently, it is easier and more economical for your doctor and his medical staff to treat you at their office rather than at home.

Therefore, if you are concerned about home treatment, there are several guidelines you can follow when asking your physician about his home visit policies.

DO:

- Ask in advance—preferably at your initial interview—about your physician's house call policy.
- Ask your doctor about emergency care *before* you need it. For example, whom should you call first: doctor, ambulance, or hospital? What hospital should you use? Which ambulance service?
- Look to the very young and the very old doctors and those in practice for themselves if you want a physician who is willing to make house calls.
- Have a friend call his doctor for you if you are new in town and need a house call.
- Expect to pay more for a house call than for an office visit. Find out how much more beforehand.
- When you telephone for a house call, tell your doctor precisely what is wrong and why the problem cannot wait or why the patient cannot come to the office.
- Pay your bills on time—not just to your own physician but to any doctor in town. Word gets around, and courtesies like house calls tend to become unavailable to those who renege or stall on their medical payments.

DO NOT:

- Ask simply, "Do you make house calls?" Rather, ask, "Under what circumstances will you make a house call for me?"
- Waste precious time trying to get a house call during a serious medical emergency. Unless your physician has told you to do otherwise, go quickly to a hospital emergency room for those critical situations in which minutes are vital.
- Expect a house call from a doctor who does not know you as a patient unless you live in a very small community.
- Abuse the privilege of getting house calls if you find a doctor who makes them willingly.[27]

Following these guidelines will assist you greatly in obtaining house call service. Physicians still treat patients at home, and it is to your advantage to find out all the circumstances under which your physician will afford you this service. In the age of the Internet, there is a new form of house call slowly beginning to emerge. It is called the virtual house call. These Internet house calls are really intended for such issues as a child's ear infection, a rash, and follow-up care for chronic ailments. It should not be used for urgent problems such as bleeding in late pregnancy or chest pain.

Proponents state that virtual house calls are meant to occur within a doctor-patient relationship that has already been established in person, and they are designed to replace unnecessary office visits but not quick phone calls or e-mails, which still will be handled for free. Patients click onto a secure Web site. If required to pay, patients provide a credit card number and answer questions about their complaint. A doctor reviews the answers and replies, generally within a business day. If the doctor decides the patient needs to come in after all, there is usually no charge for the Web exchange. Examples of such virtual house calls are Medem, a Web service initiated by the American Medical Association and other major doctor groups for which the patient pays a charge for its Online Consultant, and the First Health Group, a very large for-profit network of doctors. If you use these groups, find out whether you must pay any charges for their use.[28]

CARING FOR A RELATIVE OR A FRIEND LIVING FAR AWAY

The aging of America places more pressure on families with elderly relatives who live far away and become ill. To prepare yourself to be of the greatest assistance to that person, plan ahead. Learn as much as you can about the person's illness, whether your knowledge comes from publications, Web sites, a physician, or whatever other sources will provide you with accurate information. Remember, you also have your own emotional and physical limitations, so don't assume so many responsibilities that you harm your own health or personal situation. Don't let your act of caregiving isolate you either emotionally or physically from other people such as your friends. In fact, you may wish to think about joining a support group that can provide you with emotional balance during this period in your life. In addition, don't give up other activities that give you pleasure like hobbies, entertainment, and various forms of exercise like walking or swimming. Also, figure out what you can do to help out the elderly person from a distance like paying his or her bills. Think about the future and any potential problems that may occur. It is easier to find out about doctors, hospitals, long-term care facilities, health insurance coverage, and personal finances now before anything bad occurs later. Thus, get your elderly relative's medical information down on paper. Who are the doctors? Which hospitals are nearby? What medicine is the relative taking and when? Who will pay? What information will the relative's doctor provide you to assist you in your efforts? Exchange telephone numbers with close friends, neighbors, lawyers, clergy, and others who have contact with your relative in the event serious problems arise, so they can contact you.

Look ahead at possible living or medical arrangements should one member of an elderly couple die or a person living alone become incapacitated. The Eldercare Locator, a free service of the US Administration on Aging, at 1-800-677-1116, or on its Web site at http://www.eldercare.gov, can link you with state and area agencies on aging and other community organizations that can provide caregiving services to your relative such as homecare, adult daycare, and other services if they are needed. Therefore, look into community services that can provide those caregiving services you are not able to provide yourself. The Eldercare Locator provides information about senior resources throughout the country. Also, let the elderly persons share in advance decision making. Make sure you understand their wishes in terms of life support and care in the event of a terminal illness or coma. When in doubt, consult a lawyer as well as family doctors about procedures such as living wills in the state where the elderly person lives. Also, the chances are that in every family there is a significant person to whom a parent will listen. Sometimes it's a child, a grandchild, a neighbor, or a doctor. Whoever it is, use that person to help effectively plan and work with whoever needs help. Let your relative's doctor(s) assist you in whatever fashion possible.

THE PATIENT'S BILL OF RIGHTS

Whether you are treated at home, the physician's office, a hospital, or another location, you as a patient have a bill of rights in regard to the care your physician gives you. On June 26, 1990, the House of Delegates of the American Medical Association passed the "Fundamental Elements of the Patient-Physician Relationship." According to this document:

- The patient has the right to receive information from physicians and to discuss the benefits, risks, and costs for appropriate treatment alternatives. Patients should receive guidance from their physicians as to the optimal course of action. Patients are also entitled to obtain copies or summaries of their medical records, to have their questions answered, to be advised of potential conflicts of interest that their physicians might have, and to receive independent professional opinions.
- The patient has the right to make decisions regarding the healthcare that is recommended by his or her physician. Accordingly, patients may accept or refuse any recommended medical treatment.
- The patient has the right to courtesy, respect, dignity, responsiveness, and timely attention to his or her needs.
- The patient has the right to confidentiality. The physician should not reveal confidential communications or information without the consent of the patient unless provided for by law or by the need to protect the welfare of the individual or the public interest.
- The patient has the right to the continuity of healthcare. The physician has an obligation to cooperate in the coordination of medically indicated care with other health providers treating the patient. The physician may not discontinue treatment of a patient as long as further treatment is medically indicated without giving the patient sufficient opportunity to make alternative arrangements for care.

- The patient has a basic right to have available adequate healthcare. Physicians, along with the rest of society, should continue to work toward this goal. Fulfillment of this right is dependent on society providing resources so that no patient is deprived of necessary care because of inability to pay for the care.[29]

Another American Medical Association document addressed the fact that doctors affiliated with many health plans are paid by how economically they practice— that is, by how few costly tests, hospitalizations, or referrals to specialists they approve. If they cost the plan too much, they may be paid less or even forced to pay a penalty. Some health plan patients have complained bitterly that under this system they have been denied needed care. Accordingly, the AMA has stated:

- Physicians must not deny their patients access to appropriate medical services based [on] personal financial reward.
- Physicians must inform patients about all appropriate treatment alternatives regardless of cost and regardless of whether or not the health plan provides them.
- Physicians must make sure patients are told about any restrictions on treatment and any obligations their physicians may have to restrict patients' options.
- Physicians should promote active programs to monitor quality of care wherever they practice.[30]

HEALTH RECORDS PRIVACY RULES

Effective April 14, 2003, the US Department of Health and Human Services (DHHS) put into effect new patient health record privacy rules to improve privacy protection of patient medical records. These rules relate to *electronic medical records*, not paper medical records. In general, patients may inspect their medical records, receive a copy of their medical records within thirty days of a written request, and ask for corrections in regard to any mistakes in their medical records. Your provider may refuse to correct any mistakes but must permit you to attach your version of the corrections to your file. However, the final regulations do not require that a patient's written permission be obtained before physicians, hospitals, pharmacies, and insurance companies can handle their personal health information. The regulations also allow companies to pay health plans to market drugs to you. Instead of requiring written permission, the final rules simply specify that patients, at some point, be informed of their privacy rights by those who handle their records. So, for example, you still will not know whether hospital staff improperly looked at your medical records. As result of this new regulation, you will find in your physician's office, for example, pamphlets entitled *A Notice of Privacy Practices* for your information. These written notices are provided to healthcare consumers to explain the new patient rights that are mandated by the Health Insurance Portability and Accountability Act of 1996 (HIPAA) and to inform them about how healthcare providers and insurance plans use and disclose medical records. In general, the rules allow the sharing of information in personal medical records only to treat patients, pay bills, and carry out a broad, undefined category of "healthcare operations" such as hospital administration.

Although the provider or health plan is not required to agree to the restriction, it must abide by the limitation once it agrees with the patient's request. Moreover, consumers have the right to ask providers and plans to communicate with them only in certain ways (that is, by telephone or in writing) or at certain locations other than at home (such as work) if they do not wish to be contacted at home. Your doctor is obliged to comply with your request to send mailings to or leave voice-mail messages at such designated locations other than your home, if that is your wish.

In a hospital, your stay is not a matter of public record, so you may choose not to be listed in the patient directory. Deciding to be excluded from the hospital directory means the hospital won't give callers or visitors any information about you. But be aware that some hospitals may return your name to the directory if you even discuss your treatment with your spouse in the room. If that happens, try appealing to the hospital's privacy officer, a new position created by the law. In addition, access by employers to their workers' health information will be restricted, and psychotherapists will be permitted to keep treatment notes (so-called process notes) confidential so that insurers can no longer require seeing them to justify paying such claims. Due to legal constraints on the US Department of Health and Human Services's authority that is included in the HIPAA law of 1996, the final regulations fail to cover all medical records keepers. Health data gathered through employees' assistance programs, worker's compensation, and pre- and postemployment physical and drugs tests are not protected under this new regulation. The new law does not cover most Web sites, so be careful of sharing your medical information online. Also, be aware that some hospitals like the Beth Israel in Boston, Massachusetts, now allow patients to sign on to a Web site with a password and review their prescriptions, laboratory results, and history. Under the new federal standards, the smallest amount of information should be disclosed for specific purposes and, when possible, patients' names are to be left out.

Until now, patients' medical records have been governed by a haphazard patchwork of state laws. The federal standards will override weaker state laws but will not interfere with states that have adopted stronger policies to protect consumers. If you feel your rights to patient confidentiality have been violated under this new regulation, find out who else has looked at them and seek penalties against anyone who misuses the information. Violators of this new privacy law confront up to $250,000 in fines and ten years in prison. The law does not give you the right to sue, although some states do grant you this right. So filing a complaint with the US Department of Health and Human Services's Office of Civil Rights or your provider are the only other choices.

To learn how to file a complaint, go to the Web site http://www.hhs.gov/ocr/hipaa or telephone 1-800-368-1019. You can obtain a model complaint from

Georgetown University's Health Privacy Project in Washington, DC, at http://www
.healthprivacy.org. The nonprofit group asks patients to send them a copy of the
protest so that the organization can follow up on how well DHHS investigates
alleged violations.

THE PHYSICIAN'S OFFICE: COST CONTROL, QUALITY OF CARE, AND THEIR EFFECTS ON THE PATIENT

The internal operation of your physician's office has a direct impact on overhead
expenses.

"You know, Marian," Harry said, "I wish more people would realize that physicians also have a responsibility in holding down my medical costs. As a consumer, I can employ whatever cost-savings techniques I hear or read about in the media, but if physicians themselves don't cooperate with the public in the way they conduct their medical practices, how can my medical bill ever go down?"

Physicians who have been able to hold down operational costs can pass their
savings on to patients by not increasing fees or by keeping increases to a minimum.
The American Medical Association, in trying to help physicians control their office
expenses, and their impact on the fees they charge their patients, asks doctors:

- Does your office employ preprinted forms whenever possible to reduce the
  costs of letter writing?
- Does your office send in insurance forms promptly in order to improve its
  cash flow?
- Is your staff knowledgeable about the claims submission procedures of the
  third-party payers you encounter in your practice? A clear understanding of
  claims procedures will speed up processing and payment and will save you
  and your patients time, money, and frustration.
- Does your office deposit patient payments on a daily basis? Doing so is good
  business management.
- Do you shop around and get quotations from several companies before purchasing your office supplies?
- Does your office take advantage of bulk purchase discounts on frequently
  used supplies? And do you take advantage of all supplier discounts that many
  firms offer on promptly paid bills?
- Do you mistakenly fail to record and collect on certain types of patient
  encounters, such as hospital emergency rooms and consultation visits? Some
  physicians are slow, or even forget, to bring this information back to the office
  for billing purposes. Patients who pay for office visits may be subsidizing
  those who are never billed.

- Do you or appropriate members of your staff discuss with your patients the proper utilization of health services and, in particular, procedures followed by your office?[31]

Your physician's office operations not only affect the size of your medical bill but can also have a direct impact upon your view of the medical treatment you receive and your response to it. A survey by *Medical Economics* of patients' attitudes toward physicians and their treatments found that following factors can have a negative impact:

- Staying an undue length of time in the waiting room to see the physician after scheduling the appointment in advance.
- The booking of more than one patient in the same time slot and the "second wait" in the examining room before the examination begins. If the physician explains the reasons for the delay, the patient's irritation can be alleviated.
- Office surroundings having an impact on the patient's mood include inadequate waiting room space; temperature variations from room to room; too few creature comforts—no decent facilities for undressing and dressing and hanging up clothes, no carpeting on floor for bare feet, cold-to-touch plastic furniture, paper dressing gowns; lack of privacy for patients in the office setting; not enough time-passers such as current magazines in the reception area or examining room; an office so plush patients feel they are paying for it.
- A bill which is sent out the day of the visit and arrives at the patient's home before he does; conversely, one which arrives several months late or says "pay immediately." Patients like a system in which the bill is sent out the month of the visit, includes a return envelope, and contains clear summary of visit date, diagnosis, treatment, and charges.
- Inability of the physician to explain why certain procedures or services are so costly.[32]

The above-mentioned characteristics should not be interpreted as being representative of all physician offices or of all patients, but they are, unfortunately, all too common. Even more important, they illustrate that many factors influence the patient's feelings toward his physician and, ultimately, toward the medical treatment he receives—even if these other factors are of a nonmedical nature. Patients and physicians must both be aware of and sensitive to all the nuances if they are to improve the doctor-patient relationship and, thereby, assist in the patient's recovery.

NOTES

1. American Medical Association, Physician Master File, Chicago, IL, December 2000.

2. *Source Book of Health Insurance Data, 2002* (Washington, DC: Health Insurance of America, 2002), p. 116.

3. David Brown, "Recruiters Offer Doctors a Small Town 'Option,'" *Washington Post*, October 6, 1991, p. A3; Janet McConnaughey, "Doctors for Rural Areas Are Sought," *Washington Post*, January 30, 2005, p. A13.

4. Wayne Hearn, "Health on the Outskirts," *American Medical News*, July 1, 1996, p. 13; McConnaughey, "Doctors for Rural Areas Are Sought," p. A13.

5. US Department of Health and Human Services, *A Report to the President and the Congress on the Status of Health Professions Personnel in the United States* (Washington, DC: Public Health Service, August 1978), pp. 1V1, A6.

6. Mary Beth Franklin, "Senate Warns of Shortage of Doctors for the Elderly," *Washington Post/Health*, May 14, 1996, pp.12–14; Carole Fleck, "America's 'Forgotten' Patients," *AARP Bulletin* 43, no. 10 (November 2002): 9; Peggy Eastman, "Restoring the Inner Self," *AARP Bulletin* 44, no. 3 (March 2003): 16–17; and *Fact Sheet: The American Geriatrics Society (AGS)* (New York: American Geriatrics Society, 2001).

7. Sandra G. Boodman, "When Doctors Say They're Board Certified, What Do They Mean?" *Washington Post/Health,* July 12, 1994, p. 17.

8. Victor Cohn, "Getting the Best Emergency Room Care," *Washington Post/Health*, April 11, 1989, p. 11.

9. *Seconds Save Lives in Medical Emergencies* (Washington, DC: American College of Emergency Medicine, 2005); Medline Plus, "Recognizing Medical Emergencies," *Medical Encyclopedia* (Washington, DC: US National Library of Medicine and the National Institutes of Health, January 11, 2004).

10. Cohn, "Getting the Best Emergency Room Care," p. 11.

11. Paula Siegel, "Telephone Medicine," *Self*, November 1982, p. 40.

12. Bernard Gavzer, "Why Some Doctors May Be Hazardous to Your Health," *Parade*, April 14, 1996, p. 4.

13. "An MD Who Puts His Advice to Patients in Writing," *American Medical News*, July 14, 1978, p. 4.

14. Catherine O'Neill, "What Your Doctor Checks on," *Washington Post/Health*, August 20, 1991, p. 18.

15. Jay Siwek, "How Doctors' Assistants Can Help," *Washington Post/Health*, April 11, 1989, p. 19.

16. William A. Nolen, "Cutting Your Medical Costs in Half," *McCall's*, August 1978, pp. 78, 172; "Cervical Cancer Screening: Testing Can Start Later and Occur Less Often under New ACOG Recommendations," American College of Obstetricians and Gynecologists news release, July 31, 2003; "The Best Thing a Woman Can Do," *Parade*, September 11, 2005, p. 27; Fran Carpenter, "Help Save Your Own Life," *Parade*, September 11, 2005, p. 27; and Brenda E. Sirovich, Steven Woloshin, and Lisa M. Schwartz, "Screening of Cervical Cancer: Will Women Accept Less?" *American Journal of Medicine* 118, no. 2 (February 1, 2005): 151–58.

17. Nolen, "Cutting Your Medical Costs in Half," p. 172.

18. *Physician's Cost Containment Checklist* (Chicago: American Medical Association, November 1978), pp. 2–3.

19. Sally Squires, "Concerns about Disposable Contact Lenses," *Washington Post/Health*, November 17, 1992, p. 17; Adam Geller, "No Glasses Needed with Vision Correction," *Washington Senior Beacon*, July 2004, p. 6; and Diedtra Henderson, "Lens Implant Restores Crisp Sight," *Washington Senior Beacon*, November 2004, p. 1.

20. Sally Squires, "With Contact Lenses, Put Safety First: Ulcers on the Cornea Can Become Infected and Impair Eyesight," *Washington Post/Health*, September 26, 1989, p. 7.

21. Lauran Neergaard, "Exams Can Catch Early Signs of Vision Loss," *Washington Senior Beacon*, April 2004, p. 20.

22. Consumer Reports, "Eye Exams," *Washington Post*, November 1, 1993, p. B5; Neergaard, "Exams Can Catch Early Signs of Vision Loss."

23. Ibid.

24. Hugh Downs, "The Complete Medical Checkup: What You Need to Know," *Parade*, June 30, 1996, p. 5; Isadore Rosenfeld, "Don't Delay, Get a Checkup," *Parade*, February 11, 2001, pp. 10–12; and Dianne Hales, "Finally Better Treatment for Women (and Men Too)," *Parade*, March 7, 1999, pp. 10, 12.

25. Lawrence Galton, "How to Communicate with Your Doctor," *Parade,* February 12, 1978, p. 20.

26. Lawrence Charnas, "Be Prepared When Going to the Doctor," *Consumer Health Reporter*, November 1984, pp. 1–2.

27. "Why Doctors Don't Make House Calls," *Family Health*, July 1976, p. 68.

28. Rita Rubin, "The Virtual Doctor Will See You Now," *USA Today*, June 10, 2002, p. 1.

29. Victor Cohn, "AMA to Members: Put Patients First," *Washington Post/Health*, November 13, 1990, p. 12.

30. Ibid.

31. *Physician's Cost Containment Checklist*, pp. 4–5.

32. "Your Office and Staff, Passing Marks But . . . ," *Medical Economics*, November 26, 1976, pp. 104–31; "Fees and Income: Is Resentment on the Rise?" *Medical Economics*, November 29, 1976, pp. 66–73; and "Rapport: Where the Breakdown Begins," *Medical Economics*, November 29, 1976, pp. 9–16.

CHAPTER TWO
DENTAL CARE

INTRODUCTION

Dentistry, in contrast to medicine, is still a profession in which most dentists practice in separate, self-financed offices with their own highly expensive equipment. About nine out of ten dentists presently practice in noninstitutional settings and are involved in general dental practice. The rest of the nation's active civilian dentists are specialists. In terms of numbers, dentists rank fourth after the professions of nursing, medicine, and pharmacy. In 2000 there were an estimated 168,000 active dentists in the United States (excluding dentists in the military service, US Public Health Service, and Veterans Administration), or 60.4 dentists per 100,000 population.[1]

Although dentists generally do not use centralized treatment sources such as hospitals and other institutions, an increasing number of dentists in recent years have begun to practice in health maintenance organizations (HMOs) and other kinds of group practice. Also, in contrast to other professions, especially nursing and medicine, dentistry does not have an extensive range of allied health personnel. Dental hygienists are the only licensed or registered auxiliaries, and they perform their duties under the direct supervision of dentists. Other allied dental personnel include dental assistants and dental laboratory technicians. Another category of dental assistants found in some dental offices is the expanded-function dental auxiliary (EFDA), who is either a dental hygienist or a dental assistant whose training embraces a wide range of clinical functions and direct patient care procedures previously performed only by a dentist. This latter position is similar to that of the physician assistant and, though not yet widely used in dentistry, offers a significant potential for increased dental productivity.

While similar in some respects to the medical profession, dentistry is also significantly dissimilar. Like the profession of medicine, the geographic distribution of dentists throughout the United States is not uniform and remains a major issue in the delivery of health services. On the other hand, the process for obtaining a state license to practice dentistry is more burdensome than that for medicine since a dental license requires the satisfactory completion of both a written test and a clinical examination. Licensure by reciprocity or endorsement is also more limited for dentists than for physicians. Consequently, dentists are not as mobile. In the dental educational setting, clinical teaching facilities are essentially all located in the dental school itself. However, since the 1990s there has been a rapid proliferation of proprietary courses for general dentists and dental specialists, outside the sponsorship of a dental school. These courses are under the umbrella of continuing education courses (CEs) and are mostly in lecture format. But an increasing number also include demonstrations or patients "hands-on" (clinical) care.

HOW TO FIND A DENTIST

Given the characteristics of the dental profession both in its manner of practice and in its geographical dispersion, the patient-consumer faces a very basic question. How can I be assured that I am spending my money prudently and receiving quality dental care services? Like physician care, dental care is a highly personalized service whose quality will differ from one dentist to another. However, there are certain guidelines you can use in choosing your dentist and judging the quality of his dental services.

Ed came to know this through the many years that he had been Dr. Williams's patient. Ed knew that Dr. Williams would make sure that he came in every six months for a cleaning appointment. His secretary would contact Ed a day or so before each appointment to reconfirm. When he arrived, Ed did not have to wait to see the dentist because Dr. Williams operated his office quite efficiently. He practiced dentistry conservatively, always instructing Ed about how to care for his teeth, never suggesting expensive therapies like root canals or tooth extraction before first trying everything else to save Ed's teeth. When Ed arrived for a cleaning, Dr. Williams always checked his teeth after the hygienist cleaned them, without charging fees in addition to that of the hygienist. Dr. Williams raised his charges moderately through the years, never charging steep fees. When the time came for Dr. Williams to retire, Ed wondered what he would do. He had known only one dentist for many years. How was he going to choose another? What dental qualities should he be looking for? His options: stay with the new dentist who had purchased Dr. Williams's practice or leave and find another. If he chose to leave, what should he be looking for since each dentist is an individual with separate skills and talents—medically and in terms of personality? Ed was lucky. He stayed, and Ed was happy with Dr. Williams's replacement. The new dentist turned out to have many of Dr. Williams's qualities, both professionally and personally.

Not everyone is as lucky as Ed. If you are searching for a new dentist, follow these guidelines to find and select a dentist who meets your individual needs.

Sources of Information

Before selecting a family dentist who will provide you with regular care, you may want to visit several to determine who will best meet your personal needs. The American Dental Association has several suggestions for locating a dentist in your community:

- Ask your friends, neighbors, or coworkers to recommend dentists with whom they are pleased. If you are a member of a local dental managed plan, you will probably have to limit your search to dentists associated with the plan in order to have your treatment covered.
- Faculty members of dental schools in your geographic area may be able to recommend dentists in your community.
- A nearby hospital with an accredited dental service should be able to offer suggestions.
- Check with the *American Dental Association Directory*, which can be found in many public libraries and in all dental school libraries.
- If you have a family physician, ask who provides his dental care.
- Check with your local pharmacist.[2]

In addition, you should contact your local dental society for the names of dentists on its referral service. (However, be aware that the society almost certainly will not be able to inform you which dentists provide care of high quality and which do not.) If you use a computer, your task is easy. Going on the Internet and surfing the Web opens up a new world to you. You can search the American Dental Association Web site for a member dentist, specialist, and geographic proximity to your home or office in addition to each academy or dental specialty organization (for example, the Academy of Oral and Maxillofacial Surgeons or the American College of Prosthodontists).

Not only can you identify a dentist near you but also his/her qualifications and membership status such as board certification. If you do not have a computer, your library has computers and will assist you in your search. By using these various sources, you should be able to find a family dentist in general practice who will take a sincere interest in your oral health. As in the case of finding a physician, it makes sense to select and become acquainted with a dentist before an emergency arises. As with a physician, a dentist in private practice becomes keenly familiar with his patients, their families, and their particular needs. For example, making an emergency call in the middle of the night to a dentist with whom you are not familiar may result in emergency or definitive treatment that does not match your particular health, goals, or financial circumstances.

Definitions of Dental Specialists

A dentist in general practice is fully qualified to provide all routine care. He can also refer you to other dentists where specialized treatment is required. The following kinds of dentists provide specialized care:

Endodontist—specializes in the treatment of diseases of the inner tooth pulp and related tissues. This is also called root canal work.

Oral Pathologist—specializes in the interpretation and diagnosis of changes caused by diseases in tissues.

Oral Surgeon—specializes in the extraction of teeth and surgery of the mouth and jaw.

Orthodontist—specializes in straightening teeth and in other work relating to correcting the position of the teeth and jaw.

Pediatric Dentist (formerly called a pedodontist)—specializes in the dental problems of children.

Periodontist—specializes in treating diseases of the gum and of the tissues that surround the teeth.

Prosthodontist—specializes in making dentures, bridges, and other artificial replacements of teeth.

Public Health Dentists—trained formally in the principles of public health, this specialist may practice in a community health clinic, operate a group practice, work in public or private administration, or engage in research.[3]

Most good specialists practice only their own specialty; be cautious of a dentist who does each and every kind of dental work. The reason is that an increasing number of dentists have received a "certificate" for attending a one- to two-year residency in advanced general dentistry (AGD). A recently graduate dentist usually takes this residency immediately after graduation from dental school (the old name was "internship"). This intense training program does not make that dentist a specialist as such but provides a higher level of skill in all areas of dentistry. Many dentists who have served in the US armed forces have had this training. (In the military, the program is called "Comprehensive Dentistry.") The yellow pages of your telephone book may indicate whether a dentist limits his practice to a particular specialty. Also, the American Dental Association's *American Dental Directory* is arranged by city and state and lists the name, address, specialty school, dental school, and year of graduation of each dentist. As already noted, many large libraries keep this directory.[4]

When considering a specialist, ask what his/her training is and how frequently he/she has performed the procedure. Then ask for the names of patients you may call for a reference. To prevent dentists from selecting patients who are biased in the dentist's favor, ask for patients who fall into a narrow category such as those who are your age and sex.

HOW TO JUDGE A DENTIST'S QUALITIES

After you have obtained a recommendation from a source you believe in, call the dentist's office for an appointment. You can learn a great deal of information in the initial visit.

- *Is the appearance of the dentist and dental staff neat, clean, and orderly? Are the waiting and treatment rooms also maintained in this manner? Is the waiting room backed up, and are auxiliary personnel in evidence? Does the dentist seem to be going back and forth from one examining room to another? Are you taken care of promptly?* Note the pace of the office.
- *Is the dentist's availability in regard to both location and appointment schedule a problem? Ask about his policies in regard to emergencies—those requiring immediate care without an appointment as well as those that take place outside of office hours? Does he have a backup referral arrangement with another dentist—or an emergency referral or paging service?*

  If you can, select a dentist whose location is convenient to you so that you will not have to travel long distances to and from his office. Also, choose a dentist whose waiting time for an appointment is not unreasonable. If your appointments are not honored on a regular basis, find another dentist who does practice in this manner—taking your dental records with the permission of the dentist you are leaving. Remember, "patient records" are legally your property. The dentist is the custodian.

  He/she cannot deny giving a copy of these records (including copies of radiographs or x-rays) to you. There may be a small fee for the office staff to duplicate these records. Also, it is customary for records to be transferred from dentist to dentist to ensure safety and continuation of treatment that may still be in progress.

- *Does your dentist take a personal interest in you and your health? Does he schedule you to come in at least once or twice a year for a checkup? Does he send you periodic reminders when you are due for another checkup?*

  All these are good indicators of your dentist's competence and interest in you as a patient, that your dentist values the importance of good dental care, and that his practice is well organized. Also, have a dental checkup before undergoing major surgery. The results of an operation could be endangered if certain bacteria—which are always present in the mouth—get into the bloodstream. This point cannot be emphasized enough. We are now into an age of heart valve repairs, bypasses, and joint replacements. It is essential that your dentist know your history in this regard. Gum disease or periodontitis is now known to be a leading cause of heart valve complications and infections that may cause or lead to serious medical complications.

- *Does your dentist take a complete medical and dental history on the first appointment and thoroughly examine your teeth, jaws, gums, and the rest of your mouth and surrounding muscles, screening for cancer and other disorders? Does he update your history at each subsequent examination? Does he check your head and neck for signs of infection, such as swollen glands? Does he ask about any drug allergies or whether you have been treated for diabetes, rheumatic fever, heart disease, or hemophilia? Does he ask questions about current and recent illnesses? Does he try to prevent you from discomfort by working efficiently and gently, observing you closely, and providing you with appropriate painkillers, if needed? If you are still apprehensive, does the dentist suggest any special options to relieve it like acupuncture or other treatments such as anti-anxiety medication, nitrous-oxide/oxygen, or simply scheduling your appointment at a quiet time of your day or his/her schedule when your anxiety may be at a lower level? If an examination reveals a dental disease, does the dentist explain to you the pros and cons of a wide range of new and old technologies, such as implants, bonding, various restoration materials, and evolving approaches to periodontal disease? Does the dentist mention that more effective topical anesthetics help make your receiving Novocain a painless procedure? Or that using noninvasive, nonsurgical techniques and antimicrobial treatments can help patients treat their gum disease successfully? Or that there are new cosmetic developments whereby teeth can be whitened in an about hour or that new adhesives combined with tooth-colored fillings make it practically impossible to determine that cavities have been filled or an old filling replaced?*

My dentist recently relayed to me a story about Tina, a sixteen-year-old high school sophomore. She had recently been seen by a new dentist to correct some discolored areas of her upper front teeth (central and lateral incisors and canines). There were one or two discolored fillings present as well. The dentist described only one treatment plan—that was full porcelain veneers on six teeth. As you can guess, the cost was significant. More important, this would have involved cutting well into the front surfaces of her teeth (called tooth reduction or preparation), making a mold, and sending it out to the laboratory for fabrication of the veneers. In a young patient, the more cutting and preparation by the dentist, the more natural tooth structure is lost. In addition, in the simple act of cutting into a tooth, the closer the drill necessarily comes to the vital core or pulp of the tooth, both of which in a young patient is very aggressive and potentially damaging. Now, this may not necessarily have been bad treatment, but there are many more updated techniques and options that would have served this young patient as well or even better. After making numerous calls, and with each call becoming more educated, she came to my dentist. He ended up bleaching two teeth, replacing two discolored fillings, and, extending a whiter shade of composite resin onto the surface of one of the darker teeth. My dentist indicated that his goal was to treat each tooth with the minimum degree of "invasiveness"—an approach that would optimize the risk/benefit ratio (i.e., your goal is to seek treatment that will provide the needed benefit with the least danger or risk).

These and other procedures constitute good dental practice. For example, in conducting a soft tissue examination, including lips, cheeks, and tongue, your dentist should also be looking for oral lesions, some of which are harmless, but some of which could be cancerous. In a hard tissue examination, your dentist should be examining each tooth and the relationship between the upper and lower teeth. Be aware that dental checkups are also necessary for the early discovery of oral cancer and other diseases. Mouth cancer often goes unnoticed in its early and curable stages because pain is not always a symptom. And careful self-examination is essential. If you notice any red or white spots in the mouth that bleed or do not go away in two weeks, be sure to have them checked by a dentist. Many dentists use a simple "brush biopsy" technique, where a sample of area of concern is simply "brushed" onto a swab and sent to laboratory for analysis. On the other hand, it is a sign of poor dentistry if you have crowns, bridges, or fillings that are loose or fall off repeatedly or if you have pain, swelling, or bleeding months after a root canal was completed. Also, it is sign of bad hygiene if your dentist fixes his glasses, goes through a drawer, or writes with a pen while still wearing the protective gloves he used in your mouth.

- *Does the dentist observe or ask you whether you have observed any of the following signs of disease: bleeding, swollen, or inflamed gums; loose teeth; continual bad breath; bad taste in your mouth; pain when eating sweets or drinking hot or cold liquids; or pain when chewing? If you are a woman, ask your dentist whether panoramic dental x-rays, which show the whole skeletal jaw, can also show the beginnings of low skeletal bone mineral density, the first step toward osteoporosis? Panoramic radiographs also can show signs of calcification in blood vessels such as carotid arteries that have the potential for strokes.*

- *Does the dentist use modern equipment and treatment techniques? Remember that every dental office must meet the current OSHA (Occupational Safety and Health Administration) guidelines for sterilization and disinfection of instruments. Does he provide advice on dental care that you should follow between visits? Is he prevention oriented? Does he show you how to brush your teeth and use dental floss? Does he explain what plaque (pronounced plack) is and how to keep it off your teeth?* (Plaque is a gummy and adhesive mass of bacteria growing on teeth that can cause tooth decay and gum disease such as pyorrhea.)

- *Does your dentist offer you free information on dental health? If you are a woman, does your dentist explain how puberty, menstruation, birth control pills, pregnancy, and menopause may affect your oral health?*

You should look for a dentist who is skilled in both the treatment of oral disorders and in the latest preventive measures. For example, during a dental examination all dentists should be using a periodontal probe to detect the presence of gum disease like gingivitis. To summarize, a good oral examination as a minimum should require (1) an oral soft tissue examination (cheek, lips, and tongue); (2) a periodontal examination to examine the teeth below the gum line to detect the level of gum disease damage; and (3) a dental exam (specifically, looking or probing each tooth for the presence of tooth decay. As a preventive health measure, ask your dentist prior to receiving radiation treatment to the head or neck area or cancer chemotherapy about fluoride treatments to prevent or lessen the possibility of severe tooth decay that may occur from these procedures. As far as removing plaque from your teeth, you can test your own skill by chewing a disclosing tablet, colored with a food dye. This will "disclose" or show you where any plaque may still remain on your teeth.

- *What are the dentist's arrangements in regard to his fees? Does he give you an estimate of his fees for the treatments he is proposing to perform? Are his charges reasonable compared to other dental charges in your geographic area? Does he perform all the services for which you are billed?*

    Do not be ashamed to ask the dentist in advance about his fee schedule or payment plans and get an advance written estimate for dental work that is not routine. Competent dentists are willing to discuss their fees, give detailed explanations, itemize their bills, and describe their services in advance of treatment. Be wary of dentists who do not do so.

- *If your dentist is a specialist, is he board certified?*

    Any licensed dentist can practice as an orthodontist, periodontist, or in any other specialty even if not qualified by training or experience to do so. A dentist who is board certified in a specialty has satisfied requirements of dental training and experience that are designed to assure his competency in the field of his specialty. As already noted, the *American Dental Directory*, published by the American Dental Association, lists board-certified specialists. Public libraries may have this directory. State dental societies also maintain specialty lists. As already briefly noted, since the 1990s there has been a huge expansion in both medicine and dentistry of "CEs," or continuing education courses, available to healthcare professionals. This has been a huge boon to professionals and patients as healthcare consumers. These are both proprietary (directed by pharmaceutical companies, equipment suppliers, educational services, and study groups) or university based. As medical/dental technology has proliferated, the need to "spread the word" or to expose these new concepts to practicing dentists is necessary and a welcomed event. Course attendance is verified by providing the dentist with a "certificate of continuing education." Further advanced training with appropriate written and oral examinations may result in the title "master" or "fellow" in a particular technique, philosophy, or specialty field. A dentist who is technically not a specialist according to the American Dental Association now can attain a higher level of competency through these CE courses. There are now titles such as "esthetic and cosmetic dentistry," "sedation dentistry," "implantologist," and fellow in the Academy of General Dentistry or the American Academy of Osseointegration. A fundamental guideline still applies: Individual CE courses and CE courses leading a dentist to achieve membership or honorary titles in a society are approved by your state board of dentistry. They are mandated by protecting the public through licensure. So if your dentist indicates a special skill in a specific area, he must be able to document his training, membership, and competency.

• *Does your dentist polish your new fillings?*

This procedure enhances the appearance and durability of the fillings.

• *Does the dentist furnish technically competent treatment that results in a comfortable bite and nicely finished tooth surfaces?*

• *Does the dentist have his biographical resume in the waiting room, describing his education and qualifications? Are the dentist's dental school diploma, license, and other educational certificates in sight? Is his/her license to practice dentistry in your state on display?*

• *Does the dentist take continuing education and refresher courses in his field?*

If in general practice, is the dentist a member or fellow in the Academy of General Dentistry? Since the academy requires that dentists complete a certain amount of hours for membership or fellowship every three years, membership in this professional body is an indication of a dentist's continual commitment to education. However, a note of caution: The academy approves sponsors of courses rather than the courses themselves, and it relies on dentists to report which courses they have attended. Licensure alone is not a guarantee that a dentist will practice good dentistry over the years. Licensure is bestowed at two levels. The first level is the state or regional Board of Dental Examiners such as the NorthEast Regional Board, which covers that part of the country. This level verifies that the new graduate of a dental school has achieved competency. Without this the new dentist cannot practice at all. This is a onetime certification. Additionally, a dentist has to be licensed in a particular state. This license is either annual or biannual and only requires paying a nominal fee, but it does require a minimum of twenty-five hours of continuing education for that one- to two-year period. A dentist who passes the NorthEast Regional Boards, for example, can receive reciprocity to practice in another region such as Maryland in the Mid-Atlantic, providing, of course, he meets whatever criteria or tests that particular state may require for practice.

• *Does the dentist pay attention to your dental problems with compassion and understanding? Does he have physicians and other dentists as patients?*

• *Does your dentist maintain ethical standards of practice specified by the American Dental Association?*

• *Does the dentist use dental auxiliaries such as hygienists and assistants?*

By employing these aides, the dentist can increase his work productivity both economically and efficiently since they perform many of the less complicated dental duties.

• *Does the dentist employ x-rays in his diagnosis? Does he take a full series of x-rays before starting any treatments? Does he place a lead apron on his patients for their protection while taking x-rays? Does your dentist consider your dental x-rays to be your property or his? Does your dentist permit you to have full access to your dental records and x-rays? Does your dentist object if you request that independent qualified auditors such as his dental peers review the quality of his dental treatment (including examination of your x- rays and records)? Does he explain to you how the x-rays will help with the diagnosis?*

If you are a new patient, a dentist will probably ask that you take a full set of mouth x-rays, unless suitable ones are available from your previous dentist and you ask that they be transferred to the new dentist. Depending upon how often you visit your dentist and your dental history, you may or may not need x-rays during each visit. The American Dental Association has indicated that x-ray examinations need not be part of every dental examination. But be wary of the dentist who does not take any x-rays at all or who lets years pass by without taking screening x-rays; many dental problems cannot be detected without their use. Many others can be detected earlier with the aid of x-rays than by visual examination alone. But any unnecessary radiation is excessive radiation. And any excessive radiation is dangerous radiation. The dentist should take a full set of x- rays or a panoramic film every three to five years. The x-rays help the dentist detect cavities, some remote deposits of calculus, bone loss around the teeth, abscesses of the tooth tip, impacted teeth, retained roots, cysts, and tumors of the jawbone. A more limited set of x-rays called "bitewings" should be taken more frequently to detect cavities only.

• *Does your dentist practice in a group with other dentists or alone?*

Dentists who practice in a group are able to check on the work of other dentists, easily consult with each other, can get rid of poor dentists, deal with a greater variety of dental problems under one roof, provide for emergency care, and achieve savings in group practice that hold down dental costs.

• *Does the dentist have an appointment to a dental school's faculty?*

While there is no relationship between a dentist's teaching ability and manual skills, it might suggest that the dentist is up-to-date on the latest scientific developments in his field.

• *Does the dentist have a hospital affiliation?*

As a member of a hospital staff, a dentist has the opportunity to exchange knowledge with other dentists and physicians.

• *Does your dentist explain optional courses of treatment and the possible benefits and complications that may follow from any proposed treatment? Does he provide a written treatment plan before major procedures? Does your dentist begin some procedures such as filling or capping a tooth without informing you in advance and getting your consent?*

Under the legal doctrine of informed consent, a patient who has not been fairly advised about the risks of any dental or medical treatment has not legally consented to it. The patient, therefore, may sue a dentist for malpractice if the dentist treats him without fully and fairly explaining the risks involved. Do not hesitate to ask questions about the proposed treatment and all its possible ramifications. The law requires the dentist to obtain permission and explain his course of treatment before proceeding. Any other course of action is not only psychologically harmful for the patient but also illegal. In the final analysis, it is still your decision whether you want your dentist to perform the procedure that he is recommending.

- *Does your dentist take precautions against the spread of disease? Do all dental staff members wear disposable rubber gloves when working on patients? Do they flush water lines and disinfect suction lines? Do they wear surgical masks? Does the dentist use disposable needles? Does the dentist use disposable equipment covers such as x-ray unit heads and dental lamp handles that can be splattered with germ-filled saliva, blood, or other materials during dental procedures? Does the dental team wear protective glasses or goggles? Do patients get disposable cups to rinse their mouths? Are all nondisposable instruments sterilized after every use? Are all dental team members vaccinated against hepatitis B, the viral disease most commonly passed between dentists and their patients? Do all dental team members wear clean gowns? Do dental personnel conscientiously wash their hands between patients and after handling such items such as money, dental charts, and doorknobs?*

Ideally, the answers to all these questions should be "yes."

- *Does the dentist show you how to care for your dentures?*

If you have dentures, you should keep them clean and free from deposits that can cause permanent staining, bad breath, and gum irritation. Once a day, brush all surfaces of the denture with a denture-care product. Be sure to remove your dentures from your mouth for at least six to eight hours every day and place them in water (but never hot water) or a denture-cleansing solution. It is also helpful to rinse your mouth with a warm saltwater solution after meals and at bedtime. After a number of years, dentures may have to be relined or even replaced. Do not attempt to repair dentures at home. You can damage them or, more important, harm the tissues in your mouth.

Partial dentures should be cared for in the same manner as full dentures. Be especially careful to cleanse under and around the clasps of partial dentures. This is where germs tend to collect.

- *Does your dentist do everything possible to save a tooth? Does he encourage consultation?*

For example, if a tooth extraction is proposed, you are entitled to receive a second opinion about the extraction from another dentist. A qualified dentist will not only support such a consultation but also may advise it. When you seek a consultation, ask your dentist to send your x-rays and the results of his examination to the consulting dentist. If your health insurance plan covers dental procedures, ask the plan whether it pays for second opinions in regard to dental services. The importance of consultation is illustrated by the American Dental Association, which has stated that denture construction and repair is one of the areas abused by quacks. Dentures fitted by unqualified persons and mail-order dentures can damage mouth tissues. Poorly fitted dentures can cause serious problems—these may include eating problems, difficulty in speaking, and the destruction of bone that is needed for denture support. Some damage, such as excessive bone loss, is not reversible. Constant irritation from an ill-fitting denture, if continued over a long period, may contribute to the development of open sores and other serious lesions such as tumors. Poorly fitted dentures can cost the patient more over time when the damage they cause has to be corrected. Thus, if your dentist recommends the extraction of teeth and their replacement by dentures, consult a dental specialist in this regard. An endodontist who specializes in saving teeth can tell you whether the procedure is necessary.

In some states, denturists—the dental technicians who actually make the teeth in the lab—are allowed to provide complete denture service. Denturists not only claim they can provide the service at less cost than the dentist but that they can provide faster and better service. Unlike a dentist who must send the dentures back to a lab to make adjustments, a denturist can make changes on the spot. Some states allow denturists to practice in this fashion but stringently regulate and license the practitioners. Check with your state if it has such denturist laws. But be cautious: there are many denturists working illegally. Know your denturist's credentials and be sure your dentures fit comfortably when you have your final fitting.

Finally, remember that just as good medical care requires a trustful partnership between you and your physician, good dental care requires a cooperative partnership between you and your dentist. Look for and choose a dentist who will explain what he is doing and why and what to expect. He must be able to explain any problems you may have and tell you how to avoid these problems and prevent dental disease. He should also explain any alternate options to the treatment he is proposing. Some dentists are even beginning to practice what is called "spa dentistry." The purpose of spa dentistry is to make the patient feel as comfortable as possible in the dentist's office prior to undergoing whatever procedures he may need. Such services may include foot massages, fresh cranberry-orange bread, hot towels, neck rubs, or the lulling sounds of wind chimes that are used to distract the patient from Novocain shots or the sound of drills or the scraping noises of the hygienist's instruments. And those who practice this kind of dentistry state that they are not charging for extras because most spa services are more than covered by an increase in patient referrals and repeat business. The American Dental Association expects the number of dentists who practice spa dentistry to grow in the future. The more a patient is free of the memories of dental care as a painful procedure, the better the patient will take care of his teeth and the more frequently the patient will seek dental care to get rid of his problems. If you feel your dentist is not serving you well or making decisions in your best interest, seek another—it is your dental health that is involved and that matters the most.[5]

A DENTIST FOR CHILDREN

In reviewing the qualities one should seek in choosing a dentist or a dental specialist, some parents prefer to take their children to pediatric dentists (formerly known as pedodontists), dentists who limit their practice to the treatment of children.

"I think this is very important for our child," Diane told her husband. "You know Alice has been a thumb sucker ever since her new teeth came in, and look what her sucking has done to her mouth. Her teeth are not aligned properly and may require some kind of brace to straighten them out. Michael, you know Alice as well as I do. You just mention a visit to the dentist and she begins to scream and cry. She is terrified of going there. She does not like the drill or all the other equipment the dentist may put in her mouth. I think we should take her to a dentist who specializes in treating children. Don't forget there is as much psychology involved in making a child's dental visit as pleasant as possible as there are dental procedures. Some of the dentists in town now have music in their offices to soothe their patients' fears or special colors on walls and other soothing features in decorating their offices."
Michael replied: "A pediatric dentist may be the answer to our problem. But how do they differ from the general practitioner who also treats children?"

Since children may be treated either by those in general practices or by pediatric dentists, it may be of value to give a brief description of this dental specialty.

Pediatric dentists are especially trained to deal with the anxieties and emotions of children. In order to become board certified, these dentists, after completing their DDS degrees, must meet the required two years of additional preparation that the American Board of Pedodontists (now renamed the American Board of Pediatric Dentists) established in the early 1960s. Either as graduate students in a master's degree program or as hospital residents, they receive extensive training in child psychology, children's emergency treatment, methods for accommodating retarded and handicapped patients, current preventive dental measures, general anesthesia, and hospital procedures.

A pediatric dentist's practice is usually limited to children between the ages of two and fifteen, although he will also treat handicapped and retarded adults. It is recommended that a child's first visit occur between the ages of two and two and a half (before all primary teeth have erupted). However, some dentists believe a child's first visit to the dentist should be made by the first birthday or six months after the first tooth erupts, whichever comes first. Ask your dentist what he recommends. But most pediatric dentists prefer that parents visit them well beforehand to counsel them about their child's diet and oral hygiene homecare programs. Check with your dentist on these matters.[6] Primary teeth are as important as permanent ones, and their loss can affect a child's teeth, eating, and appearance. Baby teeth are important for chewing, speaking, and maintaining the proper space between teeth. And because the primary teeth are in close proximity to and guide the eruption of the permanent teeth, it is necessary to keep them as plaque free as possible.

According to Dr. Jed Best, a pediatric dentist and consultant to Kinder-Care Learning Centers, the largest provider of childcare in the United States, by age six, kids should be using an over-the-counter fluoride mouthwash daily. By age eight, they should be able to floss alone or under your supervision. Brushing should be performed with a child-size brush with soft, end-rounded bristles. These are less likely to injure gum tissue. Replace the brush about every three or four months. As far as electric brushes are concerned, Best says that studies have not shown that electric brushes are superior in removing plaque. However, in 2003 the Cochran Collaboration—an independent nonprofit group based in Oxford, England, that evaluates medical practices—stated that electric brushes with bristles that spin in both directions are the only kind offering an advantage over regular toothbrushes. The rest were not worse, but they were not better, either. So, for the rest, whichever brush your child is most likely to use—manual or electric—is the best choice.[7] Another way to protect against cavities in children, according to Dr. Stephen J. Moss, former chairman of the pediatric dentistry department at New York University College of Dentistry, is to have a child brush with a fluoride toothpaste after breakfast and before going to bed and to have the child visit a dentist twice a year. He also recommends vitamin supplements and mouth rinses enriched with fluoride and the application—by a dentist—of a protective resin sealant to the biting surfaces of a child's permanent back teeth when they come in. He warns against neglecting baby teeth since they lead others into the mouth.[8] Sealants, developed in the 1960s and 1970s, work by forming a thin, clear plastic coating on tooth surfaces that protect against decay by creating a barrier between the tooth and food particles or bacteria. Sealants, as already noted, are used primarily to protect against decay in molars and premolars in children. Unlike incisors and canines, which have flat chewing surfaces, molars and premolars have many pits and fissures that increase the surface area for grinding food. But they also have places where food and bacteria can be trapped and cause cavities. According to Dr. Louis W. Ripa, former chairman of the department of children's dentistry at the State University of New York's School of Dentistry at Stony Brook, dental sealants are best applied to children when permanent molars erupt, usually at ages six to eight and twelve. Most dentists and dental groups recommend sealants only through age seventeen. But Ripa says—given the increasing number of cavities dentists have seen in older teens and young adults—perhaps they, too, would benefit as well from sealants. By the time they reach their midtwenties, most people have already had most of the cavities that sealants are designed to prevent. Ripa says that sealants can reduce decay by up to 99 percent for the first two years after application and up to 62 percent four years later. How long and how well they work depends upon the skill of the dentist or the hygienist who applies them, as well as whether the teeth are treated again when the sealant begins to deteriorate. A 1983 National Institutes of Health consensus conference called sealants a safe and "highly effective" means of preventing cavities. Get your dentist's recommendation for your children. If your child has no history of cavities, then a sealant might not be necessary. If you have dental care insurance, find out whether your policy covers the cost of sealants.[9]

Another form of treatment for children may be called preventive orthodontics. For example, for a child who loses a baby tooth prematurely, there are now space maintainers that keep adjacent teeth from crowding the permanent teeth. There are also tongue/thumb guards for children whose baby front teeth have been bucked because of thumb sucking. They make thumb sucking difficult and permit the permanent teeth to come in straight. Preventive orthodontics may be an answer for preventing the need of braces later for a child.[10]

One of the most prevalent dental problems found in children today is caused by well-meaning but uninformed parents; "the baby-bottle syndrome"—rampant decay and decalcification of the primary teeth—occurs when the child has regularly been given nighttime or nap-time bottles containing fruit juices, formulas, or other sugary liquids. Dentists suggest that if a baby needs to suck on something, try a bottle of cool water or a clean pacifier. Even if it is diluted, limit the amount of juice because within twenty minutes, the acids of the juice begin working on the teeth.[11] Dentists consider this decay preventable and, if your community water supply is not fluoridated (check with your local health department) or your baby is entirely breast-fed, your dentist can tell you how to protect your children's teeth. These preventive measures may include the use of fluoride toothpaste as well as prescribed fluoride drops for infants from their birth until as youngsters they can take prescribed fluoride tablets up through fourteen years of age. Fluoride drops or tablets should be taken daily during the years when permanent teeth are forming. Fluoride gels may also be available from your dentist. In some communities, through public health programs, children, with written parental consent, can receive in school fluoride tablets and/or a weekly fluoride mouth rinsing. But, again, talk about these various preventive measures with your dentist and find out how often and for how long a period of time your child should take them. Also, be aware of bottled water. Every sports hero, young mom and dad, and children everywhere are sporting their backpacks with water attached. It's bottled water. The problem from a dental perspective is that the water is not fluoridated. This is not as critical for adults as it is for children with developing adult teeth. Again, fluoride in some form in drinking water is vital for healthy tooth structure. Ask your dentist as to how you and/or your children can compensate for the lack of fluoride in the bottled water and protect your teeth. Other measures parents can take to prevent early childhood caries include the following:

- Mothers should reduce their own oral bacterial infection through dental care and effective oral homecare during prenatal and postnatal periods. Women of childbearing age who have cavities or have many fillings are at greatest risk to infect their newborns with cavity-producing bacteria. These bacteria live on sugar that is part of the baby's diet and deposit acid against the child's tooth surfaces.

- Once babies weigh ten pounds or more, they do not require sleep-time feedings. Avoid leaving a bottle in the crib and excessive nighttime bottle and breast-feeding.
- Try comforting the child with a pacifier or a favorite toy or blanket instead of using the bottle or breast as a pacifier.
- Even before teeth appear, wipe an infant's gums with a clean, damp washcloth at least once a day. This gets rid of the bacteria from milk and the baby gets used to having his mouth cleaned. Clean a child's teeth as soon as they erupt. Again, parents should use a damp cloth or a toothbrush to clean these teeth. When cleaning, parents should be sure to check their baby's teeth regularly for any chalky white or brown spots that could be the beginning of decay.

While pediatric dentists, through their specialized training, can do much to ease a child's trauma in receiving dental care, there is much that parents can do in this regard as well. These include the following recommendations:

- Never use the dental visit as a threat.
- Avoid using words such as hurt, pain, and brave in connection with the dental appointment.
- Do not discuss your own unpleasant dental experiences in front of your child.
- Try to make the first visit sound as positive as possible, but don't overexplain or make a "big deal" out of the appointment. Leave most of the explaining to the dentist. If you are not sure how to handle the explanation, a quick preappointment phone call to the pediatric dentist should answer all your questions.
- Avoid specifics about the dental visit. For example, if you say, "the pediatric dentist is only going to count and wash your teeth," that's all the child expects to happen. But should the pediatric dentist discover something that needs immediate attention, or should his routine differ from your description, the child will be unprepared for these changes and this could result in unnecessary anxiety. Therefore, it's best to say something like, "The dentist is going to count your teeth (or whatever will be part of the visit) and then he'll see what else needs to be done." Be willing to wait for your child in the reception room and don't encourage clinging, particularly when the dental assistant or pediatric dentist comes for him.
- Be sure to tell the pediatric dentist whether your child has had any previous negative dental experiences, as well as any fears you (or others) may have either consciously or unconsciously transmitted to him.
- Friends and older brothers and sisters frequently frighten youngsters about the dentist. Try to discourage this, but if situation is unavoidable, teach your child to depend on the pediatric dentist and you for accurate information.[12]

Parents are able to choose whether to bring their child to a dentist in general practice or a specialist such as a pediatric dentist.

WHERE TO TAKE A DENTAL COMPLAINT

A patient who is careful in choosing a family dentist and always discusses fees in advance of treatments can expect to have a long-lasting, good relationship with that dentist However, even in the best relationships, problems can arise. That was true in Keith's case.

Keith had some old fillings that had been in his mouth for more than forty years. His dentist convinced him that, given their age, perhaps he should begin to consider placing crowns over some of them, especially those with cracks in their enamel. Well, Keith took the dentist at his word and had crowns, which are expensive, placed in his mouth. One day, Keith had been referred to another specialist for a dental problem not related to the crowns. In the course of his conversation with the dentist, the subject of crowns arose and Dentist B didn't think Keith needed the crowns that Dentist A had placed in his mouth. Keith was confused. Who was right? The dentist who placed the crowns in his mouth or the other specialist? Keith began feeling that the dentist who placed the crowns in his mouth did so unnecessarily so as to increase his dental income. Keith wanted to file a complaint against the original dentist, but he did not know how to go about doing it. To whom should he complain?

If a patient believes that the dentist has treated him unfairly, he should first make sure that the dentist is aware of the problem. Often a problem is simply the result of poor communication between the patient and the dentist. It is best to give the dentist the opportunity to correct the situation. Even expertly administered care will not always achieve the expected results: in such a situation the dentist will want to readminister the treatment or use an alternate procedure—or call in a consulting dentist. If a dentist overcharges you, ask him to reconsider his decision. But whatever your complaint, there are several steps you can take if you believe the dentist has not taken the appropriate corrective action. You can file a complaint with the appropriate government agency that licenses dentists. If insurance covers your dental work, find out from the insurance company whether it has access to the review committees of the local and state dental societies in order to judge and settle claim questions; if so, seek help from the insurer. Also, if your claim is serious enough, there may be grounds for suing your dentist for malpractice.

A good first step is to send your complaint to the county or local dental society. Dental societies are usually listed in the yellow pages of the telephone book under "dentists" or "associations"—or ask any dentist. You can also contact your county health department or the American Dental Association, 211 East Chicago Avenue, Chicago, IL 60611, for the address of the local dental society.

Ask the local dental society to review impartially your complaint against the dentist. The dental society, in turn, will ask you to report the details of the complaint in writing and then will assign the case to a review committee. Frequently, the next step is to assign one member of the review committee to meet individually with you and the dentist. Many times the complaint is resolved at this stage. If any problems are hard to resolve, a panel of dentists may review them, the patient is given a dental examination, and the dentist is asked to submit his treatment records. However, it should be noted that all this activity is voluntary; the dental society has no legal authority to compel either the dentist or the patient to cooperate. All parties have to be committed in good faith to resolving the problem fairly. On the other hand, it is encouraging to note that the great majority of cases brought to dental society review committees are successfully resolved and their conclusions agreed to by all parties.

Finally, remember that each state has a dental practice act—a set of laws that govern the practice of dentistry—and a state board of dentistry that is empowered to establish regulations for the practice of dentistry and the protection of public dental health. If you feel that a dentist has performed in a manner that violates the state dental laws or regulations, the matter should be brought to the attention of the board of dentistry. The same is true if you suspect a person who is not licensed to practice dentistry is performing dental procedures for the public.[13]

HOW TO PAY FOR DENTAL CARE

"I thought it was bad enough when you had to figure out how to file a complaint against a dentist. But trying to figure out how to pay for dental care is worse. I don't even know where to begin," said Muriel.

Reply: Public programs, such as Medicaid and private dental insurance, are available—also, managed dental care. In addition, dental schools provide low-cost clinics.

"The question remains, do I need it? I find so many rules and regulations to both the private and public programs that I cannot keep track of them, or even begin to understand them. I have far less dental expenses each year than medical bills. Is it really worth spending so much money for dental insurance when I generally only visit the dentist twice a year? Sometimes the cost of the premiums exceeds the total amount I spend on dental care each year. Can I be protected against dental expenses, yet spend as little as necessary for such protection?"

There are a variety of ways to pay for dental care today: public assistance programs such as Medicaid, private health insurance plans, and self-payment among them. Persons who need financial help to receive dental care can contact the local dental society for information about dental programs for which they may qualify. The dental society knows what assistance programs and dental care centers, such as dental school clinics and public facilities, are available and can help with referrals.

These dentals schools may charge low-cost fees for checkups and cleaning because care is provide by graduate dentists and dental students under the careful supervision of faculty experts.

In regard to public medical care programs, Medicare, an insurance program administered by the federal government throughout the United States, *generally does not cover dental care services.* But effective July 1, 1981, Medicare covers hospitalization for noncovered dental services where the severity of the procedure or the condition warrants hospitalization. Those who are eligible for the Medicare program are people over sixty-five years of age; disabled people who have been entitled to Social Security disability payments for two consecutive years; and people who are insured under Social Security or the Railroad Retirement system who need dialysis treatment or a kidney transplant, including those under sixty-five years of age. On the other hand, *Medicaid* is a *public assistance* program financed by federal, state, and local governments. Each state designs its own plan according to federal guidelines. In addition, the District of Columbia, Puerto Rico, and the Virgin Islands have Medicaid programs. Low-income people who fit into the following categories receive Medicaid coverage: the aged (sixty-five years or older), the blind, the disabled, members of families with dependent children, and some other children. Some states provide coverage for other groups of low-income people who, although not qualified for welfare, cannot afford medical care. This latter group is called medically needy. Because each state designs its Medicaid program to meet the needs of its own state residents and because Medicaid is subject to funding problems, states that might have covered a benefit at one period of time may no longer do so now. Consequently, ask your state or county department of public welfare whether the Medicaid program in your state covers dental care services, for children as well as for adults over the age of twenty-one. As of 2003, according to the Kaiser Commission on Medicaid and the Uninsured of the Henry J. Kaiser Family Foundation, only Alabama, Connecticut, Arkansas, Delaware, and the District of Columbia did not have dental care health benefits in their Medicaid programs. The rest of the states did have such a benefit. Dental services under Title XIX of the Social Security Act, the Medicaid program, are an optional service for the adult population, individuals age twenty-one and older. However dental services are a required service for most Medicaid-eligible individuals under age twenty-one, as a required component of the Early and Periodic Screening, Diagnosis, and Treatment (EPSDT) benefit. Services must include as a minimum, relief of pain and infections, restoration of teeth, and maintenance of dental health. Dental services may not be limited to emergency services of EPSDT recipients. States may elect to provide dental care services to their adult Medicaid-eligible population or elect not to provide dental services at all as part of their Medicaid program. Most states provide at least emergency dental services for adults, but less than half of all states provide comprehensive dental care. There are no minimum requirements for adult dental coverage.

There are certain facts that the elderly should know about dental care:

- Losing teeth is *not* a normal part of the aging process. Over 60 percent of persons age sixty-five and older have their own teeth.
- In the United States older persons are at greater risk for developing cavities than are fourteen-year-olds.
- Medicare does not pay for 96 percent of dental care.
- "Dry mouth" is a side effect of the majority of medication prescribed to persons with high blood pressure. Dry mouth can lead to tooth loss.
- If not removed, plaque begins to have a harmful effect within twenty-four to seventy-two hours.
- Persons with Alzheimer's disease may not be able to tolerate extensive dental treatment in the later stages of the disease.
- Diabetes lowers defenses for fighting bacteria throughout the body, including the mouth.
- Sixty is the average age of persons diagnosed with oral cancer.
- Serious infections of the mouth are common in cancer patients who receive radiation and chemotherapy.
- Five years is the average life span for a set of dentures.
- Dentists and dental hygienists have specially adapted tooth brushes and flossing equipment useful to persons impaired by arthritis or recovering from a stroke.
- New portable dental equipment allows the treatment of nursing homes residents and homebound persons in their own environment.

Your local dental society, dental school, or dental hygiene program can provide you with additional information about your oral healthcare concerns should you be elderly.[14]

If you are a patient in a nursing home, be aware that federal legislation, effective October 1, 1990, makes nursing homes receiving federal dollars "directly responsible for the dental care needs of their residents." Each nursing home is required to have a written agreement with a dentist to provide dental services. Nursing homes are responsible for helping residents have their damaged or lost dentures repaired or replaced. Homes are also responsible for arranging dental appointments and transportation under the legislation. There are certain steps nursing homes can take to ensure good dental care for their residents:

- All dentures (uppers and lowers) should be permanently marked—just in case they are left on a food tray or get lost.
- Staff must assume responsibility of a resident who cannot care for his/her own teeth.
- Snacks that don't stick to the teeth are preferred (avoid raisins, caramels, and excessively sweet drinks).
- Be prepared to look for warning signs when noncommunicative persons cannot tell you they have a toothache or that they have seriously bitten their tongue.

- Make sure sponge swabs are available to clean out the mouths of persons without teeth.
- Dentures must be removed at least eight hours per day to rest gums.

If you do not qualify for dental care financial assistance under Medicaid and still cannot afford to pay very much for dental care, consider going to the dental clinic of a dental school, as already noted. The care in a dental school clinic is provided by graduate dentists or dental students under the careful supervision of faculty experts. The fees charged are minimal, usually including only partial payment to cover the cost of materials and equipment.[15] In addition, free or low-cost dental checkups might be available through your child's school health program or the county health department. Also, many dentists maintain a continued relationship with their patients long after they transition to a retirement residence or nursing home. As long as your dentist maintains a license to practice in your state, most nursing homes seem to welcome these dental visits. Ask your dentist on the availability of this service for yourself or your loved ones.

UNDERSTANDING DENTAL HEALTH INSURANCE

Another method of financing dental care is through the purchase of private health insurance.

Max had a problem. He did not know whether to buy dental insurance and add additional premium costs to his other insurance.

"My dental expenses are not that much each year, and the insurance costs could exceed my yearly bills. Although I'm getting older and my teeth and gums are not in the best of shape, so far I've been lucky with minimum annual dental expenses. I don't qualify for Medicaid, I'm too young for Medicare, and there are no dental schools or clinics in my area. Should I get private dental insurance? What about joining a managed care plan? I could find a new dentist if mine is not affiliated."

While Max was weighing his options, he had the occasion to visit his dentist complaining about some sensations in his teeth that would not disappear. The dentist immediately inquired about his insurance.

"Why," asked Max? His dentist informed him that it might be necessary to extract the teeth or perform a root canal on the affected nerve.

"I will need to send you to a specialist for these procedures, and that can chalk up quite a steep bill. Even more expensive than what you would pay for annual dental insurance."

Max checked and found that his insurance policy at work permitted him to purchase dental insurance. But a note of caution: Most dental third-party (insurance) carriers have a blocked-out period of one year on costly procedures such as orthodontics and prosthodontics (crowns, bridges, and dentures), meaning they won't pay for such procedures until the waiting time has passed, namely, until the second year of the policy, and when they do pay it may be on a coinsurance basis, for example, 60 percent of the oral surgery fee and 50 percent of periodontics procedures. Emergency procedures involving acute infection such as endodontic (root canal treatment) are usually not subject to this restriction. The other issue is the annual insurance "cap" or annual ceiling on dental expenses. This is usually established at $2,500 annually. For example, in 2005 a root canal treatment of $1,000 plus a core to build up the tooth after root canal of $370 plus a final crown to protect the tooth of $950 would consume your annual maximum amount very quickly.

Like Max, it is wise to check your existing health policy to see if it provides the option of purchasing private dental insurance. While most dental costs are paid privately, dental health insurance is a rapidly growing means of payment. Today millions of American workers have dental coverage with insurance and service plans, through employee and union groups throughout the country. The key difference between dental and medical insurance is that medical insurance is generally oriented to treatment after illness strikes while dental insurance promotes regular treatment as a way to minimize serious costly problems at a later date. Dental health insurance plans vary greatly; while most plans provide for such basic and routine service as emergency treatments, examinations, fillings, x-rays, cleaning, and fluoride applications, their coverage of restorative work, oral and maxillofacial surgery, root canal treatments, prosthodontics, and orthodontics increases the cost of the premiums. If the plans include preventative benefits, they may offer to pay a higher percentage of the cost of preventative care services such as cleanings and examinations than they will pay for restorative care like fillings and sealants. Dental costs in a hospital are rarely included, nor are cosmetic treatments.[16] Therefore, find out if the dental insurance plan covers preventive as well as restorative treatment in addition to offering you the freedom of choice on selecting your own dentist.

If you do not have comprehensive dental care insurance, you still may be covered for dental care through major medical insurance plans, which are a common part of employment packages or may be held individually. These may cover some expensive procedures such as the surgical removal of impacted teeth, periodontal surgery, and some endodontic surgery such as removal of root abscesses. They also often pay for oral surgery that is required owing to a nonoccupational accident. So don't fail to investigate if your dental needs fall into any of these categories. The other and perhaps the most important issue is that "trustworthiness" that was discussed previously between you and your dentist and that has developed between both of you for many years. If accepting an insurance plan that your dentist does not participate in means you have to leave his care, you may forfeit his guidance, professional opinion, and empathy that has taken years to nurture.

Reimbursement Methods

Reimbursement methods among dental prepayment plans also vary. The most common method is the "usual, customary, and reasonable" (UCR) basis, under which individual dentists charge their usual fee for a particular service and the insurer reviews and verifies the charge. *Usual* means the fee the dentist usually charges for a service. *Customary* means that the fee is comparable to fees charged by most dentists for the service. *Reasonable* means that an exception can be made to meeting the first two criteria if the circumstances dictate it. For example, a dentist may reasonably charge more than usual for a service if the patient was uncooperative and caused the dentist extra work. The advantage of using a usual, customary, and reasonable system is that employees are covered to the same extent no matter how much fees may rise. The disadvantage is that the UCR system costs more in premiums than a table of allowances. Some "usual, customary, and reasonable" fees have a deductible amount that the beneficiary must pay before the benefit begins. Others have a coinsurance or copayment provision, under which a portion of the dental fee is paid by the beneficiary, the balance by the plan. Under a few dental insurance plans, the patient pays a decreasing share of his dental bill if he visits his dentist on a regular basis.[17]

Another dental reimbursement format is the table of allowances that lists the actual dollar limits the insurance plan will pay for each covered service. In this instance, find out whether the plan has established a total lifetime dollar limit per person for any service it covers. Under this kind of plan, you receive the specific sum the company allows in its schedule of services. Some of the criticisms of this plan are that the table of allowances is significantly lower than the fees that dentists charge, and you must pay the difference between the amount allowed for the service and the dental fee, and some policies may be more heavily oriented toward repair than dental prevention—that is, root canals and crowns are covered, checkups and cleaning are not. On the positive side, though, such plans can afford a measure of protection against unnecessary work. Under many plans, extensive treatment plans or work in excess of a specified amount are reviewed by the insurance company beforehand to determine what portion of the work will be covered. Another plus is that you may choose any dentist you want. One thing to be aware of in this type of dental insurance is calendar-year limitations. Also, remember not all calendar years extend from January to December. Some may cover from May to April. If your plan includes such a clause, you can receive benefits only up to certain dollar limits within each calendar year. If this is the case and your dentist recommends an expensive treatment plan, you and the dentist may be able to work out a schedule that extends treatment—and thereby benefits—over two years. In correspondence with the author Dr. Michael J. Tabacco, clinical professor of prosthodontics at the University of Maryland's Baltimore College of Dental Surgery, offered the following example.

Mary Jane, a forty-two-year-old mother of three, has dental insurance with an annual calendar limit of $2,500 for dental expenses. She tripped on a rug and fractured her right upper two central incisors (call them #8 and #9). One had to be extracted (#8) with a temporary partial denture placed and later an implant placed in that position; the other (#9) required root canal treatment, a post, and a crown. The estimated expenses are as follows: #8 extraction, $250; place a temporary removable denture (remember the tooth is missing and you may find it difficult to smile with one tooth out), $500; an implant placed by a surgeon, $1,700; general dentist or prosthodontist (five months later) placed an abutment, $350; and a crown, $1,100. The tooth next to it, #9, needed root canal treatment, $950, and a post-core to build up the center, $975. The total cost for this accident is financially catastrophic: $6,250. Since the "cap" is $2,500, out-of-pocket expense will be $3,850, at least. Staging treatment over two years would at least bring payments approximately into the "cap" range: Here is how it would work extending treatment over three years.

A third procedure gives beneficiaries direct payments from the company with the dental bill itself determining the amount of reimbursement. Still another format that could meet the dental payments for the above illustration is the Flexible Spending Account for medical/dental care. It is a benefit plan, established under Section 125 of the Internal Revenue Code, that allows employees to pay for certain qualified benefits (such as dental care) with pretax dollars. This means the employees' cost of these certain benefits are paid from their salary before taxes (FICA, federal, and, in most cases, state taxes) are calculated. That is, because no federal, state, or FICA taxes are imposed on the money that is placed into the account, this situation can result in lower tax liability (both for the employee and the employer) and more take-home pay. However, in a flexible spending account, the taxpayer forfeits any money that is left unused at the end of the year. You must use it or lose it; unused money will not be returned to you. Thus, in the above illustration if the employee had established a flexible spending account in year two for $2,500, for example, reducing her income tax liability by that amount, but only spent $1,700 on dental care, she would have lost the $800, which would not have been returned to her from that account. Each year you must set up a new contract and almost bet how much you may be spending for dental or medical services a year in advance, with the possibility of losing the amount you do not spend. No matter the format, many plans call for insurer's approval (precertification or predetermination) before the dentist proceeds with work exceeding a specified amount. Obtaining approval is usually not much of a problem. It takes about two weeks because the dental work has not reached the super-expensive stage as yet. You may check with your local dental sources to determine whether a program exists in your community. It may be the kind of dental plan in which you wish to participate.

Dental Cooperatives

Another kind of dental plan that has developed is similar in concept to a health maintenance organization (HMO). For an annual membership fee, which varies according to the individual or the number of family members you wish the dental plan to cover, the plan provides a specific set of dental services at fees that are lower than the prevailing community rate. The dentists who participate in the program are duly licensed and approved by the state and may practice in their own private offices rather than in a clinic. The plan is able to offer reduced dental fees because its participating dentists have formed a "buying cooperative" and purchase as a group the goods and services they require for their dental practice at prices lower than if they had purchased the same goods and services individually. The dentists are then able to pass these savings on to their patients. In addition, the program may have a peer-review system that at least annually reviews the quality of dental services provided by each of its participating dentists. The plan may serve as an alternative or a supplement to your present dental insurance. It may also be available on a group-enrollment basis at your current place of employment. You should check with your local dental sources to find out whether such a program exists in your community. It may also be the kind of dental plan in which you wish to participate.

Since insurance plans differ from each other, it is very important to understand the benefits and limitations of each. Should you require extensive dental treatment, it may be possible to extend the treatment out over a number of years in order to utilize most effectively your plan's maximum annual benefit. If you have a plan that includes a group of participating dentists who agree to accept a specified fee schedule, you can save money by using one of these dentists.

Dental Capitation Plans

Still, another type of prepaid dental insurance is dental "capitation" plans (a flat amount per member per month), which HMOs use. The capitation plans are so named because companies pay dentists on a per capita basis with the purpose of capping dental care costs. Proponents of the

---

THREE-YEAR PAYMENT PLAN EXTENSION FOR MEETING ANNUAL DENTAL CAP

YEAR ONE

Extract #8	$250
Temporary Partial	$500
#9 Root Canal	$1,700
#9 Post-Core	$375
#9 Temporary Cap	$150
TOTAL	$2,975*

YEAR TWO

#8 Place implant	$1,700
Continue to use same Partial #9	
Continue Temporary Cap	
TOTAL	$1,700*

YEAR THREE

#8 Abutment	$350
#8 Crown	$1,100
#9 Crown	$975
TOTAL	$2,425*

*Remember you will still have to keep money in reserve monthly for other dental expenses (cleaning for family and minor fillings). This illustration assumes that your plan has approved this amount from its predetermined table of allowances.

coverage say that capitation plans can profit dentists and still reduce costs for employers. Expenses can be predicted accurately, advocates say, by using insurance industry and dental industry data on average visits, treatment needs, and personnel as well as administrative costs. Using this information, proponents say, the dentists and the employer can establish a monthly fee that should preclude any losses for dentists. Additionally, such plans can free dentists from dealing with insurance forms and billings, leaving more time to care for patients. Employers, meanwhile, can save money by eliminating insurance premium payments or by paying reduced premiums in a combined capitation or fee-for-service plan. On the other hand, some dentists not associated with capitation plans say that such coverage threatens the quality of dental care. They state that if more visits occur than anticipated, dentists will have three choices: absorb the extra costs, perform fewer services, or use cheaper materials. As a consumer, make sure that you are receiving the kind of quality of care for which you are paying.

Dental Preferred-Provider Organizations

In addition to dental HMOs, another form of managed care within the dental field today is preferred-provider organizations (PPOs). There are two kinds of PPOs. One is called a single-area-fee PPO; and the other, a multi-fee PPO. Essentially, a preferred-provider organization is a combination of traditional fee-for-service and HMO. As in the case of an HMO and physicians, there are a limited number of dentists to choose from. In regard to the single-area-fee PPO, all dentists who have agreed to accept a single fee schedule for a geographic area are listed in the PPO directory with this kind of plan. Some of these PPOs are quite large. The fee schedule usually is 10 to 20 percent below the community average charge. Overall, the dentists who join the PPO have fees near or below the PPO fee schedule. Some savings are received because of dentists who lower their fees to meet the schedule. If you are a company considering a single-area-fee PPO as a benefit for your employees, look for organizations that

- have large networks in areas required by the employees;
- are willing to contract and solicit every dentist treating the company's employees;
- have significant savings (20 to 30 percent);
- reject at least 8 percent of dentists applying; and
- provide excellent phone support to employees.

The multi-fee PPO is one of the newest types of managed dental plans. It is distinguished from the single-fee PPO because it negotiates a discount from its dentists' normal fees. That is, a single-fee PPO offers one set fee rate, which, on occasion, is the same or even higher than certain dentists' normal fees. Multi-fee PPOs simply take the dentists' normal fee rates, whatever they may be, and discount them a certain percentage. The savings are assured because every dentist in a multi-fee PPO has agreed to a fee reduction, and many plans negotiate free exams as well. Other savings are achieved by a decrease in out-of-network benefits. On the other hand, multi-fee PPOs are more difficult for employers to administer because every dentist has a different fee. Patients can also be confused about what they're paying because they do not know what a dentist's fees were before the dentist agreed to the discount. Because all dentists in multi-fee PPOs agree to reduce their fees look for that multi-fee that

- evaluates its members' utilization patterns;
- utilizes a careful credentialing process when selecting dentists; and
- offers a wide range of dentists from different economic levels, providing its members with the greatest number of choices.[18]

Other Prepaid Dental Insurance Plans

Just as dental programs that are available for the consumer vary, so do their costs, depending on the type of services, the methods of reimbursement, and the company offering the plan. As inflation rises, however, so do the charges. At present many programs are covered under the Delta Health Plan system (nonprofit state dental service corporations) originally established by the dental profession. Normally, you use the services of participating dentists who have filed their fees with the plan in advance. The dentist is then paid directly by the plan on a "usual, customary, and reasonable" fee basis. Delta Plans also generally require preauthorization by one of their consultants for work in excess of a specified amount, and sometimes x-rays are required in posttreatment to see that work has been properly completed. Dental insurance is also provided by private insurance companies, Blue Cross and Blue Shield, and independent plans.

Although prepaid dental plans are still developing, they can help reduce your dental expenses but probably won't save you money if you already have an employer-provided dental insurance coverage. The dental insurance will only contribute to the fees that the prepaid plan charges you. Since the insurance plan will already be reducing your costs, the addition of prepaid plan coverage will add relatively little to your savings.[19] Also, in a prepaid plan there might be restrictions on choice of dentist and location of treatment. If you already have a dentist you like and the dentist does not participate in the plan, you may not wish to join. In addition, make sure that your dentist doesn't treat you extra quickly because your case pays less than a regular fee-for-service plan. However, prepaid dental plans may be for you if without dental insurance your own dental costs (if single) or those of your family (if married) are higher annually than would be the combined costs of annual dental insurance premiums and any personal out-of-pocket expenses you may incur for dental procedures that the insurance may not cover. To find out more about dental care and dental health insurance, go on the Internet to http://www.medlineplus.gov and search on dental health insurance.

WHAT YOU SHOULD KNOW ABOUT RETAIL DENTAL CENTERS

Retail dental centers have also begun developing in the United States.

"But, what are they and how good are they," Jack asked? "Will they be like those 'doc-in-the box' medical clinics for people just off the streets, where I've heard that the quality of care provided is sometimes questionable? The kind of clinic where the relationship between provider and patient is strictly business, not personal, and after treatment the patient may never show up again for follow-up care if the dentist who provided treatment is no longer there?"

Most providers in such centers are quick to state that quality is never compromised. They may appear in shopping mall dental centers and dental departments of established retail stores. Frequently, these dental practice alternatives are staffed by dentists who are looking for a way to beat the high cost of operating a private practice. Many large centers offer expanded hours, including evenings and weekends. Appointments are usually available within a day or two or may not be necessary at all; dental work such as bridges, crowns, and dentures may be completed in just one day. The new centers report that they can save money and charge lower fees than traditional practice by sharing office space, personnel, and expensive equipment and buying supplies in volume, although all centers are not necessarily less expensive than dentists in traditional private practice. By having a group practice work in essentially two shifts, fixed costs such as rent, equipment, and a computer to keep accounts are spread over a large number of patients, becoming significantly lower per customer. Some centers also make use of another cost-saving device—their own on-the-premises dental laboratory. Other savings occur because specialists in root canal, periodontal work, and orthodontics are often available under one roof— saving you the cost of a consultation visit. Innovations, convenience, and cost aside, the most important question is, can you obtain quality care? Many centers practice some form of self-imposed peer-group review—which means that a second opinion is obtained either before, during, or after treatment on either a spot-check or a routine basis. This review may be performed by dentists outside the clinic, by the clinic director, or by a peer-group committee. The American Dental Association advises that you, as a patient, and state agencies should judge a "discount dental clinic" by the same criteria that must apply to all forms of dental care: Is there a good doctor-patient relationship? Does the clinic place its emphasis on such a relationship or on other matters? Is preventive dentistry emphasized? Is there emphasis on continuing long-term dental care? Retail dentists are not for you if you seek a personalized service; a common complaint is that the dentist who treated you the first time is no longer there on the second visit. Some of these dental centers may be franchises in which the franchisee is provided with a standardized dental facility as well as with management, accounting, and marketing support where the charges for routine services are advertised or available for all potential patients to see. For example, the franchise company chooses, leases, and improves the site; helps to hire the staff; and creates an advertising campaign to attract the first patients. In this way, the dentist is free to concentrate on the clinical aspects of his or her practice. As already noted, the dental centers may advertise longer hours, convenient locations, accessible parking, emergency walk-in services, state-of-the-art equipment, handpicked professionals, quality care, and affordable prices. As a consumer, only you can judge the veracity of such claims.

HOW TO REDUCE YOUR DENTAL BILL

As a percentage of total health costs, dental expenses have declined from 11.0 percent in 1950 to 5.3 percent in 2000.[20] The profession has achieved this moderation in cost increases through its emphasis on preventive dentistry; frequent examinations to diagnose disorders early when they can be easily corrected rather than have extensive and expensive repairs later; greater productivity through the use of such auxiliary aides as dental hygienists and full-time assistants; and the development of modern instruments that speed up the dentist's work as well as make the patients' visits more comfortable. Another reason why dental bills have increased so slowly is that many people still pay their dental bills privately, out of their own pockets.

Steps a Patient Can Take

"When I was younger," Phil was telling a coworker, "I never thought about dental bills. I was young; I went to the dentist once or twice a year. Cost was much less than it is today and I was only responsible for myself. But now I am married. My children have to wear braces; my wife recently had a root canal; I have bleeding gums; and the bills are adding up. I know I can't escape dental bills, but how can I control the cost?"

There are a number of steps a patient may take to reduce the costs of dental care. The principal way in which patients can control their dental expenses is through good preventive care. This includes regular brushing, flossing, and professional cleanings, which can inhibit future outlays for treatment and restoration. In addition, a patient can ask as to whether there may be alternative lower-cost treatments available when a dentist proposes a particular course of care.

Another way to save money is by asking your former dentist to forward to your new dentist your x-rays and other records. Unless your new dentist believes that new x-rays are necessary, full-mouth x-rays by your previous dentist are good for three to five years.

Seek a second opinion before undergoing a costly treatment to make sure that you are receiving appropriate, reasonably priced care. This could be a useful step if a dispute arises later. Make sure you consult a dentist who has no relationship to your present dentist, informing the dentist in advance that you will not be using him or her for treatment. Your present dentist should be willing to forward x-rays and exam results to another dentist for review. Be wary if a new dentist recommends far more treatment than did your former dentist such as suggesting that many silver fillings need to be replaced by gold or many teeth now need to be crowned, though in some cases such treatment may be appropriate. Dentists can have conflicts of interest. The specialist has an interest in suggesting the extensive and complex treatment that only the specialist can provide. The general practitioner, on the other hand, may never raise the alternative of a specialist's treatment to avoid losing the opportunity to treat you himself.

Don't be afraid to ask about dental fees for a few common procedures. Most dentists will readily tell you. You can also inquire as to whether the dentist accepts credit cards or offers discounts to senior citizens. Regardless of a dentist's fees, if you are treated more than you should be, the costs will be high. Therefore, ask about a treatment plan, obtain the opinion of an independent dentist, and review your bill relative to the treatment plan, both of which should itemize treatment costs. A dentist should not make you feel uncomfortable when discussing fees and should be willing to work out a payment plan or an alternative treatment if the costs are more than you can afford.

Find out whether the dentist will give you a written warranty on major restorative work, such as a bridge or a crown. If a dentist does not provide you with a warranty, ask for a free replacement if the restoration doesn't last as long it should. Any warranty should include a description of the problem as it currently exists, the proposed treatment, expected costs, expected results, and a specified period during which the dentist will replace the work free of charge. Note of caution: It will be difficult to find a dentist who will offer such a warranty. There are a variety of reasons for this. The argument for both medicine and dentistry is that you cannot guarantee biological systems; the variables, for example, in terms of healing, body response, mouth acidity, age, wear rates, and biting forces cannot be forecast. According to Dr. Michael J. Tabacco, clinical professor of prosthodontics at the University of Maryland's Baltimore College of Dental Surgery, "In Academia we solve this problem by looking at the failures we see. These are divided into mechanical failures and biological failures. *Mechanical failures* are fractures of a newly placed crown, breaking of a solder joint, fractures of a filling, breaking of a wire clasp for a partial denture, fracture of an implant screw, breaking of a denture (assuming it is not dropped on floor). If this occurs early enough (generally within a year of service), we assume there may have been a laboratory error, structural defect, or premature metal fatigue. We give the benefit of a doubt to the patient and generally provide an unwritten guarantee to some extent. There is the possibility that the patient has a very heavy bite or is bruxing (grinding) . . . but we still give the odds to patient. On the other hand, a *biological failure* is impossible to predict or provide warrantee against. This includes the ravages of periodontal disease, nutritional factors (carbonic acids from soda, sugar intake, hard candy use), cavities (decay) level, failure of adequate oral hygiene, and, in the case of oral surgical interventions for implant placement or periodontal surgery, factors of general health, tissue response, healing ability, bone calcium densities, immune responses, systemic nutrition and absorption . . . all of these add to the dilemma of codifying a predictable result. For high-cost surgical dental treatment such as placing an implant, if failure of the implant occurs within the period of placing the implant and uncovering it (a four- to six-month period), generally, the failed implant will be replaced with a new implant, with a nominal fee, following a suitable period of healing."[21]

Consider taking advantage of any discounts and special offers your dentist may propose. Some dentists offer periodic specials on certain procedures so that patients who have been postponing dental work will make an appointment and come in for treatment. Other dentists advertise low-priced treatment packages that include examination, cleaning, and x-rays. Some dentists even offer price discounts for special groups such as senior citizens or persons on extremely limited incomes as well for cash payments in advance since this latter offer saves them time and money in collecting unpaid bills.

If you are covered by Blue Cross and Blue Shield or another insurance plan that has a maximum fee schedule for participating dentists, you will likely save money by using a dentist who participates. And if you are eligible for Medicaid, you will want to receive treatment from a dentist who participates in that program.

As already noted, consider receiving services at the clinic of a dental school. Schools offering a dentistry program can provide services ranging from examination, cleaning, and cavity repair to periodontal surgery for approximately half of what a private dentist may charge. Dental hygiene programs also offer services such as x-rays, cleaning, plaque-control training, and nutritional guidance at similar rates. Work in both cases is closely supervised by professors using the latest techniques available. The only drawback: Some clinics have a screening program and accept only cases appropriate to the learning needs of the students. And, if time is a factor, this may not be for you. Students usually work very slowly. Dental schools are in continuous need of patients; receiving dental care at these clinics seems to be ideal for retired individuals, those with evening-shift jobs, or unemployed patients. As stated, the quality of care is optimal, and your participation in the dental education is very appreciated by both students and faculty at these university centers. To find out about school clinics near you, contact your local dental society listed in the white pages of your telephone book, or send a self-addressed, stamped envelope for a list from the American Dental Association, 211 East Chicago Ave., Chicago, IL 60611.

One development which parallels medical care that is now being seen with increasing frequency is receiving your dental treatment overseas. This is particularly seen for high-cost treatment such as full mouth reconstruction, multiple bridgework, and other extended care. A brief and recent example relates to Maria, a sixty-year-old Mexican American, and Carlos, a forty-five-year-old Greek American, both first-generation Americans. They have maintained close ties with their families in "the old country." Each had numerous dental areas of missing teeth that required crowns and bridgework. Treatment plans were estimated at approximately $4,000 to $6,000. Through a Web site search, and family recommendations, dentists were found in Mexico City and Athens who were American trained, very well credentialed, and reportedly quite competent practitioners. With the encouragement of their American dentist, who provided x-rays, stone models, and a brief of what was required, these patients went back to their own countries, and the treatment was completed in a three-week period of time. They enjoyed a much-welcomed trip uniting with family members and paid for it all—trip and dental care—for one-half of the estimated fee. The downside is follow-up care and the warranty issue previously discussed.

Other low-cost possibilities are state clinics, hospital clinics, and mobile dental units. The price may be right, but one criticism is that clinic care can tend toward the fast, cheap extraction rather than more extensive tooth-saving techniques, so shop carefully in this area. Programs may also have low-income or other requirements, so check to see if you qualify. Contact your local health department or local dental society to learn what services are available in your area.

Taking Care of Your Teeth

Although dentists are attempting to control costs, there is much the patient can do. High dental bills because of tooth decay and gum diseases have a direct relationship to the way you take care of yourself. The key to reducing dental costs is preventive care. This cannot be emphasized enough. Only half the population visits a dentist as often as once a year and half this group goes only for emergency treatment. Tooth decay affects 95 percent of those who have teeth and more than fifty million teeth are extracted each year.[22] Thus, although good dentists will give top priority to teaching you the proper care of your teeth and gums, patients must make sure that they and their families receive, understand, and follow instructions for preventive dental care. The following are suggestions for taking care of your teeth:

- Most people should visit the dentist every six months. Of course, if you notice any unusual symptoms such as pain or inflamed, bleeding, or swollen gums, don't delay and make an appointment immediately.
- Fighting cavities begins in the supermarket. Remember that sugar and tooth decay go hand in hand. Look for sugar-free gum and food products.
- Coddle your children's baby teeth. Neglecting a child's first set of teeth will cost you more in the long run.
- Flossing your teeth routinely and brushing with an accepted fluoride dentifrice (toothpaste) are vital preventive measures. Using toothpastes containing sodium fluoride, sodium monofluorophosphate, or stannous fluoride can prevent caries, or cavities, the main cause of tooth loss among people under thirty-five. For extra protection after brushing, use a mouthwash containing essential oils that slow the formation of bacteria-filled plaques.
- Do not allow the accumulation and mineralization of bacterial plaque in your

mouth. Plaque is an important factor in tooth decay and is the cause of gum diseases or periodontal disease, which, in turn, can lead to the loss of the involved teeth. Unless plaque is removed within about seventy-two hours, plaque hardens (calcifies), becoming white colored tartar that darkens over time and, unless halted, can create pockets of bacteria between gums and teeth. Dentists analyze the degree of the infection by measuring the depth of these bacterial pockets with a probe.

- Be aware of the warning signs of periodontal disease. These include inflamed gums that bleed during tooth brushing (gingivitis); soft, swollen, or tender gums; pus between the teeth and gums; loose teeth; receding gums; change in the fit of partial dentures; shifting teeth; and persistent bad breath. In general, evidence is increasing that gum infection may provoke heart disease, respiratory disease, stroke, or preterm birth, and may worsen osteoporosis as a person ages and when the body's natural defenses have been lessened by any chronic disease.

- Tooth decay, according to the American Dental Association, can be reduced by as much as two-thirds in communities where the drinking water is fluoridated one part per million. This protection can last a lifetime.[23]

Be aware of the effects of soda. According to Dr. Michael J. Tabacco, "from a dental viewpoint, the sugar in soda (specifically sucrose) feeds the mouth's bacteria, causes the proliferation of all bacteria residing in the folds and crypts of the mouth, and enhances the accumulation of destructive plaque. Additionally, the carbonic acid in soda is an especially strong corrosive agent which actually cuts into and dissolves tooth enamel. Finally, the style and form with which we drink sodas sipping slowly continuously has even a worsening effect on enamel. In effect, it becomes a daylong bathing of teeth in a corrosive and sugar-filled medium. The enormous increase in calories becomes a weight-gaining issue as well. In older patients with dry mouths (already a danger factor for a high decay level), soda consumption worsens this effect." In the January–February 2005 issue of *General Dentistry*, a clinical, peer-reviewed journal of the Academy of General Dentistry, a pilot study, authored by J. Anthony von Fraunhofer, professor of biomaterials science at the University of Maryland Dental School, and Matthew M. Rogers, DDS, of the United States Air Force Dental Corps, showed that "while sports and energy drinks help athletes rehydrate after a long workout, if consumed on a regular basis, they can damage teeth." The pilot study was intended to simulate in terms of exposure time normal beverage consumption over thirteen years, which, according to the authors, is a realistic period for evaluating potential enamel attack among children and young adults. The study accomplished this simulation by continuously exposing enamel from cavity-free molars and premolars to a variety of popular sports beverages, including energy drinks, fitness water, and sports drinks, as well as noncola beverages such as commercial lemonade and ice tea for a period of fourteen days (336 hours). The study showed that there was significant dental damage associated with all the beverages tested. Listed from most to least damage to dental enamel, the result was as follows: commercial lemonade, energy drinks, sports drinks, fitness water, ice tea, and cola. While acknowledging that this pilot study accomplished its objective of determining whether sports drinks and some of the newer noncola beverages are more aggressive toward dental hard tissues, the authors also noted that more extensive studies will require a larger sample than this study included to confirm the statistically significant differences between the beverages. According to the Academy of General Dentistry, "Most cola-based drinks contain one or more acids, commonly phosphoric and citric acids; however, sports beverages contain additives and organic acids that can advance dental erosion. These organic acids are potentially very erosive to dental enamel because of their ability to breakdown calcium, which is needed to strengthen teeth and prevent gum diseases." Dental enamel is the outer layer of hard tissue that helps maintain the tooth structure and shape, while protecting it from decay. The American Beverage Association that represents nonalcoholic commercial drinks like soft drinks, sports drinks, bottled teas, waters, and juices disagreed with the study's findings, noting that dental erosion has many origins, including behavior, lifestyle, diet, and genetics. A previous study published by Professor von Fraunhofer in the July–August 2004 issue of *General Dentistry* showed that carbonated soft drinks may cause significant long-term enamel dissolution. The carbonated beverages were markedly more aggressive toward enamel than brewed black coffee, brewed black tea, and root beer. In the study root beer appeared to be the safest drink for the health of dental enamel, while noncola drinks and canned ice tea demonstrated the most aggressive dissolution of dental enamel. Tap water showed minimal enamel dissolution. Academy of General Dentistry president-elect Bruce Deginder, DDS, MAGD, stated, "We recommend altering or limiting the intake of soda and sports drinks and choosing water or low-fat milk instead to preserve enamel and ultimately to protect teeth from decay." Professor von Fraunhofer, in an interview with *WebMD Medical News*, noted that he was not trying to trash any drink. Rather, "What we are saying is, by all means drink what you want. Don't sit and sip for a long time. Rinse out with a bit of water. That will minimize the effects. The other thing to realize is that when once the enamel is gone, it's gone forever. It doesn't come back." According to Professor von Fraunhofer, it takes the mouth about thirty minutes to recover from the pH decrease (acidity increase) from food, so continuous or even intermittent sipping on a large container of a soft drink, especially one that is citrus flavored, over a long period such as working at a computer or driving over a long distance does not allow the mouth to recover, and that is why the attack on the teeth occurs.[24]

Smoking is not only potentially life threatening, but it is proven to alter microcirculation (blood supply in small arteries of mouth tissue and bone) and vascular circulation in general. Periodontal disease is worsened in smokers and the success with placing implants in smokers is decreased significantly. It not uncommon for oral surgeons and periodontal surgeons to refuse to place implants in chronic smokers.

Dental Products

The products you purchase to maintain your oral health can help reduce your dental costs. The American Dental Association states that in purchasing dental health products the best advice is the recommendation of your family dentist. Do not hesitate to ask him for his opinion on products. However, there are other things you should know to be a wise consumer of oral health products: The American Dental Association conducts a continual independent review of the most commonly used commercially manufactured dental products. The association allows products that are proven safe and effective to carry statements of ADA acceptance on their packaging and advertising. The dentist has traditionally depended upon the American Dental Association for evaluation and classification of the professional products he uses in his practice; consumers, too, can benefit from the ADA's Council on Dental Therapeutics's evaluation of fluoride toothpastes and its Council on Dental Materials and Devices's decisions on powered toothbrushes, oral irrigators, and denture adhesives. In order to maintain a product's acceptance rating, the manufacturer must adhere to the American Dental Association's advertising code. Consumer advertising for association-accepted products must be completely accurate in fact as well as in implication, and proof must be available on demand. No other health profession benefits from such a comprehensive advertising process. The American Dental Association is not a government agency and has no statutory control to regulate manufacturers. It exerts its influence with manufacturers principally by the prestige of its professional opinion. The American Dental Association's advice in regard to various oral health products is as follows:

- *Dental floss*

    Dental floss comes waxed and unwaxed. While many dentists recommend unwaxed as doing the better job of getting rid of plaque, people with tightly spaced teeth may find it easier to use waxed floss. It is important to floss every day in the manner prescribed by your dentist or his auxiliary aide in order to remove the plaque.
- *Manual toothbrush*

    Your dentist may recommend that you use a special toothbrush. The type that matches the requirements of the greatest number of people is a brush with soft multitufted, round-end bristles. Make sure that the head of the brush is small enough to reach all accessible areas in your mouth.
- *Powered toothbrushes*

    Before the American Dental Association gives its acceptance to a powered toothbrush product, its method of obtaining power, the safety in design, and various other factors are taken into consideration. According to the ADA, no one has been able to show satisfactorily that either manual or powered brushing is superior. If the patient is more thorough and consistent in his use of one type, that type should be his choice. Because of its novelty, children may find the powered toothbrush appealing and use it more often than the manual toothbrush. Persons with certain physical handicaps often find powered toothbrushes easier to use.

* *Oral irrigating devices*

According to the American Dental Association, in all instances a patient should seek the advice of his dentist on how to use oral irrigating devices. Persons with certain oral conditions can injure oral tissues with incorrect use of pressure sprays. Oral irrigating devices use a direct spray of water to remove loose particles and other materials from about the teeth. However, they cannot take the place of either the toothbrush or dental floss in getting rid of plaque, but for certain patients they are an effective additional aid to oral cleanliness. Patients with orthodontic bands or fixed partial dentures may find oral irrigators particularly helpful.

* *Mouthwashes*

Mouthwashes can temporarily freshen your breath or sweeten your mouth. However, according to the American Dental Association, mouthwashes do not remove plaque and cannot prevent decay or gum disease. In addition, the association states that commercial mouthwashes available without prescription are primarily cosmetic; unfortunately, advertisers sometimes imply more extensive benefits. The American Dental Association Council on Dental Therapeutics discourages the use of medicated mouthwashes unless their use is supervised. Offensive breath may indicate poor oral health or other bodily disorders—a mouthwash simply masks the basic problem. In general, mouthwashes can be considered to serve no greater purpose than aiding in the removal of loose food and debris.

* *Toothpastes*

The American Dental Association continually assesses commercial toothpastes. The association's Council on Dental Therapeutics permits the use of its seal and acceptance statement on products that have proven, in clinical studies, effective in reducing tooth decay. So that there is no misunderstanding, the ADA emphasizes that fluoride toothpastes are not a substitute for the fluoridation of community drinking water, which has been shown to reduce dental decay by as much as two-thirds. Used together, fluoridated water and accepted fluoride toothpaste can have a compounded value in reducing tooth decay.

Modern dentifrices are generally either paste or powder. Pastes are by far the most popular and widely used. According to the American Dental Association, some toothpaste can do more than just clean your mouth; namely, fluoride toothpaste has shown that it has proven decay preventing benefits. As far as the abrasiveness of toothpastes is concerned, toothpastes must have some degree of abrasiveness to assist the brush in removing plaque and stains. It is known that excessively abrasive toothpastes can be harmful to softer tissues of exposed root surfaces and to restorative materials. For any one individual, the most desirable toothpaste is one abrasive enough to prevent plaque and stain accumulation but not so harsh that it injures teeth or gums. Your family dentist can recommend toothpastes in the proper range of abrasiveness, based upon each patient's individual needs.[25]

Finally, it cannot be emphasized enough that a patient should consult a dentist on all matters of personal oral health. However, if you have questions concerning the general nature of dentistry and dental health, you can contact the American Dental Association, Bureau of Public Information, 211 East Chicago Avenue, Chicago, IL 60611.

NOTES

1. US Department of Health and Human Services, *Health, United States, 2003 with Chartbook on Trends in the Health of Americans* (Hyattsville, MD: National Center for Health Statistics, 2003), p. 294 (table 102).

2. *How to Become a Wise Dental Consumer* (Chicago, IL: American Dental Association, 1978), p. 3.

3. Herbert Denenberg, *Shopper's Guide to Dentistry* (Washington, DC: Consumers News Inc., 1970), pp. 124–25.

4. Ibid., p. 125.

5. *How to Become a Wise Dental Consumer*, pp. 4–5; Denenberg, *Shopper's Guide to Dentistry*, pp. 120–29; "Dentists and Dental Care," in *Washington Consumer's Checkbook* (Washington, DC: Center for Study of Services, 1990), p. 36; and "Could This Transcend Dental Medication?" *Washington Post*, April 13, 2003, p. A12.

6. Ileen Fidler, "Dentists for Kids Only," *Family Health/Today's Health* 9 (October 1977): 32; "The Myths of 'Soft Teeth' in Kids," *Vitality* 4 (2000): 10.

7. "Look Dad, No Cavities," *Washington Post/Health*, February 19, 1991, p. 18; Rob Stein, "One Type of Electric Toothbrush Tops Study," *Washington Post*, January 12, 2003, p. 10.

8. Judith Randall, "New Thinking on Tooth Decay," *Washington Post/Health*, October 18, 1988, p. 21.

9. Jeffrey P. Cohn, "Shrink Wrap for Molars: Plastic Coating Seals Teeth so Bacteria Can't Cause Cavities," *Washington Post/Health*, July 17, 1990, p. 16.

10. "The Finances of Health & Fitness," *Sylvia Porter's Personal Finance*, June 1984, p. 62.

11. Fidler, "Dentists for Kids Only," p. 32; Dianne Hales, ". . . A Tot's Teeth," *Parade*, September 15, 2002, p. 14.

12. Fidler, "Dentists for Kids Only," p. 34.

13. *How to Become a Wise Dental Consumer*, pp. 9–10; Denenberg, *Shopper's Guide to Dentistry*, p. 8.

14. *Function, Aging, Oral Health: An Overview of the Dental Issues Affecting the Health of Older Persons* (Washington, DC: American Association of Dental Schools, 1989).

15. *How to Become a Wise Dental Consumer*, p. 8.

16. Sylvia Porter, "Dental Insurance Spurring Preventive Care," *Washington Star*, June 19, 1978.

17. Ibid.

18. Robert Leaf, "Taking a Bite out of Dental Costs," *Managed HealthCare* (September 1996): 42, 44.

19. "Dentists and Dental Care," *Washington Consumer's Checkbook*, p. 38.

20. *Source Book of Health Insurance Data, 2002* (Washington, DC: Health Insurance Association of America, 2002), p. 102 (table 5.5).

21. Michael J. Tabacco, correspondence with author, May 22, 2005.

22. Sylvia Porter, "Get Better Dental Care at Lower Cost," *Washington Star*, June 28, 1978.

23. *How to Become a Wise Dental Consumer*, pp. 5–6; Annabel Hecht, "Brushing and Rinsing to Prevent Cavities," *FDA Consumer* 14, no. 5 (June 1980): 23; and Isadore Rosenfeld, "Ignore Your Gums and Your Teeth Will Go Away," *Parade*, January 25, 2004, pp. 10–11.

24. Tabacco, correspondence with author, May 22, 2005; Academy of General Dentistry news release, "New Study Indicates That Popular Sports Beverages Cause More Irreversible Damage to Teeth Than Soda"; J. Anthony von Fraunhofer, "Dissolution of Dental Enamel in Soft Drinks," *General Dentistry* 52, no. 4 (July–August 2004): 308–12; J. Anthony von Fraunhofer and Matthew M. Rogers, "Effects of Sport Drinks and Other Beverages on Dental Enamel," *General Dentistry* 53, no.1 (January–February 2005): 28–31; J. Anthony von Fraunhofer, correspondence with author, January 27, 2006; and Miranda Hill, "Which Drinks Damage Your Teeth the Most?" *WebMD Medical News*, http://my.WebMD.com/content/article/100/1015874.htm (reviewed by Brunilda Nazario, MD, and accessed February 16, 2005).

25. *How to Become a Wise Dental Consumer*, pp. 10–14.

CHAPTER THREE

TRADITIONAL
PRIVATE HEALTH INSURANCE

INTRODUCTION

In 1999 the US Bureau of the Census reported that public and private health insurance provided protection against medical expenses for 261 million Americans, but almost 43 million persons—many employed by firms that do not offer coverage, many below the poverty line—were still without health insurance coverage. Of those without health insurance, 8.5 million were children. Many of these people without coverage were poor but still not did qualify for the federal-state program of Medicaid.[1]

Private health insurance began in the United States during the middle of the nineteenth century when the first health insurance company was founded in 1847 to meet the public's need for coverage against income losses from injuries sustained in steamboat and rail accidents. Three years later another company was organized specifically to write accident insurance. By the mid-1860s coverages were available for virtually every kind of accident, and by the beginning of the twentieth century forty-seven companies were selling such insurance. Then, in the early 1900s both accident and life insurance companies became interested in health insurance. With their entry, health insurance coverage began to grow and change in the ensuing years.

In the beginning, health insurance did not stress hospital and surgical benefits. Rather, the purpose of the insurance was to protect the individual against the loss of earned income that would happen if the person was accidentally injured or contracted certain specified diseases such as typhus, typhoid, scarlet fever, diphtheria, and diabetes. Although succeeding plans covered additional diseases, eliminated medical examinations, and included surgical fee schedules, the emphasis of insurance on the loss of earned income remained until the early stages of the Great Depression in 1929. As the Depression deepened and unemployment rose, the public became increasingly aware that new methods were required to help pay for the costs of medical care. Meanwhile, hospitals were confronted with empty beds and declining revenues. These conditions led a number of teachers and the Baylor Hospital in Dallas, Texas, to develop an arrangement whereby the teachers would receive hospital care on a prepayment basis. This development had a significant effect on the insurance industry, foreshadowing the arrival of reimbursement policies for hospital and surgical care. At the same time, another form of prepayment service was starting in Los Angeles, California, where a group of healthcare providers assumed the responsibility for organizing and integrating medical services on a prepaid basis—that is, combining group practice with prepayment. This physician-sponsored organization, known as the Ross-Loos Medical Group, was the predecessor of such eminently known programs as the Kaiser Foundation Health Plan of California and served as the prototype for today's emerging medical care foundations and health maintenance organizations (HMOs).

During World War II a major change took place in the health insurance field when fringe benefits became a significant factor of collective bargaining after industrial wages were frozen. Eventually, group health insurance became part of this package. In the postwar years, three powerful forces came together to provide modern health insurance with its strongest push for growth. First, in 1948 a decision by the US Supreme Court held that fringe benefits, including health insurance, were a legitimate part of the collective bargaining process; the second was the sharply increasing cost of medical care; and the third was the capability of the private health insurers to introduce new kinds of coverage and broaden existing benefits. An important spur in the growth of group health insurance, for example, was the favorable tax treatment that group coverage received.

As the nation emerged from the Depression economy to a more affluent status, insuring organizations began to develop more extensive benefits and, in the early 1950s, introduced the most comprehensive insurance coverage yet developed— major medical expense coverage. This policy has been defined as insurance especially created to offset heavy medical expenses resulting from catastrophic or prolonged illness or injury. From its beginning, major medical has grown rapidly as families responded to the need to protect themselves against quickly rising hospital, medical, and surgical costs. Benefits levels under comprehensive major medical expense policies increased from a range of fifty thousand to several million dollars.

The rapidly developing economy in the years following World War II also led to the reemergence of protection in the form of long-term disability benefits, stressing once again the idea of income replacement during times of disability and other financial emergencies.[2]

Beginning in the 1960s and continuing through the 1990s, health insurance began to expand in a number of public and private areas. In 1965 the federal government became a major insurer when Congress enacted Medicare and Medicaid. The Medicare program (Title XVIII of the Social Security Act) provides compulsory hospitalization insurance (Part A) as well as voluntary supplementary medical insurance (Part B) to help pay for physicians' services, medical services, and supplies that the Part A hospitalization plan does not cover. But, because Medicare does not provide total comprehensive benefits, private insurers created new kinds of policies to fill in Medicare's gaps, called Medsupp or Medigap policies. By the beginning of the twenty-first century, Medicare had added two new parts. Medicare Advantage, Part C, provides coverage for managed care, and Part D represents the prescription drug benefit program in the Medicare Prescription Drug, Improvement, and Modernization Act of 2003 that President Bush signed into law on December 8, 2003. Meanwhile, Medicaid (Title XIX of the Social Security Act) is designed to share the cost of medical care between the federal and state governments for low-income persons. With federal matching funds, Medicaid allows the states to add health coverage to their public assistance programs for low-income groups, families with dependent children, the aged, and the disabled.

In addition, some large corporations began to self-insure their costs when they realized that the total health insurance actuarial experience and the costs of their large workforce remained relatively stable from year to year (except for the inflation of medical prices). Given this predictability, the companies decided that they could save money by insuring their own employees themselves by putting aside a certain amount of money to pay for their employees' claims rather than paying premiums to an insurer to take the risk. In addition, the firms themselves could administer the funds until the time arrived to pay the bill. Also, through self-insurance employers did not have to pay a premium tax and because of the Employee Retirement Income Security Act of 1974 (ERISA) were not required to comply with certain state-mandated benefits and services that insurers had to follow in covering groups. Thus, companies avoided the extra costs of these mandated benefits. However, while self-insurance became a dominant form of group coverage, employers still often turned to insurers to administer these plans: these contractual arrangements are known as administrative services only (ASO).

Once self-insurance became a choice and demonstrated that it was less expensive to leave the "community," employers began to use "experience rating"—that is, they based the premiums of the health insurance policy upon the group's own claim experience. However, much earlier commercial insurers and Blue Cross and Blue Shield plans had already begun to use "experience rating" as the major form of premium rating rather than their former method of "community rating" that reflected the risk experience of the total community, which included higher risk groups or individuals.

During this period, other kinds of health insurance plans and delivery systems also began to emerge and grow rapidly. These included health maintenance organizations (HMOs), which, if federally certified, continue to use community rating today, and these HMOs soon were followed by preferred-provider organizations (PPOs) and other hybrid arrangements (modes of health delivery through which a

sponsoring organization like an insurer, employer, or third-party administrator negotiates price discounts with providers of health services in exchange for more
patients). These groups developed in response to the rapid rise in healthcare costs
during the 1970s and 1980s. These new delivery systems (now called managed care)
offered the potential to control costs by organizing providers of healthcare into
coherent networks and by integrating the financing and delivery of medical care.
Managed-care plans coordinate a broad range of patient services and monitor care to
make sure that the care is appropriate and delivered in the most efficient and inexpensive way. By the mid-1990s and into the early twenty-first century new federal
laws like the Health Insurance Portability and Accountability Act of 1996 and the
Medicare Prescription Drug, Improvement, and Modernization Act of 2003 were
passed by Congress The latter, in part, created new health savings accounts to permit
individuals to budget for their medical expenses, and the former allowed some
degree of portability for persons losing or changing their jobs and through tax breaks
spurred the growth of long-term care insurance. Other new programs also began
emerging by the beginning of twenty-first century. In these programs providers like
physicians are being reimbursed on the basis of their performance because in providing services they attain goals of quality of care in contrast to the system that reimburses doctors, hospitals, or other providers regardless of whether they provide good
services or not or whether the patient is satisfied with their care. In requiring high
quality, the programs are trying to eliminate from the health system expensive mistakes as well as inefficiencies relating to various kinds of medical treatments and the
management of patient care. As a result, better doctors are being reimbursed at higher
fees, those in the middle with standard payments, and the worst providers receive a
reduction in fees. As pay-for-performance develops over time, the next logical step
would be to supply consumers with a shopping guide that gives them information
about their providers' costs and quality of care. As new challenges arise, the health
insurance field continues to demonstrate its innovation and flexibility to meet them.

DEFINITIONS OF PRIVATE HEALTH INSURANCE PLANS

Private health insurance is available from a variety of organizations including Blue
Cross and Blue Shield, independent plans, and commercial insurers. Independent
plans consist of employer-employee union plans, private group clinics, and HMOs,
which offer health services on a prepayment or insuring basis to the subscribing population within a given community area.[3]

At the present time, the kinds of insurance policies being written in the United
States number in the many thousands, while the combination of these policies is infi-
nite. In addition, many of these policies may contain cost-sharing provisions that
require the covered individual to pay some portion of his covered medical expenses.
These cost-sharing provisions include deductibles, coinsurance, and copayments. A
deductible is the amount of money you pay for health services before the insurance

company will pay for all or part of the remaining costs of the covered services. A *copayment* is usually a fixed amount the patient is required to pay for each medical service (for example, $10) and the insurance company pays the rest. *Coinsurance* is a policy provision frequently found in major medical insurance where the patient and the insurance company pay a designated percentage of the medical expenses. For example, an individual may pay 20 percent and his insurance program pays the remaining 80 percent under the terms of a policy. This variety can make it extremely difficult, if not impossible, for the purchaser of health insurance to compare benefits and costs wisely. However, regardless of the diversity of health insurance policies being sold, there are five basic kinds.

Hospital Expense Plans

These plans provide benefits for all or part of the costs of hospital room, board, and miscellaneous hospital services and supplies—including laboratory service, x-rays, medications, and use of an operating room. The service-type benefit plan will reimburse the full charge for semiprivate room and board. Though not too common today, other policies have a system of indemnity benefits, in which a specified amount per day is paid toward hospital room and board, which may leave you with a large bill.

Regular Medical Expense Plans

These programs provide benefits toward payment of physicians' fees for nonsurgical care given in the hospital, at home, or at the physicians' offices. Some regular medical expense plans also cover diagnostic x-rays and laboratory services. This plan is often offered in combination with basic hospitalization and surgical expense plans.

Surgical Expense Plans

Benefits are usually paid according to a schedule of surgical procedures. The policy lists the maximum benefit for each type of operation covered. The reimbursement allowance may not match the fee in full, requiring the patient to pay the difference. Sometimes the benefit is stated as reimbursement up to the "usual and customary" surgical charges in the region where the operation is performed. Usually offered in combination with a hospital expense policy, this coverage applies whether surgery is performed in a hospital or in a doctor's office.

Major Medical Expense Plans

These plans are basically catastrophic-illness health insurance and pay benefits for virtually all kinds of healthcare prescribed by a physician. The policy is often superimposed or provided as a supplement to basic protection; that is, the benefits do not begin until regular hospital-surgical or medical expense plans are exhausted, or a second kind of policy can be provided as comprehensive protection whereby both the basic and the extended benefits are integrated as a single unit.

These policies help in covering the cost of treatment given in and out of the hospital, special nursing care, x-rays, prescriptions, medical appliances, nursing home care, ambulatory psychiatric care, and many other healthcare needs. In other words, major medical coverage offers broad and substantial benefits for large, unpredictable medical expenses. The majority of major medical policies, whether written for individuals or under a group plan, are subject to some form of deductibles and coinsurance payments by the insured person. Some policies may pay the first dollar of expenses; may have a waiting period before the policy takes effect; and may exclude coverage (for a prescribed time, at least) for preexisting medical conditions. Few policies cover routine checkups for essentially healthy people, although such coverage may be possible if the doctor is investigating a particular complaint.

Loss of Income Protection Plans

Although you may not think of this kind of protection as health insurance in the traditional sense of surgical or hospital or major medical, the insurance industry has offered this kind of protection to the public for many, many years. Loss of income (or disability income) protection is designed to provide wage earners with regular weekly or monthly cash payments in the event that wages are cut off as a result of illness or accident. (Short-term policies are those with maximum benefit periods up to two years; long-term plans are for periods greater than two years.) When disability coverage is provided as part of group insurance, the benefits are usually integrated with those derived from public programs such as Social Security. The total benefits from these sources generally are established at a level that does not exceed 60 percent of earnings. Individual disability income policies usually pay a fixed dollar amount of coverage. This amount may be greater for those Social Security rejects. Individual disability income policies may take many forms and may be designed to fit the special needs of the individual policyholder.[4]

As already noted, these five basic health insurance policies have countless variations. As a result, health insurance policies are being sold that may be inadequate in terms of such basic coverage as hospitalization and lack uniform standards in regard to such areas as length of stay and surgical services. As a consumer you should be aware that these problems exist. In addition to the five basic policies and their many variations, there are also policies related to specific public programs or treatment categories.

Medicare Supplemental Insurance

Referred to as Medigap or Medsupp, this is accident and sickness insurance that supplements the hospital, medical, or surgical expenses of persons covered under Medicare.

Long-Term Care Insurance

This covers services provided on an inpatient, outpatient, or at-home basis for chronically ill, disabled, or retarded persons. Its sales began in earnest in 1985 when the number of companies selling this coverage doubled.

Dental Expense Insurance

Generally available through insurance company group plans, prepayment plans, and dental service corporations, this coverage reimburses for expenses of dental services and supplies and encourages preventive care. The coverage normally provides for oral examinations (including x-rays and cleaning), fillings, extractions, inlays, bridgework, and dentures as well as oral surgery, root canal therapy, and orthodontics. Plans usually include substantial consumer copayments, although copayments may be lower for preventive services.[5]

Thus, when you are choosing health insurance coverage for your personal needs, it is very important to be aware and knowledgeable about these traditional forms of health insurance protection.

ASKING THE RIGHT HEALTH INSURANCE QUESTIONS

"Well, Paul, it's that time of year again. I have to choose my health insurance policy. Do I want to keep what I have or change to another plan? At least we are offered choices; I don't know how a person who buys an individual policy does it. There are literally thousands and combinations of thousands to choose from. Sometimes, I feel like I am making a bet for the coming year. I hope what I am choosing is the best coverage for my family and myself and doesn't end up costing me a lot of money from my own pocket. Not only do I have to choose a policy, then there are those federal laws that affect me like COBRA and HIPAA. It sounds like animals in a zoo, but sometimes I feel like I'm in a zoo trying to figure out the meaning of all these policies. Do you even understand their language and terms? They sound so technical and legal. And, sometimes what's in the fine print is even more important than the larger print."

"Alan, maybe the best way to approach the problem is methodically. First, try to find out as much about the company selling you the policy as you can. You don't want to get stuck with medical bills if the company is out of business or fraudulent, to begin with, when the time comes to use them. Then consider the benefits. Are there any benefits or services that you need for yourself and your family that the company's policies don't cover? Look how extensively they cover benefits and what do they exclude? Then try to figure out, if you can, how much you must pay from your own pocket for items that they don't cover like sharing the costs through copay-

ments, deductibles, and other means. Can you afford to pay these out-of-pocket costs, along with their premiums? Also become acquainted with the federal laws that sound like animals in a zoo because they not only affect your ability to take your insurance from one company to another but also cover you for certain amounts of time if you lose your job or are unemployed. All these items are important to know."

"Paul, what you are saying makes sense."

As numerous and diverse as today's health insurance policies may be, the questions the sophisticated purchaser of health insurance should consider prior to purchasing a policy are even more so. First, whether you are buying a health insurance policy as an individual policyholder or through the mail or at work as part of a group, do you know the health insurance company that is selling you the policy? The following can serve as a guideline to determine this information.

The Insurance Company

Is the insuring organization a legitimate business?

Be aware that there are fraudulent health plans in this country. A health plan that claims to be exempt from state regulation is not necessarily fraudulent because most self-insured plans are legitimately exempt. Contact your state insurance department to confirm that the company is licensed to do business in your state—use its exact name—and to see if there have been complaints or problems. Also, check with the Better Business Bureau to determine whether or not the company is reputable and its agents are licensed to sell an insurance product in your state. Be wary if an agent says he does not need a license because the coverage is not insurance or is exempt from regulation. Also be careful if the agent asks you to join some organization or pay dues to receive coverage such as a union plan that is being sold but includes no other traditional union benefits. A union plan should not be available through an insurance agent. Additional signs that an agent may be defrauding you are if the agent tells you that the coverage being sold has better benefits but lower premiums than you can buy from licensed insurers, and that his company will insure everyone regardless of their age, accepting all preexisting conditions and placing no limitations on the use of coverage. Be very suspicious if you are asked to pay for an insurance policy with a large amount of money up front or to pay in cash. Never pay in cash. Ask for a receipt for all payments. The receipt should include the policy number, the date, and the name of the health plan. If you do not receive your insurance plan's documents within a specified period of time, contact the insurance company and demand proof that you are covered. Read the plan documents very carefully when you do receive them. The following is the basic con of fraudulent health plans: They enroll as many people as they can, keep them paying premiums as long as they can, and when claims become substantial or insurance regulators become aware of them, they close down and move somewhere else. One source of information to detect such plans is the Coalition against Insurance Fraud. For the coalition's scam alert on fraudulent healthcare coverage, including a list of ten warning signs and a roster of unlicensed operators, go to http://www.insurancefraud.org and click on "Consumer Info" and then "Bogus Health Plans." Another site for such information is the Georgetown University Health Policy Institute. Its Web site, http://www.healthinsuranceinfo.net, displays alerts about fraudulent insurance operations and has published *A Consumer Guide for Getting and Keeping Health Insurance.* Also, the former Health Insurance Association of America, a trade group based in Washington, DC, and now renamed America's Health Insurance Plans (AHIP), has an online *Guide to Health Insurance* at http://www.ahip.org as well as a directory of state insurance agencies. The state agencies carry lists of insurance companies approved to operate in each state. Another link to state insurance departments is the National Association of Insurance Commissioners. Go to http://www.naic.org and click on "Consumers" and then "Insurance Department Web sites." Also, find out if the National Association of Insurance Commissioners still has available a useful brochure entitled *Protect Yourself against Illegal Health Plans.*

What kind of company is selling you the health insurance?

One of the best sources of information about the health insurance company from whom you are considering buying a policy is in your public library or an insurance library: *Best's Insurance Reports Life/Health.* The higher the rating (A+ or A) the insurance carrier receives from *Best's*, the less likely the insurer is about to go out of business. You also want a AAA rating from at least one of the other major rating firms—Moody's Investors Service Inc., Standard & Poor's, or Duff and Phelps Inc. Standard & Poor's also passes out "q" ratings for insurers it hasn't examined in full—the highest being BBBq. Such a company might be an AAA if Standard & Poor's examined its books.

Also, be cautious of "multiple-employer welfare arrangements" (MEWA), which have gone out of business, often through fraud. MEWAs sign up small companies that cannot afford to purchase coverage from major insurers. Some MEWAs are legitimate, but others collect premiums and then disappear. With MEWAs, the sign of a high-risk plan is lower monthly premiums than the competition sells. Employers should not buy into a MEWA without finding out from their state insurance commission if the plan is licensed to sell there and whether there have been any complaints. Avoid new MEWAs.[6]

What about medical discount cards?

Be very careful of medical discount cards that advertise that they offer you low prices on doctor visits, hospital stays, prescription drugs, and dental care. Some cards charge administrative fees that are higher than the discount so that their coverage costs you more than if you never were protected at all. Their advertisements may use words like "benefits," "health plan," and "protection" that make them sound like an insurance plan. Also, be wary of advertisements that state that there are no age limits, include a promise to accept all preexisting conditions, and guarantee there will be no rate increases. Remember the old adage, if it sounds too good to be true, it probably is. Experts state that medical discount cards actually operate like a buyer's club. They appear to offer much higher savings than they do and masquerade as regular health insurance companies so that those who have no insurance, especially the elderly, and those who have insurance but are looking for a cheaper policy are fooled that they have a less expensive plan than their current insurance. Then, after getting rid of their current insurance plan, they find out that they have been deceived when they require insurance coverage at their neediest time.

While there are legitimate discount plans, here are some steps you can take to avoid being deceived. Carefully read the terms of the plan. For example, if you read *savings up to* 70 percent, the words *up to* can mean far less than 70 percent. Find out from your doctor, hospital, and pharmacy if they participate in the plan. If you need specific drugs and medical services, read the plan carefully to see if it covers them before you sign up. Make sure the plan covers generic drugs. Find out what the fine print says about administrative charges and ask if you can cancel the plan at any time and if your membership fee is refundable. Contact your Better Business Bureau or even your state insurance commissioner's office to find out if anyone has complained about the discounter. Conduct your business with reputable organizations. Discount medical cards such as those the AARP (American Association of Retired Persons) recommends are legitimate. However, one more word of caution: *These programs cannot replace legitimate health insurance plans, cannot even begin to cover high-cost items like various surgeries or costly hospital stays,* and if the salesperson wants you to purchase the program immediately and does not answer your questions directly when you ask them, it is time to investigate this plan to make sure it really meets your personal health needs, both physically and financially.

Is the insurance company licensed to do business in your state?
What are the problems of buying insurance on the Internet?

As already noted, make sure that the company from whom you are considering purchasing your health insurance policy is licensed to do business in your state. The quickest way to find out is to call your state insurance department. If the company is not so licensed and a dispute between you and your company occurs, your state insurance agency will not be able to help you very much with your problem.

Many Internet sites offer price quotes and policies, but be careful. Some ask for personal information. And be sure to read the fine print of the policy, since you may be required to purchase extra coverage for maternity care or prescription drugs. Many plans increase rates or reduce coverage for people with preexisting conditions. Two Internet sites that do not require sensitive personal data in order to obtain an instant price quote are http://www.ehealthinsurance.com and http://www.insure.com.

Does the insurance company have a good history of paying claims?

Ask your state insurance department or your friends if they have any information in this regard. Health insurance companies advertise in national magazines, by mail, and on radio and television—even on matchbook covers. Be careful. Find out, for your own financial protection, what kind of record they have in paying claims.

What can you do if your insurer goes out of business and you are left having to pay your medical bills yourself?

There are a number of steps you can take if your insurer goes broke and leaves you with your own medical bills. Find out whether your insurance plan has a *hold-harmless clause*. This clause prevents physicians and hospitals from demanding payment for bills that should have been paid by the medical service plans. All federally qualified health maintenance organizations have such clauses, while some states require that Blue Cross and Blue Shield and regular insurance plans have such clauses. If some doctors overlook hold-harmless clauses and bill you anyway, ask your state insurance department if you must pay. If you sign an agreement to pay when you enter a hospital, you might, in some states, give up your protection of the hold-harmless clause. Also, if your insurance agent sold you a policy from a company not licensed in your state, the agent may be liable for any bills the company defaults on. Some states hold insurance agents liable if they knew or should have known that the company was insolvent. If you work for a large company whose insurer goes out of business, the chances are good that your employer will still pay your bills. Smaller companies, however, may not be capable of doing so. Sometimes physicians and hospitals don't bill patients whose insurers fail, but that is not a guarantee, either. So look at all the possibilities, public and private, to determine whether other organizations will pay your medical bills if your insurer fails before you yourself pay them.[7]

All states now provide guaranty funds for individual policies. They cover up to one hundred thousand dollars of medical expenses (more in some states) for insurers licensed to sell in the state. Most group health plans are not included nor are multiple-employer welfare arrangements (MEWAs). In general, the funds guarantee (up to the dollar limits of state law) all your previous bills, all your present bills, and all your future bills until you find another insurer or your policy comes up for renewal, which may be anytime from the next day to a year. Beginning from the time your insurer went out of business, you have to pay premiums to the guaranty fund, perhaps at higher rate than you paid the insurer.

Why can a company either still solvent or in Chapter 11 bankruptcy terminate retiree health benefits, leaving retirees responsible for their own health coverage, either permanently or temporarily?

This situation is not supposed to happen. In the 1980s Congress passed legislation, sponsored by Senator Howard M. Metzenbaum, requiring companies in Chapter 11 bankruptcy to continue paying health benefits to retirees. However, health benefits, unlike pensions, are especially vulnerable to termination because companies are not required to "prefund" the benefits and can decide to pay out for retiree hospital and doctor bills as the expenses are incurred. As a result, many companies have generated billions of dollars in liabilities that will come due as their workers retire. Because the federal government does not insure health benefits the way it does pensions, workers have no guarantees, other than the promises of their companies, that the health benefits will be there after retirement. A major reason behind other companies that are not in bankruptcy canceling their retirees' health insurance coverage is an accounting rule that went into effect in 1993 called the Financial Accounting Standard 106, which requires companies to subtract from their profits the future costs of providing retirees' health benefits. Many businesses never estimated their future health obligations or, as already noted, didn't put aside enough to honor their health benefits promises to their retirees and few ever disclosed them. In most cases, Medicare benefits are not available until age sixty-five, and retirees who cannot continue their company health coverage often have trouble obtaining health insurance because of existing health problems. Medicaid only covers the poorest of the poor.

Does your insurance policy provide service or indemnity benefits?

The Blue Cross and Blue Shield plans provide *service benefits*, making payments directly to the providers of care, such as hospitals, rather than the patient paying the health providers and then being reimbursed by Blue Cross and Blue Shield. The payments are made on the basis of a negotiated reasonable figure rather than paying the charges of the covered services. These pay all or a share of actual costs and are adjusted as those costs change. The advantage: payments keep up with rising medical costs to some degree. The disadvantage: with inflation, premiums rise as well— or coverage is cut back.

Under an *indemnity benefit*, the health provider generally bills the patient, who submits to the insurer proof that he has paid the charges, and the patient is then reimbursed by the health insurer in the amount of the covered charges, which may be much lower than the amount charged by the doctor or hospital. Most commercial insurers operate in this way. Any uncovered expenses are paid by the patient himself. One form of indemnity benefits appears in the hospital income policy—a limited kind of health insurance that pays you its benefits in cash on a daily a basis only when you are hospitalized. The advantage: premiums of this policy remain relatively stable over the years. The prime disadvantage: payments to you remain fixed even though medical costs rise—and you pay the difference in these rising medical costs.

What is the insurance company's loss ratio?

Try to learn about an insurance company's loss ratio—the percentage of premiums the company pays back to its policyholders in the form of benefits. For example, the nonprofit Blue Cross and Blue Shield plans have a loss ratio of about 85–90 percent. This means that for every dollar paid to them, they return 85–90 cents to their policyholders. Commercial health insurance companies maintain a loss ratio of about 60–65 cents for each dollar, partly because they pay sales costs and state taxes while nonprofit organizations do not. However, the loss ratio is not the only criterion you should use in deciding upon an insurance company. Older companies may have a low loss ratio because they accept only low-risk customers. A company with a high loss ratio may not be keeping enough cash in reserve and could go bankrupt. But, in general, the percentage of returned benefits can tell you whether an insurer is selling high-value policies. Most experts agree that a good company should have a loss ratio of at least 50–60 percent. You can also ask your insurer about the loss ratio on the specific policy you are buying. The company may not be willing or able to give you the figure, but it will not hurt to ask.[8]

Can the company cancel your health insurance policy?

No health insurance coverage is of much value if it can be canceled at the option of the insurance company—perhaps because you had too many claims. You could be left with no protection just when you need it most. To avoid this, you should choose a policy that only you can cancel and for which the premium cannot be increased. This feature, of course, will add to the cost.

If you want to hold down the initial premium yet still have the right to renew, look for a *guaranteed renewable* policy. This allows the company to increase the premium at renewal time only if it does so for *all* persons owning that particular type of policy. In other words, it cannot raise your rates because of any previous claims that you, as an individual, have had. Some policies state that the company will continue insuring you as long as it continues to insure people in your state with the same kind of policy.[9]

What are the problems involved with mail-order insurance?

Mail-order health insurance is promoted in various media—newspapers, magazines, radio, and television, to cite but a few examples. Most of these policies offering hospital-surgical-medical coverage generally provide indemnity-type benefits paying cash directly to you, to be used as you wish. The benefits are usually based on the number of days you spend in a hospital, with a maximum payment per month. This kind of health insurance is also known as a hospital income policy.

Remember, according to the American Hospital Association, the average hospital stay was not more than six days in 2000. If a policy advertises it will pay $1,000 a month while you are in the hospital, that amounts to $33 a day—and if a hospital charges $900 a day, for example, the daily difference of $867 has to be made up either through your personal financial resources or through additional insurance coverage. So do not be fooled by the maximum payments advertised by mail-order insurance. Figure out exactly what it would mean to you personally if you were to be hospitalized.

When purchasing mail-order health insurance, ask the same questions discussed in this chapter as you would if buying a regular health insurance policy through an insurance agent. Especially important is the question of the company's loss ratio. Because mail-order companies often make heavy and liberal use of preexisting-condition exclusions, they deny a greater percentage of claims than other insurance companies and thus have a low loss ratio. Are illnesses as well as accidents covered? Is there a deadline for applying for the policy? Be very careful! The deadline—by stressing that you must enroll in two or three days or be denied the opportunity of buying the policy—may prevent you from making the proper inquiries in order to protect yourself against poor policy protection.

Do not rely on mail-order health insurance for basic or major medical insurance coverage. Consider it as supplementary coverage only. Study its advertisements very carefully to make sure that it is not promising more dollars than it actually will deliver. Premiums are generally paid monthly; the usual grace period is ten days. If you pay the premium weekly, the grace period is seven days. Since companies usually do not issue reminder notices, you must keep track of your payments yourself. If a policy lapses because of nonpayment, a new round of waiting periods may be reinstituted. Also, do not choose a policy because it advertises that its cash benefit payments to you are tax free. This is not unique. Most health insurance benefit payments are not taxable and this includes coverage obtained through your employer or if you are self-employed. And, unlike regular health insurance policies, premiums on this type of mail-order policy may not be tax deductible. Finally, make sure the company is licensed to do business in your state. If you have a problem with the company and it is not licensed to do business in your state, your state insurance department cannot help you very much. Be cautious! Find out as much about the company from your state insurance department or your friends or relatives as you can.

One of my medical bills was turned down by the insurance company. Is there anything I can do?

Ask the insurance company why the claim was rejected. If the answer is that the service isn't covered under your policy and you are positive that it is, call the provider—usually a doctor or hospital—and ask that he double-check the procedure code and diagnosis. (If a provider mistakenly puts in the wrong diagnosis or procedure code on the insurance claim form, your claim may well be denied. There are codes called the Current Procedure Terminology [CPT] codes. They are designated for services common in modern medical practice and that are being done by many physicians in clinical practice in multiple locations. For each service, there is a five-digit code and a text descriptor, for example, "82270-Fecal occult blood test." It is possible your physician cited the wrong diagnosis or procedure code.)

In addition, you may also ask your doctor to write a *letter of medical necessity* for you, which means that without the care in question your condition could become worse. Also, ask the company to make sure that your deductible was correctly calculated. Did you skip the essential step under your plan, such as securing a second surgical opinion or a preadmission certification? If everything is in order, ask the insurer to review the claim.[10] Make sure that you keep all written records relating to the claim—not just the denial-of-care notice but all the correspondence from the insurance company—in the event that your case escalates over time and is eventually heard by a panel of reviewers.

When you initiate an appeal, the insurance company—generally by law—must begin a timely review of your case. Federal law requires insurers to provide an appeals process if a member wants to protest the denial of a claim or, as in the case of managed care plans, a refusal to refer to outside specialists. Don't depend upon the customer service department of the insurance company that is under no legal time limit to answer your appeal when you call in a complaint. Follow up the call with a written letter in which the word *appeal* is used. Send it by certified or registered mail, overnight delivery, or fax, making sure to keep the respective receipts for your records. Send a copy of your letter of appeal to the head of personnel or human resources at your company, if applicable. Since the department actually buys medical insurance and other insurance on your behalf, the insurance company views your company, not you, as the customer. When the human resources department places pressure on the insurance company, things can happen. Also, speak with one of the nurses or medical directors who are reviewing your case for the insurance company.

If you disagree with the claim adjuster's decision on your health insurance claim, ask to talk to the supervisor. If you don't receive any satisfaction from the supervisor, ask to speak with the claims manager or even the vice president in charge of claims administration. If the company still refuses to pay, contact the state insurance commission. Provide the name of your insurance company, the adjuster, and, as concisely as possible, the reason(s) for the disagreement. The insurance commission should act as an intermediary and contact the company about your problem. Your insurer will probably pay close attention to the commission's efforts to intervene on your behalf because the commission has the power to suspend the company's right to conduct business in your state. If you don't get any satisfaction from the insurance commission's efforts, consider hiring an attorney who is knowledgeable about insurance matters. In many cases, this may lead to an out-of-court settlement because insurance companies prefer not to go to trial over claims; juries tend to sympathize with claimants. Be assertive. Don't give up or abandon critical decision-making power along the way. Conduct some research. Many medical organizations have established "practice guidelines"—suggested standards for basic care—which you will find on their Web sites. For example, if coverage is denied for a drug that is commonly prescribed after a heart attack, you could use that fact to advance your case.

To learn more about how to handle disputes with a health insurance organization, go to http://kff.org/consumerguide. The Consumers Union and the Kaiser

Family Foundation have worked together to produce an online guide that explains how to navigate from beginning to end internal and external dispute processes. In addition, the Medicare Rights Center, a private group, at http://medicarerights.org directs Medicare recipients through the appeals process; it also operates a toll-free national hot line (1-888-466-9050) to answer consumer questions. Finally, the Centers for Medicare and Medicaid Services of the US Department of Health and Human Services provides extensive detailed information on the Medicare system, Medicaid, and other federal health programs.

While filing a claim may be tedious work, the insurer depends upon the reports you and your physician file to adjust the claim. If you are filing the claim, rather than having the physician fill it out for you, you must provide the following information: when the accident or illness occurred, the date you first received medical treatment, and, for disability claims, the total number of days lost from work. If you cannot understand how to answer any question on the claim form, call the company and ask. Be sure you understand what benefits your policy covers. Most individual policies do not pay for routine checkups, so, again, be sure your doctor specifies an illness, injury, or physical complaint as the reason of treatment. A few days after you've delivered the form to your physician's office, if you are filling it out yourself rather than having the physician do so, check back and make sure he or she has mailed it in. Allow about thirty days to hear from the insurer about its decision on the claim. Remember, insurance companies are vigilant for potential fraud whether it be the consumer falsifying claims, presenting false records of employment and eligibility, or making other fraudulent misrepresentations on the application, or the provider presenting fraudulent diagnoses or dates, waiving copayments or deductibles, or billing for services not rendered.

Also, remember that some companies self-insure their employees, that is, they themselves pay the costs of their employees' healthcare under the federal Employee Retirement Income Security Act of 1974 even though an outside insurance company might administer the plan and handle all the other details. Persons in these self-insured plans have few alternatives other than their internal review process. Beyond that persons can contact the US Department of Labor, file a lawsuit, or contact specialists who resolve healthcare issues.

BENEFITS, SCOPE OF COVERAGE, AND OUT-OF-POCKET PAYMENTS

Whether you purchase your health insurance as an individual policy, through the mail, or at work as part of a group, these policies have three elements in common: benefits, scope of coverage, and out-of-pocket expenses that the health policy may require you to pay such as deductibles, coinsurance, or copayments. The following questions can help you understand your policy in regard to these three broad areas.

Benefits

How soon after family membership begins are maternity benefits effective?

Is there a waiting period? What are the benefits for normal delivery? For abnormal complicated delivery? For out-of-hospital birth? Birthing rooms? What about pre- and postbirth examinations for mother and newborn? Effective January 1, 1998, insurance companies are required by the Newborns' and Mothers' Protection Act, signed by President Clinton on September 26, 1996, to allow a minimum forty-eight-hour hospital stay to new mothers and their babies following normal delivery and a minimum ninety-six-hour hospital stay following cesarean section. Note that the act does not actually require the mother and/or newborn to remain in the hospital for these periods, only that the health plans permit the minimum stays. A mother would still be able to go home sooner if she wishes.

Also, on June 20, 1983, the US Supreme Court ruled that employers who fully insure spouses for other medical needs cannot deny or limit pregnancy coverage for them. The Pregnancy Discrimination Act, passed in 1978, protects female employees from discrimination in insurance coverage when they become pregnant. According to a ruling by a US District Court against Illinois Bell Telephone Co. in September 1982, maternity leave must be treated in the same way as any other disability absence. Companies must automatically reinstate returnees to their jobs without the qualification of whether the jobs are still open.

What prevention benefits are included?

Does the plan cover well-child care? Physical examinations and periodic checkups? On what schedule (should correspond with the recommendations of National Preventive Service Task Force or American Medical Association guidelines)? Dental care? Vision Care? Hearing Aids? Immunizations?

What special services are covered?

Does your plan cover the cost of blood needed for a transfusion? What about therapy after you get out of the hospital? If so, what is the maximum number of visits covered? Is coverage reduced or excluded for some needs, such as orthodontics, eyeglasses, and mental health problems?

General problems?

What provisions are made for out-of-area emergency care? Does the plan have a list of preferred providers? What happens if you go outside that list?

What benefits are provided for daily hospital visits by the attending physician?

Are there provisions for office or house visits?

Is a deductible payment required for these visits?

Are there provisions for concurrent services of more than one physician?

Does the policy pay for consultants' fees? Under what conditions?

What provisions are made for radiation therapy, diagnostic x-rays, laboratory tests, and anesthesia services? What about second opinions, alcohol- or drug-abuse treatment, and physical, occupational, and speech therapy? Inpatient or out-of-hospital diagnosis and treatment? Does the plan omit specific services you now require?

If you have the option, decide whether or not you want coverage for each of these services. If you are not covered for a service that you would like, it might be possible to buy supplemental coverage. Ask your employer. It is also important to know just how extensive the policy provisions are. For example, while your plan may provide payment for diagnostic tests, this may only apply if the procedures are performed in a hospital. Read the fine print to be sure.

What kinds of emergency and outpatient hospital services are covered?

Physician services, other treatments, operating and emergency room charges, x-rays and other tests, physical and other outpatient therapies, and mental health services (to fifty visits yearly)?

What kind of inpatient hospitalization services does your health insurance policy cover?

Do you have to pay a deductible? How much? Does your policy include benefits for intensive care? Are the benefits limited? What inpatient hospitalization benefits are provided? Inpatient and rehabilitation care, including semiprivate room and board, physician care, diagnostic and treatment services, physical and other therapies, medications, equipment supplies, operating or delivery or recovery room charges, drug or alcohol detoxification (with one readmission a year), and mental health services while hospitalized (how many days)? Does it pay for all high-cost services? Does it cover emergency care? Ambulance? Does the policy have any "inside limits" covering only part of the cost of your hospital room per day, obligating you to pay the rest out of your own pocket?

Are hospital benefits provided for nervous and mental disorders?

Are there deductible or coinsurance amounts? Are there benefits for psychiatric treatment in a doctor's office? In a hospital outpatient facility? By psychologists or social workers? Are there any limits on the number of days for inpatient treatment that will be paid in a given year—often thirty days is common and takes into account the average stay for most acute mental illnesses or the most common substance-abuse treatment programs. Are there dollar limits or other restrictions on coverage for services? Is there a cap on the amount spent on inpatient care over a lifetime—a fifty-thousand-dollar cap is common. Does your employer's plan require that you use "preferred providers" for mental health services who meet the employer's standards for cost and quality? Some employers are setting up networks of mental health providers that employees are encouraged to use. Providers, who are encouraged to recommend outpatient treatment, are paid a set amount under the terms of a contract with a company. Limiting the number of providers employees can use is supposed to reduce the cost of mental health benefits.

On September 26, 1996, President Clinton signed into law the Mental Health Mandate of 1996 (Public Law 104-204), effective January 1, 1998, which requires that all health plans with more than fifty participants must offer the same annual and lifetime dollar limits for treatment of mental illness as they provide for other general medical treatments of physical disorders. But nothing in the law requires employers to provide mental health coverage or even to keep the coverage they have. In addition, under this new mandate, plans will be allowed to impose different deductibles and copayments for mental illness and treatment. It is also legal for employers to limit treatment such as providing their employees no more than thirty days a year in a psychiatric hospital or twenty outpatient sessions with a therapist. Recognize that this mandate does not cover individual policies as opposed to group health plans nor does it cover the treatment of chemical-dependency cases, alcoholism, or substance abuse (although it is required for state-regulated plans in Maryland and Vermont and in Minnesota for state-regulated plans that offer mental health benefits). Plans also can treat these coverages differently and subject them to lower calendar-year or lifetime benefits. Employers may be able to gain an exemption from the mandate to provide lifetime dollar caps for mental illness equal to that of physical illness if they can prove that compliance will increase their overall plan expenses by 1 percent or more. It should be noted that few states have tougher laws than this federal act, although those laws usually don't affect the biggest companies. State-regulated group health plans must cover severe mental illness on a truly equal basis with physical illness in Colorado, Connecticut, Maryland, New Hampshire, Rhode Island, and Vermont. There is also significant protection in Maine, Minnesota, and Texas.

Are there any exclusions other than the common ones?

Some plans may exclude such expenses as cosmetic surgery that is purely by choice.

Are surgical procedures covered wherever performed?

If payment is subject to a schedule of benefits, is the schedule in line with current surgical fees in your area? What provisions are there for operations not specifically listed? Are fractures and dislocations covered? Oral surgical procedures? How much of a surgeon's bill is paid by the insuring organization? Is the cost of a second surgical opinion covered? What percent of its cost? What about cosmetic surgery unrelated to an accident?

Is coverage provided for services of a registered nurse in a nursing home?

Of a licensed practical nurse? Are nursing benefits limited to periods of hospital confinement?

Is there insurance coverage for homecare?

Short-term, long-term? Skilled nursing services (up to thirty visits for short-term or up to ninety visits for long-term care), physician visits, medications and equipment, physical and other therapies, and high-technology services?

What benefits are provided for services in an extended-care facility?

What is the maximum number of days covered? Must this follow hospitalization within a specified period of time? What is the allowance per day? Do these benefits include room and board (up to forty-five days for short-term nursing home care and up to ninety days for long-term nursing home care), skilled nursing visits, physician visits, equipment and supplies, physical and other therapies? Short-term, long-term?

Does the policy cover prescription drugs?

Any prescription drugs my doctor prescribes or only certain drugs, or only generic drugs? Does the plan allow the pharmacist to substitute a generic drug without consulting my doctor?

Does anyone besides your doctor have a say in your care?

Many plans now require second opinions for surgery and preapproval of nonemergency hospitalization and review many medical procedures for "appropriateness" before paying. Who decides these things? Who decides for how long you stay in the hospital? If your physician or you disagree, how can you appeal and who pays while waiting for an answer?

What services does your health insurance policy cover and how well?

The previous questions will enable you to determine the kinds of benefits your health insurance policy covers and any additional benefits you wish to buy. While an affordable program is not likely to cover your expenses down to the last cent, it should protect you against most of the costs of illness or injury. But also, remember, in regard to health insurance plans that have low premiums, if you cannot afford to pay the required deductibles and copayments, your savings on those low premiums may not mean very much. Besides normal hospital services and surgery, look for at least partial coverage of such expenses as diagnostic tests, prescription drugs, outpatient care, and private nursing. These benefits may be expressed in specific dollar amounts with maximum limits. This may also be true of room-and-board benefits. If so, try to find out whether these sums are realistic in relation to today's costs in your area. Older policies are almost certain to have benefits so low that you are left with a big share of the bill to pay out of your own pocket.[11]

Should you buy a "dread disease" policy?

A dread disease policy is meant to provide financial protection against a specific major disorder—for instance, cancer and heart, respiratory, or liver disease. Most insurance experts say these kinds of policies should not be purchased. It is wiser to spend your money on a good medical-and-surgical policy that pays when *any* illness strikes, including those listed herein. There are too many exclusions and limitations in a dread disease policy. Also, dread disease policy coverage often overlaps with Medicare and/or other supplemental insurance you may have. But if you insist on buying dread disease health insurance, ask yourself these questions: Do you need it? If you have basic medical and major medical policies, how much will the special policy pay in addition if the disease occurs? What are its exclusions and limitations? Does it pay for diagnostic tests and pathology reports, rehabilitation or checkups after treatment, for treatment due to complications, for outpatient or for home treatment? Many policies pay only for "definitive" and hospital treatments of cancer, not for related treatments. In times of inflation, seek a policy that pays a percentage of rising hospital bills rather than a flat fixed fee per day. Does the company readily pay its claims? What percentage of premiums is paid out in benefits? Is the company financially stable? Does the company use scare or high-pressure sales techniques? Be very wary and cautious about buying a policy from such a company.[12]

Extent of Coverage

What family members are covered under a family plan?

How much coverage do you need? What services do you or your family expect to need? Are your existing conditions covered? Are newborn babies covered from birth? To what age are dependent children covered? What is the insurer's definition of a dependent child? Are there provisions for older dependent children? For full-time students? For foster children? For children of a previous marriage living in the same or another state? Is a child covered if married?

Are your children covered adequately under your medical insurance plan?

It is a good idea to check your health insurance policy to determine at what age your children are no longer covered. A great many children are dropped at age nineteen, while some are still covered through ages twenty-three to twenty-five, if they are still your dependents, or when they stop being a full-time student, whichever comes first.

If a young person in college is dropped from the family medical plan, it is fairly simple to enroll in the college's own inexpensive group plan or the student can purchase his own plan. If your child does enroll in a college medical plan, make sure that he is not already covered under the family group plan as well. You now are paying twice (or once, if the family is covered by an employer), but no extra benefits accrue. Be aware that some students are not able to extend their parents' coverage for the years they are in college while others have trouble obtaining treatment while away from their hometown because the costs are not covered under their parents' health insurance plan. College healthcare coverage can also be complicated by the domination of health maintenance organizations and other managed-care plans that have come into being to curb soaring costs. These operations make it increasingly difficult to provide proper medical treatment for students because they frequently question diagnostic tests and treatments proposed by college physicians. Remember, while nearly all private colleges require mandatory health coverage as of 2005, more and more public colleges like the University of Connecticut, Ohio State, and all ten schools of the University of California system also are beginning to require that students have mandatory health insurance coverage before they begin their studies.

When a student goes to work and is not covered by the family plan, he or she might be able to sign up for plan offered by the employer. Again, check your own coverage to make sure you are not paying for a child who is covered at work. Also, find out if your insurance company will provide individual coverage (at added expense) when your child loses the protection of the family group plan and cannot get other group coverage. This can be important if your child develops an illness that would make it difficult or impossible to get coverage elsewhere. A number of policies will permit rolling over and conversion into individual coverage for children, without a waiting period or penalty because of a preexisting illness. Find out if such a situation is applicable to your case. A conversion plan simply means that the insurer must offer some type of plan to the college graduate.

Other options exist for college students, but at a higher price. The Consolidated Omnibus Budget Reconciliation Act of 1986 (COBRA) allows college graduates to extend their coverage under their family's plan for up to thirty-six months after graduation while paying 102 percent of the premium. For a graduate with a preexisting condition, a COBRA plan allows him or her to continue treatment.

If college graduates know they will be without work for longer than six months but don't want to go through their parents' plan, they can purchase a regular yearlong policy through the normal underwriting process. Just prior to graduation, students should ask their parents about their options on the family insurance plan such as COBRA and conversion plans.[13]

Few, if any, insurers give any formal notice when a young person is going to be dropped from a health insurance policy because of his age. Once you are dropped, you have about thirty days to qualify elsewhere or, if you qualify, to roll over into an individual policy. But if you don't know you are going to be dropped, how can you get other insurance in time? If you miss the thirty-day deadline and your child has a preexisting illness, your chances of getting new coverage for him are very limited. Even if you can obtain an individual policy with the same insurer, you will get less coverage at a much higher price. Therefore, examine your own health insurance policy in regard to your children's coverage and see that they are protected.

Does coverage provide for payment based on surgeons' and physicians' usual and customary fees?

Are there any policy limits on surgical expense payments? On choice of surgeons?

If the insured is covered under more than one contract, are benefit payments restricted?

Are there provisions for coordination of benefits among contracts? If your spouse has another plan, is that more suitable? How would that affect your benefits? (Most group policies limit benefits under two group policies to 100 percent of the amount billed.)

Can an individual apply for separate coverage after becoming ineligible for dependent coverage?

Is there a time limit on this application (e.g., 15 or 30 days)? What provisions are made for continued coverage of dependents if the primary insured is over age sixty-five? If the primary insured dies? Upon divorce or separation from the primary insured?

Are there any limitations on choice of physicians?

Does your policy place limitations on the choice of hospital or other place of care?

Is coverage provided for injuries or illnesses incurred prior to the contract's effective date?

Does coverage apply equally to healthcare services anywhere in the United States?

What benefits are available for healthcare received outside of the United States?[14]

How many days of hospital care are covered for each illness?

Does the plan limit hospital days covered? Are the covered days limited to one period of hospitalization? Are there limitations such as a waiting period on readmission to a hospital for any or the same illness? A standard rule of thumb is that to be considered satisfactory your insurance coverage should equal at least 75 percent to 80 percent of costs.

Are you covered for preexisting conditions? How soon?

Some insurance companies can get very tough about paying benefits for an illness or injury that existed before your policy was issued. These restrictions are explained in the policy and may exclude any such payment to you for as long as two years. Look carefully at the policy language. Some companies, for example, stretch the meaning of "preexisting" to cover not only previous treatment for a specific health problem but also any symptoms that should have led you to see a doctor. Do not assume that you can avoid this problem by not mentioning the earlier illness in your application. If you have a reoccurrence of this illness before the end of the period of preexisting conditions, the insurance company has ways to uncover the earlier illness. The chances are you will not be able to collect. This situation applies mostly to individual policies; group coverage is more liberal. If a company attaches a "rider" (a document that modifies or amends an insurance contract) to your policy, not allowing coverage for preexisting conditions, insist on a lower rate or try and find another company that will give you coverage. But be prepared if the companies also insist on a rider or refuse your application. They may have access to the same information as the original company as members of the Medical Information Bureau, which is a nonprofit clearinghouse that provides to its member companies medical information it may have on file about an insurance applicant. If an insurer rejects you because of health or other reasons such as age, look for insurers such as Blue Cross and Blue Shield plans that have "open enrollment" periods in which they must cover anyone who applies. In addition, a few states have programs specifically for people who can't be otherwise insured. Ask your state insurance commission whether your state has enacted such a program.

Is there a waiting period before accident benefits begin? Before coverage of certain illnesses or operations?

Are these periods acceptable in view of your family's medical history?

How many days of coverage does your policy give you?

Many hospital policies place a limit on the number of days for which you can collect benefits. This may relate to how many consecutive days you can be hospitalized or to the total number of days in the year. The average hospital stay is about six days. Disability policies may also restrict the period of time for which you can collect benefits. Or the amount may be reduced after a certain number of payments. Remember, however, that Social Security pays disability benefits after five months if it seems likely that your condition will continue for at least twelve months. Also, except in some group plans, you pay no income tax on disability income. Use these facts to help you determine your needs.

What are the exclusions in your health insurance policy?

These are the services and/or circumstances that are not covered by a health insurance policy. For example, many hospital policies do not cover private-duty nursing or convalescent stays in nursing homes. And almost no policy protects against claims arising from acts of war. But some lower-cost policies get that way by excluding coverage for things you rightfully want and need. Therefore, make sure that you read the portion of the policy where these exclusions are spelled out.

Out-of-Pocket Payments

How much is the monthly premium?

What will your total cost be each year? There are individual rates and family rates. If you go with a cheap plan but it does not pay for the benefits you need, you are not getting good value for your health insurance dollars. Consider the value of your plan versus its price. You may wish to consider that if you are young and healthy, you can go for lower premiums and higher copayments. But if you are older, have chronic medical conditions, or have young children who make frequent trips to the doctor, you may be better off with higher premiums and lower copayments.

Will your premiums rise if you become sick?

A reputable health insurance plan will not raise your premium just because you became ill.

What is the maximum you would pay out of pocket per year?

How much would it cost you directly before the insurance company would pay everything else?

Is there a lifetime maximum cap the insurer will pay?

The cap is an amount after which the insurance company won't pay any more. This is important to know if you or someone in your family has an illness that requires extensive treatments.

If your illness goes from one calendar year into the next, do you have to pay a second deductible?

Most reputable companies do not require this.

In a major medical contract, does the deductible amount apply per illness, or is it based on the calendar year?

How large is the deductible? Is the deductible for the entire family or for each person? Is there a maximum family deductible? Is a coinsurance payment required? How much? What benefits are covered, excluded, or limited? What percentage of the costs above the deductible will be paid by your major medical plan?

What is the maximum amount payable under this policy?

Does the maximum coverage apply to each separate illness or is it a maximum life-time figure for all illnesses? Can maximum benefits be restored after recovery from an illness? If major medical insurance isn't adequate, can you purchase extra cov-erage using a "piggyback" or "excess" supplemental major medical policy with a high deductible, which might be $15,000 or more, and coinsurance rate and equally high maximum payout for each illness?

Does the health insurance policy contain deductibles? And how much are they?

When you think about savings on the costs of your premium, think about the size of the deductible you are paying—that is, the amount of money which you pay for health services before the company will pay all or part of the remaining cost of the covered services. Deductibles can range from zero for basic coverage to $1,000 or more for major medical insurance policies. As with auto collision insurance, the higher the deductible, the lower the cost of the policy. When selecting an individual policy, you must decide which is most important—less premium to pay now or the possibility of having to pay a larger sum before your insurance benefits begin con-tributing to your medical and hospital bills. The general rule of thumb when com-paring policies is this: If the difference in monthly premiums over an eighteen-month period is greater than the difference in the amount of the deductible, you are better off with the policy that has the high deductible.

You have much the same decision to reach in regard to the percentage of your bills that major medical is to cover. Do you want the insurance company to pay, for example, 80 percent, with only 20 percent remaining for you to pay? Or are you willing to assume a higher percentage of these future costs in trade for lower premiums now? Does your policy contain a "stop-loss" provision? Many newer policies do while many policies sold years ago do not. This provision, while adding to the cost of your insurance, provides that after you have paid out a certain amount (such as $1,000), including deductibles and your coinsurance such as 20 percent of medical expenses, the insurance company will start paying 100 percent of the bill. If you want such protection, check your policy carefully to see exactly what it says.

Some policies will cover only a portion of your medical charges, even after you've paid the deductible. Then, once your bill reaches a certain amount, coverage becomes total. It's important to find out whether this rule applies when your medical expenses reach the specified amount or only when the portion you've been paying out of your own pocket goes that high.

What is the coinsurance rate?

What percentage of your bills for allowable services will you have to pay?

Why are health insurance premiums generally higher for women than for men?

Although health insurance policies vary from state to state and from company to company, some insurers either still increase their premiums for women in their childbearing years or refuse to cover maternity expenses. Many policies that do not have maternity coverage won't cover claims—including such complications as miscarriages or ectopic pregnancies—if they occur within the first ten months after the purchase of the policy. Vasectomies for men are routinely covered, but female sterilization sometimes is not. Although breast reconstruction is generally covered, some insurers require that it be done immediately after the mastectomy, while other operations such as prostate reconstruction or glass eye replacement can be done at any time. The industry also states that women visit doctors more than men, that they make more claims, and that their surgery costs are higher as additional reasons why their health insurance premiums are higher than for men. The insurance industry argues that pregnancy is a voluntary and planned event and therefore an event that can be budgeted. Extending coverage to include childbirth and pregnancy-related care, according to the insurance industry, would escalate the cost of health insurance. Check with your state insurance department to find out whether your state now requires that pregnancy-related coverage be included in the health insurance policies sold in your jurisdiction.[15]

GENERAL ISSUES

However, regardless of the benefits, coverage, and out-of pocket costs your health insurance policy may contain, most people receive their health insurance policies through their group plans at work and a minority have their own individual plans. Even here, whether group or individual, these plans may have some common characteristics. Most are experience rated rather than community rated and have other characteristics you should understand. As examples:

What should I know when filling out my health insurance application?

You should be very careful when filling out your health insurance application—especially your medical history—or you may have trouble collecting later. The insurance company will verify the information by contacting your credit bureau, doctor, employer, and the Medical Information Bureau (a nonprofit clearinghouse that provides its member insurance companies with medical information it may have on file about an insurance applicant). If a company has refused you insurance on the basis of inaccurate information, you can request that data from the Medical Information Bureau if it has the information on file. If you contact its disclosure office, it will inform you how to correct any inaccurate information. Write to the Disclosure Office, Medical Information Bureau, P.O. Box 105, Essex, MA 02112. If you telephone, the Medical Information Bureau is listed in the telephone directory under its initials, MIB. If you wish to learn more about how the Medical Information Bureau operates, read William B. Swarts, "A Decade of Change at MIB," *American Society of CLU Journal*, April 1977. The journal may be available in your public library or an insurance library.[16]

What is the difference between community and experience rating?

The original concept of health insurance was that all members of a community would pay into a pool to protect each member of a group against mishap. Such an arrangement recognizes the random nature of illness and accidents and spreads the risk over a large number of people: Everyone pays a little so that no one will have to pay a lot.

Up until the early 1980s, local Blue Cross and Blue Shield plans and even some commercial insurers offered "community-rated" policies, in which everyone in a particular area was charged the same rates for coverage, regardless of their personal health history. There are two kinds of community rating. *Pure community rating* most often means that an insurance carrier's rates can vary only by geographic area—the "community"—and by family type. In other words, every two-parent family in Boston insured by particular carrier would pay the same rate, but single people in Boston would pay a different rate; single people in Boston insured by different carriers would pay different rates. *Modified community rating* allows an insurance carrier to use objective demographic factors such as age, gender, and, perhaps, health-conscious behaviors, in addition to geography and family type, when setting premium rates. Under modified community rating, younger individuals and families and employers with younger workforces would pay lower-than-average rates. In either type of community rating, premium rates may not vary based on an individual's or a small group's health status, claims experience, or duration of coverage. Today, community-rated policies are difficult to find.

Instead, both Blue Cross and Blue Shield and commercial insurers use "experience rating" and base premium costs on an individual's or group's prior health claims. As a result, one major illness in a small business can lead to significant increases in health premiums for all employees. Industry critics claim that because of rising medical costs, insurers are concentrating their efforts on avoiding high-risk cases. Insurers decide who they will cover, and at what price, on the basis of underwriting, which considers each individual's or group's health status, as well as other factors, such as age, sex, lifestyle, place of residence, and occupational hazards.

Underwriting is an increasingly exacting tool that allows insurers to identify and eliminate those most likely to incur high health costs—by applying advances in genetic screening, computer analysis of demographics and medical statistics, and greater understanding of disease—and to seek out those people least likely to need more than routine medical care (a practice called "cherry picking"). Because their business is competitive, health insurers have a strong incentive—profits—to exclude people with medical problems from their rolls. The result of this free-market process is that, for a large portion of this country's workers, only those who don't need health insurance coverage can obtain it at reasonable costs. In a process experts call "adverse selection," healthy people who are low risks often elect to do without insurance to save money, while sick people tend to be willing to pay whatever they can afford for coverage. The result is that the population of healthy insured people—those who pay into the system without using it—is shrinking, raising the cost of insurance for healthy and sick people alike who stay in the pool.

What are the advantages of buying a single comprehensive health insurance policy?

Try to select a company that offers a wide variety of health service benefits. No one can foresee what kind of illness or accident may place you in the hospital—therefore you should avoid purchasing a policy that does not include as many services as you may need. Some "dread disease" policies are so limited in scope that they pay only if you contract a specific illness like cancer, and most people do not contract this illness. So try to avoid a policy that covers one specific disease and select a good general policy that covers various health adversities. In addition, try to find a company that will sell you an insurance benefit package. Purchasing one large health insurance policy is usually less expensive than buying several smaller ones; also, you avoid the possibility of paying for duplicative benefits that the insurance company would not honor. An expensive policy may not always provide good coverage—but a cheap policy will almost always be inadequate to serve your needs.

How long is the health insurance policy's waiting period?

A new health insurance policy might not become effective immediately (except for injuries resulting from accidents). There is a waiting period, usually two weeks to a month, before you can collect benefits for illness. Any sickness that starts before this waiting period is completed will not be covered. Some policies make you wait three to six months; generally, these should be avoided. Maternity benefits, of course, are a different situation. Most policies require a nine-month waiting period before these take effect. No waiting period should be longer than a year.

What are the advantages of group versus individual health insurance policies?

Health insurance is available both on an individual policy basis and on a group insurance basis. Group insurance is available through your place of employment, labor union, or fraternal, religious, or alumni associations, among other sources. For example, if you must buy your own health insurance, the general advice has been to look at your local chamber of commerce or some other kind of business group or association such as a trade group or, as already noted, an alumni association, which may offer less expensive coverage than you could purchase for yourself. Or if any member of the family is in an affinity group like real estate agents or other occupational organizations, check if there is a group policy available. If you don't know a trade group with a group health insurance plan, go to the library and look up the *Encyclopedia of Associations.* Using its index, look up associations you might be eligible to join. Each group's summary will tell you whether it offers health insurance. Associations generally offer comprehensive medical and hospital insurance. If you find that too expensive, even in a group plan, health insurers also promote two alternatives. One is comprehensive major medical insurance with high deductibles. Instead of paying the first $250 or $500 of your annual medical bills, you might pay the first $2,000 or more. The other kind is "major hospital" insurance. This kind of policy covers your bills when you are in the hospital, up to a million dollars. But you are not insured for doctor bills outside the hospital.[17]

Group health insurance usually costs less and is generally more comprehensive than an individual health insurance policy at the same price. Moreover, if you become a member of a group at your place of work, your employer will probably pay most of the premium. Group health insurance costs less for actuarial reasons. The group represents a cross section of the community—some sick and some healthy. Because of odds that most group members will not file a claim, the risk is lessened and the insurance company is likely to profit. Group health insurance has another advantage. Individuals, regardless of their physical status, are eligible for coverage most of the time at their place of work. In addition, a group policy involves sharing paperwork, agent's fees, and other management activities, which results in financial savings. When you leave the group, however, though you usually can convert to an individual policy, the price will go up, and the coverage may decline, and it is best to be aware of this ahead of time. Also, ask you employer how long your group health insurance will cover you after you leave your job.

One reason why individual health insurance coverage is more expensive is that many insurers believe that someone who has not found a group policy is likely to be a higher-risk person. Despite this fact, you might prefer individual coverage for the following reasons: an individual's policy can be designed to fit particular needs, since everyone's requirements vary to some degree. For example, if you are young, single, and in good health, your problems are different than if you had a family of five dependents. Also, individual insurance can provide "interim" protection between jobs, just as group insurance can.

Typical interims are thirty, sixty, ninety days, or more. These generally are open-enrollment plans (nonmedical exam) and have liberal preexisting-condition clauses. Find out whether your company offers this kind of insurance protection. Also, ask whether the new policy will provide uninterrupted coverage of existing conditions.

Whether you purchase group or individual health insurance, try to protect yourself against as many risks as you can on a single policy. This cannot be emphasized enough. You will get more for your money—and probably better coverage—than you would with several small limited policies, which will tend to overlap and cost more. To learn more about health insurance, the Agency for Healthcare Research and Quality, which is part of the US Department of Health and Human Services, maintains a Web site, http://www.ahcpr.gov, with good, basic information on the types of insurance available, definitions of terms, and advice on how to shop for insurance.

INDIVIDUAL POLICY COVERAGE

Because most people have health insurance coverage through their place of employment rather than individual policies, let us look first at the major issues dealing with individual coverage.

If I must buy an individual health insurance policy, how should I proceed?

If it is necessary for you to purchase an individual health insurance policy, the following suggestions may be of assistance:

- First, as already noted, don't purchase health insurance at all without making an attempt to join some kind of trade, alumni, religious, or other kind of organization that has a group plan. Premiums will probably be less expensive, benefits better, and exclusions fewer. A self-employed person or group of up to fifty workers may join the Small Business Service Bureau of Worcester, Massachusetts, which groups its members to try to purchase benefit coverage at favorable rates and with as few exclusions as possible from plans located in the applicant's locality. For information, telephone 1-800-222-3434.
- If you've just left your job, federal law, the Consolidated Omnibus Budget Reconciliation Act of 1986 (COBRA), states you may keep your former employer's

group plan—paying the entire cost yourself—for eighteen months (as of 2006), giving you an opportunity to find insurance if you can afford the COBRA premium. If you are disabled, you as a qualified beneficiary may extend the original eighteen months of COBRA eligibility for up to twenty-nine months if the qualified beneficiary is disabled as of the date of the qualifying event and remains disabled through the end of the eighteen-month COBRA period.

- Watch out for advertisements or call insurers to learn whether they offer periodic "open seasons," usually fifteen-day periods when some offer complete coverage to all purchasers without exclusions.
- If you smoke, stop. Some companies charge nonsmokers less.
- Remember that there are unreliable fly-by-night companies in the health insurance field which cite a modest rate initially and then give you a big increase later. While almost all companies raise their rates annually, seek out a good insurance broker who knows which companies offer what kind of benefits and which are most responsible about rate increases and reimbursements.
- Before you begin looking for health insurance, decide how much you can afford to pay for total healthcare each year. Because some insurers give you several choices as to deductibles and coinsurance, you can lower your monthly premium a great deal if you know how much you can pay out of your own pocket or savings.
- Plan to spend a day or more on the telephone just gathering information.
- Read the plans' literature carefully for coverage and exceptions. Don't count on anything you don't see in writing.

Following the previous steps will make it easier for you to decide and find the kind of policy you need.[18]

What is stopgap insurance and do you need it?

Health insurance policies are usually sold for one-year periods with the right to renew. However, some insurance companies offer nonrenewable health insurance policies limited to 60–180 days. This type of insurance is designed mainly for job-hunting college graduates, people between jobs, and people in new jobs who are waiting to qualify for company insurance. The short-term plan varies according to varying states' regulations, but the basic coverage is the same.

The stopgap insurance covers hospital and surgical plans, which pay a prescribed amount per day for the hospital room as well as some surgical, outpatient, and miscellaneous expenses. Major medical plans cover a broader range of expenses up to an overall limit. Check with the companies and your own insurance agent to see what benefits are offered by these stopgap plans. Like other health plans, these policies circumscribe benefits in various ways that might not become clear to you until you read the policy, so ask for a sample. The restrictions and benefits differ widely among companies, making it difficult to compare premiums. But try to comparison shop—find out whether your own insurance company now sells such a policy and what the benefits and restrictions are in each policy—using the questions already noted in this chapter as a guide.

Short-term policies are relatively inexpensive but often carry high deductible and copayments. That means you could have a lot of out-of-pocket expenses if you become sick, but if you really don't expect to be filing any health insurance claims and are looking only to prevent catastrophic expenses in case an unexpected event does occur, they may be suitable policies. Short-term policies are good if you know you are going to obtain other coverage in the near future.

Also, remember, you don't have an automatic right to renew these short-term policies. If you still need coverage, you will have to reapply and get another policy. But, be aware that if something happened to you during the previous policy and you still require care as a result, that will probably be considered a preexisting condition and will not be covered by the new policy. In addition, these policies do not cover preventive care or maternity costs. Also, if it takes longer than expected to obtain group health insurance protection with your next employer, you could find yourself without coverage and be forced to purchase a second short-term policy from another company. As a safeguard, look into the possibility of buying a regular one-year renewable policy.[19]

GROUP HEALTH INSURANCE

As far as group insurance is concerned, the insured have many questions concerning such coverage as they see their monthly premiums skyrocketing and their employers asking them to pay more and more of their own insurance costs through higher deductibles, copayments, and other mechanisms. The era when employers covered 100 percent of their employees' health insurance has gone the way of the horse and buggy. Here are some of the questions you should ask.

In a group contract, can the insured convert to another form of coverage on termination of employment?

Are there any restrictions on conversion for any circumstances? Is there a time limit?

Are claims paid promptly and fairly under your plan?

Ask coworkers with the same plan or the employee benefits personnel where you work.

Can the contract be canceled?

By whom? Under what conditions?

If both you and your husband work, are you covered by his group plan and he by yours?

If so, this does not mean that you can collect double for your medical expenses. What it does mean is that if you should become sick and find that your policy covers only part of your costs, your husband's plan may pay for the rest. And vice versa. Another option might be to trade off either your husband's or your policy for cash. Some employers may agree to this, giving you the money they would otherwise spend on your policy. It is certainly worth asking about.

Can I decide whether to be covered by my employer's health plan? What should I do if my employer does not have health insurance coverage?

In some instances, you can decide whether to be covered. Sometimes, when people begin a new job, they already have health insurance coverage—perhaps because they are included in a spouse's plan or because they are covered by a health benefits plan that they themselves have obtained (for example, through an association). Some employers will give you the choice of refusing their health benefits plan. An employer who allows employees to "opt out" will usually require that the employee state it in writing.

Often you will not be able to refuse coverage. Why? One reason is that your employer may have a contract with an insurer to provide health benefits to "all" employees. In this instance, if you are protected by your spouse's plan, perhaps you can make an adjustment (switch from family coverage to individual, if that is appropriate). Remember that the coordination of benefits rule (no coverage for more than 100 percent of your costs) applies. But realize that once you refuse coverage under an employer's health plan, you may have to show that you are "insurable" (and you may have to have a health checkup) should you change your mind later on. Getting into that plan may no longer be automatic.[20]

But if your employer does not have any health insurance, whatsoever, you have several options to protect yourself. You can look for an individual health plan; sign up for the relatively new, tax advantaged "health savings account," which was part of the law creating the new prescription drug benefit under Medicare in December 2003; or enroll in high-risk pools created by some states such a Maryland in 2002 for people who were rejected for healthcare coverage elsewhere.

If you are purchasing your own health insurance, you can locate an agent through recommendations of your home or car insurance agent, find agents on the Internet, or work with an online broker such as http://www.insure.com, which provides price quotes, explanations of understanding health insurance plans and programs, and other information related to this field. If you do not have any health insurance coverage, the information at http://www.ehealthinsurance.org can also help you with such topics as health coverage and alternatives, a health plan checklist, carrier ratings, and other information. You can also telephone an insurance company to find out if it sells health insurance policies directly to individuals. Again, check with the state insurance department to make sure that the agent or healthcare provider is licensed to do business in your jurisdiction. You should also be warned that individual policies cost more than group policies at work, their benefits such as prescription drug coverage are more restricted than group health plans, and maternity coverage may be very difficult to find. The reasons individual polices are higher priced than group insurance is that employees do not subsidize these individual plans; it is more efficient in terms of cost to purchase insurance for a group rather than an individual; insurers do the negotiating, collect the premiums, pay the insurance agents, and do the medical underwriting (underwriting is the process by which insurance companies assess an applicant's health before granting coverage). Thus, they might cover all other conditions but your diabetes, for example. Insurance companies are also more exposed to risks on individual purchasers than with employer groups, which tend to have more average distribution on health risks. Find out from your state insurance commissioner's office whether your state has "guaranteed issue" laws that require insurers to provide some kind of coverage without medical underwriting. Also, if you are seeking individual health insurance, Georgetown University's Health Policy Institute has created a state-by-state *Consumer Guides for Getting and Keeping Health Insurance* for every state and the District of Columbia on its Web site, http://www.healthinsuranceinfo.net. The guides summarize your protections and so may not answer all your questions. They are also not replacements for legal, accounting, or other professional advice.

If you cannot obtain a private health insurance policy, find out whether your state offers a "high-risk" pool for people who have been rejected for medical reasons by individual plans and do not have access to group coverage or federally sponsored health insurance. An example of one such state is Maryland for which "high-risk" pool information can be found by telephoning 1-866-780-7105.

Another idea for protecting yourself against healthcare costs is to create for yourself a Health Savings Account (HSA), which Congress established as part of the 2003 Medicare prescription drug law (the Medicare Prescription Drug, Improvement, and Modernization Act of 2003). You can enroll in high-deductible plans and establish tax-sheltered accounts to pay for benefits not covered in an insurance plan. Persons under age sixty-five can purchase medical policies in 2006 with minimal deductibles of $1,050 for a single person and $2,100 for a family to establish an HSA. These amounts are indexed annually for inflation. Each year you or your employer can fund the HSA with an amount equal to the deductible, subject to a limit, and the amount could be used to pay for health expenses or be invested. The money going in would be pretax dollars. And withdrawals for medical care would be tax free.

With an increasing number of companies either ending or sharply reducing healthcare coverage for their retirees, how can I be sure that my company will not do the same when I retire?

First, obtain a copy of your company's plan documents, which describe the benefits offered, specify eligibility, and provide other details.

Then, examine your Summary Plan Description. This describes the major features of the plan. It can be changed from year to year or contract to contract, so make sure it is up-to-date. The plan in effect on the date you retire is the controlling document—obtain a copy and keep it. There may be other documents you wish to examine such as a collective bargaining agreement or an insurance contract.

When you examine the documents, search for language that looks like a clear promise to continue benefits or provide them for a certain period. But also look for language that gives the company the right to change or eliminate them. This "reservation clause" typically will state something like: "The company reserves the right to modify, revoke, suspend, terminate, or change the program, in whole or in part, at any time." The chances are the statement will be there since companies want to avoid open-ended promises to workers and retirees. Thus, for example, the company can increase the cost of your retiree health insurance premiums very quickly. In addition, some companies limit what they will contribute toward retirees' insurance premiums. Once the employer's costs hit the limit, retirees have to pay the rest. Should this situation happen to you, ask the company what changes have happened in regard to the employees' benefits to justify the rapid increase in the cost of health insurance premiums.

When both a promise and a reservation clause are present, it is not clear what your rights will be. Some courts have refused to enforce what seemed to be a clear promise if there was a reservation clause; others have enforced a promise contained in the summary even though there was a reservation clause elsewhere in the plan documents.

Keep any other communications your company or supervisors give you. Courts sometimes take into account informal communications in deciding rights.

If you are planning to retire early, read the documents concerning terms. Special promises made in such situations can override other plan documents. And don't hesitate to look out for yourself. If you can negotiate a personal promise of health insurance for yourself and/or your dependents in retirement, do so. If your company really wishes you to leave, it may well agree. In addition, talk to experts. If you belong to a union, officials there can assist you. Or you may wish to consult a labor lawyer on these matters. Remember, there is a great deal of finances involved.

Check with the US Labor Department, Employee Benefits Security Administration, Washington, DC, to see whether there is literature available on these matters.[21]

I'm planning to keep working after age sixty-five. Will I be covered by Medicare or by my company's health insurance?

If you work for a company with twenty or more employees, your employer must offer you (through age sixty-nine) the same health insurance coverage offered to younger employees. After you reach age sixty-five, you may choose between Medicare and you company's plan as your primary insurer. If you choose to remain in the company plan, it will pay first—for all benefits covered under the plan—before Medicare is billed. In most instances, it is to your advantage to accept continued employer coverage. The employer can also offer supplemental plans that cover health services that Medicare does not cover such as routine physical examinations, outpatient prescription drugs, and most dental services.

But be sure to enroll in Medicare Part A, covering hospitalization; it can supplement your group coverage at no additional cost to you. You can save on Medicare premiums by not enrolling in Medicare Part B until you finally retire. Remember, though, that delayed enrollment will result in slightly higher Medicare Part B premium and a waiting period for coverage.[22]

In view of my impending divorce, can I still receive benefit protection from my husband's health insurance plan?

Your first step is to check or have your lawyer check the provisions of your husband's health insurance plan. Some health insurance policies may allow a divorced spouse to receive continuous benefit protection under the husband's group health insurance plan, if this privilege is part of the divorce decree. If the divorce decree says your former husband must continue to provide the same coverage you had during your marriage, some employers will allow you to remain in his group plan regardless of the rules. Employer-sponsored group coverage is generally the least expensive and most comprehensive option. If this situation is applicable to you, and your former spouse worked in a business with more than twenty employees, then you are eligible for COBRA coverage for thirty-six months, after which you could purchase insurance in the individual market. But if this situation is not applicable to you, find out how long you will be covered after your divorce is final. As already noted, most group health insurance policies will continue to cover you for a certain number of days before protection ends. Find out how many days your protection will last.

Make sure you find out whether the plan offers a "conversion privilege or policy." Converting group coverage to an individual policy must ordinarily be done no later than six months after the date of the divorce if you do not qualify for COBRA. As already mentioned, under this privilege, you have the right to convert or change your group coverage to an individual policy without undergoing a physical examination. You also can continue to receive coverage for conditions that are already present without undergoing a waiting period and either pay for the new policy yourself or reach an agreement for your former husband to pay. Many states require insurance companies to offer a divorced spouse such conversion rights, but the rights frequently are not offered automatically—you must request them from the company. Also, you are seldom told that you must make this request within a grace period to avoid losing the chance to convert. Find out what that grace period is. Therefore, before any divorce moves are made, make a note of this conversion privilege and ask your lawyer to remind you of it in case you should lose your group health insurance coverage. Also remember that not all states require insurance companies to sell a divorced spouse coverage without a physical examination. Even those states with such requirements do not usually insist that the converted policy provide you with coverage comparable to your original health insurance plan. Finally, even if you are able to obtain health insurance coverage similar to that you had under you former husband's plan, expect your premiums to be higher—largely because the cost of administering an individual policy is greater than with a group plan.[23] As already noted, in March 2001 the Supreme Court reaffirmed that ERISA (Employee Retirement Income Security Act of 1974) and the pensions and other benefits it represents overrides state law. Thus, if the employee designates an ex-spouse and, if remarried, not the current spouse as a beneficiary, then the benefits go to the ex-spouse, though the couple is divorced. Thus, when a divorce becomes final, parties should review the pensions, insurance, and other such assets and change the beneficiaries to match their intention (and whatever else they agreed to in the divorce).

FEDERAL LAWS AND PROGRAMS

As already noted, you must not only know about the insurance company from which you are purchasing the health insurance, its benefits, scope of coverage and exclusions, and payment responsibilities but also the general principles of health insurance and the implications of group versus individual coverage. In addition, you, the consumer, must also be knowledgeable about federal laws and programs that have been passed and created within recent decades that affect his health insurance protection. This section discusses some of these laws and programs.

The Health Insurance Portability and Accountability Act of 1996 (HIPAA)

**Congress passed the Health Insurance Portability
and Accountability Act of 1996 (HIPAA).
What are its important provisions and how do they affect me?**

In August 1996 Congress enacted the Health Insurance Portability and Accountability Act of 1996, effective January 1, 1997 (Public Law 104-191). One of the major purposes of the law is to protect workers from losing their health insurance coverage when they change jobs. Called portability, this means that if you are insured in your current job and you go to work for a new employer, you have the right to sign up for whatever coverage your new employer offers without undergoing a waiting period. As long as you have had a policy for at least twelve months, your insurability will be guaranteed if you join the new plan within thirty days of becoming eligible. Some insurers will require that you wait eighteen months for coverage if you enroll late. You'll get immediate coverage under your new employer's plan, including coverage for illnesses you already have had—that is, the company would be required to issue the policy without exclusions for preexisting conditions. This protects workers who are burdened with heavy medical expenses. Maybe you have chronic ailment such as diabetes; maybe you are pregnant, or your spouse is; maybe you are healthy but your spouse or one of your children isn't. Prior to this law, if you had changed jobs, your new company might not have covered these conditions right away. Under the new law, however, you will have to be covered. In addition, you cannot be charged higher premiums than someone in good health. However, this does not mean that you can take a more generous health plan with you when you go to your new employer, nor does it guarantee you insurance. If your new employer does not offer insurance coverage, portability will not assure you group coverage. But this new law gives you the right to purchase individual insurance coverage. In general, the portability provisions became effective July 1, 1997. The Health Insurance Portability and Accountability Act allows health insurers to charge what they want, even if it prices people out of their so-called guaranteed coverage.

The bill does not assist anyone without health insurance coverage now. If you have not had twelve or eighteen months of group coverage, health plans can force you to wait as long as twelve months before insuring most preexisting conditions (eighteen months if you do not join the new group right away). But this can happen only once during your lifetime. A break in prior group health insurance coverage lasting more than sixty-three days causes the qualifying period to begin all over again. There is immediate coverage, however, for pregnancy, newborns, and children placed in your home pending adoption if they've been enrolled within thirty days. Also, the insurance firms cannot discriminate against someone with a predisposition to a genetic illness. You may not receive every benefit that your new plan offers. Employers can limit you to the type of coverage you have had before. If your old plan didn't cover prescription drugs, for example, your new plan isn't required to offer it to you—even if others employees have it. Whether companies will act in this manner remains an open question. Nothing mandates what benefits the health plan has to cover. The employer could exclude certain illnesses for all employees or put a cap or ceiling on benefits. As long as premiums are paid, health insurers must renew coverage.

State and local government can choose not to participate in this law. That would free them to exclude your preexisting illnesses. Insurance companies that sell small-business plans generally have to take all buyers. They cannot reject or cancel a company that has had a lot of claims. This protection applies to firms that employ two to fifty people. There is no limit, however, to the cost of your premium. Employers can raise the group's plan copayments and deductibles as long as all employees pay the same. Insurers can also increase premiums on small plans with lot of claims. This law may not cause much in the way of additional price increases for group plans, however, because insurers can spread the risk.[24]

How does the Health Insurance Portability and Accountability Act of 1996 affect workers who leave their group plans and seek individual insurance?

If you are leaving a job for self-employment or have a job without insurance or have been fired, quit, laid off, or your employer went out of business, you can eventually purchase an individual health insurance policy under the act from any company that sells one in the state. And if you have received unemployment benefits for at least twelve weeks, the act allows you to make penalty-free withdrawals from an Individual Retirement Account to pay your premiums. If an individual has lost insurance coverage through a spouse in a divorce, then the individual is eligible for COBRA coverage for thirty-six months, after which the person could purchase insurance in the individual market. To qualify for the individual insurance, you first must come out of a group plan and, second, you must have been covered by a group policy for at least eighteen months and not be eligible for other insurance such as Medicare. If your former company employed twenty people or more, you can keep its group plan, at your expense, for at least eighteen months. You must have exhausted any benefits allowed under COBRA, the federal law that allows a person to stay with a former employer's group plan for eighteen months by paying the premium price, plus 2 percent. This coverage must be used up before the Health Insurance Portability and Accountability Act applies. If you allow group coverage to lapse and have been without protection for sixty-three days, then you could face a twelve-month wait before any preexisting condition is covered by any new insurance. Under the law, any health problem diagnosed or treated during the six months before enrollment in an insurance plan is a preexisting condition. There's no waiting period for coverage of health problems for which you haven't been treated in the last six months and which were diagnosed before then. There is no guarantee of coverage for persons who cannot pay premiums. State laws apply. If you haven't had eighteen months of group coverage and seek individual coverage rather than a group plan, you get no protection under the law. In these cases you can still be rejected for coverage or denied insurance for preexisting conditions.[25]

States have several options for arranging guaranteed, individual coverage. Each state will decide what those choices are. One possibility is bringing you into the high-risk insurance pools that exist in more than thirty states. Find out from your state insurance commissioner whether your state has established such a pool. But under this arrangement your premium costs can be far higher than the standard rate. Other state options include requiring open enrollment periods when health insurers have to take all buyers. States may require group plans to offer individual policies to departing workers. Or health insurers might have to sell policies to all qualified buyers. This law does not guarantee you coverage if you want to change from one individual policy to another; a group must be involved.[26]

Medical Expense Savings Accounts

What are Medical Savings Accounts (MSAs) and how do they work and differ from Health Savings Accounts (HSAs), Health Reimbursement Arrangements (HRAs), and Flexible Spending Accounts (FSAs)?

The basic difference between a medical savings account (MSA), later called Archer MSAs, and a Health Reimbursement Arrangement (HRA) is that the medical savings account is open to self-employed individuals and small businesses (50 or fewer employees) and the HRAs are open to large companies. Essentially a medical savings account is a tax-deferred trust or custodial account in which you set aside money to pay for routine, out-of-pocket healthcare expenses and to build up savings for your future medical costs. You or your employer contributes money to the MSA throughout the year or by making a lump-sum payment at the beginning of the year. An MSA must be paired with a major medical health plan (sometimes called a "catastrophic plan") that has a high deductible. Under the Health Insurance Portability and Accountability Act of 1996 Congress as a test established medical savings accounts as a way to pay for medical bills. From 1997 through the year 2000, insurance companies could sell up to 750,000 high-deductible policies for large medical expenses. Deductibles were established between $1,600 and $2,400 for a person and $3,200 and $4,800 for families.

The policyholder then could open a medical savings account. As noted, contributions, whether from an employer or the person, are not taxed, nor are any earnings. The maximum annual contribution is 65 percent of the insurance deductible for an individual and 75 percent for family policies. Money in the account can be withdrawn tax-free to pay most medical expenses, including premiums. After age sixty-five, it can be withdrawn for any reason. For those sixty-five and younger, withdrawals other than for medical expenses are subject to income tax, plus a 15 percent penalty.

To learn more about a medical savings account, contact an insurance agent or your employer. MSAs have been supplanted by Health Savings Accounts and, while existing MSAs can continue, new ones cannot be established. However, MSAs can be rolled over into HSAs. Distribution of medical savings accounts are governed by rules written by the US Treasury Department.

Health Savings Accounts (HSAs) were established on December 8, 2003, with the passage of the Medicare Prescription Drug, Improvement, and Modernization Act of 2003. An HSA is a savings/investment account that is allowed for an employee (or self-employed person) under sixty-five who has a high-deductible medical or insurance plan or policy to go along with it to pay for current or future medical expenses. As long as the high deductible health plan meets the requirements of this federal program, it can be an HMO, a PPO or an indemnity plan. This arrangement, sometimes called a "consumer-driven plan," is intended to encourage workers to look for inexpensive treatment and to avoid unnecessary spending.

Basically, the HSA is a combination of an IRA-like account with an insurance policy directed at only medical expenses. The HSA can be used to pay for routine medical bills and the insurance policy for larger medical expenses. But you pay a penalty in addition to income taxes if you use HSA money for nonmedical expenses before age sixty-five. After age sixty-five, you do not incur a penalty if you use the money for nonmedical expenses, but you would still have to pay income taxes on the money. On the other hand, you can continue to withdraw the money tax-free from the account for qualified medical expenses after age sixty-five. Participants choose among an array of investment options within the HSA account—that is, the money can be invested in a mutual fund, brokerage, bank account, or the like. Policyholders can establish an HSA and fund it with their own money even if they have the following kinds of health coverage: drug discount cards; specific disease or illness insurance and accident, disability, dental care, vision care and long-term insurance; employee assistance programs; disease management programs; or wellness programs as long as these programs do not provide significant benefits in the nature of medical care or treatment—and if you are eligible for VA benefits (US Department of Veterans Affairs) unless you have actually received VA health benefits in the last three months.

Except for the highest deductibles of $3,000 for a single person and $6,000 for a family, the worker and/or employer in 2006 can contribute an amount equal to the policy's others deductibles. In 2006 the worker and/or employer can contribute as much as $2,700 a year for a self-only plan ($3,000 deductible), or $5,450 for a family ($6,000 deductible). The money going in would be pretax dollars and withdrawals for medical care would be tax free. Under federal law in 2006, the insurance policy must have an annual deductible of *at least* $1,050 for an individual or $2,100 for a family. Excluding premiums, it must have annual out-of-pocket expense limits of $5,250 for an individual or $10,500 for a family in 2006. These amounts are indexed annually for inflation. It may, though, pay the entire cost of preventive care, which doesn't count as personal out-of-pocket expenses toward the deductibles, including periodic health evaluations (e.g., annual physicals); screening services (e.g., mammograms); routine prenatal and well-child care; child and adult immunizations; tobacco cessation programs; and obesity weight loss programs. The insurance also can apply copayments to preventive care services. If a person uses nonnetwork services, there can be higher out-of-pocket costs in terms of copayments and coinsurance.

An individual can use the money in an HSA account for a wide variety of medical expenses, and the money that an individual does not spend in one year can be carried over to the next year, as well as from job to job, allowing them to grow tax free. In retirement, whatever money remains in the accounts can be used to buy long-term care insurance and to pay for other qualified medical expenses. If self-employed, individuals can use their HSAs as tax shelters. They not only can write off their premiums but also can make tax-deductible deposits into their HSAs. But pay attention to their fees. Some plans may charge annual administrative fees, while other may not. The main problem with the HSAs is that the individual or family has to have the money to fund these savings accounts. So if you don't have the money to put into HSAs, they cannot help you very much. To learn more about HSAs you can go to http://www.Treas.gov and click on "Health Savings Account" or telephone 1-202-622-2960 or 1-202-622-4472 or e-mail:HSAInfo@do.Treas.gov.

Healthcare reimbursement accounts (or "health reimbursement arrangement" [HRA] in Internal Revenue Service terminology, Internal Revenue Code section 105-106) are a pot of employer-provided money that workers can use to pay medical costs not covered by health insurance or they can let the HRA monies accumulate over the years, and the funds would be available in retirement for the workers to supplement Medicare. In general, employers allocate workers an annual allowance—for example,

$2,500 for a family—to spend on medical expenses. The employer's contribution can be without limit, only defined by the employer's budget. Thus, the key difference between HSAs and HRAs is that the HRA is financed by the employer rather than the employee and any unused money belongs to the company. The Health Reimbursement Arrangement remains with the originating employer and does not follow the employee to a new employer. The employer can deduct the cost of the insurance plan as a business expense under Internal Revenue Code section 162. In regard to HSAs, employees make contributions to the HSA with pretax dollars—employers may or may not match them—and any unused money belongs to the employee. As already noted, HSA and HRA employees can expect to pay deductibles of at least $1,050 for an individual and $2,100 for a family in regard to their high-deductible health insurance plans before the health insurance plan begins to cover their bills for health services. Again, many high-deductible health insurance plans also require that the patients make coinsurance payments, which may range from 10 to 20 percent of the cost of services, after they meet their deductibles, and patients who look for care outside of the provider network can face even higher charges.

Except for the coinsurance or out-of-pocket expenses for which you are responsible, both the HSAs and the HRAs cover 100 percent of all medical expenses once the deductible has been reached. And both can pay 100 percent of preventive care costs, as already noted, which don't count as personal out-of-pocket expenses toward the deductibles. While they have coinsurance, these plans generally do not have any copayments, except in the possibility of covering preventive services as noted for HSAs. Also remember that the higher the deductible you meet, the less your health insurance premium; the smaller the deductible you meet, the higher your health insurance premium.

Also, if you are thinking of buying a high-deductible insurance plan, discuss it with your doctor. Traditionally, insurers pay all or most of a doctor's fees, with the patient making nominal payments for the visit. But under high-deductible plans, it is not often clear at the time of the office visit how much the patient will pay for that appointment. In addition, physicians are limited in their ability to discount fees to patients who are paying out of their own pockets. Patients cannot negotiate such payments because this would violate the contract physicians sign to join the insurer network. Therefore, when you are considering whether to be covered by a high-deductible health insurance plan versus a lower-deductible plan, compare the total costs of both premiums (higher and lower), and then, along with your annual premium costs, look at and add in what your annual out-of-pocket costs would be under a higher- and a lower-deductible plan. Then if you can, add in the costs if you faced a major medical problem. Which plan is better for you?

Also take into consideration the size of the provider network if you are considering a high-deductible plan because if you leave the provider network to receive care, the cost of your medical bills could increase greatly, for example, with higher copayments or deductibles. Therefore, when trying to decide between a higher- or a smaller-deductible plan, *you are a good candidate for a high deductible plan* if generally you are in good health and don't become ill because this means you won't spend as much money as comprehensive care requires, and those who go for years with minimal health spending can save a great deal of money tax-free in one of these HSA or HRA accounts; you have enough income or savings to pay for your out-of-pocket medical expenses; you know where to find cost and quality information on local health providers; and you understand how much money you must spend out of your own pocket to meet the requirements of your policy.

On the other hand, if you have a chronic illness or illnesses *you would be a bad candidate for a high-deductible policy* compared to a smaller-deductible plan because you could incur greater personal health service costs under a high-deductible plan that has a smaller premium than under a lower-deductible policy that has a higher premium. The reason is that you will pay less out of your own pocket in meeting the smaller deductible compared to paying more out of your own pocket in order to meet the higher deductible. As a result, because of these financial obligations you might delay seeking needed medical care like tests or drugs because you don't have the money to pay for them since the health insurance policy coverage only begins when you meet your high deductibles. Or a high-deductible plan might not be for you if you know you will be facing soon a major health issue; you have limited income and savings and suddenly cannot pay out hundreds or thousands of dollars in doctors, hospital, or drug bills from your own pocket; you depend upon costly medicine or multiple medicines; or you live in a community where your choice of healthcare providers is limited. Again, remember that regardless of whether a deductible is high or low, you must pay your personal medical expenses out of your own pocket first to meet the financial requirements of that plan's deductible before your health insurance begins to pay your bills.

Finally, with your high-deductible health insurance policy expect to receive bills from your provider, explanation of benefit forms, and other paper work, and if you open a tax advantage savings account, keep your receipts and be careful about your bookkeeping ability because your contributions may become mixed up with your employer's, making bookkeeping difficult throughout the claims payment process.[27]

On the other hand, "flexible spending accounts" (FSAs) are accounts through which *employees, not the employer* as in HRA, put aside their own money to pay unreimbursed health costs. A flexible spending account (FSA) is a benefit plan that allows companies to give their workers the opportunity to pay for their out-of-pocket health (medical/dental) and dependent care costs on a pretax basis, which, over time, lowers payroll-related taxes for both the employer and the employees—that is, the money you deposit into your account, which you set up each year, is deducted from your salary before it is taxed, giving you the benefit of immediate tax relief. It applies only to family members who qualify as dependents under IRS rules for income tax purposes. While there is no legal limit on the size of an FSA account, most employers establish their own maximums. The principal drawback of flexible spending accounts is the fact that employees must use the money or lose it. Employees decide at the beginning of the year how much money they think they will need, but if they fail to use it all up by the end of the year, they will lose the money, as already noted. This often leads to a splurge of late-year spending on health-related items as workers realize they have put aside too much money and consider buying something they really don't require or totally lose the money.

Again, in regard to an HRA, the company, not the employee, funds the account. HRAs were authorized by Congress in the mid-1990s. In addition, under HRAs contributions as well as withdrawals are not taxable to the worker if used for medical expenses, unused funds can be carried forward to the following year, and an employer may offer both a flexible spending account and an HRA to his employees. Some experts believe that the HRAs could also be used as single health insurance plans. An employer could contribute to the account and allow the workers to buy health insurance with the funds or pay their own costs out of the account. One model that is developing combines an HRA and high-deductible major medical insurance. The employer could offer the high-deductible plan, which could be cheaper—because, as already noted, the higher the deductible, the lower the premium—and then offer the HRA from which the employee could pay the deductible or other uncovered medical costs. Employees can draw from this account to pay for the usual office visits, diagnostic tests, and prescription drugs. But they can also use the money to buy services not covered under traditional managed-care plans, such as laser eye surgery. The plans keep the character of traditional systems that offer discounted rates for services provided in a network of doctor and hospitals. Once the employees spend the money in their accounts, they typically must use their own monies until they meet the annual deductible, ranging from a few hundred to a few thousand dollars, before coverage from a traditional plan begins. A premium is deducted from the employees' paychecks to help fund the coverage. Any allowance money left over can be rolled over to the next year, as already noted, allowing healthy workers to build, in effect, a personal healthcare bank account from which they can take monies whenever they wish and hopefully stay healthy as they evaluate whether they really need the medical care they are seeking.

The Consolidated Omnibus Budget Reconciliation Act of 1986 (COBRA)

What is COBRA and how can it protect me?

COBRA is a federal law that was enacted as Public Law 99-272 on July 1, 1986. COBRA makes it possible for employees and their spouses, and widowers and divorced spouses of covered employees, to continue their group health coverage for a period of time (up to three years). The law requires, as of January 1, 1997, that if you work for a business of twenty or more employees and leave your job or are laid off (except for gross misconduct) or lose health coverage because of reduced work hours, you can continue to get health coverage for at least eighteen months.

Also, under current law, a COBRA-qualified beneficiary may extend the original eighteen months of COBRA eligibility for up to twenty-nine months if the qualified beneficiary is disabled as of the date of the qualifying event and remains disabled through the end of the eighteen-month period. Effective January 1, 1997, the COBRA-qualified beneficiary can extend the COBRA coverage if she or he is determined to have been disabled at any time during the first sixty days of COBRA coverage, rather than the coverage requiring that the disability exist as of the date of the qualifying event. The provision became effective as January 1, 1997, as noted, regardless of whether the qualifying event occurred before, on, or after the effective date.

Another amendment to COBRA, effective January 1, 1997, makes a child born or placed for adoption during the COBRA period a qualified COBRA beneficiary. Thus, COBRA participants may be eligible to change their coverage status upon the birth or adoption of a child so that the child is covered for the balance of the continuation period.

Finally, COBRA is coordinated with the new preexisting-condition exclusion and special enrollment rules of the Health Insurance Portability and Accountability Act of 1996 (HIPAA). Under the new rules, when effective, COBRA coverage may be ended when a qualified beneficiary becomes covered under another group health plan, even if such a plan contains a preexisting-condition exclusion, unless the provision would still apply to the qualified beneficiary. This means persons who have group health insurance coverage cannot be denied group health insurance at a later date even if they have a preexisting health condition. A "preexisting condition" is a condition that is present before your enrollment date in any group health plan. Again, as already noted, if you have a significant break in your insurance coverage—sixty-three or more full days in a row—you could lose that and other protections.

In deciding whether to choose COBRA continuation coverage, you should consider all your healthcare options. For example, one valuable option that may be available is "special enrollment" in a spouse's plan, if requested within thirty days of the loss of your health coverage. This option is provided by the Health Insurance Portability and Accountability Act of 1996. However, this option is available only if your spouse is already covered by a separate health insurance policy. In addition, individuals in a family may be eligible for health insurance coverage through various state programs. For more information, you should contact your state department of insurance.

You also will be able to get insurance under COBRA if your spouse was covered but now you are widowed or divorced. If you were covered under your parents' group plan while you were in school, you also can continue in the plan for up to thirty-six months under COBRA until you find a job that offers you your own health insurance.

If you wish to continue your group coverage under COBRA, you must notify your employer within sixty days. You must also pay the entire premium, plus 2 percent of the cost of the coverage to cover administrative expenses. If you think you are being overcharged, contact the Employee Benefits Security Administration (formerly called the Pension and Welfare Benefits Administration [PWBA]). Note that group health coverage for COBRA participants is usually more expensive than health coverage for active employees, since usually the employer pays part of the premiums for active employees, while COBRA participants generally pay the entire premiums themselves, but it is ordinarily less expensive than individual health coverage. By law, an employer is required to send information within fourteen days to a former employee. If your employer refuses to send you any information or forms concerning COBRA, you or the secretary of the US Department of Labor may sue the employer to enforce this coverage. Failure to comply can result in daily fines of $100 until the problem is retroactively corrected. But if your employer goes bankrupt, there is no group health insurance, no COBRA. Once a company's group health plan is canceled, it does not have to provide a plan to connect your COBRA coverage. However, you can request a HIPAA policy that will take you with any preexisting medical conditions. But be aware these policies can be very expensive. Also, ask for a certificate of creditable coverage that shows how long you have had health coverage when leaving a job or changing your health insurance coverage because it shows how long you have had health insurance coverage. This is an important document to have if you need to show it to enroll in new group health plan or need to get individual coverage. Your employer or current insurance company is required to give you a certificate of coverage free of charge once your coverage ends or whenever you need to show proof of coverage.

Once you exhaust your COBRA coverage, you may be able to buy other health insurance under HIPAA. Some states have a conversion requirement, meaning that you must be given the option to convert to an individual policy once your COBRA coverage ends. A conversion is essentially an individual policy with the same carrier but with no preexisting medical restrictions. Also, be aware that many states have laws that allow persons to continue their insurance coverage if they work for a company with fewer than twenty people. If COBRA does not apply in your case—perhaps because you work for an employer with fewer than twenty employees—you may be able to convert your group policy to individual coverage by contacting your employer's insurance carrier directly and continuing the coverage. The advantage of doing so is that you may not have to pass a medical exam. The disadvantage, even if you are in good health, is that benefits may be reduced while premiums are higher.[28]

If you are not eligible for COBRA and you are a federal worker, check to see if you qualify for Temporary Continuation of Coverage, which is available to employees who lose their Federal Employees Health Benefits Program coverage because they leave their jobs. It is also available to divorced spouses or children who lose their family member status because they become age twenty-two or marry.

The Employee Retirement Income Security Act of 1974 (ERISA)

What is ERISA and how can it affect the kind of healthcare plan benefits I receive at work?

In 1974 the Employee Retirement Income Security Act (ERISA) was enacted into law. As a result of this law and rising healthcare costs, there was a rapid development of self-insurance health plans by various companies in which they pay their employees' doctor and hospital bills themselves, providing the companies with significant cost advantages. Self-insurance plans are not regulated by the state but rather by the US Department of Labor.

The original purpose of the law was to protect workers' fringe benefits. Although the law was aimed primarily at pensions, it has been interpreted by the courts over the years as overriding state regulation of employee health insurance plans in cases where the employer insures himself. When ERISA became law, such self-insurance was rare in corporations. Today, however, more than half of all US workers are employed by companies that self-insure, compared to only 5 percent in the 1970s, because self-insurance is less expensive than purchasing health insurance from a third-party payer. The reasons why is that self-insurance allows companies to cover only those ailments they choose to and to exclude a wide variety of coverage that state laws require of conventional insurance. In a little discussed and seemingly insignificant aside, the ERISA law at the time stated that if employers wanted to act as their own insurers—to pay premiums and pay out benefits themselves rather than using an insurance company—they would be exempt from all state taxes and regulations governing insurance. To the extent that it was discussed at all, the original intent of the ERISA health section exemption was to allow companies with dispersed operations to offer uniform health packages from state to state.

In November 1992 the US Supreme Court ruled that self-insured companies have the right to discriminate on the basis of disease in the type of health coverage they provide to employees. In the case in question, the court ruled that an Alabama music company had the right to reduce lifetime benefits for employees with AIDS from $1 million to $5,000 after an employee filed an AIDS claim. The court ruled that under ERISA self-insured companies are not subject to state insurance law requirements that would have barred such action. The company argued that its only choice was either to reduce AIDS benefits liability or cut out coverage for everyone else because the insurance costs for AIDS were so high. Although the Supreme Court decision applied to AIDS in this test case, it can apply to the benefit coverage of other diseases such as cancer as well. In addition, some large corporations have begun to combine their self-insurance system with the provision of general medical services provided by in-house medical clinics, staffed by their own doctors, or provided by contract medical firms, to lower their medical bills even more. Besides savings on drugs and tests, companies can save money by avoiding unnecessary hospitalizations through careful case monitoring and negotiating low fees with hospitals—a possibility when a firm can guarantee a hospital a lot of patients.[29]

Self-insurance is not always obvious. Your insurance documents and claim forms may bear the name of a well-known insurance company, yet you may be in a self-insured plan. The reason why is because corporations often contract with insurance or other firms as "third-party administrators," or TPAs, to process the claims. Also, the TPA arrangements do not subject the health insurance plan to state regulation. The TPA receives the claims, determines if they meet the plan's terms, and sends out the checks. However, the money is being paid by the employer; the TPA is not insuring the workers. Therefore, if you obtain coverage through your employer, find out whether the company self-insures, that is, pays claims out of its pocket, or buys coverage from an insurer.

In March 2001 the Supreme Court reaffirmed that ERISA and the pensions and other benefits it represents override state law. Also, health insurance regulation is often preempted. Thus, if the employee designates an ex-spouse as a beneficiary and not the current spouse, if remarried, then the benefits go to the ex-spouse, though the couple is divorced. Thus, when a divorce becomes final, parties should review the pensions, insurance, and other such assets and change the beneficiaries to match their intention (and whatever else they agreed to in the divorce).

The Americans with Disabilities Act of 1990 (ADA)

How does the Americans with Disabilities Act of 1990 affect the issue of pre-existing conditions and equality of health benefits with nondisabled employees?

The most immediate healthcare change that resulted from the implementation of the Americans with Disabilities Act in July 1992 has been that employers can no longer ask a potential employee about any health problems until a job has actually been offered. Questions about so-called preexisting health conditions can now only be asked during medical examinations or other tests and interviews that all prospective employees undergo after the job has been offered. If a person then has been rejected for the job, an employer must be able to show that it was for reasons other than the health cost of hiring that person.

Among other requirements of Americans with Disabilities Act of 1990 are the following:

- Disability-based insurance distinctions are allowed only if the employer-provided health insurance plan is bona fide and the distinctions are not being used as a subterfuge to evade the law.
- Employees with disabilities must be given equal access to whatever health insurance the employer provides to nondisabled workers.
- Employers may not make employment decisions about any person based on concerns about the impact on the health plan of the disability of that person or of someone else with whom that person has a relationship.

The Equal Employment Opportunity Commission (EEOC) believes that because the employer has control of the risk assessment, actuarial, and/or claims data upon which the employer may adopt a disability-based distinction relative to nondisabled workers, the burden of proof of such a decision should rest with the employer.

What about my income if I become disabled and cannot work?

Disability income insurance (also called loss of income insurance) helps replace the earnings you lose owing to a disability. Benefits during disability are limited to some portion of your regular income, such as 60 percent of a person's gross earnings at the time of purchase (typical group long-term insurance). For example, if you earn $400 a week, benefits might go up to $240 on a weekly basis.

These policies generally require that a person be totally disabled before the benefits are paid. Some policies provide benefits if an individual is partially disabled, usually following a total disability. Your policy may define total disability with one or a combination of the following characterizations: inability to engage in any gainful occupation for which you are suited by education, training, or experience; or inability to perform the duties of your occupation. The definition of disability offered in a policy is an important consideration. "Inability to engage in your own occupation" means a person could engage in another form of work and still collect full or partial benefits. It is far better than "inability to engage in any occupation," a definition that allows you to collect benefits only if you can't work at all. Read a loss of income policy carefully for the exact definition of "total disability."

Policies sometimes have waiting periods before benefits begin after the onset of the disability—these range anywhere from the thirty-first day to six months. The longer the waiting period, the lower the premium cost will be. Remember, though, the first check is usually not paid until thirty days after the waiting period. But many policies do provide benefits starting on the first day of an accident and the eighth day of an illness. Benefit periods for individual disability income insurance can range from one year to age sixty-five or even life, depending upon the contract. The longer the benefit period, the higher the premium cost. Also, remember, premiums can be reduced even further by reducing the percentage of monthly income you want to receive.

Some disability insurance policies contain a little-known benefit called "income insurance for the breadwinner's wife"; this covers the cost of household help if she becomes ill or disabled.

If you already have a disability policy, keep it. If you want to expand its coverage, just buy supplementary coverage. It pays to keep your old policy because it probably carries a lower premium, reflecting your younger age when you bought it. If your health is good, you may be able to get cheaper coverage even though you are older.

Also find out whether your disability policy will cover mental illness. If you become totally disabled as a result of a mental condition such as a nervous breakdown, many policies will pay you in full for these expenses. If your disability is only partial, your payments will normally cover up to one-half of all hospital costs.

When purchasing disability insurance, remember that the individual policy is the most expensive. Its advantages include the facts that the policy can cover you wherever you work or move and can be tailored to your needs as to the waiting time, size, and duration of your choosing. However, since work hazards can affect premiums and conditions of the policy, review your policy with your insurance carrier if you change jobs to make sure that you are still fully covered.

A group disability insurance policy purchased through your employer will cost less than an individual policy. The disadvantages of group disability insurance are that you cannot take the policy with you if you leave your job and you cannot readily convert it to an individual policy (as is possible with a group life policy). Your new employer may have a similar plan, so you should check with the company immediately. In general, if you pay premiums for an individual disability policy, payments you receive under the policy are not subject to income tax. If your employer paid some or all of the premiums, some or all of the benefits may be taxable.

Also, if you belong to a union or a professional association, you may be able to get an association disability insurance policy. Premiums are generally higher than for group policies but less than for individual ones. A limitation in many policies is that the package can be canceled even though you have been paying premiums for a long time.

To find out the best policy for your circumstances, find out whether it is non-cancelable; guaranteed renewable; optionally renewable; or cancelable. In a *non-cancelable*, generally more expensive, policy, premiums cannot be raised. In a *guaranteed renewable* policy, the insurance carrier cannot cancel but can raise premiums for a general risk class. *Optionally renewable* policies allow cancellation at an anniversary date or dates when the premium is due. Reasons for cancellation must be broad scale, never personal. *Cancelable* policies can be terminated at any time and generally without cause. Many states prohibit sale of the latter policies.

Do not purchase more policies or coverage than you need; make sure you understand the policy's maximum benefits and preexisting-condition exclusions, and check renewal rights. Disability policies requiring house confinement should not be bought. According to the insurance experts, confinement is not a valid element of the medical definition of disability. Also, buy both *accident* and *sickness* coverage. Some policies will only pay for accidents. You want to be insured for illness, too.

Monthly benefits are calculated in terms of stable, earned income at the time of purchase. Most insurers, not wanting to provide benefits so sizable that they would encourage workers to stay home, limit benefits from all sources to no more than 70 to 80 percent of monthly income. Lower-paid workers can expect to receive more of their predisability incomes, while higher-paid workers generally receive less.[30]

In an effort to improve disability insurance protection for your beneficiaries, the health insurance industry has developed several new concepts in disability coverage and they are available through major companies:

- A direct attempt is being made to help you keep up with the pace of inflation via a cost-of-living disability rider (also called "indexing") that, after a prescribed period, will increase your benefits based upon the official Consumer Price Index (CPI). Other indexed policies offer a flat guaranteed annual percentage increase. Look for CPI policies that offer a "catch-up" feature: If their maximum increase is, say, 8 percent, and in a given year the CPI increases just 3 percent, you have 5 percent left over to add to the next year's increase (that means you could get an increase of as much as 13 percent). There are certain questions you may ask in regard to a company's cost-of-living rider:
    - ▼ What is my annual premium for basic coverage?
    - ▼ How much monthly benefit can I purchase for that amount?
    - ▼ How much extra money will the cost-of-living rider cost me?

▼ What's your annual rate of increase?

▼ Is it calculated as simple or compound interest?

▼ Will I continue to receive indexing even after my benefit has doubled in size? Some policies do not stop after your benefit has doubled.

▼ Can my payments continue to be indexed even after I have reached age sixty-five? Is there a time limit to the post-sixty-five benefit period?

▼ Will I receive indexing even if I am not completely disabled?

▼ If I go back to work and then go back on disability, do I begin collecting benefits again at the previous inflated level?

▼ Is indexing of predisability income prior to a disability a standard feature?

- A special supplement rider has been developed that extends beyond the basic disability coverage of most policies. It pays an additional benefit when the insured is totally disabled but is not receiving any disability benefits under Social Security, Worker's Compensation, or no-fault automobile insurance for disability.

- "Residual" coverage also has been developed that becomes effective when there is a loss of income and a need for long-term benefits after the individual returns to his or her job on a part-time basis. Residual disability benefits provide benefits in proportion to a reduction of earnings as a result of disability as opposed to the inability to work full time. Thus, if you can work but your income is reduced because you cannot fulfill all your position's responsibilities, residual benefits can help to make up the difference in your income. A standard feature in some policies (added with rider to others), a residual benefit allows partial payment based on your loss of income generally without prior total disability. There is also the concept of "presumptive disability" in which even if you can still perform some or all of your regular job, you are presumed fully disabled and are entitled to full benefits under specified conditions, such as loss of sight, speech, hearing, or use of limbs.

- Some policies offer the opportunity to buy additional disability coverage to keep up with a rising income, without having to pass a medical examination or to submit further medical evidence of insurability.

Each of these can be obtained at moderate cost. You should find out if your insurance company offers these provisions in its disability insurance contracts—and whether they are necessary—if you are purchasing such insurance on an individual basis or as an employer. In addition, there are other questions you may wish to ask concerning a disability income policy that you are considering:

- Is the policy written to provide you with loss of income benefits if you cannot work, except on a reduced schedule? If not, can you obtain a rider at additional cost to cover this contingency?

- Does a period of disability have to precede a period of residual disability before benefits are paid?

- Does the payment of benefits depend on the reason for the disability?
- Does your policy contain a waiver of premium provision? With this clause in your policy, you won't have to worry about continuing to pay your disability insurance if disabled. Without a waiver, you would have to keep making payments throughout the period of disability if you wanted to keep your policy in force. A good waiver-of-premium provision will become effective after you have been disabled for ninety days, pay for all the premiums while you are disabled, and refund the premiums you paid during the first ninety days of disability. A poorer one will make you wait longer than ninety days and won't refund the early premiums. And some won't wave the premium unless you are totally disabled.[31]
- How long will the benefits last? A year? Until age sixty-five? To age seventy-two if still employed full time? A lifetime?
- How long can you wait before you need disability payments to begin?[32]

In determining your needs for disability insurance, be sure to take into account how long your employer will continue to pay your salary if you are not able to work; also consider how long any other income such as Social Security disability and, in a few states, state disability plan payments will continue. If you were in the military or were a civil servant, what about qualifying for government disability programs? This will enable you to calculate the right waiting periods for your needs and to better budget against loss of income. Remember, there are different definitions of disability. Be sure to ask your insurer what disability means in any policy you buy. Look for a policy that doesn't have too many restrictions on what kind of work you can do or what kind of income you want to maintain. Some policies are a lot harder on these factors than others. In this way, you will purchase the right policy at the lowest cost. Talk to several insurance agents who represent a variety of companies and read each policy carefully. It really pays to compare. Finally, before acquiring disability insurance, compute the total amount your family can get from all sources if your income should cease so that you can purchase the best set of benefits.[33]

There is no doubt that purchasing a health insurance policy may be one of the hardest and most complex decisions a consumer must make. To begin with, the market is huge: hundreds of commercial insurance companies, independent plans, and Blue Cross and Blue Shield plans. (Blue Cross pays hospital and related bills; Blue Shield pays medical-surgical bills. They are both nonprofit organizations.) Health insurance, as already noted, comes in more sizes, styles, and prices than any other type of insurance. The benefits, options, and language of policies are hard to compare. The result seems to be a fair amount of confusion on the part of policyholders. Consumers are not always sure exactly what their policies cover; because they do not understand, they complain when their policies do not live up to their expectations. It is hoped that the questions and guidelines cited in this chapter will enable you to understand your health insurance policy more clearly and assist you in purchasing the kind of policy you seek.

SEEKING MEDICAL CARE WITHOUT INSURANCE

But what should you do if you cannot afford health insurance? How can you still receive medical care for your illness? There are a number of options you may wish to consider. First, if you require medical care for your children, all states now offer health insurance coverage for children of low-income families through Medicaid or the Children's Health Insurance Program (CHIP). As part of the Balanced Budget Act of 1997, Congress created Title XXI, the State Children's Health Insurance Program (SCHIP). To address the growing problem of children without health insurance, SCHIP was designed as a federal/state partnership, similar to Medicaid, with the goal of expanding health insurance to children whose families earn too much money to be eligible for Medicaid but not enough money to purchase health insurance. SCHIP is the largest single expansion of health insurance coverage for children since the initiation of Medicaid in the mid-1960s. SCHIP offers states three options when designing the program. The state can use SCHIP funds to expand Medicaid eligibility to children who previously did not qualify for the program; to design a separate children's health insurance program entirely separate from Medicaid; or to combine both the Medicaid and the separate program options. Some states even cover parents of eligible children in low-income families who are working, the ability to do so increasing under section 1931 of the Social Security Act as well as using a combinations of state Medicaid section 1115 research and waiver demonstration initiatives and SCHIP funding authorities. In some states developing fetuses may be covered. The cost is either free or inexpensive, depending on your income and the state you live in. The insurance will pay for doctor visits, medicine, hospital care, and more, such as immunizations. As of December 2005, states had different eligibility rules, but in most states uninsured children under age nineteen whose families earn less than $36,200 a year (for a family of four) are eligible. To learn more and locate this program within your state government, telephone your state welfare or health department. In addition, you can find out what your state offers on the Internet by searching http://www.insurekidsnow.gov/states.htm or in Washington, DC, telephone toll free 1-877-543-7669.

In addition to children's health insurance coverage, if you are seeking health programs that will help you receive quality medical care free of charge, you may also go to the Web site sponsored by Unite for Sight, Inc. at http://www.uniteforsight.org. In addition to information on eye health, this Web site lists on its home page, at its Healthcare Portal, according to state, both free community-based clinics for medically underserved and uninsured persons and available free healthcare program coverage so that they can obtain quality care. Also ask your county health department or social services if there are free health clinics in your community. These clinics are staffed by doctors who volunteer their time, and they generally are located in disadvantaged areas of your community and are sponsored by state or federal governments.

Theres is also http://www.BenefitsCheckUp.org, which is one of the country's most complete online services for federal, state, and some local private and public benefits for older adults (fifty-five years and older). It contains more than thirteen hundred different programs from every state (including the District of Columbia). On average there are about fifty to seventy programs for individuals per state, including health coverage. In addition to identifying the programs from which persons may be eligible to receive assistance, the Web site also provides detailed descriptions of the programs, local contacts for additional information (typically the addresses and telephone numbers of where to apply for programs), and materials to help successfully apply for each program.

Another source for finding information about discounted or free medical care in the United States is the National Library of Medicine's MedlinePlus Financial Assistance Page at http://www.nlm.nih.gov/medlineplus—type in "financial assistance" in the search box. This site covers a number of topics, including financial assistance for the treatment of eyecare, cancer, diabetes, dental care, HIV/AIDS drugs, transplants, complementary and alternative medicine, long-term care, bleeding disorders, mental health services, Alzheimer's disease, pain, the homeless, patient care costs in clinical trials, pregnancy, and kidney failure.

For information on healthcare outside the United States, you may go to the Web sites of the International Federation of Red Cross and Red Crescent Societies, http://www.ifrc.org/address/directory.asp. There is also another Web site to find out about free or discounted healthcare that exists in foreign countries and may be found in a directory of international medical care organizations. Go to http://dir.yahoo .com/Health/Medicine/Organizations/International_ Relief_and _ Development.

Because low-income workers often have difficulty obtaining health insurance coverage through the public programs that are technically available to them, another development has occurred to make low-income health insurance available through employers. Two states, in addition to others, where this approach is working are Massachusetts and Idaho. Idaho established a "premium-assistance program," which is a subsidy program that promotes health insurance coverage by paying part of an employee's share of job-based health insurance premiums. In Idaho the program expands coverage by giving low-income workers a Health Insurance Access Card to enroll in the State Children's Health Insurance Plan, purchase individual coverage for children, or pay for employer-based family health plans. Workers in small businesses of fewer than fifty employees can use the access card to help pay for insurance. Massachusetts has a similar premium-assistance program, but the subsidy goes through the employer. In Massachusetts, for example, the state's Insurance Partnership program, working with the MassHealth Family Assistance Program (MHFAP), offers an incentive payment that encourages small businesses to offer health insurance to their low-income employees. Find out if your state has such a program to enable you to purchase health insurance if you are a low-income employee.

Going even further to protect its state's residents against the rising costs of healthcare, on April 4, 2006, Massachusetts became the first state in the nation to pass a compulsory law that requires every Massachusetts resident to have health insurance. The law requires all Massachusetts residents to be insured beginning July

1, 2007, either by purchasing insurance premiums directly or by obtaining it through their employers. The law does not call for new taxes but requires businesses that do not provide health insurance to pay an annual fee per employee. Phased in over three years, poor people in Massachusetts will be offered free or heavily subsidized health insurance coverage (the poorest having their premiums and deductibles completely paid for and those whose higher incomes are up to a specific percentage of the federal poverty level paying what they can afford without deductibles); those who are able to purchase health insurance but refuse will face increasing tax penalties until they obtain coverage; and those already insured are expected to witness a modest decrease in their health insurance premiums.

If you cannot afford to pay for hospital care, you may qualify for free or low-cost hospital care under the Hill-Burton program of the US Department of Health and Human Services. A Hill-Burton hospital is a facility that has received federal funds from this program for construction and modernization. Therefore, when you enter a hospital, look for a sign in the business office, emergency room, or admission office that says: NOTICE: *Medical Care for Those Who Cannot Afford to Pay.* Ask the admissions office for a copy of the Individual Notice. This notice will tell you what levels of income qualify for free care and what kind of free care the hospital is providing. The program only covers hospital costs, not physician bills. Once the hospital gives a certain amount of free care each year, they can stop. For more information about the program, you can contact the regional offices of the US Department of Health and Human Services in such cities as Boston, Philadelphia, New York, Atlanta, Chicago, Dallas, Kansas City, Denver, San Francisco, and Seattle. *Or you may telephone toll-free 1-800-638-0742 in any state except Maryland. In Maryland you may telephone 1-800-492-0359.*

In some states low-income persons with high medical costs qualify for their state's Medicaid program, funded by state and federal governments. If your costs are high and counted against your income, your income for medical eligibility may be low enough to qualify for Medicaid. If you become disabled, you may qualify for Supplementary Security Income.

Look at community health centers that provide both primary and preventive healthcare. They will diagnose your problem, prescribe medications, provide prenatal care, and immunize your children. To find centers in your community, go to the Internet Web site http://www.bphc.hrsa.gov and click on "Find a Health Center." Most centers provide care either free or on a sliding scale. Also, as already noted, to supplement this information, do not forget that Unite for Sight compiles information about free clinics in cities throughout the United States that provide free health services to the medically underserved and uninsured. The locations of free clinics by state are included in the information in addition to their telephone numbers and a list of their free services. Unite for Sight's Web address for the free clinics is http://www.uniteforsight.org/freeclinics.php.

Look at public hospitals that often have outpatient services available for those who cannot pay for inpatient care.

Finally, take advantage of free health screenings, free blood pressure checks, cholesterol screenings, and other services that are periodically offered in public places such as malls. With millions of Americans lacking health insurance, a new source of medical care is arriving at the mall, namely, medical clinics in retail stores. This concept hopes to capitalize on the fact that millions of Americans do not have any health insurance, must pay out of their own pockets for doctor's visits, and thus may be attracted to such medical facilities in retail stores. Their development is said to originate from a retailer's efforts to attract more customers for nonmedical shopping and thus increase business rather than the retailer establishing a medical clinic simply as another source of business revenue. Shoppers may be heading for the store to buy some items anyways and, if they already know that the retail establishment contains a medical clinic, will find it convenient to ask the clinic about that headache or cough that will not disappear. The retail clinic model is quite simple. A medical clinic is operated by an outside company in a retail store, generally is staffed by nurses and physician's assistants, and offers a limited range of basic tests and treatments at a lower cost than a doctor's office. These clinics are not the same as the stand-alone clinics that are sometimes referred to as "doc in a box." Patients never need an appointment and can visit them after regular business hours. Often the price of care is listed on a message board. The retail store clinics can operate at lower cost to patients because they have less overhead for medical office equipment, such as only needing cotton swabs, a tongue depressor, and simple laboratory work to diagnose a step throat. However, the lower overhead also means the clinics are limited in the kind of health services they can provide. Remember these retail clinics are not a substitute for the continuity of medical care a physician provides in his office or visiting an emergency room if you have an illness that requires this kind or degree of care nor should these retail store clinics be viewed as a continuous source of medical care instead of visiting a physician or a hospital when you need to visit such providers. But they do usually offer diagnoses for a predefined set of minor illness from ear infections to a strep throat to bladder infections as well as vaccinations. If you do have health insurance, find out if they accept your plan's coverage. However, if you do not have health insurance, compare their prices to what you can afford to pay because these retail clinics may be another source of access to medical care at a lower cost than a doctor's office visit and may be convenient to you in terms of their location—for example, at a mall's retail store. But also remember there is an important difference between being treated for a minor ailment and an illness that requires a doctor's attention whether in his office or, if necessary, in a hospital's emergency room. The bottom line is that a quick treatment at a lower cost at a retail store clinic may be better than no medical attention at all if the patient cannot afford to visit a doctor or an emergency room.

SOME FINAL CONSIDERATIONS ON HEALTH INSURANCE PLANNING

In summation, when planning your health insurance program, there are eleven principal points to remember.

1. Shop carefully. Policies differ widely in coverage and cost. Contact different insurance companies or ask your agent to show you policies from several insurers so you can compare them. Make sure your agent and the company he or she represents is reliable. Also, beware of high-pressure tactics by an agent or glowing promises in an advertisement. Do not be a victim of purchasing phony health insurance. Study the policy with special care before you sign up. Watch out for phony organizations that choose names resembling those of legitimate health insurance companies. Typically they advertise that rates are "25 percent to 50 percent below normal, and coverage is easy to obtain."[34] You may also be asked to join an association and write a premium check. Be careful. Also, be wary of "discount plans" that are not health insurance policies. They offer reduced rates for medical services, but patients can sometimes obtain price reductions on their own. Some are bait-and-switch scams in which promised services are not provided. Find out from the state insurance department if the company is licensed to do business in your state, whether anyone has filed any complaints against the company, and what was the nature of the complaints. To learn more about insurance fraud, visit http://www.insurancefraud.org.

2. Determine as precisely as you can what your health insurance needs are and make sure your coverage fits them. Pay special attention to "catastrophic coverage"—that is, a high-benefit major medical policy—and protection against loss of income.

3. Read and understand the policy. Know exactly what your insurance will pay for and what it won't.

4. If you pay your premiums directly, ask your insurer whether it would be cheaper to pay on an annual or quarterly basis rather than a monthly basis.

5. When you receive a policy, take advantage of the "free look" provision. You have ten days to look it over and obtain a refund, if you decide it is not for you.

6. Check to see that the policy states the date that the policy will begin paying (some have a waiting period before coverage begins) and whether any of your current or preexisting conditions will be covered.

7. Beware of single-disease insurance policies. There are some policies that offer protection for only one disease, such as cancer. If you already have health insurance, your regular plan probably already provides all the coverage you need. Check to see what protection you have before buying any more insurance.

8. Ask your state insurance commission whether your state has established a health insurance plan for its residents. Though differing in detail, health insurance plans already exist in Hawaii and other states. If you qualify, these state insurance plans may reduce your medical expenses.

9. Remember there are other disability benefit programs for which you may qualify if you don't have private disability income insurance. These include

a state's Worker's Compensation program, Veterans Administration pension disability benefits, Civil Service disability benefits (if you are a government worker), Black Lung benefits, automobile insurance (if disability results from an auto accident), State Vocational Rehabilitation benefits, group union disability coverage, private insurance (such as credit disability insurance that makes monthly loan payments when you are disabled), and the Cash Sickness programs of California, Hawaii, New Jersey, New York, Rhode Island, and Puerto Rico, which provide income replacement to residents disabled because of nonoccupational injury or illness. The benefits vary considerably among the jurisdictions. Find out from your state insurance commission whether your state has established such a program or plans to do so in the future.

10. Periodically review your insurance to make sure it is keeping up with your family's present situation as well as today's cost of care.

11. Finally, compare policies. It is possible to save money on the kind of coverage you need—just make sure you understand what you are buying.

If you have questions about a group plan, you should be able to get the answers from your employer or your union or association officer. If you have questions about an individual or family policy, talk them over with your insurance agent or contact the insurance company directly. In the final analysis, you and your loved ones will benefit from your research and planning.

NOTES

1. *Source Book of Health Insurance Data, 2002* (Washington, DC: Health Insurance Association of America, 2002), pp. 6, 11 (table 1.1).

2. *Source Book of Health Insurance Data, 1977–1978* (Washington, DC: Health Insurance Institute, 1978), pp. 7–8.

3. US Department of Health, Education, and Welfare, "Independent Health Insurance Plans in 1976," *HCFA Health Notes*, Washington, DC, pp. 2–3; and Karen Pallarito, "A Business Prescription," *US News & World Report*, July 25, 2005, pp. 38–39.

4. *Source Book of Health Insurance, 1977–1978*, pp. 22, 24.

5. *Source Book of Health Insurance Data, 1996* (Washington, DC: Health Insurance Association of America, 1996), pp. 16–18.

6. Jane Bryant Quinn, "A Poor Health Insurer Can Leave You Ill-Prepared," *Washington Post*, March 15, 1992, p. H3.

7. Ibid.

8. "Who, Me? Need Health Insurance," *Current Consumer*, January 1978, pp. 4–14.

9. US Department of Health, Education, and Welfare, *How to Shop for Health Insurance* (Washington, DC: Health Resources Administration, 1978), pp. 7–8.

10. *The Consumer's Guide to Health Insurance* (Washington, DC: Health Insurance Association of America, 1992), p. 17.

11. *How to Shop for Health Insurance*, pp. 5–7.

12. "Cancer Insurance: A Closer Look," *Good Housekeeping*, January 1979, p. 176.

13. Julia Angwin, "Gaps in Coverage after College," *Washington Post*, March 16, 1993, p. 9; Peter Weaver, "Covering the Kids' Medical Bills," *Washington Post*, November 19, 1978.

14. US Department of Health and Human Services, "Checkup on Health Insurance Choices," Public Health Service (Washington, DC: Agency for Healthcare Policy and Research, December 1992), p. 10; "A Checklist for Rating the Quality of Health Plans," *Washington Post*, November 15, 1988, p. 22; and "Does Coverage Meet Your Needs?" *Today's Health* 47 (December 1969): 54.

15. Maureen Smith Williams, "Health Insurance: The Higher Cost of Being a Woman," *McCall's*, May 1979, p. 70.

16. Carolyn Jabbs, " Health Insurance Policies Are Not All Alike," *Ms*, June 1978, p. 88.

17. Jane Bryant Quinn, "Individual Health Policies Compete with Group Plans," *Washington Post*, June 2, 1991, p. H3.

18. Victor Cohn, "Solo Insurance Hunting," *Washington Post*, November 17, 1992, p. 15.

19. "Stop-Gap Insurance," *Changing Times* 32, no. 9 (September 1978): 38.

20. *The Consumer's Guide to Health Insurance*, p. 15.

21. Albert Crenshaw, "Retiring? Don't Assume Health Benefits Are Forever," *Washington Post*, November 3, 1996, p. H6.

22. *The Consumer's Guide to Health Insurance*, pp. 16–17; Leonard Sloane, "Health Plans: A Rule Change," *New York Times*, May 28, 1983, p. 36.

23. Sylvia Porter, "Avoid Being Divorced from Health Insurance," *Washington Star*, November 13, 1980.

24. Jane Bryant Quinn, "Insurance Safety Net Still Has Gaps," *Washington Post*, August 25, 1996 (Business Section).

25. Dave Skidmore, "Understanding the Kassenbaum-Kennedy Health Coverage Bill," *Washington Post*, August 19, 1996, p. A13.

26. Jane Bryant Quinn, "Guaranteed-Coverage Law May Hurt Some," *Washington Post*, September 29, 1996 (Business Section).

27. Christopher J. Gearson, "High Deductible, High Risk," *Washington Post*, October 18, 2005, pp. F1, F4 (Health Section); *All about HSAs* (Washington, DC: US Treasury Department, November 28, 2005), pp. 8, 13, 17.

28. *The Consumer's Guide to Health Insurance*, p. 14; "Checkup on Health Insurance Choices," p. 3.

29. Malcom Gladwell, "When Health Plan Changes Leave Employees Vulnerable," *Washington Post*, August 20, 1992, pp. A1, A4.

30. *Guide to Disability Income* (Washington, DC: Health Insurance Association of America, 1995).

31. Stephen Kaufman, "Are Your Disability Benefits In Step with Inflation?" *Medical Economics* 60, no. 8 (April 18, 1983): 223, 229.

32. "Check These Features before It's Too Late," *Medical Economics* 60, no. 20 (October 31, 1983): 92.

33. *What You Should Know about Health Insurance* (New York: Health Insurance Institute, 1978), pp. 9–11; Sylvia Porter, "Shop Carefully for Disability Insurance to Cover Income Losses," *Washington Star*, February 3, 1980.

34. "Health Insurance Scam," *Parade*, December 8, 2002, p. 24.

CHAPTER FOUR

MANAGED CARE

INTRODUCTION

One of the most recent innovations in regard to healthcare financing and delivery is a concept called managed care. This idea refers to a variety of methods for financing and organizing the delivery of comprehensive healthcare through which efforts are made to influence healthcare costs by controlling the delivery of services. Thus, managed care is basically a mechanism to reduce healthcare expenditures by controlling the use of healthcare services. Managed care is an alternative to traditional fee-for-service medicine in which the independent solo practitioner has a direct relationship with the patient and decides what tests, referrals, and treatment are appropriate and in which cost has never been a primary consideration. The term *managed care* includes such organizations as health maintenance organizations (HMOs), preferred-provider organizations (PPOs), and point-of-service financing and delivery systems (POSs). The rapid growth of managed care reflects the increasing determination of employers to hold down healthcare costs by limiting their employees' options through this operational and financial concept.

Managed care plans and more and more health insurance policies that provide coverage on a fee-for-service basis include certain features of managed care. Primary care physicians are used as coordinators and managers of care. *Utilization review* and *quality assurance* are terms applied to methods of making sure that the patient receives the most appropriate, cost-effective care. The managed care plan, or the insurance company, may require that the patient obtain authorization before being admitted to a hospital, or obtain a second surgical opinion before certain types of surgery; it may also mean that the plan or the insurer will facilitate the transfer of patients from a hospital to a more cost-effective facility (if the patient no longer needs to be in the hospital but cannot be cared for at home).

Utilization review may also include "case management," an approach designed for certain challenging cases. One example would be an expectant mother who has a disease that could cause a premature delivery. Rather than hospitalizing the patient, her managed care program arranges homecare services that accomplish the same goals, namely, a full-term baby, both mother and baby in good health, and at less cost than hospital care. Thus, the purpose of managed care is to provide quality care while helping to contain the expenses of healthcare.

All segments of the healthcare industry have developed managed care organizational models or networks. These include physicians, large payers, hospital systems, large corporate entities, and joint ventures between physicians and hospitals. Each model is somewhat different depending upon the sponsoring group, but their common characteristic is that they include both the financing and the delivery of healthcare services.

The most common networks are the following:

- preferred-provider organizations (PPOs)
- health maintenance organizations (HMOs)
- exclusive provider arrangements (EPAs)
- point-of-service plans (POSs)

Although different in many aspects, all these plans have the following features: (1) arrangements with selected providers to deliver a comprehensive set of healthcare services to their members; (2) explicit standards for selecting healthcare providers; (3) programs for ongoing quality assurance and utilization review; and (4) financial incentives for members to use providers and procedures associated with the plan.[1] Despite these shared features, not all physicians will be involved in the managed care networks. The credentialing of physicians will examine not only their medical qualifications but also the cost and quality of care the physician delivers. Economic credentialing thus becomes a hard reality in terms of physician participation within the world of managed care. As healthcare reform continues to evolve, a variety of other models for delivering and financing healthcare services in cost-effective and quality-efficient ways can be expected to be established in the future.

In 2000, 80.1 million persons were enrolled in HMOs. And managed care companies now are developing specialty networks for mental health, vision, dental, chiropractic, podiatric, and physical therapy care. Sophisticated managed care principles are also being applied to other fields, such as long-term care, as well as to medical bills associated with auto liability and worker's compensation claims. The growth of managed care can be expected to continue as new variations on existing models (and new applications) evolve.[2]

The concept of managed care, especially as related to HMOs, is not new. These organizations were called prepaid group practice plans until congressional law redefined them as HMOs in 1973. The first prepaid group practice plans were established in the late 1920s. In terms of definition, prepaid group practice plans are those to which payments (premiums) are made in advance into a fund that is used to pay for an individual's health services when the need arises. Such services may be provided, for example, by a group practice. In its most basic form, group practice is a systematic relationship between physicians and dentists who are organized for the conduct of their practice. Comprehensive group practice may provide preventive, diagnostic, and curative services by family or general practitioners, specialists, and the other professional and subprofessional technical staff working as a team in a medical center, sharing their knowledge, experience, equipment, and medical records as well as pooling their income. A health maintenance organization operates as a group practice.

Federal law recognizes two kinds of HMOs: the group/staff or " closed panel" HMO in which physicians practice together, under one roof, and are either part of a medical "group," pooling their income, or are on salary and part of an HMO "staff"; and the Independent Practice Association (IPA) or "open panel" in which the physicians practice in their own offices, not in a centralized facility, and are part of an organized system of healthcare with coordination of referral and hospital care.

According to the Health Maintenance Organization Act of 1973, HMOs must provide a prescribed range of basic health services. In addition, an HMO has the option of providing supplemental services if the HMO considers it feasible, in return for a prepaid, fixed, and uniform payment. Such is the conceptual nature of a health maintenance organization.

In terms of history, the growth of prepaid group practice plans in this country during the past half century has been characterized by great controversy. Medical societies, both locally and nationally, opposed their development—often in bitter litigation. These lawsuits involved the issues of whether physicians practicing with closed-panel groups had the right of hospital privileges as well as the right of membership in medical societies.

For purposes of discussion, two kinds of group practices must be identified. Some groups consist primarily of specialists and act as referral centers. Examples of such groups include the Mayo Clinic of Rochester, Minnesota; the Lahey Clinic of Boston, Massachusetts; and the Ochsner Clinic of New Orleans, Louisiana. In the other classification, groups consist of a substantial number of personal physicians. They not only provide referral service but also comprehensive care for the patient or for the patient and his family. In addition, such group practices also may be prepayment plans to which the patient and/or his family are a subscribing member. An example of the latter group is the Kaiser Foundation Health Plans, certified as HMOs by the federal government.

The very early era of prepaid group practice predates the large-scale expansion of voluntary health insurance in this country. Most of the early attempts at group practice originated in the labor unions and industrial organizations as the only viable means of bringing a minimum of health services to workers. Typical industrial developments included the early health service programs of the railroad, lumbering, and mining industries, while medical centers of the International Garment Workers were large-scale union prototypes in this field. But these programs were poorly financed; they never really succeeded in developing the popularity voluntary health insurance has had since the end of World II. Yet these organizations, despite their lack of universal appeal, did establish excellent reputations as being providers of high-quality care through an organized system.[3] Because prepaid group practices emphasize preventive care and ambulatory services—as opposed to the private health insurance system, which stresses inpatient hospital care rather than outpatient preventive care treatments—HMO members are hospitalized at a rate of 30 to 40 percent less than non-HMO members.[4] The preventive care emphasis of HMOs allows an illness to be detected early in its more curable stages, thus reducing the need for hospital care. Because of this mode of operation, the evidence indicates that HMO-type systems significantly reduce the cost of care without lowering its quality. Through a combination of management and provider incentives, HMOs can reduce costs below unmanaged fee-for-service by about 20 percent and below managed fee-for-service by about one-half that amount.[5]

Consequently, when healthcare costs began to rise dramatically in the period following the implementation of Medicare and Medicaid in the mid-1960s through the 1970s, a reexamination of the healthcare system seemed urgent. The Nixon administration undertook such a study. In the course of analyzing the system, the administration considered HMOs as one means of containing runaway healthcare costs. After a thorough study of the concept, the government decided to promote HMOs as a major federal initiative. Thus, a series of bills was introduced in Congress in the early 1970s—one by the Nixon administration, another by Senator Edward M. Kennedy, and still another by Congressman William R. Roy. Public hearings were held on these bills, and discussions took place with representatives of various elements of the healthcare industry. Legislative language was revised, compromises achieved, and, finally, in the late fall of 1973, the Health Maintenance Organization bill was passed by Congress, and President Nixon signed the bill into law (Public Law 93-222) in December of that year.

Managed care, especially HMOs, continues to be one of this country's most important responses to escalating healthcare costs. By 2002 there were five hundred HMOs operating in the United States with total enrollment of 76.1 million persons, a decline of about 4 million since 2000.[6]

In addition to private-sector enrollment, government programs such as Medicare and Medicaid also began enrolling their members in HMOs. In 2000 the number of Medicaid enrollees in HMOs increased to 18.8 million persons, or 55.8 percent of Medicaid's 33.7 million enrollees, and the number of Medicare enrollees who chose HMOs increased to 5.8 million in 2001, or 14.5 percent of 40 million Medicare enrollees.[7]

By January 1998 the majority of HMOs were using a variety of measures to control healthcare costs: home healthcare, preventive health, and preferred provider negotiations. Other cost-control measures include risk-management programs, durable medical equipment monitoring, retrospective review admissions, discharge planning, and the usual inpatient and outpatient utilization review.[8]

One dramatic impact of the growth of HMOs and other managed care formats has been that for the first time in US history, doctors who are working as employees at large group practices outnumber solo practitioners. The shift—the crossover point took place in 1992–1993—is attributed in part to the growth of managed care, which makes it harder for solo practitioners and small group practices to negotiate group contracts. Now employee physicians outnumber solo practitioners. According to American Medical Association researchers, should these trends continue, a majority of physicians could very well be employees in the very near future, subject to increasing bureaucratic oversight, less independence in making medical decisions, and intense pressure to watch the bottom line.[9] To counter these trends, the federal government (the Federal Trade Commission and the US Justice Department) eased antitrust regulations on August 28, 1996, in order to allow physicians to join together in networks so they can provide stronger competition to managed care plans, which dominate US healthcare. In order to meet the government's guidelines, the Federal Trade Commission (FTC) and the Justice Department said physician networks—known generally as independent practice associations (IPAs) or preferred-provider organizations (PPOs)—would have to offer consumers substantial benefits through lower costs and higher quality of care. These new guidelines are expected to continue to encourage the formation of IPAs and PPOs across the country as physicians seek greater leverage over managed care plans. According to the FTC, an example of the kinds of networks that the new guidelines would allow are physicians who operate under the traditional-fee-for-service system and could form a group and set common fees if they design a system that produces high-quality care at low cost, that is, achieves clinical integration. To meet that test, physicians in the group would have to invest in technology that could exchange information on practice patterns and results. Physicians believe that physician networks will allow them to provide better care at lower cost than an HMO, which holds down costs by being more restrictive in terms of a patient's access to specialists and hospitals.[10]

IS THERE AN HMO IN YOU FUTURE?

Although you may not be acquainted with health maintenance organizations, there is a distinct possibility that there may be one in your future. HMOs are not only enrolling business and other organizational employees but also Medicare and Medicaid beneficiaries—although according to federal law Medicare and Medicaid beneficiaries cannot constitute more than one-half of an HMO's membership. The number of HMOs in the country is expected to increase in the ensuing years, spurred by private business and a federally sponsored program to reduce medical costs.

As already noted, HMOs come in various sizes and types. Some, like the Kaiser Foundation Health Plan in Los Angeles, have more than a million members; most have thousands. Some operate from a single center; in others, members are treated in a doctor's private office and the bill is sent to the HMO. There may be an HMO in your area; it might be called a foundation for medical care, a group health plan, or a community health plan.

If you are interested in joining an HMO or learning more about it, ask your local health department or county medical society whether one has been established.

In contrast to the fee-for-service medical practice of private physicians or group practice clinics, HMOs provide most of your medical care without cost, except for a monthly premium. Also, unlike private health insurance, there are no claim forms to fill out or regular major out-of-pocket expenses for medical services. On the other hand, unlike individuals who can freely choose their own physicians and hospitals under private health insurance plans, HMO members can only use those doctors (including specialists) and hospitals affiliated with the HMO, although they can freely choose among those doctors who are on its staff.

The term *health maintenance* in the title of this organization derives from its basic purpose—namely, to maintain your health by emphasizing *preventive* medical care. Because an HMO receives a fixed premium for all medical and hospital services, regardless of the amount of services used, it has an incentive to provide high-quality preventive care and not engage in excess hospitalization or perform duplicative or unnecessary tests. Studies have shown that when HMO-salaried doctors contract to deliver health services at fixed costs, they are less apt to perform unnecessary surgeries or to prescribe marginal tests or procedures that run up health bills, and overall costs are lower than in fee-for-service cases.[11] With a typical health insurance policy, the family has to pay for regular preventive care, office visits, well-baby care, immunizations, and sometimes a certain amount of hospital expenses and part of a surgeon's fee. These are all covered by the HMO.

WHAT YOU SHOULD KNOW ABOUT AN HMO

"James, what do you think? Should I or shouldn't I join an HMO? I have heard so many stories about their rationing care, impersonal attention, not being able to receive care or at least delayed care when your doctor thinks you need it, and other problems, I don't know if I should take the chance. At least under traditional health insurance, I can choose any doctor I wish and have other freedoms and am not limited to just the doctors who are affiliated with the HMO to receive HMO coverage."

"Joe, how bad can they be? Millions are joining them each year. They are still in business after all these years. They provide benefits that may not be available elsewhere. You don't get billed each time you visit a doctor like under fee-for-service medicine because the idea of the HMO is to visit as many times as you wish for a single monthly premium. This way, if you feel sick, you don't have to stay away from a doctor because you cannot pay and then become worse. You can catch your illness before it worsens and, perhaps, be able to stay out of the more expensive hospital."

"James, both these arguments seem credible. Maybe that is why I am having a hard time deciding what to do. Maybe the real problem is that I really don't even understand the concept of managed care and all its ramifications that go beyond the advertisements I have read trying to get me to join one HMO or another."

"Joe, I think that is a problem that many people have and ought to be corrected."

As already noted, health maintenance organizations and managed care represent one of the alternatives being developed to give the American consumer a choice as to how he wishes to receive and pay for his healthcare. However, because HMOs began their rapid growth in the latter part of the twentieth century in terms of government definition, many questions are being raised in regard to them, including the following.

What is managed care?

In contrast to the traditional fee-for-service system, managed care is a planned and coordinated approach to providing healthcare services. Its goal is to lower health costs without sacrificing the quality of care. Under managed care you no longer go to any doctor or hospital you wish if you want your health insurance to pay the bill. It also means that people besides you and your doctor decide what treatments you may obtain in health plans, which closely monitor and often limit treatment, both to save money and, it is stated, to improve your health.

Managed care is being applied in two forms. One is a case-by-case review and "approvals" and "denials" in traditional insurance coverage. This is called utilization review. It typically means you must obtain a second opinion before surgery, and a nurse or doctor on the telephone at a review company has to give his or her approval before you can go to the hospital, except in an emergency. The reviewer usually limits the number of days the plan will pay for hospital or mental health or other care, if it will pay at all. It may say a doctor or dentist has charged more than the plan will pay, leaving you with the rest of the bill. But more formally, *utilization review* is a collective term for the following activities:

- *Preadmission certification*, in which elective hospitalizations are evaluated against standard criteria prior to admission. The purpose of this review is to determine whether the admission, diagnostic testing, or surgical procedure is appropriate.
- *Concurrent review*, or the formal review of ongoing hospitalizations to determine whether the length of stay and any subsequent medical intervention is appropriate and consistent with good medical practice.
- *Discharge planning*, in which, to keep hospital stays to the shortest appropriate length, the HMO prearranges for care to be received after discharge.
- *Case management*, in which systematic reviews take place to identify patients who, because of the severity of their illness, are likely to require prolonged hospitalization or intensive therapy. These patients are carefully monitored to assure the most appropriate and cost-effective care is being delivered.[12]

Another form of managed care is enrollment in various kinds of restricted groups of doctors and hospitals, for example, health maintenance organizations. Thus, managed care organizations do not actually make decisions about your medical care; your doctor does. But the organizations do decide about whether a particular service will be covered and, in that way, influence the kind of care you receive. Your managed care organization determines which doctors, hospital procedures, and sometimes even which medicines are covered by your insurance plan.

Most plans have enough doctors and hospitals to provide comprehensive care and some degree of choice. If you want a particular doctor, hospital, or procedure, then it's important to pick an insurance plan that includes the one you want. The problem is that some people obtain their insurance through their employment and, thus, don't have that option. So make sure you understand thoroughly the details of your managed care contract to ensure that it is the kind of health insurance protection you seek for yourself and your loved ones.

Thus, in managed care the insurer or employer does more than pay the bills. The payer becomes involved in choosing the doctor, hospital, or other provider and in deciding what care will be provided. Patients who insist on seeing a different doctor or undergoing an unapproved procedure will have to pay more.

What is the difference between an HMO and a PPO?

A health maintenance organization (HMO) contracts with or employs a group or groups of doctors, hospitals, and other healthcare providers in a limited number of locations to deliver services to member patients under a fixed premium rate. A preferred-provider organization (PPO) is a health plan that negotiates with providers of care to give purchasers of care lower rates if their member patients use doctors from a selected list.

What are the different types of HMOs available?

There are five basic kinds of HMOs in operation. These include:

- *Staff model*. In a staff model HMO, physicians practice solely as employees and are usually paid a salary.
- *Group model*. In a group model, the HMO pays a physician group a negotiated, per capita rate, which the group, in turn, distributes among individual physicians.
- *Network (direct contract) model*. A network model HMO contracts directly with two or more independent (single or multispecialty) group practices to provide services, rather than work through an intermediary, and pays a fixed monthly fee per enrollee. The group decides how fees will be distributed to individual physicians.
- *Independent practice association (IPA)* In an IPA, the managed care plan contracts with individual physicians in independent practice or as an *Independent Practice Plan (IPP)* contracts with associations or groups of independent physicians to provide services to the plan members at a negotiated rate per capita, or flat retainer, or a negotiated fee-for-service rate. Physicians main-

tain their own offices and see patients on a fee-for-service basis while contracting with one or more plans.

- *Mixed.* A mixed model combines two or more models in a single HMO.[13]

What is a federally qualified HMO?

A federally qualified HMO is a prepaid health plan—either a group or an IPA—which agrees to meet the various requirements of the federal government's HMO law.

These requirements include the following: a stipulation of the kind of health services to be offered; a community rating (everyone, regardless of age or health status, pays the same premium); a board of directors on which one-third are HMO members; provision of medical and social services and health education to HMO members; fiscal soundness with safeguards against insolvency; inability to expel any member because of health status; and enrollment of persons broadly representative of the HMO service area.

There are also many nonqualified HMOs operating in the country that provide comprehensive health services. The difference between a federally qualified HMO and one that has not been so certified is that the qualified HMO must meet standards mandated by federal law. The nonqualified HMOs determine their own requirements and, for reasons of their own, have not chosen to obtain federal qualification.[14]

Why should I want or not want to join an HMO?

You may wish to join an HMO if you:

- want to obtain a variety of prepaid medical services under one roof
- are not satisfied with your present physicians
- need a way to find doctors, perhaps because you have just arrived in your community
- want unlimited office visits, perhaps because you have a chronic disease
- dislike the problems of filing insurance claim.
- place a high value on preventing illness and staying out of hospitals

You may not wish to join an HMO if you:

- are content with your present physicians
- dislike making appointments far ahead of schedule
- learn that the HMO in your area is known for skimping on medical care

What are the advantages and disadvantages of belonging to an HMO?

Advocates of HMO services state that the advantages of its healthcare include the following:

- One-stop medical care where comprehensive services that are efficiently coordinated are available for all family members and all conditions.
- Twenty-four hours of service, seven days a week.
- Convenient location.
- More health benefits including preventive care and follow-up for the same money.
- A physician who has ready access to your medical records and is backed up by a range of specialists providing a continuity of care.
- HMOs have little or no paperwork and do not require claim forms for office visits or hospital stays.
- Patient education services are available such as classes for persons with diabetes or hypertension.
- You can join an HMO regardless of your medical condition, provided you sign up as a member of a group. If you wish to join as an individual, the HMO may require a physical examination.
- Provision of better treatment at lower cost and lower rates of hospitalization for HMO members because of the HMO's emphasis on preventive health services compared to private health insurance policyholders who use fee-for-service medical services and the use of primary care physicians as gatekeepers to restrict access to costly specialists, tests, and hospitalizations.
- Your medical records are centralized because your doctors are all in one location. Thus, by glancing through your file folder, or, in some HMOs, your computerized case history, any of your physicians can learn about your past health problems and how other doctors treated them.
- With the removal of the burden of having to pay for each physician office visit, people tend to seek treatment earlier, often allowing a disease to be detected in its most curable stage before it worsens and possibly requires hospitalization.
- Less inferior care under the HMO system than under traditional fee-for-service medicine because it constantly reviews physicians' practices.

Critics of HMO services state the disadvantages of HMO healthcare include the following:

- You cannot choose your own doctor. You can only use those doctors who belong to the group, and the HMO may encourage physicians to see you as little as possible because the physicians are paid an established annual fee no matter how many appointments you make, so the fewer appointments a physician sees you, the less he works on your behalf and keeps expenses to a minimum. Critics say that if you require a particular treatment, ask the physician to write a letter on your behalf for that particular treatment and tell him that you would pay him for writing that letter.
- Inconvenient location. HMOs have geographic limits and aren't good for

people who travel, who have dependents in other cities, or for retirees who spend part of the year elsewhere.

- Clinic- or charity-like atmosphere. HMO care dehumanizes medicine in favor of cost savings. Read your HMO contracts very carefully for any kind of wording or clauses that either mention or imply any kind of limitations or prohibitions between patient and doctor discussing fully all available treatment options, even those not covered by an HMO. These have been called "gag rules." If there is no written material, ask whether the plan has any kind of policy in this regard for your documentation purposes. Also find out what the HMO's policy is in regard to treating a long-term illness. Are there any clauses in the contract that can lead to the loss of HMO coverage if you are being treated for a long-term illness? Is there is any kind of penalty written into the contract if you publicly complain about an HMO problem or treatment? Be aware that on February 20, 1997, former president Bill Clinton issued a directive that prohibits managed healthcare plans from imposing "gag rules" on doctors who treat Medicaid patients and in August 1998 the president announced that the administration had ordered that the 350 insurance companies who were then participating in the Federal Employees Health Benefits Program, and serving millions of federal employees and their families, eliminate "gag rules." In addition, on December 9, 1996, the US Health Care Financing Administration, now renamed the Centers for Medicare and Medicaid Services, announced that Medicare managed care plans may not prevent physicians from providing information to patients regarding all medically necessary treatment options. If you are concerned about whether or not HMO "gag rules" are allowed in your state, contact either your state insurance commission or state medical society to find out about the legal status of the "gag rule" in your jurisdiction.
- Operates on quick turnover, assembly-line basis.
- Impersonal attention is given patients.
- Involves long waiting periods prior to the delivery of health services. Or if an HMO won't pay for treatment or by mistake tells you and your physician that the treatment is not available or covered, you should be assertive; keep records of calls and letters; request a letter from your plan listing the clinical reasons why the claim was denied; ask your state's insurance office or state review board for help; or bring a lawsuit in a small-claims court. However, in June 2004 the US Supreme Court ruled that HMOs cannot be sued for malpractice in state courts by patients who obtain their medical insurance as an employment benefit. HMOs can only be sued in federal court, and all you, the patient, can recover are the payments to which you are entitled under your benefit contract. Patients have to sue in federal court because their claims are preempted by ERISA—the Employee Retirement Income Security Act of 1974—whose provisions govern disputes involving employment benefits. However, the state can force the HMO to provide the required treatment. Also, the HMO's appeal

process may be very difficult and time consuming. In addition, HMOs often develop new policies to make them more efficient but whose ultimate purpose is to reduce the kinds of treatments for which they pay.
- You must sever your relationships with your private physicians.
- You must terminate your private health insurance policy—an employer may not pay or contribute to the employees' premium. HMOs exercise more control over healthcare than fee-for-service plans. Depending upon the HMO, membership may cost more than traditional fee-for-service medical insurance and, if the policy is obtained through your employer, you may have to pay more.
- Hospitals affiliated with HMOs may not always have a good reputation. An HMO may even state that you or a loved one is "too old" to receive the best treatments available such as a complicated heart bypass operation, or if they do pay for such care, the HMO may send you to inferior centers, compared to centers that might give you better care, in order to save money. Critics state that patients should demand that the HMO put them in a particular hospital if it can save their lives and that patients or their heirs will sue the HMO if the patient deteriorates at an inferior center.
- HMOs do not always save the employer money. In some areas of the country, HMOs do not have enough patients to reduce costs over traditional fee-for-service insurance.
- Small employers often have too few workers to bargain with HMOs for discounts that are significantly lower than traditional health insurance.
- HMOs may not be cost efficient in rural areas owing, in part, to the fact that the number of doctors are so few to enable an HMO to bargain with them for lower costs.
- Some kinds of HMOs cannot grow fast enough to absorb many new members.
- Individuals—the self-employed, part-time workers, and the unemployed—do not have enough economic clout to obtain lower HMO premiums.

Remember, joining an HMO is an individual decision. Each HMO is different and should be judged upon its individual merits and demerits in terms of your personal health needs. Therefore, in examining an HMO, find out which of the previous advantages and disadvantages may be applicable to the organization you are considering. Learn as much as possible about the HMO before you make a decision. For example, some experts believe that at least 50 percent of an HMO's medical staff should consist of board-certified physicians and that not more than 20 percent of the doctors should be trained abroad. Authorities also suggests that you check upon the number of hospital days the HMO provides per year per 1,000 patients under sixty-five years of age, The number should be between 350 and 450 days. Any figure under this range can mean that the HMO is skimping on care. Also, compare the cost of the HMO with your fee-for-service medical care expenses and those of your old health insurance plan. Which is lower on an annual basis (including premiums and out-of-pocket expenses)? Finally, talk with HMO members and ask them about their treatment after hours—whether the HMO staff is helpful—and how you go about filing a complaint.[15]

What kind of health services does a federally qualified HMO offer?

A federally qualified HMO is required to offer the following basic health services:

- physician services (including consultant and referral services by a physician)
- medically necessary inpatient and outpatient hospital services
- medically necessary emergency health services
- annual short-term (not to exceed twenty visits) outpatient evaluative and crisis intervention mental health services
- medical treatment and referral services (including referral services to appropriate ancillary services) for the abuse of or addiction to alcohol and drugs ("Ancillary" means hospital services or other inpatient health program, other than room and board, and professional services.)
- diagnostic laboratory as well as diagnostic and therapeutic radiologic services
- home health services
- preventive health services (including immunizations, well-child care from birth, periodic health evaluations for adults, voluntary family planning services, infertility services, and children's eye and ear examinations, conducted to determine the need for vision and hearing correction through age seventeen)

In addition, an HMO may offer supplemental benefits if it has the staff to do so and if its members wish to purchase such services. These supplemental benefits may include:

- intermediate and long-term care facility services
- vision care
- dental care
- mental healthcare
- long-term rehabilitative services
- prescription drugs

In most cases, the monthly HMO premium will cover all health costs. However, some HMOs do charge a fee of a few dollars per visit or small fees for prescription drugs. These nominal costs are imposed to discourage unnecessary use of the HMO rather than to produce income for the organization. Check with your local HMO to find out what its policy is in regard to these administrative procedures.

What is a managed care "primary care physician" (PCP) and how do I select one?

Primary care physicians are usually doctors in family practice, general internal medicine, pediatrics, and, in some health plans, obstetricians/gynecologists who are case managers for your healthcare. If your plan requires you to select a primary care physician, be certain to choose one from the plan's directory at the time you enroll so that you can receive the care you may need. To help you decide, some plans provide new members with a directory listing the names and qualifications of the primary care physicians in the plan, and they encourage members to interview several physicians before deciding upon a doctor. Furthermore, members are free, usually at any time, to change primary care doctors within the plan. A centralized record system makes it convenient to provide the newly selected physician with the records needed to ensure continuity of care—a benefit rarely available to patients who want to change doctors in traditional private practice. When you join an HMO, the first person you may deal with is the "gatekeeper," who may be a nurse or a primary care physician and who evaluates your case and assigns a doctor. In the most rigid setup, you have no role in this decision, but, as already noted, many doctors allow patients to choose among staff doctors and select one as "their own." If you are allowed this choice, look for a doctor who makes you feel comfortable, will spend an appropriate amount of time with you, and will be on your side in a dispute with the HMO. Also, find out if you can easily get help over the telephone. Though you may be allowed this option of selecting your own doctor, certain decisions such as when to involve specialists remain within the purview of the HMO. The purpose of the primary care physician serving as gatekeeper is not only to screen patients seeking medical care but in doing so to eliminate costly and sometimes needless referrals to specialists for diagnosis and management. The primary physician is also responsible for administering the treatment and coordinating and authorizing all medical services, laboratory studies, specialty referrals, and hospitalizations, as already noted.

What is a " referral"?

Your primary care physician uses a referral to advise the health plan that you are being sent to a specialist doctor or other healthcare specialist for such services as laboratory work or x-rays. You must take the referral form with you so that the specialist can bill and receive payment from your plan. Otherwise, you may be expected to pay for the service. Some plans use an automated referral system and may issue you a card with a referral number.

What is the process of choosing a specialist in an HMO? Can you choose a specialist as a primary care physician?

Choice of a specialist in an HMO may be more limited than selecting a primary care physician who acts as a "gatekeeper" to approve specialty care. Most HMOs employ or contract with a small number of specialists in each field, and patients are usually referred by their primary care physicians to a specialist in the plan. HMO specialists are almost all board certified, but they may not be the patient's first choice. However, an increasing number of HMOs are now offering what is called "point-of-service" choices. For a slightly higher premium, members can receive care from many specialists outside the HMO's network. When they exercise that option, they usually also pay a small deductible and modest coinsurance—20 percent is the general figure. "Point-of-service" options are increasingly popular because members can enjoy the efficiency, convenience, and savings of prepaid networks for most of their healthcare, while reserving the choice to select outside specialists on those few occasions when they may need tertiary care. Even with the extra cost of "point-of-service," staff and group-model HMOs will probably be less expensive than other types of medical insurance.

How can I use the doctors I want?

Most managed care plans limit choice in some way to lower costs. A PPO gives you more leeway than an HMO but generally at higher premiums and copayments. If you do not choose from your PPO's list of contracted doctors, you will pay more in out-of-pocket expenses. In April 2003 the Supreme Court ruled unanimously that states have a right to force HMOs and other health networks to open themselves to all doctors, hospitals, and other providers who agree to abide by their terms. The ruling upholding Kentucky's so-called any-willing-provider (AWP) law was aimed directly at the economic heart of HMOs, which attempt to hold down healthcare costs by establishing limited networks.

When an HMO says a physician has been credentialed, what is involved in this process?

When HMOs establish a plan in a new area, they usually sign up any physician who will agree to their reimbursement schedule and then put the physician through their "credentialing" process. This process seeks to eliminate bad physicians—those who have not told the truth about their qualifications, lost their hospital privileges, are unlicensed, or abuse drugs. Even if a physician passes the credentialing process, that information does not guarantee a physician's competence. Once a doctor joins the network, some HMOs try to reevaluate competence through "recredentialing." Every two years or so, plans try to learn whether patients have filed many complaints, whether the physician has delivered poor care, and whether the doctor has lost hospital privileges. Many plans also examine how many and what kinds of services their physicians have ordered and investigate when the patterns of practice falls outside a typical range—ordering twice as many of a particular test as the average doctor. Good plans also search for doctors who use too few services, a sign that members may not be receiving adequate care. The basic test of recredentialing, however, is whether a plan rids itself of bad physicians. Legal complexities may hinder such efforts so HMOs try to rehabilitate them.

What is case management?

Many managed care plans now employ case managers to assist patients through treatment and recovery. In many HMOs, good planning has decreased the number of often-overused procedures such as hysterectomies. Case management is probably being used most in the field of mental health (including alcohol and drug abuse). Through early intervention and coordinated or intensive case management—that is, actually encouraging people to obtain help, then hospitalizing or even treating them over time if necessary but only if necessary—case management has done a great deal to lower healthcare costs. Case management substitutes economical for expensive care (such as sending patients to nursing homes instead of allowing them to stay in the hospital).[16]

Will HMOs cover all hospital expenses?

All hospital services are covered as long as they are considered medically necessary. Some HMOs lease or own hospitals to provide care for their members. Others just negotiate arrangements with hospitals to provide the HMO members with hospital services.

What does the fine print of the HMO policy contract state?

Do you understand in detail what a particular HMO will or will not cover since not all HMOs are federally certified? To do so, make sure you ask the HMO the following questions:

- Does the HMO cover some services you know you might need? If you are not sure, ask the HMO.
- Are any financial incentives provided to doctors that might discourage them from referring patients to specialists? Try to find out how doctors are paid. If they are paid a set fee for each patient under their care, they may have an incentive to skimp on treatment or needed tests.
- What options do you have for going outside the plan? Will it cost extra, and how much? How much of the doctor's fee will the HMO pay if you go outside the plan as a point-of-service option. If you find yourself needing a service that is not covered, or wanting to see a doctor who is not in your plan, talk with your primary care doctor. He or she can make a formal appeal on your behalf, provided that you have a good reason for your request.
- Are there any drugs that aren't covered? Has the HMO established a formulary or an approved drug list from which doctors are required to prescribe medication, usually low-cost generics or drugs that a pharmaceutical company has deeply discounted to the HMO. If you are taking medication, is it listed on the formulary? Will the plan approve the drug regimen you are on? If not, how will you receive the medication you need and pay for it? If you have special medical needs, find out how the plan will treat them and what

kinds of doctors the plan will allow you to see. If you are taking a brand-name drug, is only its generic counterpart available on the HMO formulary? Is that generic drug, in your doctor's opinion, therapeutically equivalent to the brand-name drug for purposes of your treatment?

- Are there any limits on how much enrollees can spend on drugs each year under the plan's coverage? What specifically is this financial limit?
- If the plan charges a copayment for drug refills, do members get a week's worth or a month's worth of drugs when they go to a pharmacy?
- Does the plan cover medical goods, such as wheelchairs and braces, hearing aids, eyeglasses?
- Is cosmetic surgery covered? What are the costs of extra benefits?
- Does the HMO provide out-of-service-area coverage for your children who are away from their hometown in college? How? Must a student be treated for illnesses in the HMO's own facilities even though he or she is away from the HMO service area? If there is no network in the student's region, can the student call an 800 number and get authorization to find his own doctor? Who pays? Does the plan also question diagnostic tests and treatments proposed by college physicians? If the HMO says that the college-based treatment or admission to a hospital is not proper, who pays? The college? The parent? The student?
- What operations are considered serious enough to warrant a hospital stay? (Many plans state they will pay for 100 percent of inpatient hospital stays without clarifying that members may be asked to use an outpatient facility for some surgeries.) Does the plan cover outpatient care? Is general dental care, oral surgery covered?
- What about mental health benefits? Has the HMO hired an outside behavioral firm to determine the kind and length of treatment the plan will pay for? Plans initially authorize a set number of sessions, usually eight, and therapists have to call to obtain approval for more if they believe a patient is not progressing. Does the schedule of the plan's mental health benefits meet your needs?[17]

What about chronic conditions? How will the plan treat them?

If you have a chronic illness like asthma or diabetes, ask the HMO as to what kind of outreach or monitoring program it operates. Also ask your doctor for his opinion as to whether the HMO's program can improve your health. Some plans offer special programs for members with asthma, cancer, diabetes, AIDS, mental illness, or substance abuse.

Under what conditions will the plan not pay for a visit to an emergency room?

If you and your family have a condition that could require emergency room care periodically, like a heart condition or asthma, ask how the plan pays for those visits? Does the plan use a "prudent person" standard to pay for emergency care—in other words, will it pay for anything a prudent person would have considered an emergency?[18]

Do HMOs provide quality care?

According to the federal government's HMO office, HMOs try to ensure the delivery of quality of care by:

- hiring physicians who are board certified or board eligible in their specialties and also those who are qualified to teach in medical schools or teaching hospitals.
- offering incentives for doctors on staff to continue their medical education.
- fostering a close relationship among staff doctors so they consult readily about cases.
- operating a quality-assurance program that includes peer review.
- constantly monitoring HMO medical directors for unnecessary testing and surgical procedures.
- establishing a formal grievance system so that patients can voice dissatisfaction with HMO treatment.

How can patients verify the quality of an HMO for themselves?

Determine if the plan you are considering joining has been graded by the National Committee for Quality Assurance (NCQA), a nonprofit group that accredits managed care plans. If the plan has not been reviewed, learn why and whether it will be. Submitting itself for accreditation shows that the plan cares about quality. To examine how NCQA accredited plans, whether they are HMOs or point-of-service, compare with other plans in terms of medical and service quality and to review various kinds of information to learn whether a particular plan meets your personal needs, visit http://www.usnews.com, operated by the national magazine *U.S. News & World Report.*

The NCQA accreditation process measures whether the plan has structures and systems in place to deliver good medical care—that is, whether it has a method to monitor utilization of services, a credentialing process, and a requirement that physicians follow practice guidelines. The NCQA does not measure patient outcomes—that is, whether fewer patients died because they had one procedure rather than another. Plans that come closest to meeting all the NCQA standards win a full three-year accreditation; those that meet most of the standards receive a one-year accreditation; and those that have no deficiencies that pose a risk to quality of care, obtain provisional status. If a plan does not meet with a number of standards, or has one deficiency that poses a risk to quality of care, the NCQA denies accreditation. Remember, in terms of delivering quality care accreditation is an important but not a primary or absolute standard.

In addition to accreditation activities, in July 1996 the NCQA published new guidelines, known officially as HEDIS 3.0 (for Health Plan Employer Data and Information Set). The guidelines, which replace an earlier version of HEDIS, include seventy-five treatments and preventive measures that show how well an HMO cares for its patients. The guidelines are designed primarily to help major corporations choose health plans for employees. Although not legally binding, the guidelines are expected to have a major influence since most major buyers will deal with health plans that follow the criteria.

HEDIS 3.0 established eight performance domains including effectiveness of care, accessibility and availability of care, satisfaction with care, cost of care, health plan stability, informed care choices, use of services, and plan descriptive information. The intent is that health plans will be able to standardize their measurement and performance information under these eight areas. A score card of how various health plans performed on earlier guidelines is available from an NCQA "Quality Compass" (1-202-955-5697) or you can call 1-800-839-6487 to obtain an Accreditation Summary Report for any plan reviewed during the past twelve months. An Accreditation Status List is available at that number or on the World Wide Web, at http://www.ncqa.org. Quality Compass does not assign HMOs overall grades but rates them on a scale of 1 to 5 in certain HEDIS measures where higher (or, in some cases lower) scores are clearly better. The Quality Compass also compares each plan in various measures against the top-performing HMOs and with national, regional, and metropolitan-area HEDIS averages. Accreditation status is included as well. For some HEDIS measures, experts do not agree on an optimal score. For example, most healthcare experts believe that the rate of hysterectomies in the United States is too high, but no one is certain how low the rate should be. In such cases, the Quality Compass notes whether a plan falls in the top or bottom 10 percent of all plans or in the middle 80 percent, since an HMO that performs too few procedures—or too many—could be a cause for concern. But remember Quality Compass is not perfect. Most of its data have not been audited and could include inconsistencies and errors on the performance data collected by some plans. But despite problems in the state of the art of HMO report cards today, small businesses, labor unions, and individual consumers, as well as large companies, can still see how different plans rate to some degree.

The National Committee for Quality Assurance began compiling information using the new guidelines of HEDIS 3.0 in January 1997. The guidelines, or measures as they are called, concentrate on the processes used by HMOs to provide care. The guidelines do not, however, establish a standard for treatment outcomes or results. A note of caution about HEDIS data: the data come from the plans themselves and, for the most part, are not audited by an impartial third party, do not account for differences in the health of a plan's members, and like any organizational data collection process could have inconsistencies in the ways plans measure data, differences in the quality of their data collection systems, and insufficient information to judge how well plans serve their members. So when you look at this data, small differences in report card numbers between plans may not necessarily mean that one plan is better than another.

But the National Committee for Quality Assurance is not alone in its efforts. Another organization concerned with the issue of quality is the nonprofit Foundation for Accountability (FACCT), based in Portland, Oregon. This organization also offers guidelines that focus more on the user of health plans rather than corporate purchasers, with a more outcome-related approach. The consumer should be aware that differences of opinion still exist about the definition of quality of care and that it is still a difficult concept to measure. One obstacle to obtaining comparable outcomes from different plans is that some HMOs begin with sicker patients than others. For those plans, poorer patient outcomes may not reflect inferior care.[19]

Also, find out whether there are any unresolved complaints against the plan. Contact your state insurance and consumer-affairs agencies.

What is an HMO's medical loss ratio?

Investors like plans that spend less on medical services. An HMO's efforts to reduce physician fees and medical services are reflected in a statistic known as the medical loss ratio—a measure of an HMO's medical expenditures as a percentage of the premiums it collects.[20]

How do I join an HMO?

As with group health insurance plans such as Blue Cross and Blue Shield, membership in an HMO is offered primarily through employers. Most health insurance plans offer individual memberships, but some HMOs have open enrollment periods when individuals or families can join. If after joining an HMO you believe that the organization is not delivering what you consider to be quality medical care, you have the right to end the membership and either go to another HMO or renew your subscription to your former health insurance plan.

What are my rights as an HMO patient?

As of 2002, eleven states—Arizona, California, Georgia, Maine, New Jersey, North Carolina, Oklahoma, Oregon, Texas, Washington, and West Virginia—allowed patients to sue their HMO for damages if care denied to them causes harm. As already noted, on June 21, 2004, voting unanimously, the U.S Supreme Court ruled that patients who claim that their HMOs would not pay for recommended medical care cannot sue for large malpractice or negligence damages in state court. The Supreme Court agreed with insurers, which claimed that patients could only go to federal court and then only to recover the value of whatever benefit the HMO denied. The court based its ruling on the language of a 1970s federal law, originally meant to protect employee pensions and other benefits but now applied to the managed care industry. The law, the Employee Retirement Income Security Act of 1974 or ERISA, forces the HMO patients to sue only in federal courts. The insurance industry argued that ERISA supercedes state patient protection laws or other state laws that allow medical negligence suits in local courts. The Health Administrative Responsibility Project (HARP), at http://www.harp.org, seeks to help consumers deal with these and other legal liability issues in regard to managed care when the consumer believes that he or she has been medically harmed. As of February 2006, acknowledging on its Web address that its site has gaps and perhaps even some errors, HARP states that its purpose is to be a resource for patients, physicians, and attorneys who are seeking to establish the liability of HMOs, managed care organizations, and nursing facilities for the outcomes of their decisions. HARP notes that, in its opinion, these groups are losing sight of the "quality" of care they deliver in their rush to "efficient" medical care.

In addition, forty-one states have passed measures permitting consumers to ask for an external review of an insurer's decision by independent medical experts. At least eighteen states have established state-funded ombudsman programs to aid managed care enrollees in obtaining the appropriate service. Finally, about one-half of all states have published "report cards" comparing the performances of different health plans to help consumers select an insurer. The availability of the report cards and the number of insurers evaluated, however, vary widely from state to state. For state-by-state information go to the following Web site http://www.consumersunion .org/health/hmo-review or to the Kaiser Family Foundation Web site at http://www .kff.org/consumerguide. Also, find out whether the Consumer Union or the Kaiser Foundation still has the following publication available to the public: *A Consumer's Guide to Handling Disputes with Your Private or Employer Health Plan.*

In regard to an HMO that is really performing its duties, you should have the following expectations as a patient according to one well-regarded HMO, Med-Centers Health Plan of Minneapolis, which listed these rights in its brochure for members.

- The right to quality and accessible preventive care.
- The right to efficient, courteous, and honest treatment from all staff members.
- Accountability, [which means that] every person and every administrative unit within the HMO must be both responsive to your needs and responsible for their actions. It also means the HMO must provide a means for monitoring its own actions [to assure] that it will provide quality care.
- The right to comprehensive health education, including printed information, classes, and counseling.
- The right to communicate with the HMO staff regarding the organization itself. This means you should have the opportunity to voice your concerns, make any suggestions, and, in general, provide feedback to the HMO administration. It means that if you have questions or worries, the HMO is required to respond to them promptly and thoroughly. Finally, it means that there should be available a standard grievance procedure for all HMO member complaints. If you have some problem, you should be able to present your grievance and have it dealt with appropriately and in a timely fashion.[21]

Is the HMO membership subject to cancellation?

As long as you pay the HMO's premium you cannot be dropped, even if you develop a chronic illness after joining an HMO. During the HMO's annual open-enrollment period, the plan must take all who apply regardless of health status. During the closed period, however, the HMO may refuse an applicant for any reason. At present, open enrollment is only required for those HMOs that have been operating for five years or those with fifty thousand members and no financial deficit in the previous year. Also, as of 1976 an HMO's open enrollment does not have to accept people, although they can apply, who are already institutionalized someplace else with a chronic illness or permanent injury if these conditions would economically impair the HMO. Also, can you renew your coverage as often as you like? If not, what are the guidelines that prevent you from doing so?

What can I do to learn as much as I can about an HMO?

If you are considering HMO membership, get as much descriptive literature as you can about its policies and operation. Visit the plan's headquarters; ask questions about the physician's qualifications, costs, services, and quality assurance programs; find out whether the HMO's hospital is accredited and has a good reputation; ask if there is consumer representation on the HMO governing committees; and inquire as to what the annual dropout rate for HMOs members is (it should be less than 20 percent per year).[22]

How can I judge the financial soundness of an HMO and its future economic viability?

Each qualified HMO has a provision for continued services in the event of bankruptcy. This is called protection against risk of insolvency and is mandated under federal law. Furthermore, the financial resources of an HMO are regulated by the state insurance commission. Request copies of the HMO's financial statements to see facts and figures.[23]

What is a Medicare risk HMO?

Medicare risk HMOs contracts, which originated in the 1980s, had fallen from a high of 346 contracts in 1998 to 152 in 2002, according to the Centers for Medicare and Medicaid Services (CMS). Risk plans are so named because they have assumed the insurance risk, receiving a capitated payment for each enrollee. This sum amounts to 95 percent of the average local payment for traditional Medicare. The formula assumes that an HMO's organization and delivery of care will yield at least a 5 percent savings to the Medicare program.

In addition to these risk plans, some eight hundred thousand elderly persons are enrolled in older HMO arrangements that receive straight fee-for-service payments.

Until the beginning of the twenty-first century, generous payments to risk HMOs meant that there was no shortage of HMOs willing to participate in Medicare, except in mostly rural counties where Medicare payments are often low. Because the CMS strictly regulates risks' profits, plans are forced to return their savings back into operations. Risk HMOs responded by reducing premiums and adding services such as vision checkups and annual physicals, which are not covered by traditional Medicare. In fact, in 1999, 61 percent of Medicare beneficiaries had access to plans with zero premiums according to the Centers for Medicare and Medicaid Services. By 2002 that decreased to 34 percent because the economic climate for HMOs in the Medicare + Choice (M+C) program, now renamed Medicare Advantage, had changed. Many health plans in this program began to charge enrollees higher premiums and copayments. And many reduced benefits—with half the plans that cover prescription drugs no longer paying for brand names but only lower-cost generics. As of 2003 plans with zero premiums and reasonable prescription drug benefits still operated, principally in urban areas in Florida, California, and New York. Eleven states and the District of Columbia did not have any Medicare Advantage managed care plans.

Under traditional Medicare, patients often use Medigap insurance to cover the program's unreimbursed costs, such as office visit copayments. When they join risk HMOs, they may no longer need these policies, which can save them money. While HMO marketing is basically focused on employers, risk HMOs must appeal directly to individual enrollees. Seniors who are unhappy with their risk HMOs have the option of disenrolling within a month—or even retroactively if they were deceived into enrolling. In addition, regional CMS offices monitor disenrollment rates and complaints, looking for potential problems, then meeting with HMOs to work out improvement plans. If you are an elderly person who is considering joining a risk HMO, then find out as much as information as you can about the organization that you are considering to join.[24]

But some words of caution: It is not difficult to leave an HMO if you are unhappy with the plan and want to go back to traditional Medicare; you can disenroll from the HMO and be back on Medicare the first day of the following month. But even if you get back your Medicare benefits, you, in the meantime, may have already given up your Medigap policy (insurance that covers the difference between what Medicare pays for and the actual cost of your healthcare) and be unable to buy a new one. The best time to buy Medigap insurance is within six months after you become sixty-five and apply for Medicare; during that period, you can buy a policy without meeting an insurer's health requirements. But after that "window" of opportunity of protection is gone, you could be out of luck if you are not well. People in poor health who want to leave a Medicare HMO and buy a new Medigap policy may find that no insurance company will sell them one. That can result in a frightening situation: go without Medigap protection or remain in an HMO that may not meet your medical needs.

Be very cautious when signing up with a Medicare HMO. Understand everything you need to know about the plan in regard to your own medical needs. You don't want to find yourself in a situation where you not only have an HMO not meeting your medical needs but also cannot find protection in the private sector because you had chosen an HMO rather Medicare program coverage.

If money is not very important and you can afford a Medigap policy, you may be better off initially staying in Medicare, and if you need chronic care treatment such as the necessity for a home-health aide or know you will require nursing home care in the future, HMOs are not the option for you.

On the other hand, if you have high prescription drug bills, then an HMO that covers part of those costs may be worthwhile. But you have to understand the details of the HMO drug program. Compare it with the new Medicare prescription drug benefits that became effective on January 1, 2006. Are they the same? Not similar? And if not similar what are their differences and how may these differences affect your own drug needs both therapeutically and in terms of costs? Which programs will cost you more in drugs expenses over the long term? Some HMOs may have financial limits as to how much they will pay out or count copayments in different ways so that you have a smaller benefit than you had hoped. As already noted, through formularies, some also restrict the drugs your doctor can prescribe in a manner that makes it hard to remain on your present drug regimen.

Only you know your personal situation best and what is the best kind of health insurance plan for you—an HMO or Medicare. Beneficiaries can compare 2003 year details of plans in their county (if any) on the Health Plan Compare site at http://www.Medicare.gov or by calling 1-800-633-4227.[25]

Do Medicare beneficiaries who are members of HMOs need supplementary insurance?

The Medicare beneficiary would be covered as any other HMO enrollee and would not require additional health insurance. HMOs actually provide much broader coverage than Medicare. According to federal law, not more than one-half of an HMO's membership can be comprised of Medicare and Medicaid beneficiaries.

Does the federally certified HMO have a mechanism that allows its patients to voice their complaints?

Each federally certified HMO is required by federal law to have a realistic workable grievance procedure as part of its operational mechanism. In an HMO, you have to take particular care that your concerns are listened to, whether they be about referrals, appointments, or other issues that bother you. The first person you should go to with your problem is your doctor or nurse practitioner or the manager at your HMO clinic. You can then go to higher officials if need be. Find out whether the HMO has a specified ombudsman or patient representative to listen to your complaints. Is there any arrangement for appeal or review of any differences over your treatment or coverage? Can you influence HMO policies in any way? To find out ask other members.

You should be aware that effective January 1, 1990, the Joint Commission on the Accreditation of Healthcare Organizations established new standards for complaint procedures, requiring:

- an effective mechanism exist for receiving complaints.
- patients be informed about the mechanism and about their right to file a complaint.
- the organization respond to significant complaints, and take appropriate action.
- a patient not be penalized for filing a complaint.[26]

Can an HMO member transfer from one HMO to another?

Circumstances vary. Check with your employer and/or local HMO(s) for details.

What are social health maintenance organizations (SHMOs)?

Social health maintenance organizations (SHMOs) are very few in number and are demonstration projects of the Centers for Medicare and Medicaid, US Department of Health and Human Services. Established in 1984, they now operate in Long Beach, California (SCAN Health Plan); Portland, Oregon (Kaiser Permanente); Las Vegas, Nevada (Health Plan of Nevada Plus); and Brooklyn, New York (Elderplan). They may lay the basis for future public-private access initiatives involving doctors and hospitals.

Since their establishment, they have provided acute and long-term care services to senior citizens under a single cost-effective insurance and delivery system. SHMOs fill the omissions in Medicare and most private insurance, including HMOs, by providing extra benefits, such as prescription drugs and up to a specific dollar amount for community-based long-term care benefits. The programs have a reimbursement system similar to that used by HMOs holding Medicare risk contracts with the CMS. SHMOs draw from an insurance risk pool created through monthly capitated payments from Medicare and Medicaid, enrollees' premiums, and copayments for expanded chronic-care benefits. Medicare pays into the pool monthly rates set at 100 percent of what would have been spent on beneficiaries in the local fee-for-service system. Medicare risk SHMOs receive only 95 percent of that amount. Providers and managers each receive a negotiated share of the pool. The ceiling on revenues gives managers and providers an incentive to minimize expenses. Thus far, their experience has demonstrated that the SHMOs have become skilled at limiting the opportunities for providers to shift patients into more expensive forms of care, which is one of the reasons Medicare costs keep going up.[27]

Does the HMO premium have to be paid all at once?

No. The HMO annual premium is paid on a monthly basis.[28]

How much is an HMO's monthly premium?

The premiums vary from one region of the country to another and from state to state within the regions. Also, the premiums for single individuals would be lower than those for families.

If the HMO allows you to receive as many medical services as you need with only a monthly premium and allows you to make as many visits as you want without charging you for each visit, how can an HMO operate successfully?

An HMO makes a profit by reducing uncalled-for hospitalization, avoiding needless diagnostic tests, and not performing surgical procedures that are not necessary. As a member of a prepaid health plan, it is in the financial interest of the HMO to keep you well. For example, if you do not get a flu shot, you may end up in the hospital with pneumonia. The cost would far exceed your annual premium and the HMO would lose money. Keeping you well by emphasizing preventive care is how an HMO budgets its costs. On the other hand, an insurance company is only responsible for reimbursement for care—not the availability and access of healthcare or the delivery of services.[29]

What happens if you become ill outside the area that the HMO services? Will the HMO cover the cost of such care?

An HMO does cover emergencies outside of its service area regardless of whether you are in the United States or abroad. Find out what percentage of the costs the HMO will pay.

When you become a member of an HMO, do you have the freedom of choice as to doctors and hospitals?

Your HMO membership only covers services provided by physicians associated with the plan, although you may change doctors within the HMO plan itself. Services by any outside physician would not be reimbursable unless accepted by the HMO or the physician. The same applies to the hospital; only the one affiliated with the HMO would be reimbursed. This does not mean you cannot go outside the plan to other physicians or hospitals, but you may have to pay for their services. This payment would be in addition to your HMO costs if you are still a member at the time of these outside visits.

If one of your children becomes ill at school and you are not home, will the HMO pick up the child if the school nurse calls?

No. However, in certain emergency situations, the HMO might pay for the ambulance.

If your area has a physician shortage and there is no HMO in your area, and you wish to establish such a plan, where do you begin?

It can take up to three or more years before an HMO plan becomes reality—one year for a feasibility study, a second for planning, and the third for initial development (hiring staff, buying equipment, erecting buildings). Usually, HMOs are started with a nucleus —for example, a group of physicians, a hospital, a community health center. If such a core group does not exist in your community and you wish to establish an HMO, contact the Office of Managed Care, Centers for Medicare and Medicaid Services, (an agency of the US Department of Health and Human Services) in Baltimore, Maryland.[30]

Whom do I call with questions about my health plan?

Ask your health benefits officer at work, or call your health plan directly with any questions. Your health plan's customer service telephone number is usually printed on your insurance card.

How can I learn more about HMOs and find out if an HMO exists in my community?

You can write to the Office of Managed Care, Centers for Medicare and Medicaid Services, US Department of Health and Human Services, Baltimore, Maryland.

It is very important that you become knowledgeable about health maintenance organizations because a strong drive by government, labor unions, and private business to establish these organizations has made them a major alternative to the way healthcare is presently being delivered under the fee-for-service medical system. Although HMO monthly premiums may be slightly higher than conventional health insurance premiums, depending upon where you live, out-of-pocket healthcare expenses have generally been shown to be lower. Such HMO savings occur because under most conventional insurance policies you must pay a deductible plus a percentage of all charges over the deductible. This is not applicable to HMO operations. In addition, as noted previously, the preventive care approach of the health maintenance organization will save you money over the long term as well.

HMOs AND YOUR RESPONSIBILITY AS AN EMPLOYER

"Ken, I'm just a small businessman. I don't have the resources of a General Motors or any other large corporation to study the pros and cons of HMOs or PPOs or other forms of managed care for my employees compared to traditional health insurance. I'm just trying to find the best insurance not only for them but also for myself so that I can keep these people employed and not have rising health costs affect the profit

margin of my company. I see what health insurance costs can do to the bottom lines of larger corporations where their profits are impacted and they have to lay off employees. Yet, at the same time, I know I have legal obligations to my employees in regard to offering them HMOs and PPOs as an alternative health benefit, but I am not sure what these obligations are. I have too many other responsibilities in operating this business to be an insurance expert, too. And I want to know enough to make sure that I understand what the managed care representative is telling me is also best for my employees and the economic viability of my business. I also want my employees to understand what these plans are all about and pick the plan that is best for them. An employee who does not have to worry about medical bills has one less worry on the job and can be more productive and, through such increased productivity, help increase the profits of my business. Therefore, what should I tell my employees when they ask about my company's health insurance coverage and are interested more in managed care than in being covered by traditional health insurance?"

"Milt, I think you should become acquainted with the general obligations you have in presenting HMO or other managed care coverage to your employees because they need as much information as they can receive from both you and the managed care companies to make an informed choice in terms of health insurance coverage, be it HMOs, preferred-provider organizations (PPOs), other forms of managed care, or traditional health insurance."

Membership in an HMO is primarily available through your employer. For example, in January 1979, as a result of approval by the US Civil Service Commission, a group of Blue Cross and Blue Shield–sponsored health maintenance organizations began to operate as a network, offering the same benefits at the same rates to government employees enrolled in the Federal Employee Health Benefits Program. Yet, despite such marketing advances by HMOs, employers generally still do not understand the implication of the federal law that requires them, under certain circumstances, to offer an HMO option to their workers. Accustomed to dealing with either Blue Cross and Blue Shield or a commercial health insurer, corporate health benefits mangers must now, if the company's employees are dispersed around the country, negotiate with dozens of HMOs, with new requests appearing regularly as more HMOs are qualified by the US Department of Health and Human Services. Therefore, in order to understand the responsibilities of your business firm in offering HMOs as an alternative health insurance option to your employees, the following questions are of importance.

What is dual choice?

Dual choice means that employers, under certain circumstances, are required to offer their employees *qualified HMOs* as an alternative to indemnity health or service benefit insurance plans, in accordance with the requirements of Section 1310 of the HMO Act of 1973 (Public Law 93-222).

A qualified HMO is one that provides basic and supplemental health services to its members in accordance with the act and meets other requirements relating to fiscal soundness, marketing practices, grievance processes for members, continuing education for staff, and membership representation on the HMO board of directors.

As an employer, under what conditions must I offer HMOs as an alternative choice to other kinds of health insurance programs?

The HMO law applies to all employers subject to section six of the Fair Labor Standards Act of 1938 (minimum wage laws) who also meet the following conditions:

- There are twenty-five or more employees in the company.
- There are at least twenty-five employees living in the service area of the HMO.
- The firm currently offers and makes financial contributions to a health benefits plan.
- The HMO has presented a valid request to be included in the health benefits plan of the company.

Which employees are eligible for HMO membership?

All full- and part-time employees and their dependents who live in an HMO's enrollment area and who meet the employer's requirements for participation in the employer's health benefits plan are eligible for membership.

What constitutes a valid request by an HMO that it be included as an alternative choice to the health plans offered by my company?

To be valid, the "approach" from the HMO to the employer must include:

- evidence that the HMO is qualified
- a current financial report
- a description of the service area and dates when services will be provided
- a description of the location of facilities, including dates and hours of operation
- a proposed contract between the HMO and the employer
- sample copies of marketing brochures and membership literature
- the identity of the staff and the ownership of the HMO and the physicians who will provide the services
- a statement of rates for various categories of membership
- a statement of the capacity of the HMO to enroll new members and the likelihood of any limitations on such enrollment in the future
- an indication of the *type* of HMO, either "group/staff" or "Individual Practice Association"

The type of HMO, that is "group/staff" or Independent Practice Association (IPA), represented by any one request is important, for ultimately the employer is required to offer one of each if both kinds approach him with requests. The employer may be required, therefore, to offer a "triple" choice: the company's original health insurance plan, a group/staff model, and an Independent Practice Association HMO plan. But if the employer receives a written request from more than one qualified HMO of the same type, such as three IPAs, and they all serve the same area, the employer may choose which HMO to offer. On the other hand, if the employer is approached by more than one qualified HMO of the same type, *and* the additional HMO(s) have a unique service area not duplicated by the other HMO(s), *or* if the other qualified HMO(s) have closed their enrollment period, then the employer must offer each HMO only to those employees (25 or more) who live in the unduplicated service area of the additional (HMOs).

What categories of employers must offer an HMO option to their employees?

The federal HMO law requires two categories of employers: those who have collective bargaining agreements with their employees and those who do not.

What defines a binding offer from the HMO to the employer?

To be binding, the offer by the HMO must be received by the employer within a variable but prescribed time frame:

- For employees covered by a collective bargaining agreement, the employer must receive the HMO offer at least 90 days before the expiration date of the contract.
- For employees covered by a health benefits contract or an employer/employee contract, the employer must receive the HMO offer at least 180 days before the expiration or renewal date of the contract.

What are the employer's obligations when the HMO offer is received within the specified time frame?

Assuming the HMO offer appears within the specified time and manner, the employer's obligations are to make the offer to employees covered by the collective bargaining agreement when the new contract is negotiated, or on the anniversary date of the contract if it has no fixed term, or at the reopening of the contract negotiations. For other employees, the offer must be made when the existing health benefits contract is renewed, or at the anniversary date of the contract if it has no fixed term, or when a new health benefits contract is negotiated.

How much time is allowed for the HMO to present its program to an organization's employees?

In addition to a ten-day group enrollment period, the employer must assure that employees are given the opportunity to make an informed choice. The federal HMO law requires that the HMO be given "fair and reasonable" access to employees for thirty days for the purpose of explaining the HMO, with the minimal requirement being that access includes an opportunity to distribute brochures, relevant descriptive material, and announcements of meetings.

What kind of monetary contribution must the employer make on behalf of his employees?

The federal HMO law requires only that the employer pay to the HMO an amount equal to the cost to the employer of the health benefits plan provided under the terms of the collective bargaining agreement or the employer/employee contract. If the HMO premium is less than the employer's contributions to his other health plans, the employer is not required to pay more than the HMO premium, which may be shared by the employer and employee or paid entirely by the employer.

How do an employer's responsibilities under ERISA affect an HMO offering?

According to a ruling by the US Department of Labor and the US Department of Health and Human Services, employers are relieved of their fiduciary responsibilities under ERISA (Employee Retirement Income Security Act of 1974) when offering a federally qualified HMO. In addition, employers are not required to offer their retired employees the option of joining a qualified HMO. However, ERISA does permit an employer to examine and approve the HMO's marketing materials.

What is the ultimate responsibility of the employer under the federal HMO law?

The HMO law, as amended, and its accompanying regulations, make the HMO offer subject to the collective bargaining process. The employer, upon being approached by an HMO, must make the HMO offer to the bargaining representatives in accordance with the requirements of the National Labor Relations Act. If the union accepts the offer, the HMO option is then made to the employees covered by the collective bargaining agreement. If the union rejects the HMO alternative, your obligation to the union is satisfied. However, the employer still has the responsibility for making the HMO offer to nonorganized employees.[31]

In response to the growing demand by American business to know more about health maintenance organizations and how these organizations can improve the health of their employees as well as reduce their health expenses, there are now private organizations whose interests pertain to these matters. These include the National Business Group on Health (50 F St. NW, Washington, DC 20001; Tel:

1-202-628-9320; Web site: http://www.wbgh.org) and America's Health Insurance Plans (601 Pennsylvania Ave. NW, South Building, Suite 500, Washington, DC 20004; Tel: 1-202-778-3200;Web site: http://www.ahip.org).

If you have any questions pertaining to health maintenance organizations as operational entities or do not understand any part of the federal HMO law, the aforementioned organizations can help you find the answers. For example, the America's Health Insurance Plans (AHIP) is the national trade association to which HMOs, PPOs, and similar managed healthcare plans belong.

The necessity for such groups is underscored by the fact that more and more business organizations have organized their own HMOs; R. J. Reynolds in Winston-Salem, North Carolina, successfully established its own HMO in the late 1970s; Deere & Co. of Illinois also embarked upon such a venture, as had the United Automobile Workers Union in cooperation with Ford, Chrysler, and General Motors in Detroit, Michigan.[32] Consequently, there are not only HMO trade associations to which you can turn for advice but business corporations as well as who have gained actual experiences in establishing and operating these new modes of healthcare delivery. Obtain all the information you require about HMOs, and you will benefit in terms of improving and maintaining the physical and financial health of your employees and yourself as a consumer-patient.

THE RIGHT HMO FOR YOU: SOME QUESTIONS

In summary then, there are a number of questions you can ask to determine whether a particular health maintenance organization is the correct health plan for you.

Costs

- Ask friends, relatives, or neighbors who have had health problems how their plans have responded.
- Consider what you and your family want most from a health plan and what you and your employer can spend on it. If you have a family physician, gynecologist, or pediatrician who you want to stay with, seek his or her advice. Find out what plans he or she belongs to. If you have a favorite nearby hospital, see what people there recommend.
- Make sure you understand exactly what services are covered and at what price. The plans all list the monthly or biweekly costs of coverage, but they also may require patients to pay a portion of the charges for specific treatments—called copayments. Also, find out if there is a deductible that you must pay before insurance coverage starts. Remember, as a general rule, the higher the deductible, the lower the premium.
- What is the yearly total for monthly fees? How does it compare with other HMOs in your area? How does it compare with traditional fee-for-service health insurance?

- Are there copayments for office visits, emergency care, prescribed drugs, or other services? How much?
- What share of premium costs do you and your employer pay?
- What is the deductible for each family member?
- Is there a lifetime limit on benefits you receive such as medical tests, surgery, mental healthcare, homecare, or other support offered?
- What if you need services that are not covered by the HMO?
- Does the plan allow you to be treated by someone outside the network if you prefer and at what extra cost?
- Is the plan financially stable or in danger of going out of business? Ask for copies of financial statements about the HMO's operations.

Coverage

- Determine exactly what the plans covers. Think twice if it does not cover a wide variety of preventive services, such as immunizations as a low-cost way to prevent disease; well-baby care, prenatal care, mammograms and pap smears as screens for breast cancer and cervical cancer; and tests for cholesterol problems and diabetes. Does it cover preexisting illnesses such as cancer or heart attacks? And if you have a predisposition to a genetic disease, make sure it is covered. Is there coverage for physical examinations? What about coverage for home healthcare, hospice care, dental care?
- Does the plan offer preventive care? What are your benefits for mental or emotional care, vision and dental care, and for rehabilitation and organ transplants? Are there any limitations on medical tests, surgery, homecare, or other benefits?
- Are medications covered? What pharmacies must you use?
- What medical equipment does the plan cover?
- What long-term care is provided?
- What about mental health benefits? Many plans have reduced the scope of their mental health benefits in response to rapidly rising costs, and patients often pay greater out-of-pocket expenses for mental illness treatment than for physical ailments. This may include coverage for such important treatments as drug and alcohol addiction or marriage counseling.

Care

- In terms of organizational quality is the HMO accredited by the National Committee for Quality Assurance (NCQA) and/or the Joint Commission on the Accreditation of Healthcare Organizations (JCAHO). If not, does the HMO plan to apply for accreditation from either or both organizations? How soon?
- Is there an effective quality assurance program approved by a competent outside organization?

- Which hospitals are in the plan and who chooses where you will be hospitalized? Are they known for high quality? Find out what hospitals the plans uses. If you are very ill or have a chronic illness, can you go to a teaching hospital, which generally provides more sophisticated treatments for complex illnesses? If you must have a heart bypass operation, find out whether the plan insists that patients go to a hospital that performs two hundred or more procedures a year, where your chance of recovery is twice as good as in a hospital that does fewer operations.
- Will you often be seen—either before or instead of the doctor—by a nurse-practitioner or a physician's assistant. If you are dissatisfied with this arrangement, find out whether you can then see a doctor. Also, learn about a plan's or particular doctor's practice before making your choices.
- Who are the plan's doctors? How does the plan choose its doctors? Who will your doctor be? Is he or she board certified (by a specialty examining board)? Many good doctors are not certified, but this is one test of excellence. You can check your doctor's certification claims by calling the American Board of Medical Specialties, Evanston, IL, 1-847-491-9091 or 1-866-275-2267.
- Is your doctor unhappy with the plan? Why? Payment problems? Utilization constraints? If your doctor is unhappy, you may wish to choose another plan or another insurance choice if you have one. You can change HMOs at the next open enrollment.
- Ask your doctor how he or she receives approval for treatment decisions and referrals to specialist. How difficult is it to consult a specialist? If you learn that the doctors have to go through many bureaucratic procedures to practice medicine, seek out a plan that gives the physician more freedom.
- Are there many doctors to choose from? Do the doctors admit patients to university medical centers? How are they paid? Are there incentives to encourage doctors to skimp on care? Ask if a plan allows doctors to discuss their pay and whether they earn bonuses by withholding expensive treatments and tests. Can they inform you fully about the range of treatments available for your problem, even if some are not covered by the plan?
- Do you select your physician from a list of contract physicians or from available staff of a group practice? Which doctors are accepting new patients? How hard is it to change doctors if you decide you want someone else? Most plans make it fairly easy to change physicians at any time, although some may not have a large selection of primary care physicians to choose from. Other plans make it harder to change medical groups. Some plans limit changes to twice a year to discourage doctor changing and encouraging continuity of care. Look for a plan that offers a wide range of medical specialists to handle unusual or dangerous medical illnesses or allows members to go outside the plan at little or no cost to get such care if the plan does not include needed specialists.
- Ask if the plan encourages continuing education for its doctors, nurses, and

other healthcare personnel. Aside from medical competence and proficiency, try to learn as much as you can about the plan's physicians:

▼ Do they treat their patients humanely?

▼ Do they manage their time efficiently?

▼ Do they use costly resources economically but effectively? For example, do they prescribe drugs when needed but not if other measures will work?

▼ Do they work well with the plan's other personnel?

▼ Do they contribute to the plan by working in committees and contributing ideas and contribute to their neighborhood or community outside of the plan?

These various factors are indicators of quality physicians, aside from medical competence, and contribute toward making the health plan of your choice a good plan to join.[33]

- Does the health plan have any recent surveys of patient and doctor satisfaction it can show you?
- How long do you have to wait typically for services such as gynecological and eye examinations?
- Is the plan growing? Find out whether the percentage of members who have dropped in the past year is out of proportion to that of other plans in the area (but remember, some populations are highly mobile; this could distort the figure).
- What is your employer's opinion of the plan? What experiences has your employer had with different plans?
- Are complaints and grievances handled expeditiously? Is your wait on the telephone for service or answers to your questions very long? (It should be brief.) If a receptionist is impolite with you over the telephone or hesitates to give out information, seriously consider whether you want to go to that doctor. While the rapid increase in the number of health plans and different forms they require has placed additional stress on the doctor's office staff, receptionists still should be responsive to a patient's questions.
- Do you have to wait long in the doctor's office? Is it easy to get an appointment? How long does it take to make an appointment with your primary care physician? If it routinely takes more than a week, the doctor may be too busy and it pays to shop around some more. How far in advance must routine visits be scheduled? In some HMOs, it's only a few days. It shouldn't be more than a week or two for nonurgent problems; no more than a few weeks to see a specialist.
- Have you visited the plan's facilities to see how they actually treat patients as opposed to television commercials and whether you feel comfortable in that setting? See if they have evaluations by patients that you can examine.
- Are you willing to have your care coordinated and authorized by a primary care doctor?
- Is the HMO staff friendly, compassionate, and helpful?

- What specialties does the plan have? Obstetricians, gynecologists, pediatricians, dermatologists, or whatever? What are the procedures for seeing a specialist and obtaining a second opinion? Also, remember, in 2002 the Supreme Court upheld an Illinois law giving patients the right to obtain an independent doctor's ruling when the HMOs deny benefits for particular procedures or medications. In that case, the court held, five to four, that the Illinois law was a regulation of insurance, and thus exempt from the 1973 HMO law. How hard or easy is it to be referred to a specialist outside the plan? Check the process for getting a referral to a specialist. Do you have to visit your primary care physician each time or can it be done over the telephone? Find out the extra cost of going to a specialist who is not part of the network or plan.
- What happens if you or a family member is out of the country or traveling in the country or if you have a child in college and you, a family member, and/or your child need care? Does the plan cover a child in college?
- Is the HMO federally qualified (this can be a plus, although a good HMO need not necessarily be federally qualified); or has the HMO been accredited by the National Committee for Quality Assurance?
- How managed is a plan's managed care? For example, does it require an approval before patients can check into a hospital, continuing review of hospital stays, case management substitute for expensive care (such as sending patients to a nursing home instead of letting them remain in a hospital), and use of a primary care doctor as "gatekeeper" to approve specialty care.
- Does the plan have an appeal or grievance procedure for dissatisfied patients? How quickly does it work? [34]
- As a matter of precaution against future contingencies, you may want to establish a savings fund if someday you need to go outside the plan for care because you cannot obtain the kind of care you need from the plan, especially if you cannot get a point-of-service option from your employer. In this fashion, finances will not hinder you from receiving the kind of care you need and that the HMO may not be able to provide.

Convenience

- Where are the facilities located in your community that serve HMO members? How convenient to your home and workplace are the doctors, hospitals, and emergency care centers that make up the HMO network? No matter how low the price, it doesn't pay to join a plan that doesn't have doctors or facilities near where you live or work. This is especially important if you have young children, who are likely to require more frequent office visits than healthy adults.[35] Can you easily get help over the phone?
- Are the hours of the plan convenient?
- Can you access after-hours, urgent, or emergency care easily? What arrangements does the HMO have for handling emergency and after-hours care?

Nights, weekends, holidays? What's the HMO's reimbursement policy on emergency treatment? Some plans refuse to pay unless they are true emergencies. Thus, the patient must decide if an internal burning sensation is simply indigestion or a heart attack or whether a headache is sign of stroke or sinusitis. You need to be assured of telephone numbers to call nights, holidays, or weekends for medical advice and, if necessary, directions on where to go for emergency treatment. In serious emergencies, however, you should be able to go the closest hospital, or whatever hospital a rescue service takes you, and still be covered. Thus, find out what happens if you are seriously ill and must call in an outside doctor not affiliated with the HMO or if you are in a serious accident and rushed to a hospital that has no contract with your HMO. Who pays the bills—you or your HMO? These are important concerns for which you should seek answers.[36]

Before you join a health plan, talk to several members or call the National Committee for Quality Assurance (NCQA) at 1-800-839-6487 or visit its Web site, at http://www.ncqa.org, to determine whether the plan has any rating or has given its accreditation to the plan you are considering joining. Also, if you need any additional information in handling HMO problems, as already noted, you may visit the Web site of the Health Administrative Responsibility Project, at http://www.harp.org.

OTHER FORMS OF MANAGED CARE

Preferred-Provider Organizations (PPOs)

PPOs are financing and delivery systems that combine aspects of standard fee-for-service indemnity health insurance plans and HMOs. Basically, a PPO is a group of doctors and hospitals that negotiates a contract with a company, union, or insurance firm to provide medical services for reduced fees. In return, the provider, that is, a doctor and/or hospital, is promised increased patient volume and prompt payment. Hospital and admitting physicians find PPOs an attractive mechanism in which to participate because they believe that they can increase their patient base (in the case of hospitals maintain occupancy rates in areas where HMOs and hospital review programs are reducing hospitalization), improve outpatient business, alter their patient mix, protect their existing patient base, maintain their traditional form of payment of fee-for-service, and obtain more extensive hospital privileges, and they view PPOs as an effective means of competing with other alternative delivery systems for the same patients. Because competition for patients is very keen, providers are willing to negotiate discounts with insurers or others who are establishing PPOs. In addition, as hospitals themselves manage more and more of their own care, PPOs provide hospital administrators with a mechanism to follow and measure practice patterns and costs of care.

Like HMOs, PPOs have a limited number of doctors and hospitals from which to choose. The networks or panels of providers have contracts with the PPO to provide medical services and to be paid, according to a negotiated fee schedule. When you use those healthcare providers (sometimes called "preferred" providers, other times called "network" providers), most of your medical bills are covered. When you go to doctors in the PPO, you present a card and do not have to fill out insurance claims forms. There may be a small copayment such as $10 or less for each visit. For some services, you may have to pay a deductible and coinsurance. Ideally, healthcare providers are chosen for their efficiency, and the system monitors its own activities to assure that care is efficiently provided. Thus, through a PPO the patient has a choice of geographically dispersed providers, first-dollar coverage (frequently), and the potential of improved quality of care through the establishment of utilization/quality review mechanisms.

Various kinds of organizations may sponsor a PPO. If the organizations are provider-based, they may constitute hospitals, multihospital networks, physician networks, or hospital/physician joint ventures. If the PPO is sponsored by an insurer, it may be a commercial insurance company or a Blue Cross and Blue Shield plan. In a joint venture situation, the sponsor can be an insurance carrier and hospital network. Entrepreneurial-based PPOs are sponsored by investors, third-party administrators, or brokers. Purchaser-based PPOs include employers, employer coalitions, and unions. Self-insured employers can contract directly with providers on negotiated fee-for-service arrangements because self-insured employers are considered underwriting risk-sharing vehicles under most state insurance laws. If providers wish to market their services as a PPO to employers who formerly subscribed in group health plans and do not qualify for self-insured status, an underwriting organization, such as an insurance company, must enter into the contractual arrangement between the provider and employer to assume the risk. By 1999 there were 1,079 operating PPOs, covering 106.8 million eligible employees in the United States.[37]

In practice, a PPO works like this: A company offers the plan to its employees as an option. They do not have to sign up for it or may not have to contribute to its upkeep. When they require medical care, they are free to make a choice. Under the company's traditional health insurance plan for which they pay a certain percentage of the premium, they can go to their own doctor but usually must pay a deductible and certain percentage of the bill. Or they can select any doctor in the PPO network, for which the deductible is waived, and, as already noted, a nominal fee of $10 or less may be charged. For hospital and emergency room services, they pay a certain percentage of reduced charges.[38]

Freedom of Physician Choice

A PPO is distinguished from an HMO by two important points. First, physicians are not at financial risk for patient care. All the insurance portions of healthcare—the setting of premiums, the processing of claims, the absorption of losses—are still handled by the insurer. Second, patients are not locked into using the PPO physicians or hospitals. They can use any provider they want—but deductibles and copayments are usually waived if they use a preferred provider. The patient can leave a preferred provider physician at any time. On the other hand, an employee who joins an HMO must receive care from HMO doctors in order to have his or her expenses covered. Typically, a PPO is one part of an insurance plan, and each time, as already noted, an insured seeks healthcare, that person can choose to receive it from a preferred provider or from any other providers, usually at a higher cost to that individual. In addition, HMOs operate on a capitation basis, while PPOs operate on a fee-for-service system. Thus, when a PPO is part of a health insurance plan, the employer pays its insurance company fixed monthly premiums, and each visit to a healthcare provider is paid through the traditional reimbursement mechanism. If a PPO is to be successful in reducing healthcare costs, it can choose one of two basic approaches: The PPO can choose physicians and hospitals known to be conservative and presumably cost effective in delivering care if it has a method of identifying such cost-effective physicians, and/or it can rely on utilization control mechanisms designed to eliminate unnecessary services and modify medical practice styles that many have.[39]

Typically, a patient in a PPO network is given a list of physicians to choose from. As with an HMO, most PPOs require that you select a primary care doctor. Many PPOs are implementing a "gatekeeper" approach, requiring approval by a primary care physician of all key referral and hospitalization decisions. Thus, the doctor monitors your health. If you need more extensive treatment, the primary care doctor can refer you to a specialist or a hospital in the PPO network. However, these steps can be taken only after review by the PPO. In some cases, the primary doctor may make the decision on treatment or hospitalization if he or she determines that the case meets a certain set of medical standards, called protocols. In other situations, the doctor must check with the PPO. The protocols, which are drawn up by outside experts, differ from one PPO to the next. In many cases, the reviewer has some flexibility. If the doctor recommends eight days of hospitalization and the protocol calls for three days, the reviewer might allow five days, based on the doctor's description of that individual case. Rulings can be appealed to a higher reviewer, usually a physician. The negotiated rates with providers such as physicians are usually acceptable because, as already noted, the rapid turnaround on claims payment offers an attractive cash flow; participation in the PPO increases the provider's patient volume and is intended to be an effective way of competing with other alternative delivery systems for patients; and the PPO design creates a minimal financial risk for providers.

Most PPOs cover preventive care. This usually includes visits to doctors, well-baby care, immunizations, and mammograms.

In a PPO, you can also use doctors who are not part of the plan and still receive some coverage. At these times, you will pay a larger portion of the bill yourself (and also fill out the claims forms). Some people like this choice because, even if their doctor is not part of the PPO network, it means they don't have to change doctors to join a PPO.

In summary, PPOs have six characteristics in common:

1. Formal contractual arrangements with a provider panel. A limited grouping of physicians and hospitals agrees to a negotiated schedule of specified discounted fees. There is no prepayment or capitation amount paid to providers, unlike HMOs. Regional PPOs are becoming more popular because of their ability to offer easy access to providers over a large geographic area; also, many employers with multiple sites are seeking regional and even national contracts to eliminate the need for numerous contractual arrangements to secure a PPO option for their employee/subscriber population.
2. Marketing programs are directed at purchasers as opposed to consumers. Consumers are not locked into those providers, but if they receive services through the listed providers, copayment and deductibles are eliminated and/or benefits increased.
3. Benefit levels are flexible.
4. Emphasis on cost efficiency. Usually includes a program of utilization review and a management information system that provides cost and use data for employers and trust funds. Strong utilization management programs should significantly change utilization patterns of care, not simply the pricing of services provided.
5. Relatively low administrative costs.
6. Rapid turnaround on claims, so that providers are paid very quickly.[40]

Deciding If a PPO Is for You

In considering whether you should join a PPO, you should ask the following questions to determine whether the PPO is the kind of system through which you wish to receive medical care. These include:

- *Are there many doctors to choose from?* Who are the doctors in the PPO network? Where are they located? Which ones are accepting new patients? Are your doctors in the plan's network? How are referrals to specialists handled? Is there a PPO provider directory available for the public? How does the plan select its physicians?
- *What hospitals are available through the PPO?* Where is the nearest hospital in the PPO network? What arrangements does the PPO have for handling emergency care?
- *What services are covered?* What preventive services are offered? Are there limits on medical tests, out-of-hospital care, mental healthcare, prescription drugs, or other services that are important to you? Does the PPO provide annual physicals, chemical dependency programs, lifestyle screening, transportation, vision care, well-baby care, wellness programs, home healthcare, and equipment rental?
- *What nonmedical services does the PPO provide?* Does the PPO provide administration of ancillary facilities, service to a physician's office staff, data-

processing services, marketing, education, training, and service to physician office staff?

- *What will the PPO plan cost?* How much is the premium? Is there a per-visit cost for seeing PPO doctors or other types of copayments for services? What is the difference in cost between using doctors in the PPO network and those outside of it? What is the deductible and coinsurance rate for care outside of the PPO? Is there a limit to the maximum you would pay out-of-pocket for care delivered through a PPO? Is there a limit on your out-of-network payments each year?

- *How can I influence my company's choice of health plans?* Make sure that the health benefits officer in your organization knows you have preferred doctors and hospitals and ask that your preferences be considered when your company chooses a health plan. Give your employer feedback about your positive and negative experiences with the providers in your health plan.

- *What are the elements of the PPO's Utilization Review and Quality Assurance Program?* Such a system may include a set of medical standards for providing certain kinds of services: a mechanism for determining whether the care is medically necessary; preadmission certification; concurrent and retrospective review of patient records; a referral authorization mechanism to control the use of services through a gatekeeper approach; a system for reviewing the use of ancillary or other healthcare services such as pharmacy or nutrition; and procedures for facilitating second surgical opinions and using less costly services such as homecare and same day surgery. Methods of utilization control vary widely among PPOs. Some are hospital initiated; some are buyer influenced (such as employers' private sector review); some are monitored by third-party administrators (referral authorization) and claims review, initiated by a third-party administrator, and conducted by a physician review committee.

- *Who is marketing the PPO plan to your organization?* Because the PPO option is incorporated in an employer's existing indemnity plan, various kinds of groups may market this option such as brokers, benefits consultants, and insurers. What is their reputation? Reliability? Experience? Knowledge of the PPO product? How do their costs compare with other groups marketing similar alternative delivery systems?

- *How does a PPO differ from a PPA?* A PPA is a preferred provider *arrangement*. The concept refers to an agreement between healthcare providers and another organization or group of organizations (such as insurance companies or employers) to provide medical services at negotiated fees to certain groups in return for prompt payment and increased patient volume. In contrast, a PPO generally indicates an *actual organization* of providers, while a PPA basically *suggests that a contractual agreement has been made*, but there is another legal entity formed as a result of the agreement. The providers enter into a contract directly with the insurers, employers, or other organizations.

Exclusive-Provider Organizations (EPOs)

This form of managed care is a derivation of the PPO in that it is an attempt to avoid the middleman such as health insurers (including HMOs), who may take 25 percent or more of the healthcare dollar. In this arrangement, the healthcare providers deal directly with buyers of healthcare services. Providers typically are reimbursed on a fee-for-service basis according to a negotiated discount or fee schedule. Medical services that are delivered by providers who are not affiliated with the EPO are not covered, so people belonging to an EPO must receive their care from affiliated providers or pay the entire cost themselves. In this latter sense, an EPO resembles an HMO. Usually, at the beginning of the plan year, individuals must decide whether they wish to use an EPO-type organization.

Point-of-Service Plans (POSs)

Point-of-service plans, sometimes called HMO-PPO hybrids or open-ended HMOs, combine the features of both HMOs and PPOs. POS plans use a network of selected participating providers who are under contract. Enrollees choose a primary care physician, who controls referrals for medical specialists. If enrollees receive care from a plan provider, the employee pays little or nothing out of pocket as in an HMO and does not file claims. Care delivered by nonplan providers will be reimbursed, but enrollees must file a claim and pay significantly higher copayments and deductibles. The basis of provider reimbursement may be fee-for-service or capitation; however, there are usually financial incentives for providers to avoid overutilization of services.

Managed Premium PPOs (MPPPOs)

A managed premium PPO introduces an element of risk sharing by and between the purchasers and providers of care. Although the providers are paid on the basis of fee-for-service, a part of their fees is withheld and returned to the purchasers of care if the providers cannot control the utilization of health services. Likewise, the fees paid to the providers are often discounted on the basis of the volume of services delivered by the purchaser under a contractual arrangement with the providers.

As cost-containment pressures continue, and as these alternative delivery systems try to increase their market share, each tries to make its system more attractive. Often that means borrowing features from other systems. It is likely that this hybridization will continue, and it may become increasingly difficult to characterize a particular managed care delivery system as adhering to any particular model.[41] Another aspect of managed care relates to mental health. As a result of the increase in cost and utilization of mental health treatment, the rate of cost increases in this area has been higher than that of other medical costs during the past decade. Presently, more than 73 percent of employers have employee assistance programs

(EAPs) as utilization management programs for mental health cases or management for mental health, and alcohol- and drug-abuse cases.[42]

DECIDING UPON A PPO AS AN EMPLOYER

In deciding to choose a PPO as a method of insuring its employees, a company may wish to take into consideration the following points in negotiating with a PPO:

- Are the operators of the PPO experienced and reputable and the medical professionals qualified and certificated?
- Does the PPO have a computerized system to monitor, review, and control all the practices of participating providers?
- Are the providers carefully screened by their peers before acceptance and is there a formal procedure for terminating unsatisfactory members?
- A company's size and number of employees must be considered in order to identify whether a PPO is correct for it. One consideration is to consider the added cost of administering the PPO plan in addition to the firm's current fee-for-service and/or health maintenance Organization (HMO) employee offerings. What is the proportion of costs relative to the employee that the employer must bear? Is this financial responsibility acceptable to both the employer and employee in view of the financial status of the company? Is there less expensive health insurance coverage available?
- The PPO should provide geographically convenient hospitals and physicians. If employees must travel long distances to use a provider, the company risks losing employee participation, money, and time.
- An organization that has facilities in more than one location should consider a "wide area" PPO. Insurance carriers, as well as independently established PPOs, are developing the necessary resources and capabilities to affiliate with other established PPOs throughout the country.
- Define the scope of services. A comparison should be made between a company's current health benefits package of medical services and those services offered in the proposed PPO plan.
- Select the payment methodology.
- Coverage benefits to be offered to the firm's employees under the contract should be presented as an incentive to participate in the PPO. Develop appropriate employee participation incentives. If the firm decides to include a PPO in its benefits package, it is suggested that the employees' acceptance of the new program be monitored. There isn't going to be much of a cost savings if the employees do not participate.
- Include stringent utilization controls. The built-in safeguards should be examined to assure long-term cost effectiveness through constant claims review by the PPOs, a private-sector claims reviewer or a hospital-contract reviewer

who reports to the medical staff's utilization review committee. Insist on timely, accurate, and adequate data. A PPO should spend a great deal of time reviewing utilization control. Without having in place an effective utilization review system, any PPO discount should be considered with caution because it can be more than offset by the increased utilization of member services. For example, if a PPO offers a 15 percent discount through its participating providers, but then increases utilization by 20 percent over what it would have been without the PPO, the purchaser contracting for PPO services is spending more on healthcare rather than less.

- Determine provider selection (and retention) criteria. Be aware that many private indemnity insurance companies also offer PPOs as well as do hospitals, physicians, and entrepreneurs. Any organization that is considering a PPO should also consider the following points in choosing the right PPO for it and its employees.

  ▼ Determine provider risk-sharing levels.

  ▼ Clarify any provisions relating to worker's compensation and subrogation.

  ▼ Does the PPO upon request provide documentation of its financial viability and list of contracted healthcare providers? Review any insolvency and reinsurance clauses.

  ▼ Include a "hold harmless" clause to protect employees.

  ▼ What is the PPO's previous experience with claims processing, timely claims payments, and actuarial experience?

  ▼ Does the PPO have liability/malpractice insurance to cover the client firm in the event of an adverse court judgment resulting from a policyholder's suit?

  ▼ Beware of entrepreneurial salespersons offering PPOs at low prices and not much else. Is the PPO registered with a regulatory agency (e.g., the Department of Insurance or the Department of Corporations)? Check with the appropriate agency to assure proper licensure and to determine if there are any complaints on record.

  ▼ Reserve the right to terminate the agreement on short notice.[43]

However, an insurer or employer can establish its own PPO. It can be to the economic advantage of an employer to establish a PPO since a PPO can cost the employer less than traditional health insurance to cover the workforce, especially those employers whose healthcare insurance costs have been escalating very rapidly over the recent past. The cost savings come from the price discounts and utilization review negotiated with the preferred providers. Employers whose claim utilization experience indicates that their workforce has been using a great deal of services from high-priced providers are the most likely candidates to achieve large health insurance premium savings. To accomplish this, they would have to create their own guidelines for determining those providers who are to be included in the arrangement and contract with the appropriate physicians and hospitals. However, the legal complexities of today's evolving healthcare system and issues such as antitrust law require the knowledge and skills of those who are familiar with all the previous complexities in establishing a PPO since the organizer is merging the practice of medical care with insurance. For example, one of the key issues regarding antitrust law is price fixing. The fact that PPOs may reduce competition because the same discounted fees are negotiated with many insurers or employers may be seen as price fixing. However, the position of federal agencies, thus far, has been the development of PPO activity rather than its constriction. Employers are attracted to the design of most PPOs, which provide some combination of the following: improved benefits, waiver of copayment or deductibles, or better accessibility to services. The nonbinding feature allows some employees to search for a satisfactory personal physician if they have no established physician ties, and it enables employees to shop selectively for benefits when services are needed.

A number of steps are involved in developing a PPO. These include:

- Development of an adequate network of providers whose location and character depends upon the population to be treated such as geriatricians for the elderly or pediatricians for children.
- Must choose and find physicians whose manner of practice is cost effective and whose professional skills are excellent, while providing the proper incentives to attract providers to join the PPO network as well as negotiating the price discounts that physicians and hospitals will provide to PPO members.
- Must create utilization review controls to help ensure that medical care delivered by physicians and hospitals are cost effective. But the problem must be resolved that the providers practice by the utilization review standards.
- Aside from issues relating to physician practice, accreditation, hospital staff privilege arrangements, licensure, appropriate liability and malpractice insurance, and other administrative details must be arranged.
- Data-processing systems must be established so that the care provided can be followed to ensure that the most cost effective treatment is being delivered.[44]

A great deal of work and negotiations are necessary to establish a network of providers who provide quality care, are willing to discount their fees, and follow utilization review controls. To encourage employees to accept this PPO healthcare option, employers should explain to their workforce the reasons for the PPO plan, identify the preferred providers, and then explain the differences in reimbursement for the preferred provider and nonpreferred provider. However, if such efforts result in a reduction of healthcare costs but an increase in the quality of care you are purchasing for your employees, the effort will more than pay for itself over time.

TRENDS

PPOs have become increasingly popular as replacement products for fee-for-service operations or as alternatives to more restrictive HMOs. The inclusion of worker's compensation coverage, together with group health insurance in managed care settings, has enabled PPOs to provide "twenty-four-hour coverage" for some clients. Hospital-based PPOs often serve chiefly to expand the number of providers and invade the self-insured market and small payer groups. At the beginning of 2001, about 93 percent of employees were enrolled in HMOs, PPOs, and POS (point-of-service) plans. This proportion of all workers covered by some form of managed care plan has increased very greatly from the 58 percent covered in 1993. The group market share of the various managed care plans differs by firm size and region; as an organization's size increases, employees are more likely to be offered coverage in managed care plans. PPOs claimed the greatest market share at 48 percent. HMOs actually declined in market share from 31 percent in 1997 to 23 percent in 2001. POS plans increased the most in market share, from 17 percent in 1997 to 22 percent in 2001. Conventional plans continued to decline to 7 percent in 2001 from 18 percent in 1997.[45]

THE FUTURE

The rapid growth of managed care is an indicator of how serious major employers and insurers have become to stem the rising costs of healthcare services in this country. Insurers increasingly realize that unmanaged fee-for service indemnity plans do not contain the mechanism to control costs. As a result, many insurers have made major efforts to develop and sustain comprehensive managed cares systems. National managed care firms (defined as firms operating HMOs in two or more states, including commercial insurers that meet this criteria), along with Blue Cross and Blue Shield plans, will continue to account for a majority of all HMOs and represent an overwhelming majority of Americans enrolled in managed care plans. As the healthcare field continues to evolve in this country, new organizations or derivatives of managed care will continue to develop to meet the ever-demanding needs of a growing but aging American population, whether the problems be related to costs, quality of care, or other issues. These societal and healthcare issues will continue to demand resolution as the twenty-first century progresses.

NOTES

1. Stanton N. Smullens, "An Overview of the Changes in Health Care—Part 1," *Contemporary Surgery for Residents* 3, no. 2 (March/April 1995): 22; *Source Book of Health Insurance Data, 1995* (Washington, DC: Health Insurance Association of America, 1996), p. 28.

2. US Department of Health and Human Services, *United States, Health, 2000, with*

Adolescent Health Chartbook (Hyattsville, MD: National Center for Health Statistics, 2000), p. 364 (table 145).

3. Jordan Braverman, "Group Practice Prepayment Plans—Universities Give New Impetus to Old Concept," *Journal of the American Pharmaceutical Association* NS9, no. 11 (November 1969): 564.

4. Stanley S. Wallack, "Managed Care: Practice, Pitfalls, and Potential," *Health Care Financing Review/1991 Annual Supplement*, p. 28.

5. Ibid., p. 30.

6. US Department of Health and Human Services, *Health, United States, 2003, with Chartbook on Trends in the Health of Americans* (Hyattsville, MD: National Center for Health Statistics, 2003), p. 339 (table 132).

7. US Department of Health and Human Services, *Health, United States, 2000, with Adolescent Health Chartbook*, pp. 364 (table 145), 361 (table 143); *Source Book of Health Insurance Data, 2002* (Washington, DC: Health Insurance Association of America, 2002), p. 60 (table 3.5); and Earl Dirk Hoffman Jr., Barbara S. Klees, and Catherine A. Curtis, "Overview of the Medicare and Medicaid Programs," in "Medicare and Medicaid Statistical Supplement, 2001," *Health Care Financing Review* (Washington, DC: Centers for Medicare and Medicaid Services, 2002), pp. 4, 279 (table 74).

8. *Source Book of Health Insurance Data, 1999–2000* (Washington, DC: Health Insurance Association of America, 2000), pp. 60–61.

9. "Employee Physicians Outnumber Solo Ones," *Washington Post*, August 21, 1996, p. A2.

10. Stuart Auerbach, "Doctors Gain More Freedom to Form Health Networks," *Washington Post*, August 29, 1996, p. B13.

11. Iver Peterson, "Automakers and U.A.W. Initiate Low-Cost, Pre-Paid Health Plan," *New York Times*, February 13, 1979.

12. *The Fundamentals of Managed Care* (Washington, DC: Health Insurance Association of America, October 1991), p. 9.

13. *Source Book of Health Insurance Data, 1995*, p. 31.

14. Sylvia Porter, "Health Maintenance Organization Groups Gain Support," *Washington Star*, December 26, 1978.

15. Sylvia Porter, "HEW Presses for More HMOs," *Washington Star*, June 28, 1978.

16. Victor Cohn, "Can Managed Care Work?" *Washington Post/Health*, September 15, 1992, p. 12; Victor Cohn, "Choosing a Health Plan," *Washington Post/Health*, November 12, 1991, p. 14.

17. Trudy Lieberman, "How Good Is Your Health Plan," *Consumer Reports* 61, no. 8 (August 1996): 38.

18. Trudy Lieberman, "What You Can Do: Managing Managed Care," *Consumer Reports* 61, no. 8 (August 1996): 33; David Segal, "A Closer Look at Plan English," *Washington Post*, March 27, 1996, p. F1.

19. Stuart Auerbach, "How Can Patients Judge Their HMOs?" *Washington Post*, August 6, 1996, p. 7; "Picking a Managed Care Plan," *Washington Post*, June 25, 1996, p. 14; Lieberman, "How Good Is Your Health Plan," pp. 33–34; and Rita Rubin and Katherine T. Beddingfield, "Rating the HMOs," *U.S. News & World Report*, September 2, 1996, p. 57.

20. "Can HMOs Help Solve the Health-Care Crisis," *Consumer Reports* 61, no. 10 (October 1996): 32.

21. Victor Cohn, "Making Your Health Plan Work for You," *Washington Post/Health*,

November 28, 1989, p. 8; Jill S. Brown, "Managed Care Enrollees Gain Ground," *AARP Bulletin* 43, no. 2 (February 2002): 6 –7.

22. Midge L. Schildkraut, "Prepaid Health Plans: Can They Save You Money?" *Good Housekeeping*, February 1979, p. 244.

23. Porter, "HEW Presses for More HMOs."

24. Leigh Page, "Medicare HMOs Winning Over Seniors," *American Medical News*, February 12, 1996, p. 30.; Patricia Barry, "Medicare HMOs Charging More . . . ," *AARP Bulletin* 43, no. 11 (December 2002): 8; and "Medicare and Medicaid Statistical Supplement, 2001," in *Health Care Financing Review* (Washington, DC: Centers for Medicare and Medicaid Services, 2002), pp. 281 (table 76), 288 (table 83).

25. "Can HMOs Help Solve the Health-Care Crisis," pp. 30–31; Barry, "Medicare HMOs Charging More . . . ," p. 8.

26. Cohn, "Making Your Health Plan Work for You," p. 9.

27. Paul J. Kenkel, "Social HMOs: A Reform Idea on the Rise," *Modern Healthcare* 23, no. 6 (February 8, 1993): 26–28.

28. Porter, " HEW Presses for More HMOs."

29. Sylvia Porter, "More HMO Questions: How Do They Differ?" *Washington Star*, December 27, 1978.

30. Sylvia Porter, "The HMOs . . . Finally Their Time Is Now," *Washington Star*, December 31, 1978.

31. Janice Ross, "Attacking Health Benefit Costs," *Pensions World* 8, no. 11 (November 1978).

32. US Department of Health, Education, and Welfare, *Administration Promoting HMOs to Nation's Largest Corporations* (Washington, DC: Health Services Administration, November 7, 1977), p. 3.

33. Victor Cohn, "A Health Plan That Draws Praise," *Washington Post*, September 15, 1992, p. 12; US Department of Health and Human Services, *Checkup on Health Insurance Choices*, Public Health Service (Washington, DC: Agency for Heath Policy and Research, December 1992), pp. 11–12; and "Before Picking a Health Plan, Get Plenty of Information," *Washington Post/Health*, November 7, 1995, p. 17.

34. Victor Cohn, "Choosing a Health Plan," *Washington Post/Health*, November 12, 1991, p. 14.

35. "Before Picking a Plan, Get Plenty of Information," pp. 17, 19.

36. *Healthy Decisions* (Washington, DC: Georgetown University Medical Center, Fall 1996), p. 1; Victor Cohn, "The Right Choice," *Washington Post/Health*, November 18, 1986, p. 12; and Donald Robinson, "How Well Do You Know Your HMO?" *Parade*, February 5, 1989, p. 13.

37. *Source Book of Health Insurance Data, 2002*, p. 51.

38. Thomas J. Murray, "PPOs: Answer to Soaring Medical Costs," *Dun's Business Month* 123, no. 11 (December 1983): 117.

39. "Competitive Market Spawning PPOs," *American Medical News*, May 7, 1982, p. 7.

40. *AAFMC Bulletin* (Potomac, MD: Association of IPAs and Other Physician Sponsored Health Plans, March 25, 1981), p. 1.

41. *Source Book of Health Insurance Data, 1995*, pp. 31–33.

42. Ibid., p. 34.

43. John Edleston, "Some Thoughts on Selecting a PPO," *Behavior Today*, January 9, 1984, p. 4; *Health Insurance Answer Book* (Greenvale, NY: Panel Publishers, 1986), p. Q-227A; and Murray, "PPOs: Answers to Soaring Medical Costs," p. 118.

44. *The Health Insurance Answer Book*, pp. 115–17.

45. *Source Book of Health Insurance Data, 2002*, p. 53.

CHAPTER FIVE

MEDICAID AND MEDICARE

INTRODUCTION

The concept embodied in the Medicaid program, namely, government responsibility for the medical care of the needy and medically indigent, can be traced as far back as the colonial period when common law established that the care of the poor—including medical care—was essentially a function of local government. Common law held that no government should allow its citizens to perish from starvation, sickness, or exposure merely because they were poor and, generally, assigned the responsibility for "poor relief" to the smallest political unit, whether it was the village, town, city parish, or county. With the arrival of our national independence, this concept was incorporated into our state constitutions and statutes.

In the nineteenth century, state governments gradually began to assume some administrative responsibilities for helping the poor and actually began to provide care, based on need, to certain groups of the poor who until then had been only the responsibility of local government. Thus, government assistance according to category of need began. This activity was not only inspired by humanitarian motives but also by the very high costs of providing special care to only a few persons in any one special category in a single locality. These categories generally included the sick, the deaf, and the insane. The division of responsibility between state and local governments essentially continued until the 1930s. State and local governmental responsibility for the medical care of the indigent was carried out either through public institutions employing salaried physicians or by the purchase of medical care from private physicians. In most of the larger local jurisdictions, however, city or county hospitals usually provided such medical services. In addition, a large number of physicians and voluntary hospitals gave the poor free services or reduced-payment care.

As far as Medicare is concerned, the concept of a government-sponsored health insurance program can be traced as far as back as the early 1900s when interest developed in establishing a national compulsory health insurance program in the country. In fact, national health insurance had been one of the major planks in Theodore Roosevelt's Progressive Party platform in 1912. In the 1930s the government renewed its interest in the subject when President Roosevelt appointed a committee to study the issue of government health insurance. Although the committee eventually recommended health insurance legislation in 1935, President Roosevelt did not include any such proposal in the Social Security Act. The president and some members of the committee felt that the inclusion of such legislation would jeopardize the prompt passage of the Social Security legislation with its other extremely important provisions of old-age and unemployment insurance.

The Social Security Act of 1935 established a categorical public assistance system in which the federal government shared with the states the cost of providing maintenance to the aged who were needy, the blind, families with dependent children, and subsequently the permanently and totally disabled. The Social Security Act did not make any special provisions for medical assistance, but it included the cost of medical care in the individual's monthly assistance payment for which federal participation was available. Without any restrictions on how to spend their payments, many welfare recipients neglected their personal medical care—often because states set the overall payment level so low that it was not enough to pay even for basic food and shelter. This situation continued until the 1950s when congressional legislative action attempted to correct it. Beginning in 1950 Congress passed a series of amendments to the Social Security Act that expanded the definition of public assistance to include money for "vendor payments"—that is, direct payments by the state to physicians, nurses, and healthcare institutions, rather than to the welfare recipient himself. This change created an administrative framework for a welfare medical program. By 1958 the federal government was not only sharing in cash payments but also in a separate category of medical payments to those who met a state's definition of being "needy." As of 1960 most of the states made vendor payments in federally aided categorical assistance programs, and many states, in calculating their cash payments to welfare recipients, also allowed for the purchase of some items of medical care.[1] Despite this expanded federal and state effort, however, the need of the indigent for healthcare was so great that most states could only finance a few services. Efforts continued through the Kennedy and Johnson administrations during the early 1960s to improve the financing of medical care for the elderly and the poor through the Social Security system. Then Congress enacted the Social Security Amendments of 1965. President Lyndon B. Johnson signed this new legislation into law on July 30, 1965, thereby adding two new titles to the Social Security Act—Title XVIII, known as the Medicare program, and Title XIX, known as Medicaid.

MEDICAID

Program Definition

Medicare and Medicaid help many older persons with medical bills. Nearly all persons aged sixty-five years and older are eligible for Medicare, while needy, low-income elderly persons may also be eligible for Medicaid—a *public assistance* program financed by federal, state, and local governments. All states, as well as the District of Columbia, Puerto Rico, and the Virgin Islands, have Medicaid programs.

Medicare is a federal government program that is the same all over the country; Medicaid is a federal-state partnership under which benefits vary from state to state.

Whether or not a low-income older person is enrolled in Medicare, he may also be eligible for Medicaid. For senior citizens not eligible for Medicare, Medicaid helps pay for a wide variety of hospital and other medical services. For elderly persons already enrolled in Medicare, Medicaid often pays for services not covered by Medicare, such as eyeglasses and long-term nursing home care. For instance, in 2006 Medicaid may have paid

- the first $952 of inpatient hospital costs in each benefit period;
- the first $124 per year of approved medical charges;
- the remaining 20 percent of approved medical charges not covered by Medicare;
- Medicare Part A (hospital insurance) coverage for certain low-income disabled people who lose Medicaid coverage because they return to work; and
- the $88.50 monthly premium for Medicare Part B (medical insurance).

Thus, Medicare and Medicaid are interlinked. State governments can also buy into the hospital insurance plan of Medicare (Part A) for the medically needy by paying its coinsurance and deductible amounts as well as buy into the supplemental medical insurance plan of Medicare (Part B) by paying its monthly premium.

Eligibility

A state determines whether an individual or family is eligible for Medicaid according to its definition of need, within certain federal government limits. However, in general, low-income people in the following categories qualify for Medicaid coverage:

- the aged (sixty-five or older)
- the blind
- the disabled
- families with dependent children and some other children

Some states provide coverage for other groups of low-income people who do not qualify for public assistance programs but still cannot pay for medical care. These people are known as "medically needy." In addition, Medicaid also must cover children under the age of six who meet a state's AFDC financial requirements or whose family is at or below the federal poverty line; recipients of adoption assistance and foster care under Title IV-E of the Social Security Act; and all children born after September 30, 1983, in families whose income is at or below the federal poverty level (they must be given full Medicaid coverage until age nineteen). Coverage was phased in so that, by the year 2002, all poor children under age nineteen were to be covered as well as pregnant women whose family income is below the federal poverty level (services to the women are limited to pregnancy, complications of pregnancy, delivery, and three months of postpartum care) and special protected groups (these are usually individuals who lose their cash assistance because of the cash program's rules, but who may keep Medicaid for a period of time such as persons who lose AFDC or SSI payments because of earnings from work or increased Social Security benefits; and two parent, unemployed families whose cash AFDC assistance is limited by the state). These families are protected and provided a full twelve months of Medicaid coverage.[2] Check with your local public assistance or welfare office to see whether you qualify for the Medicaid program under the guidelines established for the previous public assistance categories or as a medically needy recipient.

In August 1996 President Clinton signed into law the Personal Responsibility and Work Opportunity Act of 1996 (Public Law 104-193), otherwise known as welfare reform. The welfare reform law continues Medicaid as an entitlement to families on welfare and continues coverage for one year for people who leave welfare to go to work. However, the law does change Medicaid in one major respect since it replaced the categorical program of Aid to Families with Dependent Children (AFDC) with the Temporary Assistance for Needy Families (TANF) program, effective July 1, 1997. In place of AFDC, states establish their own assistance programs, funded by annual federal payments, instead of the opened-ended federal funds they have received in the past. States can determine who is eligible and for how long, although federal benefits cannot be used to provide benefits for more than five years over a lifetime. The law reduces food stamps and Supplementary Security Income (SSI) to legal immigrants who have not become citizens. States must decide whether to continue Medicaid and cash payments to poor immigrant families.[3]

On February 8, 2006, the president signed the Deficit Reduction Act of 2005 into law (Public Law 109-171). The new law is expected to push states to tighten the work requirements for women on assistance under the TANF program.

Benefit Coverage

Medicaid pays the full cost of covered services, which, as a minimum, include the following:

- inpatient hospital care
- outpatient hospital services
- prenatal care
- other laboratory and x-ray services
- services furnished by nurse midwives to the extent authorized by state law
- skilled nursing facility services for persons over twenty-one years of age
- physician services
- early and periodic screening, diagnosis, and treatment services (EPSDT) of children under age twenty-one
- home healthcare services for persons eligible for skilled-nursing services
- family planning services and supplies
- rural health clinic services
- pediatric and family nurse practitioner services
- certain federally qualified ambulatory and health-center services

Also, in many states Medicaid pays for such additional services as dental care, prescribed drugs (as a result of the president signing the Deficit Reduction Act of 2005 into law on February 8, 2006, Medicaid is reducing payments for prescription drug benefits to combat inflated prescription drug markups and is requiring its recipients to pay new copayments and deductibles for expensive drugs and emergency room visits for nonemergency care), intermediate-care facility services, optometrist services and eyeglasses, clinic services, hearing aids, and prosthetic devices, as well as other diagnostic screening and rehabilitative services. Ask your local health or public assistance department what medical services are covered by the Medicaid program in your state; also find out whether your state Medicaid program pays for the cost of second surgical opinion programs. Since September 1978 the federal government has encouraged state Medicaid programs to offer this service so their recipients would have the opportunity to seek a second opinion prior to consenting to elective surgery. In some states the Medicaid program even pays the full cost for a third surgical opinion. With certain exceptions, a state's Medicaid plan must allow recipients freedom of choice among participating providers of healthcare. States may provide and pay for Medicaid services through various prepayment arrangements, such as a health maintenance organization (HMO). In general, states are required to provide comparable services to all categorically needy eligible persons. There are two important exceptions.

- Health services identified under the EPSDT program (early and periodic screening, diagnosis, and treatment services) as being "medically necessary" for eligible children must be provided by Medicaid, even if those services are not included as part of the covered services in that state's plan.
- States may request home- and community-based services "waivers" under which they offer an alternative healthcare package for persons who would otherwise be institutionalized under Medicaid. States are not limited in the

scope of services they can provide under such waivers so long as they are cost effective (except that, other than as a part of respite care, they may not provide room and board for such recipients).

On February 8, 2006, when President Bush signed into law the Deficit Reduction Act of 2005 (Public Law 109-171), a new mechanism for financing Medicaid health services was established. It is called the Health Opportunity Account (HOA) and is being tested as a demonstration program for the next five years, 2006 to 2011, in up to ten states.

These accounts would be similar to the Health Savings Accounts that are attached to high-deductible health insurance plans, which were created with the passage of the Medicare Prescription Drug, Improvement, and Modernization Act of 2003.

Some critics are concerned that these accounts would require low-income Medicaid beneficiaries to meet a high deductible before their standard Medicaid benefits would pay for their health services, while supporters of HOAs believe the accounts will reduce the use of unnecessary services and increase the likelihood the Medicaid recipients will use less costly services. In general, once beneficiaries have met the deductible, Medicaid coverage would begin, and Medicaid recipients would be required to pay the regular copayments and other cost-sharing charges that Medicaid requires. States would make contributions of specified amounts for adults and children into these accounts with matching funds from the federal government in order to help Medicaid beneficiaries pay the healthcare costs that they would incur before the Medicaid coverage begins. However, states would not be required to fully offset these Medicaid costs. As a result, some Medicaid recipients, especially those in poorer health who spend all the monies in their HOA accounts but still have not met their deductibles, could face substantial increases in their own out-of pocket costs, which could discourage their using the medical services that they need—that is, after spending all the monies in their HOA accounts before meeting their deductibles, they themselves would have to pay the full costs of the health services they receive in the uncovered financial gap that exists between the state's contribution and the level of the deductible. If Medicaid recipients become ineligible for Medicaid because of changes in their income or resources, they can still keep 75 percent of the funds in these Health Opportunity Accounts. The demonstration project does not have to be statewide and would permit states, at their option, to allow beneficiaries to reimburse certain providers at higher rates than under Medicaid, such as those providers who do not participate in the Medicaid program; to use Medicaid dollars to pay for medical services that federal law does not permit Medicaid to cover; and even to pay for nonmedical services, specified by the state, such as beneficiaries' tuition expenses and job training. Particpation in the demonstration project must be voluntary on the part of Medicaid recipients. The demonstration project excludes those who are sixty-five years or older, the disabled, pregnant women, and those who have been on Medicaid for less than three months. Check with the Medicaid program in your state to find out if it is establishing Health Opportunity Accounts, the conditions of participation, and how they affect you as a Medicaid beneficiary.

After five years this demonstration project could become permanent, unless the secretary of the US Department of Health and Human Services determined that each of the state demonstrations was not successful, and the secretary, without further review by Congress, could extend the demonstration project to all states.

Become knowledgeable about Medicaid service coverage and qualification standards in your state; this will enable you to obtain medical care at a time when you may not be able to afford its costs.

In addition to Medicaid, there are alternative financial mechanisms to cover the cost of an elderly person's healthcare. These include the following:

- Adult children who pay for more than half of their elderly parent's care can claim the parent as a dependent and get a tax deduction.
- Sometimes a lawyer can arrange "personal care contracts" that transfer assets to family members who help an elderly individual even after he is admitted to a nursing home.
- An aging person's assets can be transferred into an annuity that pays him or her a steady annual income. However, annuities generally carry penalties if they need to be withdrawn, such as paying for nursing home care in the first seven years.
- Flexible spending accounts permit adult children to pay for some of their parents' care with pretax money.
- A revocable family trust can keep property out of probate when an elderly person dies. This is significant because some states place liens on property during the probate process to recover Medicaid funds spent on an elderly person's care. An adult child might require what's called durable power of attorney to administer a parent's estate.
- Long-term care insurance is generally geared toward people who are many years from requiring professional assistance. But some insurers will write long-term care policies for reasonably healthy people in their seventies and eighties—though the policies can be quite costly by then. Some insurance companies also offer policies that will return to the heirs the premiums paid by elderly people who died before they required professional care.

For more information about paying for the healthcare of elderly persons, other than Medicaid, and the options that are available to you, you may check with the Internet site of the National Academy of Elder Law Attorneys at http://www .naela.org.

MEDICARE

Enrollment and Eligibility

"Ruth, I know this hard to believe, but I was in my midtwenties back in 1965 when Medicare became law and here I am about to join its ranks. Back then, Medicare seemed so far away. It was a program for the elderly, my grandparents. I never paid attention to it, and after all these years I still don't know much about it except for a few of its benefits like hospital care or physician services. I don't even know if I qualify for it."

"Joseph, you have nothing to worry about. It is not as difficult as it may seem to understand this program."

Medicare is available to nearly everyone who is sixty-five years of age or older (exceptions: certain aliens and criminals, in addition to a few federal government workers for whom benefits are limited). In 1973 Medicare protection was extended to certain people under sixty-five: those who have permanent kidney failure (renal disease) or who have been entitled to Social Security disability benefits for at least twenty-four consecutive months or Railroad Retirement disability benefits for at least twenty-nine consecutive months. Included are disabled workers and disabled widows and widowers between fifty and sixty-five, and people age eighteen and over who draw Social Security benefits because they became disabled before reaching twenty-two years of age.[4] Medicare, like Medicaid, is administered by the Centers for Medicare and Medicaid Services located in the US Department of Health and Human Services.

Original Medicare consists of two programs. Part A, the hospital insurance plan, can help pay for medically necessary inpatient hospital care and, after a hospital stay, for inpatient care in a skilled nursing facility and for care in your home by a home health agency. Part A's hospital insurance plan automatically covers people who are entitled to retirement, survivor, or disability benefits under Social Security or the Railroad Retirement system and is free except for various deductibles and coinsurance charges. Others may purchase this coverage, which as of January 1, 2006, costs $393 a month. Individuals over sixty-five years of age who do not have at least ten years of work experience covered by Social Security, the Railroad Retirement system, or Medicare-covered government employment do not get automatic Part A coverage. Many of those people are state, local, and municipal workers and teachers who often have access to other healthcare plans through their former employers or unions. Some may be immigrants who didn't work long enough in this country or people who always worked for cash and never paid into the Social Security system.[5] The increase in the Part A premium (if you have to pay a premium) is 10 percent no matter how late you enroll for coverage. Part B of Medicare is the supplemental medical insurance plan, which is purchased on a voluntary basis. This part of the Medicare program pays doctors' bills and some other charges. An individual must enroll to be eligible to participate in Part B of Medicare. As of January 1, 2006, the cost of this supplemental medical insurance plan was $88.50 per month. As a result of the Deficit Reduction Act of 2005, which President Bush signed into law on February 8, 2006, starting in 2007, the highest income seniors, those whose incomes begin at $80,000 a year, will pay a higher Medicare premium than those earning less than that amount. If you do not enroll in this plan when you become eligible for it, you can enroll at a later date, but the premium will be higher by 10 percent for each year of delay and you will have to pay this extra 10 percent for the rest of your life. Under certain circumstances you can delay your Part B enrollment without having to pay higher premiums. If you are age sixty-five or over and have group health insurance based on your own or your spouse's current employment, or if you are disabled and have group health insurance based on your current employment or the current employment of any family member of your choice:

- you may enroll at any time while you are covered by the group health plan; or
- you can enroll during a special eight-month enrollment period that begins the month the employment ends or the month you are no longer covered under the employer's plan, whichever comes first.

If you do not enroll by the end of the eight-month period, you will have to wait until the next general enrollment period, which begins January 1 of the next year.

After you qualify for the hospital insurance program (Part A) of Medicare, you will receive a health insurance card that shows you are covered. If you have medical insurance protection (Part B), the same card will show that you have this Medicare coverage as well. Keep this card with you and always show it to the hospital, skilled nursing facility, home health agency, physician, or other persons providing you with health services.

The Medicare program contains a transitional provision under which some individuals who attained the age of sixty-five before 1974 and lack the necessary work credits to qualify for either Social Security or the Railroad Retirement program may nevertheless be able to obtain free hospital insurance under Part A. Ask your local Social Security office whether you qualify for this health insurance coverage if you think these circumstances apply to you.

If you qualify for the Medicare program because of Social Security or Railroad Retirement eligibility, the protection you receive will last as long as you live. If you wish to enroll under the medical insurance plan (Part B), you can pay the premiums yourself or have the money deducted from your Social Security check. New applicants can enroll in Part B from January to March of each year with the coverage becoming effective on July 1 of that same year. Also, the Omnibus Budget Reconciliation Act of 1980 (Public Law 96-499) repealed that part of the Medicare law which formerly permitted an individual to reenroll in Part B only once during his lifetime.

At the time of eligibility, you will be notified by mail and automatically enrolled for both the hospital insurance and the supplemental medical insurance if you have previously applied for Social Security retirement and dependents' coverage. Consequently, you must inform your Social Security office if you do not want to be covered by Part B. If you plan to keep working after age sixty-five, you have to apply for Medicare. This can be done at any Social Security office.[6]

If you do not qualify for the free hospital insurance program but decide to purchase it, you must buy the medical insurance plan as well. On the other hand, if you decide you only want to purchase the medical insurance plan without purchasing the hospital insurance plan, you can do so.

The Medicare program was never meant to cover every health expense of the elderly. As healthcare costs continue to rise rapidly, Medicare is able to cover less and less. Medicare's benefits were intentionally limited to minimize the program's costs and discourage abuse, although Medicare's history has proven that the reverse has taken place thus far. It is important for present and future Medicare enrollees and their family members who one day may care for them to realize that Medicare is not a comprehensive health insurance program; it is designed mainly to relieve people aged sixty-five or older of the major part of the medical costs owing to hospitalization, surgery, and lengthy periods of recovery. Booklets are available from your local Social Security office and other organizations that explain the complexities of Medicare in great detail. Some good references are the following:

- *Your Medicare Handbook*
    This booklet, available *free* from your local Social Security office and from the Centers for Medicare and Medicaid Service's offices in Baltimore, Maryland, 21244-1850, outlines the basics of the Medicare program for consumers. It explains what Medicare covers and does not cover, how to submit insurance claims and where to send them, your rights of appeal, events that can end your Medicare protection, and other matters of great importance to you.
- *Medicare Coverage of Kidney and Kidney Transplant Services*
    This booklet describes various aspects of kidney treatment such as home dialysis and kidney transplant surgery and what Medicare's hospital and medical insurance does and does not pay for, including payments for beneficiaries covered by an employer group health plan, home dialysis supplies, equipment support services, blood, and other elements of the kidney treatment program.
- *Medicare and Other Health Benefits: Your Guide to Who Pays First*
    If you have Medicare and also have other health insurance, you need to know which health insurance pays first. This booklet tells you about some of the cases where other health insurance pays first. It discusses Medicare and work-related illness and injury such as Worker's Compensation; Black Lung; Medicare information for veterans where you can choose treatment under either the Department of Veterans Affairs (VA) or Medicare but not be covered by both programs for the same treatment; Medicare and the former CHAMPUS program (the Civilian Health and Medical Program of the Uniformed Services) now called TRICARE that covers civilian hospital services

MEDICARE
HOSPITAL INSURANCE PROGRAM—PART A

PROGRAM BENEFITS PART A	MEDICARE COVERAGE PART A	PATIENT PAYS PART A (2006)	REMARKS
Hospital Care	First to 60th day	First $952 in costs	Recalculated each year
	61st to 90th day	$238 per day	Recalculated each year
	91st to 150th day	$476 per day	Recalculated each year—after 90 days in hospital Medicare patient has 60 reserve hospital days that can be used anytime but once used are gone for a lifetime
	Ends after 150th day of hospital care	For all hospital care services	
Psychiatric hospital care	First to 190th day	Initial deductible and daily cost sharing	Limited to 190 days of care in patient's lifetime
Skilled nursing home care	First to 20th day	Nothing	Must be Medicare-participating hospital for at least three consecutive days prior to transfer to nursing home
	21st to 100th day	$119 per day	
	Ends after 100th day	For all nursing home care	Custodial care, private duty nursing, and first three pints of blood in nursing home not covered
Homecare	Unlimited home health visits in 365-day noncalendar year—Medicare pays entire cost of visiting nurses (part time), physical therapy and speech therapy services, medical supplies, and appliances (but not physicians)	For other home healthcare services such as housekeeping and full-time nursing care.	Patient can qualify directly for homecare without prior hospitalization
Hospice care	Up to 210 days or more	Up to $5 per prescription drug and 5 percent of inpatient respite care	Covers some non-Medicare benefits

and civilian doctors, suppliers, and other providers; and Medicare and No-Fault or liability Insurance.

Other subjects include Medicare and skilled nursing home care, homecare, ambulance services, mental health benefits, hospice care, coverage outside the United States, diabetes supplies and services, clinical trials, Medicare savings program, second opinions, and other topics.

Since deductibles, copayments, premiums, and other cost-sharing items in the Medicare program are periodically changed, these booklets on Medicare will enable you to understand the program and how such changes will affect your financial situation. However, because the rules and regulations of the Medicare program are complex, it is necessary to understand the general framework of the program if the details of the program are to be understood within their proper context.

Medicare's Hospital Insurance Plan (Part A)

Part A of Medicare is primarily a hospital insurance program. On being admitted to a hospital that participates in Medicare, you become personally responsible for the first $952 in costs (the deductible effective as of January 1, 2006). This deductible can sometimes be paid at a later date. From the first through the sixtieth day of hospitalization, the *Medicare program pays all the following covered services above the $952 deductible*:

- a semiprivate room (2 to 4 beds)
- all meals, including special diets
- regular nursing services
- costs of special care units such as intensive care and coronary care
- drugs furnished by the hospital during your stay
- laboratory tests included in your hospital bill
- x-ray and other radiology services, including radiation therapy billed by the hospital
- medical supplies such as casts, splints, and surgical dressings
- use of appliances such as wheelchairs
- operating room and recovery room costs
- rehabilitation services such as physical therapy, occupational therapy, and speech pathology services[7]

However, when you are a patient in a hospital that participates in the Medicare program, *the hospital insurance plan (Part A) of Medicare cannot pay for the following services:*

- personal convenience items you request such as a television, a radio, or a telephone in your room

- private duty nurses
- any charges above the hospital's semiprivate room rate, unless you need a private room for medical reasons
- the first three pints of blood you receive in a benefit period (However, if you are covered by a blood donor plan, it can replace the first three pints of blood for you. Or, you can arrange to have someone donate blood for you. A hospital or other facility may not charge you when you have arranged for replacement of the first three pints of blood for which Medicare does not pay.)[8]

If the patient's spell of illness exceeds sixty days in the hospital, then the patient must pay, effective January 1, 2006, $238 per day from the sixty-first through the ninetieth day and the government pays the rest.

If the patient must remain in the hospital more than ninety days, then each Medicare enrollee has sixty reserve hospital days that can be used at any time. Effective January 1, 2006, the patient pays $476 per day and Medicare pays the rest. Once used, the reserve days are gone forever. However, sixty days after leaving a hospital or other qualified facility such as a skilled nursing home (including the day of discharge), you are eligible for a new benefit period and can start fresh with the previous benefit coverage.

You can have under the Medicare program as many benefit periods as you need. Again, a benefit period begins when you enter a hospital and ends when you have been out of a hospital or skilled nursing home facility for sixty consecutive days.

The hospital insurance program (Part A) of Medicare is usually only good in hospitals that participate in the Medicare program. However, about two-thirds of the cost of emergency treatment in a hospital that does not participate in Medicare will be paid by the program if the hospital is the closest one equipped to handle the case and if delaying the patient's treatment can be dangerous.

Psychiatric Care

Part A can pay for up to 190 days of care in a Medicare-participating psychiatric hospital during your lifetime. Once you have used these 190 days of psychiatric care, however, the hospital insurance plan of Medicare cannot pay for any more days during your life. If you are a patient in a psychiatric hospital when you become entitled to Medicare, there are additional limitations on the number of hospital days that Medicare will pay for. Consult your local Social Security office to find out what these limitations may be. Psychiatric care provided in a general hospital is not subject to the 190-day limit. Also, Medicare's hospital insurance can help pay for the inpatient hospital and skilled nursing facility services you receive in a participating Christian Science sanatorium if it is operated, or listed and certified, by the First Church of Christ Scientist in Boston, Massachusetts.[9] You can get more information on these matters at any Social Security office.

Skilled Nursing Home Care

Part A pays for extended care in a skilled nursing home as well as for part-time skilled nursing care at home. The program works in the following manner. After your stay in a Medicare participating hospital for at least three consecutive days, not including the day of discharge, Medicare helps pay up to one hundred days of extended care in a skilled nursing facility, provided that the nursing is certified as being connected with the illness that placed you in the hospital. Skilled nursing care is defined as that which "can only be performed by, or under the supervision of, licensed nursing personnel." As with hospital coverage, the nursing home benefit pays the charges normally associated with these facilities. Medicare pays the first twenty days of nursing home care in full. For the remaining eighty days, as of January 1, 2006, you pay $119 per day and Medicare pays the rest. Eligibility for Medicare coverage in a skilled nursing home depends upon the fulfilling of five conditions:

1. You require daily skilled nursing or rehabilitation services that can only be provided in a skilled nursing home.
2. You were previously in a hospital for at least three consecutive days, not including the day of discharge, as already noted, before entering the skilled nursing facility.
3. You require additional care for a condition that was treated in the hospital or arose while you were receiving care for a condition treated in the hospital.
4. You are admitted soon after leaving the hospital—generally within thirty days. Also, if you leave a skilled nursing home and are readmitted within thirty days, Medicare will cover you without your having to return to the hospital for a new three-day stay.
5. A medical professional certifies that you need skilled nursing care.[10]

Finally, please note that *Medicare does not pay for custodial care in a nursing home*, such as help with bathing, dressing, eating, taking medication, or having dressings changed for noninfected conditions, but it does pay for meals and semiprivate rooms.

Home Healthcare

Medicare's Part A hospital insurance program also provides for unlimited homecare nursing visits by skilled paramedical personnel. Medicare Part A (or Part B if you don't have Part A) pays the entire bill for covered services as long as they are medically necessary and reasonable. Coverage is provided for the services of skilled nurses, home health aides, medical social workers, and different kinds of therapists (physical, occupational, and speech-language). The services may be provided either on a part-time or an intermittent basis, not full time. Those benefits can include therapy, skilled medical services, and supplies and equipment provided by home healthcare agencies. Besides paying for healthcare services, the home health benefit also covers the full cost of some medical supplies and 80 percent of the approved amount for durable medical equipment such as wheelchairs, hospital beds, oxygen supplies, and walkers. The home healthcare visits must be made within a 365-day noncalendar year. A prior stay in a hospital is not required to qualify for home healthcare, and you do not have to pay a deductible for home health services. The hospital insurance program pays the entire cost of visiting nurses, physical therapists, and other health workers (except doctors). Medicare pays for home healthcare when the following four conditions are met:

1. You require intermittent skilled nursing care, physical therapy, or speech language pathology.
2. You are confined to your home.
3. Your doctor determines that you need home healthcare and sets up a plan for you to receive care at home.
4. The home health agency providing the care participates in Medicare.[11]

Check with a home health agency to learn the conditions under which you can receive home healthcare services under Medicare's Part A hospital insurance program. You can find a Medicare-approved home health agency by asking your doctor, your hospital discharge planner, or by looking in the *Yellow Pages* under "home healthcare."

Blood Coverage

You may require blood as part of a covered inpatient stay in a hospital or a skilled nursing facility—whole blood, units of packed red blood cells, or blood components. If so, Medicare will help pay the costs, including the costs of processing and administering it.

You must either pay for or replace the first three pints of blood each year—this is the annual blood deductible. You can replace the blood you use yourself or have another person donate on your behalf.

Both Part A and Part B of Medicare cover blood, and to the extent you meet the three-pint deductible under one part you do not have to meet it under the other part.

Hospice Care

Another benefit available under Part A is hospice care if you are terminally ill. You can elect to receive hospice care rather than regular Medicare benefits for the management of your illness.

Hospice care may be provided by either a private organization or a public agency for up to 210 days, or even longer in some cases. Emphasis is on providing comfort and relief from pain. While the Medicare hospice benefit primarily provides for care at home, it can help pay for inpatient care as well as for a variety of services not usually covered by Medicare, including homemaker services, counseling, and certain prescription drugs.

Medicare pays nearly the entire bill for hospice care. There can be a copayment of up to $5 for each drug prescription and 5 percent of the Medicare-approved payment amount per day for inpatient respite care. Respite care is short-term care given to a hospice patient by another caregiver so that the usual person or persons who regularly assist with hospice care can temporarily rest. The amount you pay for respite care can change each year.

Medicare pays for hospice care when the following three conditions are met:

1. Your doctor certifies that you are terminally ill.
2. You choose to receive hospice care rather than the standard Medicare benefits for the illness.
3. The care is provided by a Medicare-participating hospice program.[12]

If you choose hospice care and later need treatment for a condition other than the terminal illness, you can use Medicare's standard benefits. When standard benefits are used, you must pay any deductibles and coinsurance.

Medicare's Voluntary Medical Insurance Plan (Part B)

Premiums, Coinsurance, and Deductibles

Part B of Medicare is the voluntary medical insurance program to which you pay monthly premiums. This plan helps pay for physician and surgeon services both in and out of hospitals. The voluntary medical insurance plan pays 80 percent of the Medicare-approved amount for specified medical expenses. The patient pays the rest plus a $124 deductible. The $124 is not charged more than once a year. Medicare determines what the approved amount is. Beginning in 2005, this deductible will increase annually, indexed to the growth in Part B spending. Beginning in 2006, individuals with incomes greater than $80,000 would pay a larger premium. The size of the premium would increase on a sliding scale, topping out at 80 percent of Part B costs for people with incomes over $200,000.

Physician Assignment

The basic question to ask when seeking medical services is: Will your physician or surgeon accept the Medicare *"assignment"—that is, will he accept as his fee what Medicare will pay without charging you any additional amount?* If so, your out-of-pocket expenses will be limited to the annual deductible of $124 or more, plus 20 percent of the doctor's charges. If not, your out-of-pocket expenses will include the deductible amount of $124, plus 20 percent of the physician's Medicare charge, plus that portion of the physician's Medicare charge in excess of Medicare's definition of

MEDICARE
VOLUNTARY MEDICAL INSURANCE—PART B

PROGRAM BENEFITS PART B	MEDICARE COVERAGE PART B	PATIENT PAYS PART B (2006)	REMARKS
Physicians' and surgeons' services as well as other medical services	80 percent of reasonable charge as determined by Medicare or its agent	First $124 of expenses (not charged more than once a year) plus 20 percent of all charges above $124	Voluntary monthly Part B recalculated each year

Other medical services include outpatient hospital services such as x-rays and tests; outpatient physical therapy and speech therapy; outpatient dialysis treatments; artificial limbs and eyes; limited dental surgical care and chiropractic care; certain colostomy care supplies; rental or purchase of medical equipment; and approved ambulance services if other modes of transportation are a potential health hazard |
Homecare	Unlimited visits per calendar year—pays 100 percent of reasonable charges	All services not covered by the program	Like Part A of Medicare (hospital insurance) no prior hospitalization is required to qualify for benefit.
Independent physical therapists	$1,740 maximum per year	Rest of charges	
Outpatient psychiatric services	50 percent per year	Rest of charges	

an approved amount. Medicare's system for paying physicians is based on a national fee schedule. The schedule, which went into effect on January 1, 1992, assigns a dollar value to each physician service based on work, geographic variation in medical practice costs, and malpractice insurance costs. The fees that appear on the schedule are the Medicare-approved amounts for services covered by Part B. Under the Part B payment system, each time you go to a physician for a covered service, the amount Medicare will recognize for that service will be taken from the national fee schedule.

There is a limit on the permissible amount a physician who does not accept assignment can charge you for Medicare-covered services. For example, if you read in Medicare literature that the most nonparticipating physicians can charge you is 115 percent of the Medicare fee schedule, this really means that a nonparticipating physician cannot charge you more than 15 percent higher than the Medicare-approved fee amount. This is a federal law. Any physician overcharges must be refunded. In some states the limits are even stricter. For example, in Pennsylvania, Massachusetts, and Rhode Island physicians must accept assignment, and they must accept assignment for low-income people in New York and Vermont. In New York physicians are limited to charge 10 percent above the Medicare-approved fee schedule—not the national 15 percent. Be a wise consumer and find out from your insurance carrier or your state insurance commissioner's office what the percentage, if any, might be in your state. This problem is called "balance billing" because the physician bills patients for the balance that is left after Medicare pays its share. Also, remember, if a doctor asks you to sign a waiver agreeing to pay more than Medicare allows, the Centers for Medicare and Medicaid Services states that such waivers have no legal effects and the waivers are not enforceable.[13]

The following example illustrates a comparison of your share of the cost for the same service provided by a participating physician who accepts Medicare assignment and by a nonparticipating physician who does not accept Medicare assignment where the limit a nonparticipating physician can charge is 115 percent of the Medicare fee schedule in a given year.

If you went to a *participating physician* for a service for which the fee schedule amount was $100, the physician would accept that amount as payment in full. Medicare would pay $80 and you would be responsible for $20, assuming you had already met the Part B $124 deductible. You would not have to pay any more than that amount of $20.

For the same service provided by a *nonparticipating physician*, the fee schedule amount would be $95, not $100, since nonparticipating physicians are reimbursed at 95 percent of the fee schedule amount Medicare-participating physicians are paid. Medicare then would pay 80 percent of the $95 bill or $76, leaving you with a balance of $19 to cover the remaining 20 percent of the fee schedule amount of $95 ($76 + $19). However, since nonparticipating physicians who do not accept assignment can also legally charge 15 percent more than the fee schedule amount, in this case of $95, the physician can add another $14.25 (15 percent of $95) to your bill, bringing your total out-of-pocket costs to $33.25 (that is $19 + $14.25), assuming you have also already paid your $124 deductible. You would not have to pay any charges over $33.25. Thus, as you can see, the physician who accepts Medicare assignment is less expensive ($20) than the physician who does not ($33.25).

To find out what the limiting charge is for a particular service, you can contact your Medicare carrier. Also, look at the *Explanation of Medicare Benefits* (EOMB) form that the government publishes and that you receive whenever a Medicare claim goes through. See whether it lists the maximum fee your doctor can charge you and compare it with the fee you are being charged. If you think your physician has exceeded the charge limit, you may want to contact the physician first and ask for a reduction in the charge or a refund. If you cannot satisfactorily settle the issue with the physician, you can call the Medicare carrier that processes your claims and request an investigation. If it appears to the carrier that you were overcharged, the carrier will contact the physician and ask for a refund of any overpayments you may have made. Sanctions can be imposed against any physician who knowingly and willfully, and on a repeated basis, charges Medicare beneficiaries more than the legal limit. Besides the charge limitation mandated by federal law, some states, as already noted, also limit physician charges.

You should also be aware that any physician who provides you with services that he or she knows or believes Medicare will determine to be medically unnecessary and thus will not pay for is required to so notify you in writing *before* performing the service. If written notice is not given and you did not know that Medicare will not pay, you cannot be held liable to pay. However, if you did receive written notice and signed an agreement to pay for the service yourself, you will be held liable to pay.

Benefits

Medicare's voluntary medical insurance plan helps pay for a number of medical services. Most of these are subject to the annual deductible of $124 plus 20 percent of the physician's reasonable charge. *The following benefits are covered under Part B:*

- Physician's services anywhere in the United States (in the doctor's office, the hospital, your home, or elsewhere) including medical supplies furnished by a doctor in his or her office, services of the office nurse, and drugs administered as part of your doctor's treatment that you cannot administer yourself. Beginning in 2005 Medicare also expanded coverage of implantable cardioverter defibrillators (ICDs) to patients who are at risk but have not as yet suffered fatal heart rhythms provided the patients agree to release details about their cases to a database shared by physicians in which the patient's confidentiality will be preserved. Until now Medicare has covered the ICD devices in patients who have already suffered fatal heart rhythms.
- Outpatient hospital services for diagnosis and treatment in an emergency

room or outpatient clinic of a hospital. Medicare reimburses in full (without deductible or coinsurance) diagnostic tests performed on an outpatient basis in the outpatient department of a hospital or a physician's office *if they are carried out within seven days of the patient's admission to the hospital.*

- Diagnostic tests and clinical laboratory procedures that are part of your medical treatment such as blood tests, urinalysis, and more.
- X-rays or other radiation treatments and pathology services.
- Medical supplies such as surgical dressings, splints, casts, therapeutic shoes, (covered once a year) and arm, leg, back, and neck braces.
- Artificial limbs and eyes, including eyeglasses (one pair after cataract surgery with an intraocular lens). Medicare pays in full for the standard replacement lens in cataract surgery. During surgery the cataracts are removed and a permanent lens is implanted that permits patients to view distant objects clearly. Patients can also upgrade to another option that not only replaces the cataract-clouded lens but can correct for presbyopia (the loss of the ability of the eye to focus on near objects). However, Medicare recipients will have to pay the difference in cost between the two kinds of surgery.
- Breast prostheses following a mastectomy and other prosthetic devices.
- Blood after the first three pints.
- Certain colostomy care supplies such as ostomy bags and other supplies such as surgical dressings, splints, casts, some diabetic supplies, as well as braces for the arm, leg, back, and neck.
- Rental or purchase of medically necessary durable medical equipment such as a wheelchair or oxygen equipment for use in your home.
- In addition to the services of practitioners such as clinical psychologists, social workers, and nurse practitioners, limited outpatient psychiatric and chiropractic services and dental surgery are covered. Effective July 1,1981, Medicare also covers services performed by dentists *if* those same services are presently covered when performed by a physician. Medicare also covers hospitalization for noncovered dental services where the severity of the procedure or the condition warrants hospitalization.
- Home and office services by licensed and Medicare-certified physical therapists, with certain payment limitations.
- Approved ambulance services if other modes of transportation would present a health hazard as well as emergency care. Medicare covers paramedic intercept services in rural areas and may cover nonemergency ambulance services if any other means of transportation is not advisable and the patient has a written statement from his/her doctor certifying in advance the medical necessity of ambulance transportation.
- Hepatitis B, flu, and pneumococcal vaccine shots (Public Law 96-611). Medicare pays in full for the vaccination with no patient deductible or coinsurance. If the US Center for Disease Control proves the vaccine ineffective, then the US secretary of health and human services can discontinue the program.

- Physician services outside the United States in a qualified Canadian or Mexican hospital when you live in the United States and a hospital in one of the countries is closer to your home than the nearest American hospital. Medicare also pays for services in Puerto Rico, the Virgin Islands, Guam, and American Samoa.
- Unlimited homecare visits by skilled paramedical personnel, if you are not covered under Part A of Medicare. However, in order to qualify for home health visit benefits, all four of the following conditions must be met: part-time skilled nursing care, physical therapy, or speech therapy is necessary; a doctor has determined that you need home health services and has set up a plan for home healthcare; you are confined to your home; and the home health agency providing services is participating in the Medicare program. Also included is coverage for durable medical equipment supplied by a home health agency.
- Services related to the treatment of plantar warts (warts on feet).
- Optometrists' services in connection with treating the condition of aphakia (absence of the natural lens of the eye).
- Kidney dialysis and kidney transplants.
- Heart, lung, pancreas, kidney, and liver transplants in a Medicare-approved facility under limited circumstances as well as limited immunosuppressive drug therapy with extended coverage available for transplant patients including some end-stage renal dialysis patients.
- Physician's service in preparing a reasonable supply of antigens, including forwarding a supply to another physician or rural health clinic or administration. Also, very limited outpatient prescription drugs such as oral cancer drugs.
- Comprehensive outpatient services in rehabilitation facilities, including physician services, nursing care, physical therapy, occupational therapy, speech pathology, respiratory therapy, social and psychological services, prosthetic devices, drugs and biologicals, supplies, appliances, equipment, and other items that are necessary for the rehabilitation of the patient.
- List of outpatient surgical procedures established and considered "safe" and "appropriate" by the secretary of the US Department of Health and Human Services when the procedures are performed in an ambulatory surgical center, the outpatient department of a hospital, or in a physician's office. Physicians accepting assignment for performing these procedures in the previous locations are reimbursed 100 percent of the permissible charge.

The following preventive services:

- Cholesterol and bone mass measurements for certain people who are at risk for losing bone mass.
- Prostate cancer screening for all men age fifty and older, including a digital

rectal examination (once every twelve months) and Prostate Specific Antigen (PSA) test (once every twelve months).

- Diabetes self-management training (if requested by your doctor or provider) and services including coverage for glucose monitors, tests strips, and lancets for all people who have diabetes (insulin users and nonusers). Also, medical nutrition therapy for those with diabetes and those with renal disease.
- Colorectal cancer screening for all people age fifty and over, but with no age limit for having a colonoscopy. Services include a fecal occult blood test (once every twelve months that Medicare pays in full), a flexible sigmoidoscopy (once every forty-eight months), a colonoscopy (once every twenty-four months if you are high risk for cancer of the colon), and a barium enema that doctors can substitute for a sigmoidoscopy or colononoscopy. The deductible for the colorectal screening tests that Medicare covers is waived as a result of President Bush signing into law the Deficit Reduction Act of 2005 (Public Law 109-171) on February 8, 2006.
- Glaucoma screening.
- Mammogram screening. Mammograms to screen for breast cancer are covered once every twelve months for Medicare women forty or older (you also get one baseline mammogram between thirty-five and thirty-nine) and Medicare pays 80 percent of the charges.
- Pap test and pelvic screening. Pap smears for detection of cervical cancer are covered once every thirty-six months, except for certain women at high risk who can get one more frequently. (Once every twelve months if you are high risk for cervical or vaginal cancer, or if you are of childbearing age and have had an abnormal Pap smear in the preceding thirty-six months.) Pap smear and pelvic examination also includes a clinical breast exam. You don't pay anything for the Pap smear laboratory test, but for the Pap smear collection and pelvic and breast examinations you pay 20 percent of the Medicare-approved amount (or a set copayment amount) with no Part B deductible.
- Beginning January 1, 2005, new beneficiaries who enrolled in Medicare after that date are covered for an initial onetime wellness physical examination within six months of the day they first enroll in Medicare Part B. All beneficiaries are covered for screening blood tests for early detection of heart disease (one cardiovascular screening every five years) and screening tests for diabetes (two diabetes screenings every year). The tests will be free with no copayments or deductibles. Also, coordinated care for persons with chronic illness is also covered. Some of the new benefits administered through a subsidized physical exam for new enrollees include height, weight, and blood pressure measurements; vision and hearing tests; problem drinking and depression screenings; and injury prevention services. In addition, as a result of President Bush signing into law the Deficit Reduction Act of 2005, as already noted, preventive screening for abdominal aortic aneurysms for beneficiaries at risk during a "Welcome to Medicare" physical exam is now provided.

- Beginning in 2005, Medicare pays up to four counseling sessions for beneficiaries who smoke or have smoking-related diseases or take certain medications. If the four counseling sessions do not help, then smokers can get a second round of counseling.
- Outpatient physical and occupational therapy including speech pathology services you receive as part of your treatment in a doctor's office; as an outpatient in a Medicare participating hospital; or in a skilled nursing facility, a Medicare-approved clinic, a rehabilitation agency, a public health agency, or a home health agency if these services are furnished under a plan that is established and periodically reviewed by a doctor.[14]

Also, Medicare announced in July 2004 that it now recognizes obesity as an illness, a change in policy that may allow millions of overweight Americans to make medical claims for treatments such as stomach surgery and diet programs. With this change in policy, beneficiaries will be able to request a government review of medical evidence to determine whether Medicare can cover certain treatments for obesity. Although Medicare and Medicaid programs cover sicknesses caused by obesity—including type 2 diabetes, cardiovascular disease, several types of cancer, and gallbladder disease—until Medicare declared obesity as an illness, weight-loss therapies were often denied Medicare coverage.

Exceptions to the 80 Percent Coinsurance Coverage

We have already noted that as soon as you have satisfied the $124 annual deductible in reasonable charges for covered medical expenses, the medical insurance program (Part B) will pay 80 percent of the reasonable charges for any additional covered services you receive during the rest of the year. There are several exceptions to this general rule:

- While you are a hospital inpatient, the medical insurance plan pays 100 percent of the reimbursement (with no deductible) to radiologists and pathologists who agree to accept the Medicare assignment for their services. The medical insurance plan pays 100 percent of the reasonable charges for home health services (with no deductible). In addition, Medicare pays 100 percent for clinical laboratory services such as blood tests, urinalysis, fecal occult blood tests, Pap smear laboratory tests, flu and pneumonia shots if the health provider accepts assignment, and 75 percent of the Medicare-approved amount if colorectal screening is performed in an ambulatory surgical center or hospital outpatient department. Also, Medicare pays 20 percent for all outpatient physical, occupational, and speech-language therapy services. There is no coverage limit for these therapy services provided by a hospital outpatient facility. But, if provided at another type of outpatient setting as of January 1, 2006, there is a $1,740 limit per year for physical and speech-language therapy services combined and $1,740 limit per year for occupational therapy services.

- Physician's psychiatric services on outpatient basis are limited to 50 percent of the fee schedule on an outpatient basis if the services are medically necessary.[15]

Reasonable charges of physicians are updated annually, but increases in prevailing charges from year to year are limited by an "economic index" formula that relates fee increases to actual increases in the cost of maintaining a medical practice and raises in general earning levels. This formula does not limit the amount a doctor may charge a patient; it only limits the amount Medicare can pay.

Benefits Not Covered

"Ruth, I now have a sense of what Medicare's Part A Hospitalization Insurance covers and the benefits under Part B's Voluntary Supplemental Medical Insurance plan, but I see that Medicare has a lot of gaps that I will either have to pay for myself or purchase some kind of Medigap insurance policy to cover these gaps."

"Joseph, many people purchase Medigap insurance, but as a warning, to get the most for your Medigap premium dollar, make sure that whatever policy you review or purchase covers those specific benefit gaps."

While the Medicare program gives substantial help in paying medical bills, the program was not meant to be comprehensive. Medicare is not free:

- It does not pay for everything.
- It does not pay 100 percent of the cost of all services it covers.
- Medicare is not accepted by everyone who provides health services.

The gaps in Medicare insurance coverage have caused more than half of those eligible for the program to purchase private health insurance in order to supplement their Medicare coverage. Unfortunately, many of the public are still unaware of the kinds of medical services for which Medicare pays and does not pay. As a result, the elderly spend billions of dollars annually on private health insurance to supplement their Medicare coverage, some of which are wasted on uneconomical or duplicative insurance. In order to avoid buying worthless health insurance policies from unscrupulous insurance agents, ask your insurer if the policy he is selling will cover *the following gaps in the Medicare program as of January 1, 2006:*

- Does the policy pay the $952 deductible you must meet before Medicare starts paying for the first 60 days of your hospital stay?
- Does the policy pay the $238 per day that Medicare does not cover if your hospital stay lasts from 61 to 90 days?

- Does the policy pay the $476 per day that Medicare does not cover if you have to stay in the hospital for 91 to 150 days and must use some of your "lifetime reserve days"?
- Does the policy help you in the rare instance in which you have been in the hospital 150 days and can no longer receive Medicare coverage for your stay?
- Does the policy help you if you need more than 190 days of psychiatric care in a Medicare-approved psychiatric hospital during your lifetime for which Medicare does not pay?
- Does the policy pay the $119 per day that Medicare does not cover between the twenty-first and the one hundredth day you stay in a skilled nursing facility?
- Does the policy help you out if you have been in a skilled nursing facility for 100 days and no longer can use Medicare coverage, which stops after 100 days?
- Does the policy pay the $124 annual deductible for which you are responsible under Medicare Part B?
- Does the policy pay the 20 percent of reasonable charges or a set copayment amount—for medical, durable medical equipment, and surgical bills; outpatient hospital services; ambulatory surgery center facility fees for approved procedures, diagnostic tests, and other benefits—that is not covered under Medicare Part B? These include preventive services such as bone mass measurements, colorectal screening, diabetes services, mammogram screening, Pap smear collection and pelvic and breast examinations, prostate screening, and Hepatitis B shots, as well as other services such as all outpatient physical, occupational, and speech-language therapy services; the first three pints of blood you receive as an outpatient; and then the 20 percent you pay of the Medicare-approved amount for additional pints (after the deductible) unless you or someone else donates blood to replace what you use.
- Does the policy cover charges or portions of charges that Medicare may not consider to be an approved amount?
- Does the policy help you out if you need to pay more than 50 percent of a psychiatrist's fee schedule on an outpatient basis if your service is medically necessary?
- Does the policy help you out if you need to pay 25 percent of the approved amount for colorectal cancer–screening procedures if performed in an ambulatory surgical center or a hospital outpatient department?
- Does the policy cover the following benefits that Medicare does not cover?
    - ▼ Custodial care.
    - ▼ Hearing aids and examinations related to fitting, prescribing, or changing hearing aids.
    - ▼ Routine dental care and dentures.
    - ▼ Routine annual physical examinations and tests directly related to such examinations.

▼ Acupuncture treatments and cosmetic surgery.

▼ Eyeglasses and routine related eye examinations. (Eyeglasses are only covered if you need corrective lenses after a cataract operation.)

▼ Private duty nurses.

▼ Extra charges for a private room for which Medicare will not pay unless it is medically necessary.

▼ The costs of prescription drugs outside the hospital that Medicare Part B does not pay for which now come under Part D of the new Medicare prescription drug program. (Medicare Part B does not pay for prescription drugs that can be self-administered by the patient.) The exceptions include certain drugs furnished to hospice enrollees, drugs that you cannot administer yourself that are provided as part of physician's service, special drugs furnished during the first year after an organ transplantation, and erythropoietin for certain home dialysis patients. *Beginning, January 1, 2006, Medicare began to cover out-of-hospital prescription drugs under Part D with the Medicare patient assuming out-of-pocket costs.*

▼ Full-time home nursing care.

▼ Supportive devices and routine foot care.

▼ Immunizations (except for Hepatitis B, pneumococcal, and flu vaccine) for which Medicare will not pay unless required because of an injury or immediate risk of infection.

▼ Services of homemakers, naturopaths, Christian Science Practitioners, and immediate relatives or members of your household. (Note: Naturopathy is a system preserving health by means of a simple diet, regular exercise, and the avoidance of drugs. It is based on the principle that natural processes will keep the body in health if they are given a fair chance instead of being constantly thwarted by unnatural foods, customs, and medicines. The strictest naturopath objects to all medicines and even to food grown with the aid of artificial fertilizers.)

▼ Meals delivered to your home.

▼ Comfort and convenience items in your hospital or skilled nursing facility room.

▼ Orthopedic shoes, unless they are for therapeutic purposes.[16]

Be very careful when examining a policy that is supposed to supplement your Medicare benefits. Although they may use different terms, most health insurance policies exclude the same kinds of coverage and services as Medicare. Make sure you understand the health insurance terminology used in the policy. "Medically necessary," "customary charge," and other terms in a private health insurance policy may mean that you are not purchasing the coverage you seek for the actual charges you incur or services you are provided.

Just because an insurance plan is well known, do not consider it to be the best. Some of the lesser-known policies offer better coverage. Compare the amount of money you have paid or will pay in premiums with the maximum benefits you can receive from the private health insurance policy. You may find that, while you have paid several hundred dollars in premiums annually, the policy will pay only $100 toward that foot surgery you need.

Do not be deceived by policies that offer up to $50,000 or more in hospital protection. Remember, in most cases you would have to be in the hospital for "medically necessary" services for several months or more in order to benefit from these fantastic offers—such lengthy hospitalization are rare.[17]

Purchasing Supplemental Medicare Insurance

In addition to the previous questions, the following guidelines can help prevent fraud when you are buying supplementary Medicare insurance. Blue Cross and Blue Shield and many commercial insurance companies sell good supplementary Medicare insurance, known as "wraparound coverage" because it is designed to fill in certain Medicare gaps as related to deductibles, copayments, some health services, and supplies. But the supplementary insurance rarely pays physician fees exceeding Medicare limits.

In 1990 Congress passed a law to regulate the sale of Medicare supplemental ("Medigap" or "Medsupp") insurance. Under the law, all companies that offer insurance to supplement Medicare must offer a "core" package of basic benefits, and they must provide consumers with understandable outlines of coverage that are comparable in language and format to help in comparison shopping. The law also limits insurance carriers to a maximum of nine additional coverage packages that go beyond the core plan or a total of ten packages. Except in Massachusetts, Minnesota, and Wisconsin, there are ten standardized plans labeled Plan A through Plan J. In other major features, the law:

- Forbids insurers to deny coverage or charge higher rates to anyone purchasing a policy within six months of becoming eligible for Medicare part B benefits.
- Forbids "preexisting-condition" exclusions, waiting periods, and probationary periods when a policy is purchased to replace an existing one and the new policy's benefits are similar to that of the old one.
- Requires the Medigap policies be guaranteed renewable.[18]

In 1995 Congress passed a law that requires that when a consumer is sold a policy that duplicates some Medicare or Medigap benefit, the insurance agent has to notify the buyer of that fact. Also, such policies must pay all the stated benefits regardless of other coverage. This rules out what is known as *coordination of benefits*, the practice of having one insurer refuse to pay in cases where there is multiple coverage. Coordination of benefits is widely used to keep policyholders from double dipping and receiving more than their costs, but in the past it has also meant that consumers sometimes got little or nothing from a policy that duplicated Medicare.[19]

Thus, to help you purchase quality policies, the following guidelines are additionally offered:

Understand exactly what Medicare covers and the gaps for which you must pay.

With the previous listing of Medicare coverage and the questions you should ask in regard to its gaps, make any insurance agent you deal with show you—gap by gap—what his company's policy covers that Medicare and your existing policies do not. Then check the policy yourself to make positively sure that what he says is correct.

Consider your income status.

If you receive a fixed income, do not buy the most expensive policy. You need a policy that you will be able to afford in future years as prices rise. The cost of most policies will increase as Medicare changes; some policies cost more as you become older. You also need to leave enough for health costs that neither Medicare nor insurance covers, such as medical checkups and eyeglasses.

Do you have your own emergency fund?

Start a health emergency fund of your own. There will always be some out-of-pocket expenses associated with an illness or injury, even with Medicare and a sound supplemental health insurance fund. If possible, keep your emergency fund in a joint savings account so someone else has access to it in the event you are incapacitated.

Did you receive an Outline of Coverage?

Make sure the insurance agent gives you an Outline of Coverage, a summary of benefits written in plain language.

Exercise caution about purchasing a "dread disease" policy.

These often provide duplicative coverage to Medicare or fail to provide needed coverage; have many benefit limitations; fail to cover many conditions resulting from cancer treatment such as infection, diabetes, pneumonia, and loss of hair; and may pay for certain benefits only when the patient is hospitalized—but much cancer treatment is provided on an outpatient basis. It is best to buy a comprehensive policy that pays for all diseases or accidents including cancer. Some states, such as Connecticut, New Jersey, New York, New Hampshire, and Massachusetts, have banned the sale of cancer insurance. Find out from your state insurance commissioner whether your state has banned the sale of such insurance.

What about cancer insurance as supplemental insurance?

Cancer insurance is only considered as supplemental insurance to the degree that the benefits payable are not paid by Medicare. Cancer-only policies, however, do not qualify as Medicare supplement policies.

Be careful of hospital indemnity income policies.

Although premiums stay relatively stable over the years, these policies pay so many dollars a day after you have been hospitalized for a certain period. Remember, most hospital stays are quite short and you pay the difference between your hospital's daily cost and the health insurance plan's payment. With hospital costs rapidly escalating, make sure you can afford the difference. Indemnity policies also set fixed rates for surgery and other procedures, no matter what the actual charge may be.

Try to select a policy with a high (or no) upper limit on long-term hospitalization.

You can be hospitalized for 150 consecutive days and still receive Medicare payments. Because your chances of being in a hospital for a longer stay are extremely small, the portion of an insurance premium to cover such a contingency is very small. Therefore, make sure you are insured against major expenses, also known as catastrophic coverage.

Look into policies that return the most in benefit coverage for each premium dollar you pay.

As previously noted, the Blue Cross plans usually pay back about 85–90 cents for each dollar of premiums paid in while commercial insurance companies average about 60–65 cents for each dollar. As a result, some Blue Cross policies may be more comprehensive as well as cheaper than some commercial plans. By comparing the kinds of benefits you wish to buy among Blue Cross and commercial plans you can estimate any potential savings.

Investigate the health insurance plans offered by your present or former employer or union.

Some group health plans permit participants to continue coverage after age sixty-five and after retirement. Because Medicare pays a significant portion of an elderly person's medical costs, the premium to continue such policies can be relatively small.

Do not purchase any health insurance on the spot.

Dishonest insurance salesmen will say anything to sell you a health insurance policy. Their objective is to catch you off guard and to leave fast. Before you sign anything, ask to see a sample policy, not just a brochure. Ask the insurance agent for his business card and tell him you will call him if you decide to buy the policy. Do not, under any circumstances, give a check to the salesman who minutes before was a total stranger. Also, do not cancel any existing health policy merely because one salesman says his is better.

Do not drop one policy and buy another with similar benefits merely because the second one looks a little better or is a little less expensive. You could lose or delay benefits under a new policy because of waiting periods or preexisting condition limitations.

Don't drop your Medicare Part B coverage even if you have enough supplemental coverage.

Part B premiums are subsidized by the federal government, which means that you get more for your dollar than through any other approach. Private health insurance is designed to dovetail with the Medicare program, not compete with it.

Do not buy policies with unreasonable waiting periods or tough restrictions on preexisting conditions.

Read this section of your policy very carefully, if it is included, and get expert advice if you don't understand it. Some insurance companies will not honor or pay for a legitimate claim if they feel they can find a preexisting condition as an excuse to avoid payment and as a cause of your illness. Frequently, a company also will not pay for medical coverage of an illness or injury that existed for two years prior to the issuance of the policy—but they may do so after a specified time, such as one or two years after the policy issued. Do not be misled by the phrase "no medical examination required" or you can't be turned down because of age because the use of preexisting-condition clauses makes it unnecessary to require a physical examination and there may be a long waiting period before preexisting conditions are covered, or the policy may never cover them. Avoid over-the-telephone solicitations for once-in-a lifetime offers, maximum protection policies offering minimum payments, and any offers requiring you to send in a cashier's check or money order immediately or you lose the opportunity. Many sales pitches are designed to make consumers embarrassed to ask questions. Don't ever buy an insurance policy until you are satisfied with the answers you get. Beware of attempts to lead you into thinking a mail solicitation is from the federal government. Some companies issue official-looking emblems, envelopes, and stationary. If you think the solicitation is from the federal government, call your local Social Security office and find out for sure.

Be careful about claim forms.

Claim forms should be made out carefully and completely. If they are not, delays in processing may cost you money and concern.

Do not forget nursing home coverage.

Coverage of skilled nursing home services, either in a nursing facility or at home, is available under Medicare and some insurance policies—if you meet the qualifications—to help you avoid the high cost of hospitalization.

Take advantage of working past age sixty-five.

If you continue to work past age sixty-five, you and your Medicare-eligible spouse may choose to remain covered by your employer's group health plan. Check with your employer for the advantages of doing so.

Are you eligible for other coverage?

Check for other coverage. For example, are you eligible for Medicaid? If so, you do not need Medicare supplemental insurance. Does your former employer provide coverage? If so, talk to the personnel or benefits office to determine whether you need to purchase additional health insurance. There is a good chance you may not.

How much health insurance do you really need?

Do not purchase more insurance than you really need. There are better ways to spend your money than purchasing premiums that duplicate or overlap other insurance coverage. In addition, don't be misled by endorsements by celebrities or the use of official-sounding company names. Many of these policies sound inexpensive but offer little protection. Have someone you trust examine and evaluate the policies in regard to your own needs before you purchase any.

Should you purchase more than one policy to supplement Medicare and have both of them pay for you?

That depends. You should examine the policy carefully before you buy it to determine if its coverage is reduced if you have other insurance. It is in your own best interest to avoid insuring yourself too much. That occurs when benefits exceed actual medical expenses. Obviously, the benefits payable under a second policy are available to cover expenses not covered by either Medicare or your first Medicare supplement policy and such could be extensive. If your benefits are not adequate, try to purchase only the additional coverage you need. Remember, if you have two or more policies that cover the same medical expense, each may pay only a portion of the bill. Don't expect full payment from both.

If you do not understand what you are getting, have an expert such as a lawyer, an accountant, or a financial planner review the policies. (If you seek help from a financial planner, be sure you know how he or she is paid—many sell insurance on commission, a fact that may bias their advice.)

Be sure the health insurance company is licensed to do business in your state.

If it is not and if there is a dispute between you and the company, your state insurance department will not be able to help you. But your state insurance department will be able to tell you if the company has a state license. Companies selling accident and health insurance or hospitalization insurance advertise in many places including national magazines, by mail, on radio, and on television—even on matchbook covers. Be careful. Ask your state insurance department if it has had any reason to take action against the company and whether or not the company has a good or bad history of consumer complaints in terms of paying claims. Know the meaning of various terms used in the insurance policy. Some mail-order policies define the word "hospital" in such a way that the definition disqualifies for payment many hospitals in the country.[20]

Check your state insurance department for information about the kind of consumer protection you will receive with a particular policy.

Use your state insurance department for information about a supplemental Medicare policy.

Check your state insurance department for information about the kind of consumer protection you will receive with a particular policy.

Try to purchase an insurance policy that the company cannot cancel.

Choose a policy that is cancelable only at your option. And try to get a policy, if possible, in which the premium cannot be increased (a feature for which you pay more). An alternative is to buy a *guaranteed renewable* policy, which allows the health insurance company to increase the premium at renewal time, but only if it raises the premium for all owners of that kind of policy. The advantage to you in this situation is that you cannot be assessed more because of claims you, an individual, have filed. Also, the company cannot cancel the policy as long as you pay the premium. However, if you purchase an *optional renewable* policy, it is up to the company to determine whether or not the policy is to be renewed. The policy cannot be cancelled until the expiration date on the policy, but after that the company can refuse to continue, and you will be without coverage.[21]

Read your policy very carefully.

Remember that because the insurance company only has to pay benefits that it put in writing in the policy itself, you must read your policy very carefully as soon as you receive it. If what the policy says is not the same as what the advertising, the agent, or the outline of coverage led you to believe, decide whether you are satisfied with the benefits in the policy. If you are not satisfied, you may want to reject the policy within any "free look" time shown on the front of the policy. You may also want to alert your state insurance department about the problem.

Where do you keep your health insurance policies?

Keep your health insurance policies in one place that is readily accessible and tell those people close to you where they are. Then make a list of the policy numbers and the companies that issue them in case the originals are lost or misplaced. Also, review your health insurance policies to make sure that inflation has not outdistanced the benefits.

Find out whether your doctor accepts assignment under the Medicare supplemental policy.

Inquire whether your doctor accepts assignment, which means that the doctor agrees to hold his or her fees down to the level approved by Medicare. This will save you money even if you do not have insurance to fill the gaps in Medicare coverage. If you do buy a Medicare supplement policy and your doctor accepts assignment, you can save money on your insurance because you would not need to buy one of the more expensive policies that pay above Medicare's permissible fees on your doctor bills. Some doctors, called "participating doctors," have agreed to accept assignment for all their Medicare patients. Area Agencies on Aging and Social Security offices have lists of participating doctors. Ask your physicians and surgeons about their fees and how they are paid. In April 1996 new regulations went into effect compelling physicians in HMOs to provide a summary of their HMO financial incentive plan on request. Doctors who refuse are subject to fines.[22]

Watch out for the deductible.

Even though the Medicare Part B deductible is $124 per year, be aware that some insurance companies may charge more than $124 per year for a rider to cover the Part B deductible.

Understand the meaning of a deductible.

If you decide to purchase a policy with a $200 initial deductible, make sure you understand what that means. It does *not* mean that your policy will begin to pay after your doctor bills add up to $200. It means your policy will begin to pay when you have paid $200 worth of Medicare allowable doctor bills after Medicare has paid its 80 percent.[23]

Are nursing home benefits included in supplemental health insurance policies?

Generally, this benefit is not included under Medicare supplement and hospital indemnity policies, but such coverage would be provided under long-term care policies. Most policies are not intended to cover long-term custodial care. If the nursing facility provides "skilled care," benefits may be provided. Many insurance companies are responding to the growing demand for nursing home long-term care insurance. A number of options exist in this area.

Is private-duty nursing in the hospital included in any supplemental policies you are considering?

Check the policy carefully. This option is available in some policies.

Take advantage of the "free look" provision.

As already noted, check for a "free look" provision. All companies give you thirty days to review the supplemental policy—it is required. If you decide you do not want it, send it back to the agent or company within the thirty-day period and you will receive a refund of all you have paid in premiums.

Be sure to pay your insurance bill on time.

Always pay your insurance premium when it is due; do not wait for the company to remind you. If the company fails to remind you and you do not pay on time, you could either lose your policy or have to start a new waiting period for existing illnesses.

If after purchasing your health insurance policy you feel you have been cheated, there are ways to correct the situation. A reputable company and insurance agent will help you. An unscrupulous company and agent will not. Report your problem to your state insurance commissioner and to your local district attorney and state attorney. If any part of the transaction involved the use of the mail, call your local postmaster and tell him you want to complain about possible mail fraud. Make and keep copies of all relevant correspondence and send them to your senators and representatives in your own state capital and in Washington, DC. Finally, send your complaints and grievances to the Select Committee on Aging, House of Representatives, Washington, DC 20515 and to the Special Committee on Aging, US Senate, Washington, DC 20510. These sources may enable you to correct whatever problems you may have.

Coverage of Second Opinions

On occasion your doctor may recommend surgery for the treatment of a medical problem. In some cases, surgery is necessary. But there is increasing evidence that many conditions can be treated equally well without surgery. Because even minor surgery involves some risk, you may wish to obtain the opinion of another doctor before making your decision.

Medicare pays the same way for a second opinion as it pays for other doctor services, provided that you are seeking advice for the treatment of a medical condition that Medicare covers. If the first two opinions conflict with each other, Medicare will help pay for a third opinion. You can ask your own doctor to refer you to another doctor for a second opinion. Or you can call your Medicare carrier and ask for the names and telephone numbers of doctors in your area who provide second opinions. Or you can call the Centers for Medicare and Medicaid Services toll-free telephone number, 1-800-638-6833, to locate the name of a nearby second opinion specialist.

Medicare Coverage of Nonphysician Services

Most of the physician services for which Medicare pays must be provided by either a doctor of medicine or a doctor of osteopathy. Under very limited circumstances, Medicare can help pay for the services of chiropractors, podiatrists, dentists, and optometrists. However, Medicare's coverage can be very restrictive. For example, there is only one chiropractic service for which Medicare pays. That is manipulation of the spine to correct a dislocation that can be shown by an x-ray. Medicare does not pay for an x-ray performed by a chiropractor.

When you are in doubt about whether Medicare covers a particular service, call your Medicare insurance carrier. The carrier can also tell you whether Medicare will pay for services provided by a medical professional who is not a physician. In some cases, Medicare covers the services of certified registered nurse anesthetists, certified midwives, nurse practitioners, physician assistants, clinical social workers, and clinical psychologists. The coverage is limited, so ask your Medicare carrier to find out whether Medicare will pay for the kind of service you require.

Medicare Coverage of Special Health Facilities

In addition to paying for care in a hospital or a skilled nursing facility, Medicare also pays for a variety of services provided at special kinds of healthcare facilities.

- *Ambulatory Surgical Centers*: Part B of Medicare helps pay for certain types of surgery performed at a Medicare-approved ambulatory surgical center. This kind of surgery does not require a hospital stay.
- *Rural Health Clinics*: Various services delivered at rural health clinics are also covered. These clinics serve areas where the population is sparse. Medicare

pays for services provided by the doctors, nurse practitioners, physician's assistants, nurse midwives, clinical psychologists, and social workers who are part of the clinic. In addition, Part A of Medicare helps pay for care in critical access hospitals (CAHs), which are small facilities that give limited outpatient and inpatient services to people in rural areas.

- *Comprehensive Outpatient Rehabilitation Facilities (CORFs)*: Part B of Medicare covers services at a comprehensive outpatient rehabilitation facility if they were prescribed by a doctor and the facility participates in Medicare.
- *Community Mental Health Centers*: Under certain conditions, Part B of Medicare helps pay for outpatient mental healthcare that community mental health centers or hospital outpatient departments provide. These are specially qualified programs that provide partial hospitalization for mental healthcare. Check with the program you have chosen to determine whether it meets the conditions for Medicare payment.
- *Federally Qualified Health Centers*: A full range of services can be received at federally qualified health centers. These facilities are principally community health clinics, Indian health clinics, migrant worker health centers, and health centers for the homeless. They are generally located in inner-city and rural areas and are open to all Medicare beneficiaries.
- *Certified Medical Laboratories*: Laboratory clinical diagnostic tests are covered when provided by a certified medical laboratory that participates in Medicare. The laboratory must accept assignment of your Medicare claim and cannot bill you. Part B pays all the charges. (In Maryland only, you can be billed for 20 percent coinsurance for hospital outpatient tests.)[24]

If you have any questions concerning Medicare coverage of the services these various facilities provide, call your local Social Security office or your insurance carrier who pays your Medicare bills to the appropriate providers.

The Medicare Savings Program for Low-Income Medicare Beneficiaries

If you are a Medicare beneficiary with a very low-income and few assets, you might qualify for state assistance in paying your medical bills. This Medicare Savings Program was previously known as the Medicare Cost-Sharing Program or the Medicare Buy-In Program. The three component of the Medicare Savings Program include:

- The Qualified Medicare Beneficiary (QMB) program
- The Specified Low-Income Medicare Beneficiary (SLMB) program
- The Additional Low-Income Medicare Beneficiary (ALMB-Q-I1) program

The Qualified Medicare Beneficiary program pays Medicare's monthly Part B premiums, and for certain elderly and disabled persons who are entitled to Medicare Part A (hospital insurance) the Part A and Part B deductibles and the coinsurance if you use Medicaid participating providers. If you do not go to Medicaid-participating providers, you will be responsible for Medicare deductibles and coinsurance. If you have Medicare Part A and are paying the premium for the Part A hospital insurance plan, the Medicare Savings Program may also pay the Medicare Part A premium. Your income must be at or below the national poverty level and your savings and other assets cannot exceed $4,000 for one person or $6,000 for a couple. Assets include items like money in a checking or savings account, stocks, or bonds. You generally cannot buy Medicare supplemental insurance (Medigap) if you have QMB and/or Medicaid, but you can qualify for Medicaid spend-down. In some states, the Medicaid program can purchase Medigap for you and pay your premiums on your behalf, thus enabling you to go to providers who do not participate in Medicaid.

Persons with Medicare can apply for all three programs at their local Department of Social Services (*not* their Social Security agency). You can have both Medicaid and QMB at the same time. You can also have both Medicaid and SLMB at the same time.

As already noted, Medicaid covers medical care for persons who have very low income. For people who have Medicare, Medicaid acts as a secondary payer that may cover prescription drugs, long-term nursing home care, and other benefits. Medicaid criteria for limits on income and assets differ from state to state and county to county. But the criteria are generally lower than the income and asset limits for QMB. Persons who have Medicare and whose incomes are higher than the Medicaid qualification limit, but who also have high out-of-pocket medical costs, may be able to obtain Medicaid coverage through the Medicaid spend-down program in which they reduce the financial worth of their assets to meet the Medicaid eligibility criteria.

The monthly income limits for the QMB program vary from state to state. Check with your own state Department of Social Services to find out what the monthly income limits are in your own state.

The Specified Low-Income Medicare Beneficiary (SLMB) program is for persons entitled to Medicare Part A and whose incomes are slightly higher than the national poverty level. The program pays only your Medicare Part B premium for those with assets up to $4,000 per individual or $6,000 per couple. Again check with your state Department of Social Services to find out what your state's monthly limits are.

For those who qualify, the *QI-1S program* is a Medicaid program for beneficiaries who need help in paying for Medicare Part B premiums. The beneficiary must have Medicare Part A and limited income and resources and not be otherwise eligible for Medicaid. For those who qualify, the *Medicaid program pays full Medicare Part B premiums only.* For those who qualify, the *QI-2S* program is a Medicaid program for beneficiaries who need help in paying for Medicare Part B premiums. The beneficiary must have Part A and limited income and resources not otherwise eligible for Medicaid. For those who qualify, *Medicaid pays a percentage of Medicare Part B premiums only.* For more information contact your state or local Medicaid, public welfare, or social services office. You can find the number in the telephone directory under "State Government."[25]

Paying Medicare Claims

When the time comes to pay your Medicare bill, examine it very carefully to make sure you are being charged only for those services rendered. If you feel that you are being charged for a service that you did not receive, call this to the attention of the institution or individual who provided the service. If you have further problems in this regard, report the matter to your local Social Security office or your insurance carrier.

Part A and Part B of Medicare have their own unique systems for paying claims (bills) for covered services and supplies provided to Medicare beneficiaries. Medicare claims and payments are handled by insurance organizations under contract to the federal government. The organizations that handle claims from hospitals, skilled nursing facilities, home health agencies, renal dialysis facilities, and hospices are called "intermediaries." Other insurance organizations handle Medicare Part B claims and are called "carriers." The names and addresses of the carriers are listed in the back of the *Medicare Handbook*, which may be obtained from any Social Security Administration office, or by calling 1-800-772-1213.

Medicare Part A: Hospital Insurance

It is not necessary for you to submit claims for payment under the hospital insurance program (Part A) of Medicare—the plan that covers hospital, nursing home, and home healthcare. Medicare pays its share of the costs directly to the providers of these services. The intermediary will send you a Benefits Notice showing what was billed, Medicare's portion of the bill, and what you are responsible for paying. All questions about charges and payments should be directed to the intermediary. The intermediary's address and telephone number appear on the notice.

Appealing Medicare Claims Decisions and Quality Improvement Organizations

As far as appealing decisions made by providers of services on your hospital insurance claims, you should be aware of the following information. In many cases the first written notice of noncoverage you will receive will come from the provider who delivered the services (for example, a hospital, a skilled nursing facility, a home health agency, or a hospice). The notice of noncoverage from the provider should explain why the provider believes Medicare will not pay for your services. This notice is not an official determination by Medicare, but you can ask the Medicare program for such official determination. If you do ask for an official determination, the provider must file a claim on your behalf to Medicare. When you receive the official determination, you can appeal the determination if you disagree with it.

When you are admitted to a hospital that participates in Medicare, you will be given a document entitled "An Important Message about Medicare: Rights, Admission, Discharge, and Appeal." The message contains a brief description of your state's Quality Improvement Organizations (QIOs), formerly called Professional

Review Organizations (PRO), and the name, address, and telephone number of the QIO in your state. Also, it describes your rights to appeal. QIOs are selected and paid by the federal government to review the hospital treatment of Medicare patients. Each state has a QIO to oversee the review of inpatient services in its area. These organizations have been given authority to conduct reviews of patient cases before, during, and after hospital admissions. QIOs use physicians and nurses to provide this review service. A US Court of Appeals has upheld a 2001 review finding that doctors used by the QIO cannot block the release of their review findings.

QIOs make determinations about hospital care and ambulatory surgical center care. A main function of a QIO is to review records seeking "elective" nonemergency surgery. QIOs also try to reduce admissions for procedures that can be performed safely and effectively on an outpatient basis such as cataract operations and certain types of foot surgery. The QIOs decide whether care provided to Medicare patients is medically necessary, is provided in the most appropriate setting, and is of good quality. When you disagree with a QIO decision about your case, you can appeal by requesting a reconsideration. Two things can happen with a QIO reconsideration: either the QIO will decide that Medicare will pay for some or all of the services, or it will confirm that the initial denial was correct and appropriate. The QIO's decision will be presented to you in writing. It should contain:

- the basis for the QIO's decision;
- a statement explaining which costs, if any, you will be responsible for paying; and
- a statement about your further appeal rights, including information on the proper procedures.

You should note that with a QIO decision that denies you hospital admission, you:

- must receive written notice of the QIO decision;
- must receive information about having your case reconsidered;
- have the right to request a priority review;
- have the right to submit additional information to support your case; and
- must receive written notice of the results of the reconsideration.

Then, if you disagree with a QIO decision upon its reconsideration and the amount in question is $200 or more, you can request a hearing by an administrative law judge. Cases involving $2,000 or more can eventually be appealed to a federal court.

In the case of elective or nonemergency surgery, either the hospital or the QIO may be involved in preadmission decisions. If the hospital believes that your proposed stay will not be covered by Medicare, it may recommend, without consulting the QIO, that you not be admitted to the hospital. If this is the case, the hospital must put the decision in writing. If you or your physician disagrees with the hospital's decision, you should make the request to the QIO for immediate review. You must make your request, by telephone or in writing, within three calendar days after receipt of the notice.

Appeals of decisions on most other services covered under Medicare hospital insurance (skilled nursing facility care, home healthcare, hospice services, and a few inpatient hospital matters not handled by QIOs) are handled by Medicare intermediaries. If you disagree with the intermediary's initial decision, you have 120 days from the date you receive the initial decision to request reconsideration. The request can be submitted directly to the intermediary or through Social Security. If you disagree with the intermediary's reconsideration decision and the amount in question is $100 or more, you have 120 days from the date you receive the reconsideration decision to request a hearing by an administrative law judge. Cases involving $1,000 or more can eventually be appealed to a federal court. To find your state's Quality Improvement Organization on the Internet, go to http://www.cms.hhs.gov/qio and click on "Directory."

Medicare Part B: Voluntary Medical Insurance

Under the voluntary medical insurance program (Part B) of Medicare, claims are paid in two ways. Physicians and suppliers can accept the Medicare assignment and, thus, are paid directly by the insurance carrier who acts as an intermediary between the health provider and the government. As already noted, the carrier pays 80 percent of that amount; the patient pays the rest. If your doctor accepts an assignment and the carrier pays him 80 percent of your bill, make sure that the physician does not bill you again for these services; he can only bill you for the 20 percent difference and no more. If a physician does present you with duplicate billing, notify the insurance carrier so that the insurer can straighten this matter out. You should not be paying twice for the same service. On the other hand, physicians and suppliers who refuse Medicare assignments are not bound by such agreements. They can charge you up to a specified limit established by Medicare. Medicare will pay the provider 80 percent of that charge, and you are responsible for paying the physician or supplier the rest of the bill. Make sure you find out whether your physician accepts Medicare assignments. The fees of doctors who refuse assignments are not necessary unreasonable, but there is less chance of being overcharged by a physician who accepts Medicare assignments.

There are occasions when healthcare providers who do not participate in Medicare are required by law to accept assignment of a Medicare claim. For example, all physicians and qualified laboratories must accept assignment for clinical diagnostic laboratory tests covered by Medicare. Physicians also must accept assignment for covered services provided to beneficiaries who are enrolled in the Qualified Medicare Beneficiary Program. These are low-income individuals whose Medicare monthly premiums and at least some of the Medicare deductibles and coinsurance amounts are paid by the state Medicaid program. This assistance is generally available to individuals with annual incomes at or below the federal poverty level. If you think you qualify for this assistance, you should file an application for Medicaid at a state or local office—not a Social Security Administration or other federal office—that serves people on Medicaid. The income and asset figures are somewhat higher for Alaska and Hawaii.

Medicare law also requires physicians who do not accept assignment for elective surgery to provide you with a written estimate of your costs before surgery if the total charge will be $500 or more. If the physician does not give you a written estimate, you are entitled to a refund of any amount you paid in excess of the Medicare-approved amount for surgery.

Submission of Medicare Part B Claims

In submitting Medicare claims, a form called "A Patient's Request for Medicare Payment" is used. The form is available from all Social Security offices, insurance carriers, and most physicians and must bear the claim number on your Medicare card. Doctors and suppliers who accept Medicare assignments submit the form to Medicare after you, the patient, complete and sign Part I and they complete Part II. For your information, when an itemized bill is submitted to Medicare for provider payment, it must include:

- the date you received services;
- the place where you received services;
- a description of the services;
- the charge for each service;
- the doctor or supplier who provided the services; and
- your name and your health insurance claim number, including the letter at the end of the claim number.

If your bill does not include all this information, your payment will be delayed. It is also helpful if the nature of your illness (diagnosis) is shown on the bill. To check upon the accuracy of such information, ask your medical providers what they will charge and what you will be expected to pay out of your own pocket for their services. To make sure the dates of services provided are correct, keep accurate records of your healthcare visits. Before any medical insurance can be paid, your record must show that you have met the yearly deductible. The names and addresses of the insurance carriers to which the forms should be sent is included at the end of *Your Social Security Handbook*, available from your local Social Security office. Also, remember that as of October 1, 1981, *you cannot apply medical expenses incurred during the last three months of a calendar year toward the $124 Medicare (Part B) deductible of the following year as you could do in the past.* In other words, if you incur covered medical expenses under the medical insurance plan (Part B) of Medicare during the last three months of a calendar year, you can apply these medical expenses only toward your Medicare Part B deductible of $124 for that same year. Your Social Security office can tell you more about the changes in this carry-over rule.

Regardless of whether your doctors or medical suppliers accept assignment of a claim, they are required by law to submit the claim for you within a year after providing a service. To prevent medical suppliers from defrauding Medicare, ask your physician if he or she ordered medical equipment for you and do not conduct business with door-to-door salesmen or telephone marketers who tell you that the services of medical equipment are free if you would give them your Medicare identification number. They bill Medicare for goods or services that were not needed or ever ordered. However, if your doctor or medical supplier did provide a legitimate service, the claim is submitted to the insurance carrier that serves the area where the covered service or supply was provided, not necessarily the carrier or insurer for your state. If for some reason the claim is not filed as required, it can still be sent to the carrier as long as it is sent before the close of the calendar year following the year in which the service was furnished. If the service was furnished in the last quarter of the year, the claim can be submitted until the close of the second year following the year in which the service was furnished.

After your physician or supplier submits your Part B claim, the Medicare carrier will usually send you an "Explanation of Medicare Benefits." Carefully review it. This statement details the action taken on the claim. For services of a physician, this notice shows

- what services were covered;
- what charges were approved;
- how much of the charges was credited toward your $124 annual deductible; and
- the amount Medicare paid and what you owe.

For other Part B services, the notice shows similar information. If you believe payment was made for a service or supply you didn't receive, or the payment is otherwise questionable, you should write or call the carrier that handled your claim. To prevent providers from defrauding the Medicare program, never sign blank insurance claim forms and never give total authorization to a medical provider to bill for services you received.

Appealing Medicare Part B Claims

If you do not agree with any decision concerning your hospital claim or other benefits, you have the right to appeal it. Your "Explanation of Medicare Benefits" form indicates why your claim was denied or not paid in full, and it also tells you exactly what appeal steps you can take. If you decide to file an appeal, ask your physician or medical care provider for any additional information related to the claim that might be helpful to you in challenging the payment decision.

A request for review along with any additional information must be filed with the insurance carrier within six months of the date payment was denied. After the request is filed, the insurance carrier will review the payment decision and provide you with a written explanation of the review determination. It has been the policy of the Medicare program that if a dispute is not resolved to your liking and $100 or more is involved, you can request a formal hearing on the matter with the carrier's hearing officer. If you still disagree, and if Medicare's payment on a fully allowed claim would be $100 or more, you can request a hearing with the insurance carrier. After a hearing with the insurance carrier, there is no Medicare provision for further appeal. Also, if you disagree with an insurance carrier's hearing officer's decision and the amount in question is $500 or more, you have sixty days from the date you receive the decision to request a hearing before an administrative law judge of the Social Security Administration. Cases involving $1,000 or more can eventually be appealed to a federal court. Do not hesitate to challenge any decision. Valid claims are sometimes rejected because of misunderstandings or pressure on Medicare personnel to reduce costs.[26]

Medicare Advantage Part C (Managed Care)

The preceding sections explain how the original Medicare program works if you receive your benefits through the traditional-fee-for-service system (pay-as-you-go) delivery system. As a Medicare beneficiary, you also have the option of receiving physician and other healthcare services through coordinated care plans that have contracts with Medicare under the former Medicare+Choice, or Part C, now renamed Medicare Advantage, such as competitive medical plans (CMP) and traditional health maintenance organizations (HMOs). Competitive medical plans are a kind of managed organization created by the Tax Equity and Fiscal Responsibility Act of 1982 (TEFRA) legislation to facilitate the enrollment of Medicare beneficiaries into managed care plans. CMPs are organized and financed much like HMOs, but they are not bound by all the regulatory requirements HMOs must meet.

To choose Part C you must be enrolled in Medicare Part A (Hospital Insurance) and Part B (Voluntary Medical Supplementary Insurance) and continue to pay the monthly Part B premium as well as live within the service area of the Medicare managed care plan. Medicare managed care plans are not available in all areas of the country. *In addition, you must not have end-stage renal disease (ESRD) to enroll in Medicare Part C—that is, permanent kidney failure requiring dialysis or a kidney transplant.* In addition to your Medicare Part B premium, you may also have to pay a monthly premium to the managed care plan when you enroll. Medicare Part C gives you five new options in terms of the arrangements you wish to make in paying for and receiving healthcare services. These include health maintenance organizations (HMOs), preferred-provider organizations (PPOs), provider-sponsored organizations (PSOs), private fee-for-service plans (PFSPs), and medical savings accounts (MSAs). For those under sixty-five years of age, the Medicare Prescription Drug

Improvement, and Modernization Act of 2003 created, beginning in 2006, health savings accounts (HSAs). In terms of definition:

- A *Health Maintenance Organization* (HMO) is an organization that provides a wide range of comprehensive healthcare services for a specified group at a fixed periodic payment made in advance by or on behalf of each person or family. The HMO can be sponsored by the government, medical schools, hospitals employers, labor unions, consumer groups, insurance companies, and hospital-medical plans.
- A *Preferred-Provider Organization* (PPO) is a financing and delivery system that combines aspects of standard fee-for-service indemnity plans and HMOs. Basically, a PPO is group of doctors and hospitals that negotiate with a company, labor union, or insurance firm to provide medical services for reduced fees. Unlike HMOs, PPOs operate on a fee-for-service basis and patients are not locked into using the PPO physician or hospitals. They can use any provider they want, but deductibles and copayments are waived if they use a preferred provider.
- A *Provider-Sponsored Organization* (PSO) is affiliated hospitals and doctors who operate a plan and assume the financial risk. The PSO, which does not include an insurance company, receives a fixed monthly fee from Medicare to assume the risk in providing such care.
- A *Private Fee-for-Service Plan* (PFSP) is an insurance plan that pays providers directly without a network. Services received under the PFSP are independent of the services received under Medicare. Patients can also receive services from other providers who accept Medicare. The plan reimburses doctors, hospitals, and other providers on a fee-for-service basis at a rate determined by the plan, not at the Medicare rate. Providers can also charge the patient more than 115 percent of the Medicare approved charges.
- *Medical Savings Accounts* (MSAs). Thus far, only 750,000 can enroll in this option that Congress established in the 1990s. Individuals purchase a health insurance plan with a deductible. After the individual's or a family's medical expenses exceed the deductible, the MSA pays 100 percent of Parts A and B expenses. In addition to the monthly tax deductible premium paid by the individual, Medicare pays the MSA plan the difference between the monthly premium and the enrollee's capitation rate (the amount that would be paid to an HMO). Funds can be carried over to the next year.
- *Health Savings Accounts* (HSAs) Beginning on January 1, 2006, as a result of the Medicare Prescription Drug, Improvement, and Modernization Act of 2003, a new health savings account was created for persons under sixty-five who have high deductible health insurance policies (at least $1,050 for singles and $2,100 a year for a family) and who can shelter income from taxes. Individuals younger than sixty-five years of age, employers, or family members would make pretax contributions equal to the deductible, up to a maximum of

$2,700 a year for individuals and $5,450 for families in 2006. The insurance plan also must limit the person's total out-of-pocket expenses to no more than $5,250 annually for an individual or $10,500 for a family. No one can deposit money after age sixty-five. However, so-called out-of-network charges do not count toward out-of-pocket expenses. The money deposited in the HSAs is deductible from taxable income. After sixty-five years of age, earnings and distribution also would be tax free, provided the money is used for qualifying health expenses, defined as costs incurred to diagnose, cure, treat, or prevent disease, including insurance premiums, doctor visits, prescription drugs, laser eye surgery, and long-term care, but not cosmetic surgery except when it cures an ailment such as reconstructive surgery after an accident or operation. Money in HSAs can also be used for dental expenses and orthodontia. Otherwise, funds withdrawn from the account and not used for medical expenses would be subject to income taxes with an additional 10 percent penalty. The HSAs and the flexible spending accounts (FSAs) many employers offer at work are similar to each other. Both allow workers to save their own money, on a pretax basis, to pay medical expenses that occur during the year. The biggest difference between FSAs and HSAs is that any money that is not spent in an FSA at year's end is lost, whereas money in an HSA can accumulate from year to year. The money saved in an HSA can be provided by the employer, the employee, or a combination of both. Whoever makes the contribution can take the tax deduction. While you can contribute to both an HSA and an FSA at the same time, you cannot use funds in both accounts to pay for the same medical expense. You can first pay medical expenses with FSAs, and then when the FSA is used up, you can use the HSA to pay for the same qualifying medical expenses. Should you die with money left in an HSA, and you have a surviving spouse, the account can be transferred directly to the survivor, without distribution or immediate tax implications. HSAs can be set up by employers or by individuals. Employers can establish HSAs for workers in conjunction with a health insurance plan. Or individuals with a high deductible plan can establish an HSA separately. In addition to insurers, mutual funds and banks may also establish HSAs in the future.

Disease Management Plans

Also, Medicare is working to create specialty plans, such as a Disease Management Plan, which are new ways to provide more focused healthcare for some people. These Medicare specialty plans are designed to give you all your Medicare healthcare, as well as more focused care to manage a disease or condition such as congestive heart failure, diabetes, or end-state renal disease. The goal is to provide your healthcare in an efficient, effective, high-quality manner. To find out if any Medicare specialty plans are available in your areas, call 1-800-Medicare (1-800-633-4227). TTY users should call 1-877-486-2048.

Operations of Managed Care Plans

In view of your various choices under the Medicare Part C option, it is very important that you understand how the operations of managed or coordinated care plans affect you as a patient. In a coordinated care plan, a network of healthcare providers (physician, hospital, skilled nursing homes, and others) generally offers medical services to plan members on a prepaid basis. Services usually must be obtained from the professionals and facilities that are part of the plan. Once you have signed up with the HMO, you cannot go back to your former doctor—or to a specialist of your choice—and expect Medicare to pay the bill. It won't, unless the doctor belongs to the HMO group or your HMO approved the visit. You generally must receive all covered care through the plan or from healthcare professionals to whom the plan refers you or else, as already noted, the plan will not pay. Depending upon how the plan operates, services are usually delivered at one or more centrally located health facilities or in the private practice offices of the doctors and other healthcare professionals who are part of the plan. Most managed care plans permit you to choose a primary care doctor from those that are part of the plan. If you do not choose a doctor, a physician will be assigned to you. Your primary care doctor is responsible for managing your care, admitting you to a hospital, and referring you to a specialist. You are allowed to change your primary care doctor as long as you choose another primary care doctor affiliated with the plan. If you enroll in a plan that has a contract with Medicare, a Medicare claim will seldom need to be submitted on your behalf. In fact, if you are in a managed care plan, you generally do not need a Medigap policy. But if you have a Medigap policy and decide to enroll in a plan, you may want to keep it because it could be of value to you if you leave the plan and return to fee-for-service medicine. If you previously had a Medigap policy but dropped it while in the plan or never had one before you joined the plan, you might not be able to buy the policy of your choice, especially if you have a health problem. Remember, when you join a coordinated care plan, Medicare pays the plan a set amount and the plan provides your medical care. Additionally, instead of paying Medicare's deductible and coinsurance as you would under fee-for-service care, most coordinated care plans charge enrollees a monthly premium and nominal copayments. You must also continue to pay the Part B premium to Medicare. Usually there are no other charges no matter how many times you visit the doctor, are hospitalized, or use other covered services.

Risk versus Cost Managed Care Plans

Before you join a managed care plan, find out whether the plan has a "risk" or "cost" contract with Medicare. There is an important difference.

- *Risk plans* have "lock-in" requirements. These requirements mean that you generally are committed or locked into receiving all your covered healthcare through the plan or through referrals by the plan. In most cases, if you receive services that are not authorized by the plan, neither the plan nor Medicare will pay. The only exceptions all Medicare-contracting plans recognize are for emergency services, which you may receive anywhere in the United States, and for services you urgently need when you are temporarily out of the plan's service area. A third exception offered by a few risk plans is called the "point-of-service" (POS) option. Under the POS option, the plan allows you to receive certain services outside the plan's provider network and the plan will pay a percentage of the charges. In return for this flexibility, expect to pay at least 20 percent of the bill.

- *Cost plans* are plans that do not have lock-in requirements. They receive payment from Medicare based on the enrollee's use of HMO services. If you enroll in a cost plan, you can go either to healthcare providers affiliated with the plan or go outside the plan. If you go outside the plan, the plan probably will not pay, but Medicare will. Medicare will pay its share of the charges it approves. You will be responsible for Medicare's coinsurance, deductibles, and other charges, just as if you were receiving care under the fee-for-service system. Because of this flexibility, a cost plan may be a good choice for you if you travel frequently, live in another state part of the year, or want to use a doctor who is not affiliated with a plan.

To enroll in a managed care plan as a Medicare beneficiary:

- You must have Medicare Part B and continue paying Part B premiums.
- You must live in the plan's service area.
- You cannot be receiving care in a Medicare-certified hospice.
- You cannot have permanent kidney failure at the time of enrollment.

All plans that have contracts with Medicare must have an advertised open-enrollment period of at least thirty days once a year. Plans must enroll Medicare beneficiaries in the order of application. You cannot be rejected because of poor health. Also, carefully consider the advantages and disadvantages of plan membership if you travel a lot or live in another state for part of the year. Plans must provide coverage for a fixed period of time when you travel. Also, remember that if you enroll in a plan and later move out of the plan's service area, you will have to disenroll and either return to fee-for-service Medicare or enroll in plan that serves your new location. Because each plan is different, your benefits and premiums probably will not be exactly the same if you enroll in another plan. To change from one managed care plan to another, simply enroll in the other plan as long as it has a Medicare contract. You are automatically disenrolled from the first plan.

Most plans serving Medicare beneficiaries are required to provide all Medicare hospital and medical benefits available in the plan's service area. Some plans also provide benefits beyond what Medicare pays for, such as preventive care, prescription drugs, dental care, hearing aids, and eyeglasses for little or no extra fee. You don't pay Medicare's deductibles and coinsurance.

If you are a member of an HMO or a competitive medical plan with a Medicare contract, your HMO/CMP will make decisions about your coverage and payment of services. Your appeal rights are similar to the rights of Medicare beneficiaries under traditional fee-for-service Medicare. Also, federal law requires HMOs and CMPs under contract to Medicare to provide a full, written explanation of appeal rights to all members at the time of enrollment and at least once a year thereafter. If you are a member of an HMO or a CMP and you have not received a written explanation of your appeal rights, you should request one from your organization's membership office.[27]

Summary of Your HMO Medicare Rights

As a Medicare patient of an HMO, you have certain rights. These include the following points:

- As an HMO enrollee, you have the right to the same benefits and services available under traditional Medicare.
- If you believe you require care that your HMO refuses to provide you, you are entitled to appeal the HMO's denial of services. You also have the right to know how your plan pays its doctors, and the plan must tell you in writing. You also have the right to know whether your doctor owns all or part of a healthcare facility. For example, if you are referred for a blood test to a laboratory that he or she owns.
- If your HMO refuses to cover emergency services, or urgent care services you receive outside of the HMO's service area, you have the right to appeal.
- If your HMO does not have a physician in its network who can provide you with the Medicare-covered service you require, the HMO must arrange and pay for you to see an out-of-plan doctor. You also have the right to choose a women's health specialist from your plan's list of doctors for routine and preventive healthcare services.
- If you are not satisfied with the care the HMO is providing you, you are entitled to file a grievance with the HMO; you also have the right to disenroll from the HMO and return to traditional Medicare at any time. The change occurs on the first day of the month following the HMO's receipt of your written notice.[28]

In addition, on November 25, 1996, the Healthcare Financing Administration (now renamed the Centers for Medicare and Medicaid Services) notified health maintenance organizations, which enroll Medicare beneficiaries, that patients are entitled to full medical advice and counsel by their physicians on all medically necessary treatment options. The agency that manages Medicare said that Medicare enrollees are entitled to "advice and counsel from their physician on medically necessary treatment options that may be appropriate for their condition or disease." The agency stated that in such a situation a physician may not be limited by the HMO in counseling or advising the beneficiary. The letter states that "contractual provisions that limit a physician's ability to counsel or advise a Medicare beneficiary are a violation of the law." [29] The letter was initiated because of accusations that HMO rules or "gag" provisions in contracts are preventing doctors from providing full advice to patients in situations where the HMO may not wish to provide certain treatments in order to save money even though they may be a serious medical choice. These are very important rights you have as a Medicare member of an HMO, and you should not forget them if you ever become dissatisfied with the quality of service the HMO provides you.

Medicare Part D (Prescription Drug Benefit)

"Norman, do you understand this new prescription benefit under Medicare? I once thought that if Congress added this benefit to Medicare its cost would have been included in my monthly Medicare premium like all my other benefits under Part B medical insurance and not be a separate premium by itself. Now I find myself facing the possibility of paying three premiums under Medicare. First, my monthly premium, a premium for the drug benefit plan, and then a premium for my Medigap insurance plan to cover the gaps in my Medicare coverage since I don't belong to an HMO or a PPO. I know HMOs in the Medicare program cover prescription drugs even though the federal government doesn't require them to do so. But if I join a group that is like an HMO and doesn't cover drugs, I will still need prescription coverage and will have to choose a Part D plan to do so. I will still pay three premiums: Medicare, the HMO-like plan, and the prescription drug plan. I'm not even sure if I want managed care. I like picking my own doctors as I have always done under the old fee-for-service system. I don't even understand the language these drug plans use, 'doughnut holes,' 'creditable' plans, 'preferred' pharmacies, formulary 'tiers,' and other words. By the way, what is a formulary? It sounds like what my mother used to feed me when I was a baby. The government says all the information I need to know is located on computer Web sites. I'm in my seventies. I don't even know how to use a computer. Everyday my mail is filled with brochures from companies asking me to sign up. I heard on TV that there are about forty or fifty companies alone in my city that are trying to sell this drug benefit to senior citizens. Do I have to sign up for this program? If do sign up, how can I tell the legitimate companies from the frauds? What do I do about my drug discount card that I have been using up to now? Then, the experts say in choosing a plan compare the current prescription medicines you are taking with the drugs the plan is covering. I'm not a doctor or a pharmacist. How can I tell if a different version of my drug is on the list that is just as good as the one I am presently taking? What will happen to me if it isn't on the list? I can't even pronounce the names of some of these drugs. Do you think my former employer can help me as a retiree to pay for some of these costs? I have so many questions

about this program that I don't even know where to begin. Would you please explain how this whole drug program works because I'm afraid I may make the wrong decisions and in the end harm my own health because I'm unable to understand what this program is all about."

"Daniel, let me explain the ins and outs of this program. And if you have any friends who qualify for public assistance or are retired from the military, the information will help them as well."

"Norman, I'd really appreciate that."

On November 25, 2003, the US Congress gave final approval to add a prescription drug benefit to the Medicare program, beginning on January 1, 2006. President Bush signed the bill into law on December 8, 2003, as the Medicare Prescription Drug, Improvement, and Modernization Act of 2003 (Public Law108-173). *This is a voluntary insurance program* that everyone can join if they are enrolled in the original Medicare program (with either Part A or Part B coverage) no matter what their income may be, or a Medicare Cost Plan, or a Medicare private fee-for-service plan that do not cover prescription drugs. You do not have to take any physical examination for this coverage nor can the program turn you down for health reasons. In addition, *you do not have to sign up and enroll in this prescription drug program if you do not wish to do so.* As already noted, this is a voluntary prescription drug insurance program. Again, for purposes of definition, a Medicare cost plan is a kind of HMO. In a Medicare cost plan, if you receive services outside of the plan's network without a referral, your Medicare-covered services will be paid under the original Medicare Plan (Parts A and B), except your cost plan does pay for emergency services or urgently needed services outside the service area. A private fee-for-service plan is a kind of Medicare Advantage plan (Part C) in which you may go to any Medicare-approved physician or hospital that accepts the plan's payment. The insurance plan, rather than the Medicare program, decides how much it will pay and what you will pay for the services you receive. You may pay more or less for Medicare-covered benefits. You may have extra benefits that the original Medicare plan (Parts A and B) does not cover. Despite the establishment of this Part D prescription drug program, Medicare Part B will continue to cover drugs such as those administered in a hospital or a doctor's office as it has in the past.

Enrollment Rules

Historically, in 2004 and 2005 recipients entitled to Medicare benefits or enrolled in Part A or Part B of Medicare and not entitled to medical assistance for outpatient prescription drugs or for discounts cards because they were enrolled in Medicaid were able to purchase a prescription drug discount card, which could not exceed $30 a year and that the US Department of Health and Human Services estimated would provide a savings of 10 to 25 percent.

When the Medicare prescription drug benefit program became effective on January 1, 2006, the Medicare Approved Prescription Drug Discount card program began to be phased out and officially ended on the day your Medicare Part D prescription drug plan began to cover you as a beneficiary, or on May 15, 2006, whichever date came first. If you signed up by December 31, 2005, your Medicare prescription drug coverage began on January 1, 2006. If signed up after January 1, 2006, your coverage would begin on the first day of the month following the month you enrolled. May 15, 2006, was designated as the last day you could sign up for the Medicare Part D plan without being penalized unless you qualify for an exception. Except for some circumstances, the penalty is a more expensive premium. For each month you delay in signing up for the Part D prescription drug coverage, an extra 1 percent of the initial monthly premium in 2006 is added to your own premium, and the increase is permanent as long as you have Part D coverage. In other words, for purposes of example, if the monthly premium in your state or region for a Part D prescription drug plan that you are considering joining is $50 per month in 2006 and you wait twelve months before you enroll in the Part D prescription drug plan, you will be paying an extra 12 percent penalty, that is, 1 percent for each of the twelve months, or an extra $6 (12 percent x $50) added to your premium. So instead of paying a premium of $50 per month, as an example, assuming the premium has not changed twelve months later, you will be paying $56 ($50 + $6) a month. But whether or not the initial premium has increased, the $6 added to that initial monthly premium is a permanent increase or penalty. In 2006 the actual average national monthly premium was estimated to be $32 a month, or $384 per year. Also remember the average national monthly premium is only an average of the cost of all the premiums being offered in the country. Some premiums are less than $32 a month, and others are more than $32.

If you do not enroll in the prescription Part D drug program by May 15, 2006, the next open-enrollment period for Medicare beneficiaries is November 15–December 15, 2006. If you must change prescription drug plans before that time (for example, you move from the area your plan covers) or your plan ceases to provide services or you move into a nursing home, you can choose another prescription drug plan at that particular time.

Creditable Coverage

You should also find out if any prescription drug plan coverage you now have is *creditable*—that is, is it as good or even better than the new Medicare program benefit. If your plan is creditable, you can sign up for the Medicare Part D drug plan anytime after May 15, 2006, without the 1 percent monthly penalty being added to your monthly premium and as long as you sign up for the Medicare drug coverage within sixty-three days after losing your previous prescription drug coverage. This nonpenalty rule is also true for persons who are enrolled in the US Veterans Administration health program and the US Department of Defense's TRICARE-for-Life program for military retirees and dependents because both programs are considered better than Medicare's standard plan coverage. In addition, your employer, union, or any other third party that helps pay for your prescription drugs had to tell you by November 14, 2005, whether your coverage under its prescription drug plan is "creditable." On the other hand, remember if your current prescription drug coverage is not as good as the standard Part D drug plan, you can still keep your non-creditable plan coverage, but the 1 percent penalty for each month of delay beyond May 15, 2006, will be added to your premium, as already noted, when and if you decide to enroll in the Medicare drug program after that date. Also, your employer, union, or other third party must tell you whether or not Medicare's prescription drug program will affect your current prescription drug coverage with the organization. Among its options, your organization can do the following:

- Maintain your current drug plan coverage. But you must find out, as already noted, if your current drug plan coverage is at least as good ("creditable") as the Medicare Part D drug benefit program.
- Offer you coverage through a new Medicare drug program. But you must sign up for this new plan in order to remain under your employer's drug coverage.
- Offer you drug coverage that supplements the Medicare drug plan by paying all or part of your out-of-pocket expenses.
- Drop their drug coverage—maybe helping you pay part of the cost of your premium or not helping you at all.

Transitional Prescription Drug Card Discount Program, 2004–2006

In regard to the transitional prescription discount cards themselves whose coverage ends on May 15, 2006, for those who do not sign up for the Medicare prescription drug plan by that date, critics have stated that the card does not account for inflation in drug prices. So if you plan to use your Medicare prescription drug discount cards until May 15, 2006, the following information is relevant to your situation. Unlike other discount cards available during this period, participants can only sign up for one card. If the discount card–eligible individual is enrolled in a plan under Medicare Part C, Medicare Advantage (e.g., Medicare HMO or managed care) and that plan offers an endorsed discount care program, then the individual may enroll in that particular plan.

In general, the cards are likely to have offered different discounts for different drugs made by different pharmaceutical companies. Some cards may offer "open formularies," which means they will include discounts on all drugs. Others will discount only certain drugs. You can use non-Medicare discounts (e.g., from pharmacies) as well, but not for the same prescription. Participants will have to choose a card based on which card matches best with their prescription drugs.

Remember just because a card is endorsed by Medicare does not mean it offers the best price. Savings programs at your pharmacy might save you more than the card would. Also, remember that you cannot use a card at any pharmacy. Each sponsor will specify which pharmacies accept its card. Some will also offer mail order, if that is more convenient for you, and you can compare the costs of purchasing prescription drugs through mail order versus, for example, from your local pharmacy. None of the cards can be used to buy drugs from other countries. So, based on the prescription medications you are taking, investigate which card, if any, is best for you.

By typing in your zip code, you can find pricing information as well as services offered by each card sponsor in your geographical area posted and updated on the Medicare Web site (http://www.Medicare.gov). This information also is available from the Medicare helpline (1-800-MEDICARE or 1-800-633-4273). A principal problem is that prices and prescriptions covered by a card may change at any time, but the law says participants can choose a different card only during the annual enrollment period except under exceptional circumstances, such as changing residences and moving outside the program's service areas. The cards issued by various companies such as insurance companies, wholesale and retail pharmacies, and companies that manage pharmaceutical benefits for other organizations can charge different annual fees and different prices for the same medication until the full Medicare program becomes effective in 2006.

Beneficiaries eligible for both Medicaid and Medicare ("dual eligibles") are not charged the premiums or deductibles or the card enrollment fee of about $30 but pay a $3 copayment per prescription for brand-name medicine and $1 for generics. Copayments are waived for those in nursing homes. In addition, these patients do not face any gap in their drug coverage after drug expenditures reach $2,250.

Beneficiaries with incomes below $12,569 for a single person ($16,862 for married couples) were able to get up to $600 a year for prescription drugs in 2004 and 2005, plus the remainder of what was not used in 2004, as long as they had less than $6,000 in assets, other than their house. They pay no premium, no deductible, and no $30 card enrollment. They will pay $2 for generics and $5 for brand names and nothing above the catastrophic limit. In addition, these patients did not face any gap in their drug coverage after drug expenditures reached $2,250. The subsidy is to be phased out between $12,123 and about $13,500 in yearly income and end at 150 percent of the poverty level. People who have drug coverage through Medicaid, a former employer or any other group health plans, or the military are not eligible. To apply, just ask whoever is offering you the card.

Watch out for fraudulent or fake prescription discount cards. Don't agree to purchase any card that does not carry the official logo with the words "Medicare approved" or costs more than $30. Never give out your Medicare, Social Security, credit card, or any other bank information to anyone who may telephone you or who comes to your door to sell you a card. If a company telephones you, ask for written material and an application, or write down the company's name and the details of its offer and find out how you should contact the company, if you wish, after you have done your research and read the material. You can check out legitimate prescription drug discount card sponsors by going to the Web site http://www.Medicare.gov, as noted previously, or by calling 1-800-633-4227 or 1-800-MEDICARE. Once again, remember, companies offering Medicare-approved cards are not allowed to tele-market their cards or go door-to-door to sell them. If approached by someone this way, beware of sharing personal information with him or her.

Another good site to check out information relating to prescription drug dis-count cards as well as other information relating to Medicare is the following Web site: http://www.medicarerights.org. Also, report any scams to the Medicare fraud hotline at 1-800-447-8477. Finally, make sure you need a Medicare discount card. If your income is less than the previously mentioned income thresholds of $12,569 for a single person or $16,862 for a married couple, then you are eligible to receive the low-income discount card that will give you $600 toward your drug costs and you should get this card. But if your income is higher than these income thresholds, you may obtain greater savings through either drug discount programs such as the state assistance programs (State Health Insurance Assistance Program [SHIP]) and drug company programs. Check out both sources.

Part D Medicare Drug Benefit Administration

Beginning on January 1, 2006, multiple private insurance companies approved by Medicare will administer the Medicare prescription drug benefit. In addition to stand-alone plans, Medicare beneficiaries can also join an HMO or a PPO plan (Medicare Part C called Medicare Advantage) that offers prescription drug coverage in addition to their other health benefits, if you like and want managed care. All Medicare Advantage managed care plans (except Medicare private-fee-for-service plans) must offer at least one choice that includes prescription drug coverage. On the other hand, if you like fee-for-service plans and wish to remain or change to a tradi-tional Medicare fee-for-service plan, which offers a variety of health benefits, then you may wish to consider enrolling in a stand-alone prescription drug plan, if you choose to enroll in a private-fee-for-service plan that does not include drug cov-erage. *But remember, you can only choose a combination of both a managed care plan and a prescription drug stand-alone plan if the managed care plan does not cover prescription drugs. If you are enrolled already in a Medicare Advantage plan that covers you for prescription drugs, be aware that by also enrolling in a stand-alone prescription drug plan (Part D) as well, you would automatically transfer yourself out of your Medical Advantage plan (Part C) and back into traditional Medicare (Parts A and B). You cannot join a Medical Advantage plan (Part C) as well as stay in traditional Medicare at the same time.*

If you decide to join a prescription drug plan, you will receive its prescription card, which you will bring to your pharmacy or send the card's number to a mail-order prescription drug service. In this manner, *the pharmacy can tell if you have met your deductible or what your copayments might be or whether you are in that por-tion of the program benefit gap (called the "doughnut hole") that Medicare does not cover.* To keep track of these costs, the prescription drug plan must send you a monthly statement. There will be national plans that will provide coverage to people in all states and regional plans that will be available only in certain areas. While all these prescription drug plans meet or exceed a Medicare-established standard package as defined by Congress, and, depending upon the plan, require written disclosures, each plan can differ in its coverage options, how it establishes costs (different premiums, different copayments, which are defined as a specific dollar amount for each prescription, or coinsurance, which is defined as a percentage of the prescription price, different drug prices), and in where you can buy your prescription drugs since the pharmacies that accept the plans will also vary.

Payments according to Drug Levels or Tiers

Most plans will have three or four levels (known as "tiers") of copayments or coinsurance, rising from the least expensive generic drugs at the lowest level or tier, through "preferred" brand-name drugs (on the formulary) at the second level, to "nonpreferred" brands (drugs listed on formulary but at a higher copayment than preferred drugs' tier) at the third level, to rarer high-cost drugs on the fourth level, for which you may pay a coinsurance amount rather than a copayment. In the context of the discussion about the Part D prescription drug program, a formulary is a list of certain kinds of prescription drugs that a Medicare drug plan will cover subject to limits and conditions. Plans cannot change the premium or deductible you pay between January 1 and December 31 of each year. But the copayment you pay can change during the year if a drug is moved from one tier to another tier. Plans can also change all charges for the year 2007 and in each future year. Also, you may receive more coverage and pay less out of your own pocket through a special part of the Medicare drug coverage program called Extra Help (full coverage) if your income and personal savings are limited, or if you are in a state pharmacy-assistance program, or if your employer or union coverage supplements Medicare. If you live in the US territories—Puerto Rico, Virgin Islands, Guam, American Samoa, and the Northern Mariana Islands—the Extra Help program is different from that in the states and you will also have fewer Medicare drug programs from which to choose.

Selection of Pharmacy

You should find out whether the pharmacy you presently use will be part of your drug plan's preferred or nonpreferred network (preferred pharmacies offer lower prices). Many plans will use mail-order services that will deliver the drugs to you. Plans must make ninety-day supplies of medications available through pharmacies in their network as well as through mail order. Therefore, make sure that the drugstores and pharmacies that are part of the network of the prescription drug plan that you are considering joining are convenient for you or that you can order prescription drugs by mail, if you wish. Because of possible conflicts of interest, pharmacists cannot help you choose a Part D plan because they could select a plan favorable to their own pharmacy rather than to you.

Design of Prescription Drug Benefits

The various insurers who are seeking to sell you their prescription drug plan may differ from each other in the way they design their benefits, but the overall value of their benefits must be same as the basic benefits of the Medicare standard prescription drug plan. For example, a plan may offer a lower deductible ($100), rather than the standard Medicare plan's $250 deductible, and higher copayments than does the basic standard benefit. A plan must cover at least two drugs in each class of medications (a group of drugs, e.g., similar drugs addressing a similar problem or used to treat the same condition, like statins for high cholesterol) and most of the drugs in six classes: antidepressants, antipsychotics, anticonvulsants, antiretrovirals to treat HIV and AIDS, immunosuppressants, and cancer drugs. But the plans won't have to cover all drugs, and they will be permitted to change the drugs they cover at any time. However, plans must inform you of these changes at least sixty days in advance of the changes if the changes involve prescription drugs that you currently use. Each plan has its own list of preferred drugs (a formulary), and the list of drugs differs from plan to plan since not every drug is available on every plan. The prescription drug program does not cover over-the-counter drugs as well as those medications that the law forbids Medicare to cover, such as drugs for weight problems. Each plan itself, rather than the federal government, negotiates the prices of drugs with pharmaceutical companies on your behalf. When you pay for drugs within the plan, you have access to discounted drugs. Medicare prescription drug plans will cover both brand-name and generic drugs. People who sign up for a Part D plan will be able to change plans only once each year. Monthly premiums will vary, as already noted, but some plans have premiums less than $20 a month and others are higher than the national average cost of $32 in 2006. You can have your premiums deducted from your Social Security check or pay the premiums on your own directly to your Part D Medicare drug plan. Married couples do not receive any special benefits under this program. Each spouse pays his or her own premiums, copayments, deductibles, and other personal out-of-pocket costs for medications and will reach each level of coverage according to the rate each incurs prescription drug expenses over each calendar year.

Before deciding whether the Medicare prescription drug program is for you, review your current health insurance coverage.

- Are the prescription drugs that you currently take covered by the Part D Medicare drug plan?
- What are your current out-of-pocket prescription drug costs?
- Make a list of the name, dosage, and cost of the prescription drugs you use. Different Medicare prescription drug plans, as already noted, will cover different prescription drugs.
- Compare your current prescription drug regimen—that is, all the prescription drugs you are now taking—with the list and coverage a Medicare Part D plan

offers. Which is better for you? Is it a Medicare Part D plan or your current prescription drug plan, if you are enrolled in one.

Therefore, if you enroll in Part D, select a plan that covers the drugs you are taking. If the plan you want does not cover all the drugs you use, ask your doctor if you can change prescriptions. If the doctor decides there in no substitute for your current medication, he or she can request that the Medicare drug plan cover the prescription drug(s). All plans must have an appeals process. However, before giving you an exception, a plan may require that you try a drug on its formulary (drug list) that is similar to the prescription drug that you are now taking and that is not included on its formulary in order to determine whether the prescription drug on the plan's formulary is equally as effective in treating your medical condition as the medication you are currently taking. To find out whether cheaper alternatives would meet your medication needs, the Consumers Union posts on its Web site a list of "Best Buy" drugs, which might serve as a starting point for such a discussion with your doctor. Click on http://www.crbestbuydrugs.org or http://www.crbestbuydrugs .org/drugreports.html. Also, Medicare has a Web site tool (Medicare Prescription Drug Plan Finder) at http://www.Medicare.gov that allows the Medicare beneficiary to choose the plan that is best for the person by comparing specific plans and taking into account where they live, the types of drugs they routinely take, and how much they are willing to pay in premiums and deductibles. As already noted, beneficiaries can receive drug coverage in two ways: through new separate stand-alone insurance plans or policies for drugs alone or through private health plans like managed care (Medicare Part C—Medicare Advantage) that also provide the rest of their medical care, including prescription drug coverage. As already noted, these latter plans include HMOs, preferred-provider organizations (PPOs), which encourage the use of certain doctors but allow patients to go elsewhere if they pay extra, private fee-for-service plans, which allow patients to see any doctor, or another type of health plan that provides the rest of their care. Thus, you would have to change doctors *only* if you chose to get drug coverage by joining a health maintenance organization or a preferred-provider organization that does not include your current doctor(s) in its provider network or if your own doctor(s) stops accepting Medicare.

Drug Plans and Your Employer

Employers who continue to provide drug coverage to their workers and retirees will be subsidized by the federal government, as long as their plan is as good ("creditable") as Medicare's. If you receive a statement from your company that says that your drug plan is "creditable"—again, meaning that it meets Medicare national standards—you don't have to enroll in Medicare Part D. Make sure you retain these company statements because they will serve as proof that your employer's drug plan was as good as Medicare's and will allow you to avoid a late-enrollment penalty if you sign up for Medicare Part D at a later time. *But if you join Part D anyway while working for your current company, your organization will remove you from your company's drug insurance plan and possibly may even cancel your medical insurance.* Check with your organization's human resources department as to whether you would lose your medical insurance if you enrolled in Part D. Employers that offer equivalent Medicare drug coverage for retirees would receive tax-free subsidies. Employers could also offer subsidies for premiums and cost-sharing assistance for retirees who enroll in Medicare drug plans. But be aware that you employer has the right to change or drop retiree health and drug benefits at any time.

Individual Health Insurance Policy Coverage

If you presently have an individual health insurance policy that is neither a group policy nor a Medigap policy, you can still keep this kind of individual health policy and enroll in a Part D Medicare drug plan as well. But, like employers, unions, or other third-party organizations, your insurer must tell you whether your individual health insurance policy is "creditable" or not, because, as already noted, this fact of whether or not it is as good as the standard Medicare prescription drug program in terms of value will determine whether or not you pay a premium penalty should you enroll after May 15, 2006, in the Part D Medicare drug program. If you join a Medicare drug program, you can use your individual insurance policy to supplement the Medicare coverage. If you find yourself in the $2,850 coverage gap where the standard Medicare program itself does not cover or pay for the costs of any prescription drugs, any payments your insurer makes would not count as part of your annual out-of-pocket expenses of $3,600 that would make you eligible for the catastrophic drug coverage, which begins at the $5,100 level of your annual drug expenses. *But ask your Medicare drug plan if it will cover any part or all of that $2,850 gap if you pay a higher insurance premium.*

Buying Prescription Drugs from Foreign Countries

Remember that if you purchase prescription drugs from outside the country, such as from Canada, those personal drug expenses will not count toward your annual out-of-pocket cost limit of $5,100 in drug bills that qualifies you for the Medicare program's catastrophic drug coverage because Medicare plans do not cover drugs that are purchased from other countries. In fact, the United States has a ban on drug reimportation because the Food and Drug Administration has stated that it cannot assure the safety of these medications. But this fact did not stop, by 2004, a number of states, like Minnesota and New Hampshire, and municipalities, like Springfield, Massachusetts, from defying the federal law so that they could help their residents obtain cheaper drugs from Canada and Europe. Medications from abroad are not considered as "creditable" coverage. Although it may be technically illegal, the Food and Drug Administration will not prosecute individuals who import small quantities of prescription drugs from Canada for their use (limited to a three-month supply).

But the FDA, as already noted, warns those people that the drugs may not be safe and advises them to contact their doctors. So if you lose your foreign sources of drug supplies and join a Medicare plan after May 15, 2006, until which date you could have joined the Medicare prescription drug program without being penalized, a premium penalty of 1 percent, as already noted, for each month you delayed enrolling would be added to the plan's premium at the time you do join.

Other Sources of Drug Payment Assistance

Should you be receiving free drugs from a pharmaceutical manufacturer's patient-assistance program, you can continue to receive them and still enroll in the Medicare prescription drug program, but only as long as the drug manufacturer keeps operating this program for Medicare beneficiaries.

The federal government will guarantee drug coverage in any region of the country that does not have at least one stand-alone drug plan and one private health plan like an HMO or a PPO. In other words, if a region lacks one or both kinds of plan, the government will still guarantee that drugs are covered in that particular region.

Out-of-Pocket Drug Costs for Medicare Beneficiaries

As already noted, under the standard Medicare prescription drug program, the average national monthly premium estimate in 2006 was $32 a month, or $384 per year, with some plans offering premiums below that amount and other above for their drug coverage. After the beneficiary meets the $250 deductible, Medicare insurance would pay 75 percent of the drug costs up to $2,250 (or $1,687 with the patient paying the remaining $563 out of his own pocket). Should you then incur annual drug costs between $2,250 and $5,100, you will pay the total amount of $2,850 out of your own pocket under the national standard Medicare drug plan because the Medicare program does not cover this cost gap. That is a gap that is built into the program. When your annual drug costs or expenses reach $5,100 or more, the Medicare program will pay 95 percent of your drug bill and you will pay the remaining 5 percent out of your own pocket at this catastrophic cost level. In other words, once you accumulate $3,600 in annual drug bills out of your own pocket, your catastrophic drug coverage begins under the Medicare program. The $3,600 expense limit *does not include* the cost of your monthly premium for the Part D prescription drug plan but *does include* deductibles, copayments, any out-of-pocket expenses you pay for drugs during the $2,850 gap, and any payments a friend or a member of your family made in buying drugs for you, as well as any charitable groups or a state pharmacy-assistance plan that did the same. *But in all instances, only payments for those drugs that your plan covers, including exceptions you receive, count toward the $3,600 limit.* If you purchase drugs elsewhere, just send your receipts to the plan. *Payments that are not included in the $3,600 out-of-pocket* *expense limit include your premiums, as already noted; personal costs for drugs that your plan does not cover; payments an employer, union, or other third-party payer like the federal government or your own insurance plan makes; and drugs that you buy from Canada or other foreign countries.*

Looking at this another way in terms of personal out-of pocket drugs costs, if your monthly prescription drug premium payment matched the Medicare national average of $32 a month (and many premiums are also above and below that amount among the many prescription drug plans) *the Medicare beneficiaries will have to pay out of their own pocket,* as an example, $384 in drug benefit premiums per year ($32 national average drug premium per month in 2006 x 12 months). In addition, you will pay a $250 deductible, plus $563 (25 percent) of the first $2,250 in drug costs, plus the next $2,850 between $2,250 and $5,100 in prescription drug expenses because the insurance does not pay or cover prescription drug costs between these two financial levels, and, as a minimum, at least another 5 percent of all succeeding drug costs after reaching the $5,100 level in annual drug expenses. In other words, the beneficiary will spend out of his pocket almost $4,000 that not only includes his monthly premiums but also a deductible, shared coinsurance, and the gap where no coverage exists until he reaches the $5,100 level in drug expenses, at which point he will still have to pay 5 percent of drug costs beyond that $5,100 financial level. But not everyone will fall into the $2,850 gap. Employers and state pharmacy-assistance programs may give their enrollees extra coverage to narrow or fill in the gap. So will some Medicare drug plans, probably with higher premiums. In other words, your drug expense may be large enough to get you into the coverage gap of $2,850 but not high enough to get you out, so some plans will cover some or all of those costs for the previously mentioned higher premium, perhaps covering both generic and brand-name drugs or generics themselves. But if your expenses are very high, any additional coverage you receive from a plan will not count toward the $3,600 out-of-pocket spending limit and can slow down the start of the catastrophic drug coverage that begins when you reach that personal $3,600 limit in drug expenses, excluding premium costs. One of the methods you can use to slow down your arrival at the $2,850 gap is using generic drugs or less expensive brand-name drugs that have lower copayments and will make your initial $2,250 coverage last longer. But you should ask your doctor if he would recommend your taking such drugs for your medical condition since your physician knows your health best and is the one who must prescribe the medication that treats you best. And people on limited incomes who qualify for extra assistance will receive coverage throughout the year, as well as have Medicare pay most of the cost.

Other Drug Benefit Program Options

But there is a possible loophole to reduce your drug expenses further under this law. If your state has a pharmacy program that provides drug coverage to its residents and this state program continues when the Medicare prescription drug benefit is effective in 2006, then it is possible that your state could pay only the premiums, deductibles, and copayments for the Medicare drug benefit. The state could pay these out-of-pocket costs for you until you reach the $3,600 threshold for catastrophic coverage. Then, Medicare will begin paying as much as 95 percent of the costs of drugs. As already noted, your out-of- pocket costs can also be paid by family members, a pharmacy assistance program, or a charity.

As far as military retirees or veterans are concerned, their drug benefits would not change under this law. As already noted, military retirees and their dependents who are enrolled in the TRICARE-for-Life program, which offers generous drug coverage, can decide to stay in it. Veterans can also continue to obtain low-cost drugs under the Veterans Affairs health system if they are enrolled in it.

Medigap Policies with Prescription Drug Coverage

In addition, *the new law will not allow you to have both the Part D Medicare drug benefit and a Medigap policy* (supplementary insurance that covers benefit gaps in Medicare coverage) *that includes drug benefits.* If you presently have such a Medigap policy, you can choose to keep it instead of changing to Medicare drug coverage, but if you later decide to change you would incur a late-enrollment penalty of 1 percent per month for each month of delay in signing up for Medicare Part D. (You can keep an ordinary Medigap policy plan, without drug benefits, but it cannot be used to fill in the gaps in the Medicare drug coverage.) However, other kinds of supplementary coverage—for example, retiree benefits from former employers— could be used to fill in these gaps. After January 1, 2006, no new Medigap policies will cover prescription drugs, but people who already have them will be allowed to continue them indefinitely.

In summary, if you have a Medigap plan that pays for prescription drug coverage you can (1) *keep your current Medigap plan* but drop its prescription drug coverage and sign up for a Part D plan; (2) *choose another Medigap* plan that does not cover drugs so that you can sign up for a Part D plan; or (3) keep your current Medigap plan *with prescription drug coverage.*

Medicaid Prescription Drug Coverage

If Medicaid was paying for your prescription drugs, after December 31, 2005, Medicaid no longer covered your drugs if a prescription drug plan covered the same drugs. Rather, your prescription drug benefits now come under Medicare Part D. If any elderly Medicaid recipient did not select a Part D plan by December 31, 2005, then Medicare chose a plan for that person. But the problem is that the program may not cover the drugs you take, and you will have to go back to your own doctor to get a prescription for a different drug or change your prescription drug plan to another Part D plan that does cover your drugs. If you decide to go into a new plan, you will have to fill out a new application and that will take time to get into a new plan.

Dual Eligibles for Medicare and Medicaid

If you are eligible for both Medicare and Medicaid, a "dual eligible," you will be transferred into the Medicare program, though you will have very low copayments and low costs or no premiums at all. Also, you will receive continuous treatment all year and avoid the $2,850 gap in the program in which others will have to pay the $2,850 costs out of their pockets. Depending upon your state, Medicaid may pay for other out-of-pocket costs such as drugs that Medicare does not cover. Dual eligibles must understand that Medicare will be their primary coverage and Medicaid or other assistance programs, like AIDS Dying Assistance Program (ADAPS), will be the secondary payer. If dual eligibles do not sign up for a plan and are assigned a plan by Medicare, then there is no guarantee that they will receive a plan that covers their drugs.

Supplementary Security Income and Other Public Assistance Programs

If you are receiving Supplementary Security Income (SSI), Medicare Part D will cover you as well. Supplementary Security Income is a monthly benefit paid by the Social Security Administration to people with limited income and resources who are disabled, blind, or age sixty-five or older. SSI benefits provide cash to meet basic needs like food, clothing, and shelter. SSI benefits are not the same as Social Security benefits. If an SSI recipient does not choose a Part D plan by May 15, 2006, then Medicare will choose a plan for that person. Those already enrolled in Medicaid or a Medicare Savings Program or who receive Supplementary Security Income automatically qualify for assistance (in most cases, no premium and deductible, or no payments for catastrophic drug coverage and reduced copayment for brand-name or generic drugs). If you do not have Medicaid, a Medicare Savings Plan, or SSI, but your income and assets are limited, you should apply for help through the Social Security Administration, using the agency's print or online application at http://www.ssa.gov. A Medicare Savings Program refers to a public benefit in which the state pays for out-of-pocket Medicare costs, such as premiums, deductibles, and copayments. The coverage varies according to income. There are special rules under Medicare Part D for members of this program. Three Medicare Savings Programs include Qualified Medicare Beneficiary (QMB), Specified Low-Income Medicare Beneficiary (SLMB), and Qualified Individual (QI-1). When you apply through the Social Security Administration, the amount of assistance for which you will qualify varies depending upon how your annual income compared to the federal poverty level and how many assets you own (not including your house or automobile). Many people in nursing homes will not pay anything for drugs. If you cannot obtain all the drugs you need or cannot afford to pay for them, Medicaid programs in some states will continue to supply drugs that a Medicare drug plan does not cover. Some state pharmacy-assistance programs will pay all or some out-of-pocket expenses. If you don't qualify for these previous programs, you may receive similar or better coverage from your pharmacy-assistance program. Otherwise, you can sign up for regular Medicare coverage.

More specifically, if you are single (which is defined as someone who is separated or your spouse's confinement in a nursing home is permanent) and you earned $14,355 a year or less with assets totaling no more than $11,500 or are married with an annual income as a couple of $19,245 or less with assets totaling no more than $23,000 in 2005, then you are probably eligible to get assistance for some of Medicare's Part D prescription drug costs. If your 2005 income for a single person was $12,919 or less with assets totaling no more than $7,500 or your annual income was $17,320 or less for a married couple with assets totaling no more than $12,000, then you qualified automatically for assistance. Income includes any money you receive from employment, Social Security, retirement benefits, alimony, rental properties, dividends, worker's compensation, and other sources. But income does not include cash or credit you received by taking out a reverse mortgage on your property where a lender pays the homeowner cash for equity in the home. The loan is repaid when the borrower sells the home, moves, or dies. Your assets are defined as resources like bank accounts, investments, life insurance policies, and extra real estate. Your assets do not include the value of your home, the property your home stands on, personal possessions, automobiles, cemetery plots, or some earned income. Higher incomes are permitted if you have dependent relatives living with you. If you think the total amount of your assets will be too high to qualify for these programs, the Social Security Administration does not prevent you from spending down your assets or giving away some savings to reduce them below the limit in order to qualify. When you apply, the only assets that matter are what you have. But spending down your assets may impact upon your eligibility for other programs (such as Medicaid), should you require them in the future. If you received an application for limited-income assistance, fill it out. If you didn't receive an application and you think you might qualify, go (or send someone) to apply at your local Social Security Administration office, which manages the limited-income benefit or at any one of the state health insurance assistance program (SHIP) offices. You can telephone 1-800-772-1213 or go online to http://www.socialsecurity.gov, or contact your local Medicaid office at http://cms.hhs.gov/Medicaid. Anyone is permitted to apply for you including a family member, friend, caregiver, legal representative, social worker, or SHIP counselor and can fill out a printed or online application and even sign on your behalf. In order to fill out an application, you will have to know your Social Security number and financial information. If you have insurance, you may have to ask your insurer how much money you would receive if you cashed in the policy at the present time. A married couple will be automatically signed up. If your application is not accepted, you still may qualify for additional assistance from your state. Some state programs have higher income limits or may not require assets. A SHIP counselor can advise you.

Organizational Assistance in Understanding Medicare Part D

If you need additional help in understanding the Medicare Part D prescription drug program, the Web site http://shiptalk.org lists the contact numbers of each State Health Insurance Assistance Program for individual counseling in regard to the Part D program. The Eldercare Locator (tel: 1-800-677-1116), a public service of the US Administration on Aging, can help you find information about the Medicare prescription drug program and assistance in your community at its Web site, http://www.eldercare.gov. The nonprofit Medicare Rights Center in New York City (tel: 1-212-869-3850), on its Web site, http://www.Medicarerights.org, has brochures and fact sheets, especially the work sheet titled "How to Compare Medicare Prescription Drug Plans," Two new organizations, Medicare Rx Education Network and Medicare Today—consortiums of professional groups, nonprofits, and healthcare providers—have also established Web sites to help people understand the Medicare Part D drug benefit. Visit them at http://www.medicarerxeducation.org and http://www.medicaretoday.org. Essentially, you are looking for a drug plan that covers the drugs you use at the lowest possible cost and at a pharmacy that is convenient to you. You can always sign up for another plan if your drug requirements change over time. Another effective way to compare drug plans is through the Drug Plan Finder tool on the official Medicare Web site at http://www.medicare.gov. (Click on "Compare Medicare Prescription Drug Plans" on the Web site's homepage and follow the instructions.) If you do not have computer access to the Internet, you can obtain the same details by calling Medicare's hot line at 1-800-633-4227 or the AARP at 1-888-687-2277 for community sources of help.

Prescription Drug Plan Scams

Finally, be alert to prescription drug plan scams. The federal government is not marketing Part D prescription drug plans over the telephone, so don't respond to anyone who says he or she is from Medicare and is trying to sell you something. Unless you are the one who initiated the telephone call to the plan, do not enroll in any plan over the telephone and don't let anyone force you to sign up. If you are not sure who is contacting you, telephone Medicare, at 1-800-633-4227, to confirm the name and telephone number of the plan that telephoned you. Depending upon your personal circumstances, you can enroll between November 15, 2006, and December 15, 2006, and perhaps you can sign up even after that date with or without incurring any penalties, depending upon the status of your drug coverage—that is, whether it is creditable or not creditable when compared to the standard Medicare prescription drug plan. Also, never pay anyone any money to sign up for a plan either, and if anyone informs you that the Medicare law requires that you enroll and that you will lose your Medicare coverage if you do not sign up, these statements are not true. Do not believe that person. These are voluntary drug insurance plans. It is still your choice as to whether you wish to enroll. Never give your Social Security or credit card number or Medicare identification number or bank account number to anyone who says he or she must have it in order to tell you about a plan. Only give your insurance/Medicare identification number to those who provided you with prescription drug or other medical services. If someone visits you at your home selling offers on prescription drug coverage, be suspicious of that salesperson and if you visit that salesperson at another location, try to have someone accompany you so he or she can hear the salesperson's speech. Do not pay for drug coverage on the Internet. While you can enroll in plans over the Internet, plans are not allowed to collect any payments over the Internet. Do not believe anyone who tells you that a plan offers free coverage because legitimate plans, with few exceptions, do require premiums, deductible, or copayments. Report potential scams to your state insurance department or to the State Health Insurance Assistance Program, http://www.shiptalk.org, or telephone the Medicare hot line at 1-800-633-4227 to locate your closest SHIP office where trained counselors can give you help free of charge.[30]

Private Companies versus Medicare

Also, beginning in 2010, traditional Medicare would face competition from private plans in six metropolitan areas in which at least two private plans enroll at least 25 percent of the Medicare beneficiaries. For those who remain in traditional Medicare, premiums increases would be capped at 5 percent a year and waived for low-income seniors. The competition would last six years. This experiment is known as "premium support." This experiment would abandon traditional Medicare that pays whatever it costs to provide a specific list of services to everyone who is eligible. Instead, Medicare enrollees would get a set sum to buy coverage each year, regardless of whether they stayed or left the traditional Medicare program. The sum, which could be higher or lower than the current Medicare premium, would vary depending upon region and insurer. In some instances, beneficiaries might have to use their own money if the private plan's premiums were higher than the sum they were given. In other cases, the premium might be lower, and the beneficiaries would receive rebates. The purpose of this experiment is to determine who does a better job covering Medicare enrollees, the government or private insurers. The theory behind this experiment is that private insurers would bid against each other for government work, leading to greater efficiencies, lower premiums, and better benefits to enrollees at a lower cost to the government, thereby ensuring, according to the theory, Medicare's survival. The critics say that the competition could destroy Medicare because the private insurers would insure only the youngest and healthiest beneficiaries while the sickest and costliest patients were funneled into Medicare where premiums would rise.

Drug Formularies

Finally, and it cannot be emphasized enough, when you are considering different Medicare Part D plans that offer drug benefits, they will be permitted to create formularies—lists of drugs a plan decides to cover. The new law states that each plan's formulary must include at least two drugs for each disease category. If a drug prescribed for you is not covered, your physician can request coverage because of medical necessity. If that is refused, you can appeal. If the appeal is denied, you would have to pay the full cost of that drug. One concern is that plans will be permitted to change the drugs on their formularies at any time during the year, whereas enrollees can change plans only once a year. Also, HMOs, in addition to providing generic drugs, will be required to cover brand-name drugs for Medicare recipients. Each HMO that decides to offer the drug benefit in 2006 must carry some, but not all, brand-name drugs in each disease category—and offer an appeal process for those who require access to drugs that are not in the formulary. Before joining an HMO or any other private Medicare option, you should inquire what brand-name and generic products are covered and what the copayment will be.

Summary of Basic Part D Prescription Drug Principles

When you are considering the many and diverse prescription drug plans that are seeking to enroll you, there are some basic principles that you must remember that are common to all plans and that can influence your decision. These include the following:

- *If you have been told by your employer, union, or insurance company that your present coverage of prescription drugs is "creditable,"* that is, is as good if not better than the standard Medicare national prescription drug plan, you can sign up for the Medicare plan at any time after May 16, 2005, without having to pay any premium penalty if you enroll within sixty-three days of leaving your former plan. Does you current employer plan to keep its current plan, purchase a Part D plan in its place, or help you financially to cover some of the gaps in your Part D plan? If you are a retiree, how does your former employer's decisions in regard to prescription drug coverage affect you? Also, does the plan provide coverage when traveling, if you need it?
- *What prescription drugs are you taking now?* Are these drugs included on the Part D plan's formulary (drug list)? If they are not listed, does your doctor think that those drugs on the list are equally effective in treating your medical condition? If not, does he think he can successfully appeal to the plan to place your drug on the plan's formulary? Which plan(s) offers the most affordable copayment prices for the drugs you are taking?
- *What pharmacies are participating in the plan's network?* Are there any such pharmacies in your community? Convenient to you or far away? Are the pharmacies in your community members of the Part D plan's network at lower drug costs or out of the plan's network at higher drug costs? How do you feel about having your prescriptions filled at a particular pharmacy?
- *What is the plan's monthly premium?* Average national premium in 2006 for

the Medicare Part D prescription drug program was estimated at $32 per month. How does your plan's premium compare? Remember, in addition you are also paying out of your monthly budget a monthly premium for Medicare itself, which was $88.50 in 2006, or, if enrolled, possibly a separate premium for Part C Medicare Advantage plans. If you keep a Medigap policy that has or does not have prescription drug coverage because you are not enrolled in Part C's Medicare Advantage managed care plans, you will also have to pay a monthly premium for that Medigap policy as well. So you can be paying three separate premiums: the original Medicare (Parts A and B) monthly premium, a Medigap monthly health insurance premium if you have such policy with or without prescription drug coverage, and a prescription Part D drug stand-alone plan insurance premium, or as an alternative a Part C Medicare Advantage plan premium if you join a managed care plan to receive your prescription drug coverage as well as the other health services it offers.

- *What is the plan's deductible?* Is it the same, lower, or higher than the $250 deductible in the Medicare standard prescription drug plan?
- *For the first $2,250 in yearly drug costs*, you pay 25 percent, or about $563 out of your own pocket.
- *For the next $2,850 in yearly drug costs*, you pay this amount totally out of your own pocket unless other public programs, your employer, or others help you out. In view of different coverage gaps in prescription drug plans—for example, some cover deductibles while others do not—which plan(s) can you afford?
- *After you reach the $5,100 level in drug bills on a yearly basis*, of which $3,600 came out of your own pocket, you continue to pay 5 percent of a drug's cost out of your own pocket while the federal government pays the rest at this catastrophic level.
- *If you are in a Medicare Advantage HMO that offers drug coverage and you also sign up for the Part D prescription drug plan, you will lose your HMO coverage and be placed in the traditional fee-for-service Medicare program.*
- *If you have a Medigap policy with prescription drug coverage* and you sign up for a Part D prescription drug plan, you will lose your drug coverage under Medigap. If you do not like the Part D plan that you joined and decide to return to traditional fee-for-service Medicare, you will not be able to get this Medigap prescription drug coverage back. Medigap policies with prescription drug coverage stopped being sold on January 1, 2006, so you could find yourself in traditional fee-for-service Medicare without drug coverage under these circumstances.
- *If you are on Medicaid or eligible for Medicare and Medicaid, SSI,* or other similar assistance programs, check with your state agencies, like public welfare, that are responsible for such programs to determine your income eligibility, extent of coverage, and other matters related to your buying prescription drugs.

These are some of the basic principles that you must consider when choosing a drug plan, whether it be part of an HMO's benefit structure as in Medicare Part C or a stand-alone prescription drug plan in Medicare Part D. The variations of these plans are many and diverse, and the economic and medical circumstances of each Medicare beneficiary are different. But these are the essential elements you should consider in trying to decide which plan is best for you.

When Other Insurance Pays before Medicare

Some people who have Medicare also have group health and other types of coverage that may make Medicare secondary payer on their health claims. Medicare is the secondary payer for individuals:

- Who are aged sixty-five or older and working with coverage under an employer health plan.
- Who are aged sixty-five or older and who are covered by a working spouse's employer group health plan.
- With coverage under automobile, no-fault, or liability insurance.
- With kidney failure, for up to the first eighteen months of Medicare entitlement, if they have coverage under their own employer group health plan (EGHP), or if the coverage is provided them because they are the spouse or dependent of an individual with group health plan coverage.
- Who are disabled and qualify as an "active individual," if they have coverage under their own large group health plan (LGHP), or who are disabled and have coverage under the LGHP of an employed family member.

If you fit into one of these categories, your medical and hospital bills are first submitted for payment to the other insurer. Medicare, as the secondary payer, might pay some or all of the charges for services that are not fully paid by the primary payer.

Medicare and Employer Health Plans

If you are age sixty-five or older, or have a spouse of any age who works, and your own or your spouse's employer has at least twenty employees, federal law requires that the employer's group health plan offer you the same health benefits under the same conditions as the plan offers younger workers and their spouses. Also, as already noted, an employer group health plan may not pay benefits that are secondary to Medicare for Medicare-covered items and services. This also applies if you or your spouse is self-employed and covered by a plan through association with a firm that has twenty or more employees. This description of employer health plan coverage does not apply to Medicare beneficiaries who have permanent kidney failure. Individuals under age sixty-five with permanent kidney failure who have

DECISIONS ON ENROLLING IN MEDICARE PART D PRESCRIPTION DRUG PROGRAM

ENROLLMENT QUESTIONS

Enrollment is voluntary

Are my brand-name and generic medicines on the plan's drug list? If not, can my doctor get them on? Or must I try plan's drugs first?

Should I join an HMO or a PPO with Rx drug coverage or not? I cannot join both Part D plan and HMO or PPO at the same time.

Should I keep my Medigap with Rx drug coverage or join a Part D plan and keep Medigap without Rx drug coverage?

My employer or union Is it keeping its current Rx plan? Is it buying a new Part D Rx plan? Is it dropping its Rx coverage? Will it help me with Part D financial gaps?

Is my pharmacy in the plan's network or not? If not, is plan's Pharmacy convenient to me? Can I use any mail-order services? Will there be any savings? On mail-order services? Between plan and nonplan pharmacy? How much for each drug I take?

Is my current plan "creditable"? If not, I pay a premium penalty with late enrollment.

COSTS QUESTIONS

What is my plan's premium? The Part D national average premium is $32 (in 2006).

Is there a deductible? Medicare's national standard plan is $250

Are there Rx drug copayments? How much? Coinsurance? Can I afford them?

Drugs purchased from foreign countries—not counted as out-of-pocket costs.

I personally pay $563 of the first $2,250 in yearly drug costs— Medicare pays the rest. Are there any public or private resources to help me cover my $563?

I personally pay the next $2,850 in yearly drug bills—Medicare pays nothing. Are there any public or private resources to help me pay the $2,850?

I personally pay 5% of yearly drug costs over $5,100—Medicare pays 95%. Are there any public or private resources to cover my 5% of the payments?

My yearly drug costs are—— How much am I willing to spend a year? Will Part D save me any money?

If I am in Medical Savings Plan, Medicaid, or SSI, I must pick my own plan or the government will pick a plan for me by May 15, 2006. This might include minimal cost sharing like low copayments, possibly no premiums and no deductibles, and other features.

employer group health plan coverage should obtain a copy of the Centers for Medicare and Medicaid Services (CMS) publication concerning *Medicare Coverage of Kidney Dialysis and Kidney Transplant Services.* If you have reason to believe that your employer's plan is not providing you with the same benefits extended to younger workers, or if you employer's plan is paying benefits secondary to Medicare, you should bring this to the attention of the insurance carrier that handles your Medicare claims.

If you are under age sixty-five and entitled to Medicare-based disability, and you or a member of your family works for an employer who has one hundred or more employees, federal law prohibits the employer's health plan from denying you coverage because you are disabled and have Medicare. Furthermore, the plan is not permitted to offer you coverage different from that offered nondisabled individuals or to offer you health insurance benefits that are secondary to Medicare for Medicare-covered items and services. If your employer's plan is denying you coverage, offering you different coverage, or paying benefits that are secondary to Medicare, notify the insurance carrier that handles your Medicare claims.

You may accept or reject the plan offered by your own or your spouse's employer. If you accept the employer plan, it will be your primary plan.

The following questions should clarify your circumstances in regard to employer health plans.

- *If I accept the employer plan, how does it affect my Medicare coverage?*

    If your employer plan does not pay all the charges, Medicare may pay secondary benefits for Medicare-covered services. That is, it can help pay some of the expenses not paid by the employer plan. If you are not already entitled to Medicare hospital insurance (Medicare Part A), you should apply for it. It can supplement your employer plan.

    Whether you wish to enroll in or keep Medicare medical insurance (Medicare Part B) will depend on how fully the employer plan covers the doctors' and other health services that Medicare medical insurance covers. You need to consider whether the secondary benefits Medicare medical insurance would pay are worth the cost to you.

- *Isn't there a penalty for signing up late for Medicare Medical Insurance (Part B)?*

    Not in all situations. If you are covered under an employer plan from the time you are first eligible for Medicare, special rules give you seven months to enroll in Medicare medical insurance beginning *when you stop working or drop the employer plan,* whichever happens first. However, if you expect work to stop or the employer plan coverage to end within the month you reach sixty-five or during any of the three following months, you should inquire immediately at your Social Security office if in doubt about enrolling in Medicare medical insurance.

    Therefore, although there is normally a penalty for those who sign up after age sixty-five for Part B, those who have been working and have had employer-sponsored insurance escape that penalty if the insurance is still in force when they enroll or has just ended, such as when someone over sixty-five retires and, thus, leaves the employer-sponsored plan and joins Medicare Part B. The imposition of a penalty is to discourage people from waiting to sign up for Part B coverage until they need such protection. The purpose is to have everyone contribute to the premiums so as to share the risk and keep the cost of the premium down. If only the sickest seniors enroll in Medicare Part B, the costs for Part B would be higher. As already noted, the penalty is waived for those who have employer-provided insurance, however, recognizing that they are saving Medicare money by getting most of their insurance protection outside of Medicare. (This is why such employer coverage is treated as "primary"—that is, the first in line to pay hospital and other bills.)[31]

- *What if I don't want the employer plan?*

If you don't accept your own or your spouse's employer plan, Medicare is your primary payer. This also applies to disabled individuals who do not accept their own or a family member's plan. But if you make that choice, the employer plan cannot pay supplemental benefits for Medicare-covered services. You must buy your own supplemental health insurance or "Medigap" plan, if you feel you need such additional protection.

Even if you don't accept your own or your spouse's employer plan and Medicare is your primary payer, your employer or your spouse's employer can offer health insurance protection for healthcare services that are not covered by Medicare (such as hearing aids or routine dental care).

- *What do I do about filing claims if I have employer plan coverage?*

Claims should be filed first with the employer's group health plan and then with Medicare. You should give the hospital, doctor, or any other supplier of covered services the necessary information about the employer plan (name, policy number, and other relevant information) and inform them that the employer plan should be billed first.

If, for any reason, your doctor or supplier does not submit claims to the employer plan, send your own personal claim first to the employer plan or ask your personnel office to help you. If the employer plan does not pay in full for services Medicare covers, enclose a copy of the employer plan explanation of benefits with your claim to Medicare for secondary benefits.

If you have questions or need additional advice about Medicare eligibility or benefits, contact your nearest Social Security office or the Medicare insurance carrier that handles your Medicare claims. (If you are entitled to Medicare under the Railroad Retirement system, contact your nearest Railroad Retirement Board district office.) For information on your private group plan coverage, consult your employer or your spouse's employer.[32]

Advance Directives

All adults in hospitals, skilled nursing homes, and other healthcares settings have certain rights such as the right to confidentiality of their personal and medical records and to know what treatment they will receive.

But you also have another right. You have the right to prepare a document called an "advance directive." In one type of advance directive, you state in advance what kinds of treatment you wish or do not want if you ever become mentally or physically unable to choose or communicate your wishes. In a second type, you authorize another person to make those decisions for you if you become incapacitated. Federal law requires that hospitals, skilled nursing facilities, hospices, home health agencies, and health maintenance organizations (HMOs) serving persons covered either by Medicare or Medicaid give you information about advance directives and explain your legal choices in making decisions about medical care.

The law is intended to give you greater control over medical treatment decisions. However, remember that state laws governing advance directives differ. The healthcare provider is required to give you information about the laws concerning advance directives for the state in which the provider is located. If you reside in another state, you may wish to gather information about your state laws from another source such as the office of the state attorney general.

An advance directive can be a living will or a durable power of attorney for healthcare; either document allows you to give directions about your future medical care. It is your right to accept or refuse medical care. Advance directives protect this right if you ever become mentally or physically unable to choose or communicate your wishes owing to an accident or illness such as having irreversible brain damage, being in a permanent coma, or having a terminal illness that may lead to brain damage and loss of consciousness.

Advance directives can help you, your family, and your physician. They protect your right to make medical choices that can affect your life; help your family avoid the responsibility and stress of making difficult decisions; and assist your physician by providing guidelines for your care.

Advance directives can limit life-prolonging measures when there is little or no chance of recovery by making your wishes known about cardiopulmonary resuscitation, intravenous therapy, feeding tubes, respirators, dialysis, and pain relief. Advance directives can even state your wishes regarding donating specific organs or your entire body.

A Living Will

As already noted, there are two kinds of advance directives. One is a *living will*, which is written instructions that explain your wishes and become effective while you are still alive as a patient. It is called a living will because it takes effect while you are still living. Most states have their own living will forms, each somewhat different. It may also be possible to complete and sign a preprinted living will form available in your own community, draw up your own form, or simply write a statement of your own preferences for treatment. You may also wish to speak to an attorney or your physician to be certain you have completed the living will in such a way that your wishes will be understood and followed.

A Durable Power of Attorney

The other kind of advance directive is a *durable power of attorney*, which is a document signed, dated, and witnessed that allows you to name a person (called a proxy) to make decisions for you if you become unable to do so. Such a proxy may be a husband, a wife, a daughter, a son, or a close friend. You can specify if your proxy is allowed to make decisions about healthcare, legal matters, or finances. You can also include instructions about any treatment you want to avoid. Even if your state does not currently recognize living wills, you may want to use one in addition to a durable power of attorney. This combination may express your wishes as completely and specifically as possible. Your state may have special forms for you to use.

Preparing Advance Directives

To create advance directives, check the laws in your state regarding living wills and durable powers of attorney. Put your wishes in writing and be as specific as possible. Sign and date your advance directives and have them witnessed and notarized, if necessary, in your state. Keep a card in your wallet stating that you have advanced directives (and where to find them). Give a copy to your physician to be kept as part of your medical records. Discuss your advance directives with your family and friends. Give copies to a relative or a friend who is likely to be notified in an emergency. Finally, review your advance directives regularly and make changes as necessary, informing your physician, family, and proxy of any changes. If you use a durable power of attorney, be sure to give a copy to your proxy. Remember, you can always change or cancel your advance directives. Any change or cancellation should be written, signed, and dated in accordance with state law, and copies should be given to your doctor or others to whom you have given copies of the original. In some cases, you may even cancel them orally. Also, remember you do not have to prepare an advance directive if you do not want one.

If you wish to cancel an advance directive while you are in the hospital, you should notify your doctor, your family, and others who may need to know. Even without a change in writing, your wishes stated in person directly to your doctor generally carry more weight than a living will or durable power of attorney, as long as you can decide for yourself and can communicate your wishes. But be sure to state your wishes clearly and that they are understood.

If you require assistance in preparing advance directives, or if you would like more information about them, you may contact a lawyer, hospitals, hospices, long-term care facilities, or your state attorney general's office. Having an advance directive may make your medical treatment easier for you, your family, and your physician.[33]

Using Medicare to Reduce Medical Costs

Medicare has proven to be an invaluable public program. It has enabled many millions of elderly to obtain quality medical care at a time in their life when their medical expenses may be at their highest while their income may be at their lowest. Yet, there are ways to use Medicare to reduce your personal medical expenses even more. According to one authority:

- If your physician does not accept a Medicare assignment, consider switching to another doctor who does. Your medical bills are likely to be lower.
- Always make certain that doctors, other healthcare professionals and organizations, and the services they provide have been approved for Medicare payments.
- Do not use your Medicare reserve days if you have private health insurance that will pay for a hospital stay longer than ninety days. Remember, once you use a reserved day you never get it back during your lifetime. Also, Medicare only gives you sixty reserve days in total. You will automatically begin using reserve days after ninety days in a hospital unless you tell the hospital in writing beforehand that you do not wish to use them.
- Do not reject the voluntary medical insurance program (Part B) of Medicare because you have to pay the premium. The premium is a unique and valuable bargain. The premium only pays a fraction of the cost; the rest comes from federal funds, which come from your income taxes.[34]

Remember, Medicare was created to help pay your medical bills and to lessen for you the burden of high medical costs. Knowing what Medicare covers and does not cover, supplementing these gaps with proper private health insurance benefits, and using Medicare program to save further expenses will do much to make your "golden years" a time free from the anxiety of high medical costs.

NOTES

1. *A Commission Report: Intergovernmental Problems in Medicaid* (Washington, DC: Advisory Commission on Intergovernmental Relations, September 1968), pp. 3–4.

2. US Department of Health and Human Services, *Brief Summaries of Medicare and Medicaid* (Washington, DC: Healthcare Financing Administration, June 30, 1993), pp. 21–22.

3. "Clinton Signs Welfare Reform amid Turmoil," *Washington Post*, August 23, 1996, p. A17.

4. "What Medicare Will (and Won't) Do for You," *Changing Times* 33, no. 1 (January 1979): 40.

5. "For Some, Buying into Medicare Is a Bargain," *New Haven Register*, April 28, 1993, p. 11.

6. "What Medicare Will (and Won't) Do for You," p. 40.

7. US Department of Health, Education, and Welfare, *Your Medicare Handbook* (Washington, DC: Social Security Administration, February 1978), p. 13.

8. Ibid.

9. "What Medicare Will (and Won't) Do for You," p. 41.

10. US Department of Health and Human Services, *Your Medicare Handbook, 1996* (Washington, DC: Healthcare Financing Administration, April 1996), p. 10.

11. Ibid.

12. Ibid.

13. Jane Bryant Quinn, "U.S. Begins to Clamp Down on Medicare Overcharges," *Washington Post*, December 20, 1992, p. H3.

14. US Department of Health and Human Services, *Your Medicare Handbook, 1996*, p. 14; US Department of Health, Education, and Welfare, *Your Medicare Handbook*, pp. 9–11; US Department of Health and Human Services, *Medicare and You, 2005* (Washington, DC: Center for Medicare and Medicaid Services, September 2004), pp. 25–33; David Glendinning, "CMS Finalizes 1.5% Increase, Adds New Patient Benefits," *American Medical News*, November 22/29, 2004; and Isadore Rosenfeld, "Medicare Good News for 2005," *Parade*, January 2, 2005, p. 10.

15. US Department of Health, Education, and Welfare, *Your Medicare Handbook*, p. 10.

16. Alice Loeb Green, "Your Legal Advisor," in *Age in Action* (Charleston: West Virginia Commission on Aging, January–February 1979), p. 6.

17. Ibid.

18. Albert B. Crenshaw, "'Medigap' Insurance Laws Revised," *Washington Post*, November 4, 1990, p. H9.

19. Albert E Crenshaw, "Changes in 'Medigap' Law Revive Duplicate Coverage," *Washington Post*, February 5, 1995, p. H1.

20. Jean Dietz, "Selecting Medigap Insurance," *Boston Globe*, October 2, 1986, p. 75.

21. Peter J. Ognibene, "Don't Get Caught in the Medicare Trap," *Fifty Plus* 19, no. 4 (April 1979): 21–22; *Health and Accident Insurance for Older Adults: Do You Know What You're Getting?* (Charleston: West Virginia Commission on Aging, May 1978), pp. 7–13.

22. "Buyer Beware," *Secure Retirement*, May/June 1996, p. 8.

23. Beverly Fisher and Adinah Robertson, "Preparing a Guide for Senior Citizens in the Health Insurance Maze," *Clearinghouse Review* 18 (June 1985): 119.

24. US Department of Health and Human Services, *Your Medicare Handbook, 1996*, pp. 17–18.

25. US Department of Health and Human Services, *Your Medicare Handbook, 2005* (Washington, DC: Centers for Medicare and Medicaid, September 2004), p. 46.

26. US Department of Health and Human Services, *Medicare and Your Physician's Bill* (Washington, DC: Healthcare Financing Administration, 1992), pp. 4–5, 7; Ognibene, "Don't Get Caught in the Medicare Trap," p. 42.

27. US Department of Health and Human Services, *Your Medicare Handbook, 1996*, pp. 19–20.

28. *Medicare Health Maintenance Organizations: Your Rights, Risks, and Obligations* (Washington, DC: National Committee to Preserve Social Security and Medicare, 1996).

29. Spencer Rich, "Medicare Warns HMOs Not to 'Gag' Doctors," *Washington Post*, December 7, 1996, p. A8.

30. "On Your Mark . . . Get Set . . . ," *AARP Bulletin* (September 2005): 18–20; Karen Westberg Reyes, "Medicare Medicine: The Basics," *AARP Bulletin* (November–December 2005): 35, 36; Barbara Ruben, "Drug Plans Will Be Free or Low Cost for Some," *Washington Senior Beacon* (October 2005): 38; Elaine Povich, "You Make the Call," *AARP Bulletin* (October 2005): 31; Patricia Barry, "Medicare Drug Coverage: The Basics," *AARP Bulletin* (November 2005): 19–26; and US Department of Health and Human Services, *Medicare and You, 2006* (Washington, DC: Centers for Medicare and Medicaid Services, September 2005), pp. 1–3, 39–54, 88–89.

31. Marilyn Moon, "Your Health Coverage," *Washington Post/Health*, October 31, 1995, p. 27.

32. US Department of Health and Human Services, *Medicare and Employer Health Plans* (Washington, DC: Healthcare Financing Administration, 1989); US Department of Health and Human Services, *1990 Medicare Program Highlights* (Washington, DC: Healthcare Financing Administration, 1990).

33. US Department of Health and Human Services, *Medicare and Advanced Directives* (Washington, DC: Healthcare Financing Administration, 1992).

34. Ognibene, "Don't Get Caught in the Medicare Trap," p. 40.

CHAPTER SIX

SURGERY AND SECOND OPINION SURGICAL PROGRAMS

INTRODUCTION

Surgery is a serious medical procedure. Whether the operation is major or minimally invasive, no surgery is risk free. Since at least the 1970s, there has been a national debate about how many operations in the United States have been performed unnecessarily. The US Congress, the US Department of Health and Human Services, academia, as well as other groups have been studying this issue. These studies have raised questions as to whether every hysterectomy, tonsillectomy, lower-back-pain procedure, cesarean section, and other operations were and are really necessary. The number of surgical deaths that have been projected nationally from operations that these studies have defined as being unnecessary has raised alarms. For example, in 1976 the US House of Representatives Subcommittee on Interstate and Foreign Commerce released a report titled "Cost and Quality of Healthcare: Unnecessary Surgery," which alleged that during 1974 about 2.38 million unnecessary operations were performed in the United States, resulting in 11,900 deaths and expenditures of $3.92 billion.[1] The American Medical Association (AMA) disagreed with the subcommittee's findings and the procedures, data, and definitions used, claiming that data from limited regional studies had been extrapolated to include all surgical procedures performed in the United States. Similarly, the American Medical Association in 1978 disagreed with the findings of another congressional study. In that year, the same subcommittee issued a report titled "Surgical Performance: Necessity and Quality," which stated that during 1977 unnecessary surgery took more than 10,000 lives and cost the American public more than $4 billion. Of the nearly twenty-one million operations performed in the United States in 1977, sixteen million were elective nonemergency procedures, while about two million were estimated to have been unnecessary.[2] In regard to both studies, the American Medical Association stated that unnecessary surgery cannot be defined, while for purposes of its own study the House subcommittee defined unnecessary surgery as cases where other appropriate medical treatment was not tried first. According to the subcommittee report, many tonsillectomies performed during 1977 were not needed and could have been avoided with little hazard to the child, while many hysterectomies done for reasons of birth or cancer prevention are inappropriate and should not be performed.[3] Then, in 1985, the US Senate Special Committee on Aging reported that tens of thousands of Medicare patients received unnecessary cataract, gallbladder, prostate, back, hernia, or other surgeries.[4] By the 1990s, the US Agency for Health Care Policy and Research (AHCPR), now renamed the Agency for Healthcare Research and Quality (AHRQ), was again warning that not all surgical procedures like cataract operations and surgeries for lower-back pain may be necessary, while other studies questioned whether surgeries such as cesarean sections, gum surgery, surgery for sleep apnea, and radical mastectomies for cancer were being overused. A background statement to an advisory opinion, dated February 2003, of the code of ethics of the American Academy of Ophthalmology on unnecessary surgery and related procedures noted that unnecessary surgery is that "which is clearly unjustifiable when the risks and costs exceed the likely therapeutic benefits to the patient based on the patient's lifestyle requirements. No one factor alone can determine whether a particular surgery is unnecessary; instead the patient's quality of life must be taken into account. Unnecessary surgery is not an isolated clinically observable phenomenon. A cataract operation on an 85-year-old man who reports that he sees just fine for his needs might be unnecessary, while a similar cataract in a 55-year-old bus school bus driver might require surgery. . . . For ethical purposes the term 'unnecessary surgery' should be applied only where (1) in an individual case there is a decision to perform surgery that is beyond the range of reasonable judgment in light of the patient's needs and is substantially inconsistent with accepted professional standards for determining the need for surgery, or (2) there is a pattern or general practice of performing surgery in what would generally be considered marginally justifiable cases." [5] By 2005 the US Agency for Healthcare Research and Quality still had not developed a standardized definition for the concept of unnecessary surgery.[6] Thus, unnecessary surgery continues to be a problematical issue as it had been in decades past. The reason for the lack of a standardized definition for unnecessary surgery is that medicine is still an art as well as a science and the decision to perform surgery oftentimes may be gray rather than clearly black or white. For example, Dr. Elizabeth Morgan, a plastic surgeon and the author of *The Complete Book of Plastic Surgery: A Candid Guide for Men, Women and Teens* raises the following thought-provoking questions in regard to this issue: "Is surgery unnecessary," Dr. Morgan asks,

- if there are differences of opinion as to whether the surgery should be performed?
- if there are differences of opinion as to what surgery should be done?
- if there are differences of opinion as to whether medical or surgical care is best?
- if surgery is effective but has a high complication rate?

- if surgery is safe and effective but too costly to be affordable?
- if the surgery has been largely outdated and is rarely necessary?
- if the surgery has been replaced for most patients, but not all, by medical care or minor radiological interventions?
- if the original surgery has evolved into a less invasive operation?
- if the surgery is known to have some excellent results but a high failure rate?
- if the surgery is contraindicated for specific group of patients but not for most?
- if the surgeon and hospital overcharge for the surgery?[7]

These previous situations are not as clear in determining whether surgery is unnecessary as when surgery is outdated and never necessary or when there is no medical indication for the surgery but it is performed for the surgeon's benefit.

Medicine as a science is continually evolving. The necessity for performing surgery on a medical condition in the past may have been replaced by nonsurgical, medical treatment or by radiological intervention in the present. A good illustration of such medical progress is the Cooperative Studies Program of the US Veterans Administration. This program has found the following:

- Which medical treatment for enlarged prostate works best so that men no longer have to undergo surgery with all its inherent risks and side effects (*New England Journal of Medicine*, August 22, 1996, included a critical evaluation of medications for the treatment of symptomatic, benign prostatic hyperplasia [BPH]).
- Patients treated with chemotherapy and radiation rather than with surgery for advanced throat cancer can keep their voice boxes (*New England Journal of Medicine*, June 13,1991, included a comparison of nonsurgical treatment versus surgery for the disease). Watchful waiting can be an acceptable alternative to surgery for patients with moderately benign prostate enlargement (*New England Journal of Medicine*, January 12, 1995).
- Heart drugs worked for most veterans in stopping chest pain, in studying whether giving coronary bypass surgery right away was better than giving heart drugs to patients who have chest pains because of blockage in their arteries. Only a small number of people with blocked arteries did better with surgery. Thus, although surgery does help a small number of patients who have very bad hearts, most do not need surgery right away and can be given drugs to stop their chest pain.[8]

Because yesterday's acceptable surgical treatment for a medical condition may have been replaced with noninvasive medical or radiological interventions today, it is important that you, as a patient, be aware of this medical progress and ask your physician if there are noninvasive medical treatments available for your condition rather than surgery. For example, the US Agency for Healthcare Research and Quality, the American Medical Association, and America's Health Insurance Plans have established a National Guideline Clearinghouse on the Internet. This National Guideline Clearinghouse makes clinical practice guidelines available to the public in regard to the medical treatment of various diseases. Its Web address is http://www .guideline.gov. On March 15, 2005, the *British Medical Journal* (*BMJ*) launched a new guide for patients that sets out the best treatment for sixty of the most common medical conditions. Devised by the *British Medical Journal*, it is based on evidence from thousands of research studies and is being made available through the British National Health Service (NHS) Direct Web site; the advice service for patients is at http://www.besttreatments.co.uk. In some cases, the guide says it cannot recommend any treatment because of a lack of good evidence that anything works. While the information at this site is available only within the United Kingdom, if you are in the United States, BestTreatments information is available to members of http://www .MyUHC.com (United HealthCare) and is offered by subscription as part of http:// www.ConsumerReportsHealth.org. In addition, the American College of Surgeons, at http://www.facs.org, also provides publications on various issues related to surgery.

Unless a surgery is specifically lifesaving, many doctors now tend to address a medical condition with medication. They follow an injury with watchful waiting or operate with as little invasiveness as possible. "You always have to define the degree of a disease and what you mean by 'unnecessary,'" according to Ismael Nuno, director of cardiac surgery at Los Angles County–USC Medical Center. "If a patient has coronary heart disease amenable to medical therapy or balloon therapy, we'll try that. If not, the illness must be corrected surgically."[9]

Oftentimes, the demand for surgery that studies may consider unnecessary or overdone not only arises from a patient's personal desires but also from the manner in which local specialists practice, which might not always be in the patient's best interests. From the patient's perspective, some women prefer cesarean sections rather than going through the painful labor of childbirth. From the physician's viewpoint, a cardiac surgeon might recommend bypass surgery for blocked coronary arteries rather than less invasive angioplasty, defined by the Cleveland Clinic as an invasive procedure during which a specially designed balloon catheter with a small balloon tip is guided to the point of narrowing in the artery. Once in place, according to definition, the balloon is inflated to compress the fatty matter into the artery wall and stretch the artery open to increase blood flow to the heart.[10] It should be noted that some angioplasty procedures also use a stent to help keep the artery open. But, it should be noted, many health insurance programs no longer will authorize the most overdone procedures without compelling clinical reasons, second opinions, or a regimen of nonsurgical treatment, initially. But Dr. Nuno, who is also president of the American Heart Association, Western States Affiliate, warns that "cheaper" and "noninvasive" procedures are not always better. According to Dr. Nuno, "consumers must understand that nothing is free. You can go for a lesser procedure and still wind up dead because of complications. Or you can have surgery and go home safe and sound."[11]

In view of the alleged performance of unnecessary surgical procedures, many questions arise for the patient-consumer. How can I make sure I need surgery? How can I get a second opinion? A "second opinion" is when another doctor gives her or his views about what you have and how it should be treated. Will I offend my physician if I tell him that I want another opinion? How do I look for a medical specialist who will give me another surgical opinion and how will I pay for it when I receive it? When should I ask for a second surgical opinion? What are the advantages of receiving it?[12]

The doctor's words were direct. "Ever have surgery before?" The patient was silent, trying to comprehend what was happening to him. "The problem," said the doctor, "is when your chronic condition becomes active, it scars the tissue of your organ that has now made contact with another. When the organ becomes scarred, the tissue becomes like glue and sticks to another organ. In medicine it is called 'two organs in communication with each other' when they should not be. In your case, the contact has created an opening, a fistula, between both organs. Material, which is flowing between the two, should not be contaminating the second organ as is presently taking place. The only way to resolve the problem is by surgically separating both organs and putting a collar of fat around one so they can never again make contact."

"Is there any guarantee that the collar of fat will always keep them separated?" asked the patient?

"Unfortunately, no," replied the doctor. "Right now only an operation can alleviate your current problem."

"But my other doctor told me that medication can help close the opening between the two organs."

"In nine out of ten cases medication does not work."

"I would like to try."

In his case, the medication did work.

Surgery is a serious business. No one wants to have an operation unless there is no other satisfactory way to handle a medical problem. But as a science, medicine is not exact. Doctors do not always agree on the correct medical treatment to follow. That does not mean that they are incompetent or that they are not concerned about doing what is best. It only means that there can be differences of opinion about the best way to treat a patient. Most doctors approve of patients getting a second opinion and will help you obtain it. Physicians have scientific instruments available today that will help them guide you in your eventual decision to have or not have surgery. One of these instruments is a PET (positron emission tomography) scan. PET scans work by using glucose (a form of sugar) that contains a radioactive atom. The substance emits tiny atomic particles called positrons. Unlike most imaging tests, which give views of the shape and size of internal structures only, PET scanning provides information about their metabolic activity. A special camera records the precise location of the positrons as they leave the body. PET scanning is becoming widely used to determine the spread of cancers of the breast, colon, rectum, and ovaries in addition to lung cancer. Another instrument available to physicians is the computed axial tomography (CAT) scanner, which combines a computer with an x-ray machine to give a three-dimensional view of the human body and often precludes the necessity for exploratory surgery. Third, another instrument is the magnetic resonance imaging (MRI) scanner, which also takes three-dimensional, cross-sectional pictures of the body, but it does not emit radiation. Instead, it obtains its images by means of radio waves and magnetic fields. The MRI has virtually replaced myelograms for the diagnosis of spinal-disk problems and gives more precise and complete pictures of the brain for diagnosing tumors and other neurological problems. It is also used in other parts of the body, including the pelvis, neck, knee, and for certain conditions. A myelogram is an x-ray examination performed by a radiologist to enable your doctor to detect abnormalities of the spine, spinal cord, or surrounding structure. The myelogram examination helps your doctor in making a diagnosis. The radiologist interprets the information from the procedure and reports it to your doctor, who, in turn, will discuss the report with you. Essentially, a small amount of radiographic contrast, a dye that can be seen on an x-ray, is injected into the sack that contains the nerve roots in the spinal canal. This allows the radiologist to take a series of x-rays on which the nerve roots are outlined. In this manner, any abnormalities within the spinal canal can potentially be visualized to aid in the diagnosis of certain spinal problems.

Physicians regularly seek second opinions when they are facing surgery. If you are open and honest with your physician, he/she will be open and honest with you. When you have received the opinions of two doctors, you should have enough information to decide whether you want surgery. Remember, it is still your decision. You are entitled to have your family physician and surgeon explain all the possible alternatives to surgery as well as all the complications that might result from an operation. In fact, a physician who fails to inform you about the risks of surgery may find himself subject to a possible malpractice suit. Under the legal doctrine of informed consent, a patient who has not been fairly advised about the risks of surgery has not legally consented to it. Therefore, the patient may sue for malpractice any physician who operates on him without fairly disclosing the risks. Consequently, as a patient-consumer you should become aware of the conditions under which you should seek a second surgical opinion.

WHEN TO SEEK A SECOND SURGICAL OPINION

Surgical operations are performed under a variety of conditions. Sometimes surgery must be performed on an emergency basis—as in the case of acute appendicitis—or surgery may be chosen or sought on an elective basis. *Most second opinion programs define elective procedures as those that are deferrable*—meaning, presumably, that the patient won't suffer serious consequences if the operation is postponed or not done at all. As already noted, examples of elective surgery include tonsillectomies and hysterectomies. The Medicare program also distinguishes between elective and emergency surgery. For *Medicare purposes, elective surgery is defined* as surgery that can be scheduled in advance, is not an emergency, and, if delayed, will not result in death or permanent impairment to the health of the patient. To be considered as an emergency, the conditions for which the surgery is needed must meet the definition of emergency medical conditions as specified in Section 1903 (v)(3) of the Social Security Act. This section of the act defines *emergency medical condition* as "a medical condition . . . manifesting itself by acute symptoms of sufficient severity (including severe pain) such that the absence of immediate medical attention could reasonably be expected to result in: (A) placing the patient's health in serious jeopardy, (B) serious impairment to bodily functions, or (C) serious dysfunction of any body organ or part."[13] Again, even the choice of the word "elective" can lead to different interpretations of its meaning. According to Dr. Elizabeth Morgan, a plastic surgeon, "elective surgery can mean surgery scheduled on a regular working day rather than done as an emergency. Or elective surgery can mean surgery done to improve physical difficulties, such as a hip replacement, as opposed to surgery done to improve psychological difficulties, such as breast enlargement. Elective surgery can mean there are various good options, medical or surgical or both, to choose from. Finally, elective surgery is commonly used by an insurance company to mean it refuses to pay." In questioning its usage by most second opinion surgical programs, Dr. Morgan raises the following issues: "To define 'elective surgery' as an operation that if not done leaves the patient without 'serious consequences,' requires a definition of who decides that there aren't any and what 'serious consequences' are: does it mean longevity, physical function, psychological function, physical form, freedom from pain or earning power, all these or something more?" Whichever definition you use, whenever nonemergency surgery is recommended, you should, if possible, obtain a second opinion.[14] Although surgery may be necessary, there is always the possibility that alternative treatments exist for your illness. According to Dr. George C. Crile, emeritus consultant in surgery at the Cleveland Clinic and an internationally recognized authority in the treatment of breast cancer and thyroid disease, there are three types of inappropriate operations a patient should know about. These are:

- operations in which surgery is not a proper treatment for the disease. This may be because there is no disease (as in the case of most tonsillectomies) or because the disease could be better controlled by no treatment or by medical intervention.
- operations not suited for the individual because of his or her age or physical health or both.
- rare or dangerous operations that may be inappropriate because the surgeon is not trained to perform the operation expertly.[15]

Consequently, when nonemergency surgery is recommended and you do not know what alternative treatments are available, look for a medical specialist and seek a second opinion. Dr. William A. Nolen, the distinguished surgeon-author, has listed some of the times when you should get a second opinion. These include:

- If a physician should ever tell you that you have an illness that is inevitably terminal. You lose nothing by seeking another opinion. Ask your own physician to recommend someone else, preferably a doctor who has spent much of his career treating or researching this particular ailment or related diseases.
- If you are informed that you have some rare disease, one that you never heard of. You will probably be more willing to accept this diagnosis if another physician confirms it. In such a circumstance, your physician will probably advise that you see another doctor so that this opinion may be confirmed—or disputed, if that should prove to be the situation.
- If, after two or three months of treatment, your symptoms have neither lessened nor disappeared. In such a case, you may wish to obtain another doctor's opinion as to whether you are receiving the correct diagnosis and treatment. If your physician initially explained to you that you will require several months of treatment, then make sure you are not being impatient. But if you honestly think that you are not making sufficient progress, Dr. Nolen advises that you seek a second opinion.
- If you truly believe that your doctor is neglecting you, either ask for a second opinion about your condition or find another doctor. A dissatisfied patient makes for an unhappy doctor-patient relationship, and neither party wants this kind of situation.
- If you have gone directly to a surgeon about your problem. As a general rule, Dr. Nolen suggests that it is best to go to a surgeon only when you are referred by primary care physicians—a family practitioner, an internist, or, in the case of children, a pediatrician. If you have gone to a surgeon directly, in all probability he will ask a primary care physician to talk to and examine you before surgery. If he does not, Dr. Nolen suggests that you find a primary care physician yourself. Your medical doctor may be aware of physical conditions your surgeon overlooked and should know and approve of the operation you are to have and, usually, should participate in the pre- and postoperative management of your case.
- If you have doubts about your surgeon's competence and judgment. Never let a surgeon operate on you if you do not believe in his ability. Do not be fearful to seek a second opinion because you think you may offend the surgeon. Most surgeons will prefer not to operate on a patient who lacks faith in them; under such circumstances, with few exceptions, surgeons will be happy to refer you to someone else. Dr. Nolen believes that if your surgeon is the kind who is so insecure that he resents a request for a second opinion, then you ought to have another doctor anyway.
- If your surgeon has not persuasively explained to you the need for the operation—provided, of course, you have asked him to do so. There are many operations in which the benefit to be gained by surgery is not always obvious. Such examples would include tonsillectomies and adenoidectomies, as already noted. Dr. Nolen warns, however, that doctors can honestly differ

with each other about the benefit to be gained from an operation. Medicine and surgery are not exact sciences.

- If, in your opinion, your doctor does not discuss all the alternatives open to you—not only medical treatments as opposed to surgical but also the various types of surgical treatments available.
- If your doctor thinks a second opinion is advisable. There are times when a doctor is faced with a difficult diagnostic case and will either advise his patient to seek a second opinion or, if the patient wishes, call in another surgeon whose opinion he respects as a consultant.[16]

Dr. Nolen estimates that most of the time the family physician, the patient, and the surgeon, if surgery seems indicated, can reach a satisfactory decision regarding the best treatment. But in those cases where you, the patient, are not satisfied with one doctor's or one surgeon's opinion, then you are advised to seek another. The ultimate decision is yours.

HOW TO FIND A MEDICAL SPECIALIST

There are several ways to find a specialist in order to obtain a second surgical opinion. You can ask your physician to refer you to another doctor who is a specialist. The most common mistake people make is to stop consulting their personal physicians. Perhaps they want to save money, or perhaps they think their family doctors are not experts on surgery. Whatever the reason may be, they are neglecting to use their most helpful resource. Your own doctor can do many things for you, such as:

- find the right surgeon for your problem and personality
- prepare you for the consultation
- verify that the surgeon practices at a good hospital
- recommend surgeons for second and third opinions
- help you sort out conflicting opinions
- evaluate what the surgery will accomplish
- determine whether you have other medical problems that would interfere with the success of the surgery
- offer continuing care should your surgery cause postoperative medical problems[17]

Depending upon the nature of the services required, you may also contact a local medical, dental, osteopathic, or podiatric society in your area for the names of surgeons who specialize in the field in which your illness or injury falls. Also find out from these societies or your state health department whether your state has established a Web site detailing a physician's profile such as a physician's education, any legal action taken against the physician, and other data. For example, the governor of New York signed into law the New York Patient Health Information and Quality

Improvement Act of 2000 to make it possible for all citizens of New York State to obtain information about physicians. To seek such information on the Internet, New York residents can click on http://www.nydoctorprofile.com. Find out if your state has a similar program or Web site. Your state medical society or the state agency that licenses physicians may be able to help you in this regard or, perhaps, be able to direct you to a group who may know.

If you are eligible for Medicaid, you can contact your local welfare office. If you are covered by Medicare, you can call your local Social Security office, listed in your telephone directory under US Government, Department of Health and Human Services.

You can also locate a specialist by calling, toll free, 1-800-633-4227 or TTY 1-877-486-2048 (for the hearing impaired). These telephone numbers were established by the US Department of Health and Human Services. These hotlines will direct patients to local referral centers and operate twenty-four hours a day, seven days a week. Each state has at least one referral center.

Referral Centers

- Employees at referral centers will be knowledgeable and conversant with medical terminology and specialties and ready to assist patients who are not certain about the type of physicians they need.
- Patients' confidentiality will be protected.
- Referral centers will encourage the patient to request that the first physician transfer pertinent medical records and information to the consulting physician. This is especially important when such records include the results of timely, expensive, or high-risk laboratory tests; if patients were not aware that medical records could be transferred, they might not seek a second opinion because they might not want to repeat costly or uncomfortable tests. However, referral centers will not insist that patients request the transfer of their records since some patients do not want to tell their doctors that they are seeking a second opinion. If patients do elect to have records transferred, they will have to sign a legal release allowing their physicians to do so since the doctor-patient relationship is legally confidential.
- Patients will be informed, where possible, which physicians accept Medicare and Medicaid payments for their consulting services.
- Referral centers will not make appointments for patients.[18]

Any of the aforementioned sources will give you the name of the organization nearest you, which has the names of medical specialists from whom you can obtain a second surgical opinion. To maintain impartiality, no specialist giving a second opinion in this government-sponsored program is permitted to perform the recommended surgery, and you as a patient are under no obligation to follow the opinions offered.

QUALIFICATIONS OF SURGEONS

In selecting a surgeon, as a consumer-patient you can take several steps to assure yourself that the physician has the medical skills and qualifications you are seeking to the extent that it is possible to make such determinations. First, find out whether the surgeon is board certified in his specialty. The physician receives certification after he/she takes a vigorous oral, written, and clinical examination. You can find out whether your physician is board certified by asking your local county medical society or by using the *Directory of Medical Specialists* that is available in most public or medical school libraries. Physicians who are osteopathic surgeons may be certified or accredited by a specialty board in some states or by their own Osteopathic Board of Surgery. Remember, there are competent surgeons who are not board certified. Taking or seeking board certification is a voluntary act on the part of the physician; the fact that he sought and obtained such a certification of his own volition speaks very positively of his medical proficiency. Consequently, if your physician is not board certified, or if he performs surgery though not trained in a surgical specialty, check him out very carefully. Remember, doctors who are not surgeons can perform operations, while the nation's surgeons may not have enough work to keep them busy as the number of doctors increases in the country.

In addition to board certification, try to determine whether your physician is a fellow of the American College of Surgeons. If physicians are fellows, they may use the letters FACS after their names. The college emphasizes continuing-education programs and maintains very high membership qualifications to keep out less competent surgeons. You can find out whether a surgeon is a fellow by asking your local county medical society, by consulting the *Directory of Medical Specialists*, or by writing directly to the American College of Surgeons, 633 North Saint Clair St., Chicago, IL 60611.

Aside from noting board certification, the *Directory of Medical Specialists* will allow you to learn about other aspects of the surgeon's background, thus enabling you to judge his competency. For example, it will inform you of the physician's medical school, location of residency training, length of medical practice, and other vital biographical information. In addition, ask your local county medical society if it publishes physician directories—or plans to do so. These would contain the previous information (in regard to surgeons as well as other kinds of medical practitioners) as well as such details as office hours, fee schedules, honors (if any) received in medical school, house calls in the case of nonsurgical specialists, and other important data. Also, ask your family physician or other doctors who they use when they require surgery. The greatest compliment to a surgeon is when he is used by a doctor or his family. In this manner, you as a patient-consumer can to some extent obtain a profile of the physician who will be performing your operation and the kind of medical skills that physician possesses.

HOW TO OBTAIN A SECOND SURGICAL OPINION

"I'm really upset about this operation," Tom told his wife. "How can I tell if it's really necessary? I've read plenty of horror stories. Some surgeons operate when it isn't necessary. The doctor's diagnosis can be completely wrong. I've heard stories about surgeons who mistakenly operated on the wrong body parts. How can I find another doctor for a second opinion, or even pay for it? I don't personally know any surgeons, nor do I want my doctor to think I am going behind his back. If he thinks I don't trust his diagnosis, he may be angry and I don't want to lose him. Even if I find another surgeon right now, I don't know what kind of questions to ask him. I'm not trained in medicine, and the situation is so upsetting. What if I ask all the wrong questions? I don't want to appear foolish. I'm simply in a quandary." Lucky for Tom, his wife had studied up on his condition and on the operation itself and was able to allay his fears.

You can obtain a second surgical opinion with or without the knowledge of the original physician who recommended surgery. But if you do tell the first doctor that you wish to obtain a second surgical opinion, ask that your medical records be forwarded to the second physician. This may avoid your taking the same tests again. When you visit the second physician, tell him the name of the surgical procedure your original physician recommended and what diagnostic tests were ordered. If the second physician agrees that surgery is necessary and the best form of treatment, he will usually not perform the surgery himself but will refer you back to the first doctor. On the other hand, if the second doctor disagrees with the first physician and you are still not sure about your final decision, you may wish to obtain a third opinion from still another physician. If the first and second physicians were both specialists, your family doctor is probably the individual with whom you will want to discuss the optional courses of action. But if the first doctor you consulted was your family physician and the second physician was a specialist, then you may wish to obtain a third opinion from yet another specialist. (Many insurance policies will cover a third consultation.) In handling a second or even a third opinion consultation:

- Be completely honest with the second or third doctor and explain your reasons for wanting another opinion.
- Tell the second or third doctor what procedure was recommended and why.
- If you do not agree with or like the original recommendation, explain why.
- If you disliked the first surgeon, just say so.

As already noted, you will not offend most physicians if you seek a second or even a third surgical opinion. Ethical physicians do not want to force surgery or any other kind of treatment on their patients. They want their patients to be reassured that their advice and judgment is best for the patient—a reassurance that can come from a second opinion. If the second opinion agrees with the first physician's judgment, then you have the assurance that the recommended surgery is necessary. The second opinion provides you with the information that gives you confidence in your final decision. On the other hand, if as a result of the second opinion you decide not to have surgery, you avoid the risks, costs, and discomfort usually associated with a surgical operation.[19]

In seeking a first, second, or even third opinion as to whether you should undergo surgery, make sure that you are given the answers to the following basic questions:

What operation is being recommended? Why?

Ask your surgeon to explain the surgical procedure. For example, if something is going to be fixed or taken out, find out why it is necessary to do so. Your surgeon can draw a picture or diagram and explain to you the activities involved in the procedure. Can the operation be done in different ways? One way may require more extensive surgery than another or another may be less damaging. What is the mortality rate of the operation? Ask why your surgeon wants to perform the operation one way compared to another.

Why is the operation necessary?

There are many reasons to have surgery. Some operations can alleviate or prevent pain. Others can lessen a symptom of a problem or improve some body function. Some surgeries are performed in order to diagnose a problem. Surgery can also save your life. Your surgeon will tell you why the procedure is being done. Make sure you understand how the proposed operation fits in with the diagnosis of your medical condition. To make sure you understand the operation, repeat to the surgeon in your own words what the surgeon just told you.

What are your surgeon's qualifications? Is he/she board certified? A fellow of the American College of Surgeons?

As already noted, you will want to know that your surgeon is experienced and qualified to perform the operation. Many surgeons have taken special training and passed exams given by a national board of surgeons. Ask if your surgeon is "board certified" in surgery. That means a physician has completed the training or residency period required before he or she can even take a specialty board examination. Many well-qualified, newly practicing surgeons are just waiting to take the exam. The fact that a surgeon is not board certified is not an indication that he or she is not an excellent surgeon. But board certification at least says that this surgeon was once judged qualified by surgical peers. Some surgeons also have the letters FACS after their names. This means they are fellows of the American College of Surgeons and have passed another review by surgeons in their medical practice. The surgeon has passed a thorough evaluation of both professional competence and technical fitness. Fellows are board-certified surgeons or, in unusual circumstances, have met other standards comparable to board certification.

Are there alternatives to surgery?

Sometimes surgery is not the only solution to a medical problem. Medicines or other nonsurgical treatments, such as a change in diet or special exercises, might assist you just as well—or more. Ask your surgeon or primary care doctor about the benefits and risks of these other alternatives. You need to know as much as possible about these benefits and risks to make the best decision. One choice may be "watchful waiting," in which both you and your doctor check to see whether your problem improves or worsens. If it becomes worse, you may need surgery right away. If it becomes better, you may be able to postpone surgery, perhaps indefinitely.

What are the benefits of having the operation?

Ask your surgeon what are the advantages of having the operation. For example, a hand surgery may mean that you can move your fingers with ease again. Find out how often this kind of surgery helps your kind of problem and how much.

Ask how long the benefits are likely to last. For some procedures, it is not unusual for the benefits to last for only a short time. You might need a second operation at a later date. For other procedures, the benefits may last a lifetime. When asking about the benefits of the operation, be realistic. Sometimes patients expect more than may be possible and are disappointed with the outcome or results. Ask your doctor if there is any published information about the outcomes of the procedure.

What are the risks of having the operation? Are there any possible effects or complications? What are the postoperative consequences?

In addition to benefits, no operation is free of risk. This is why you need to consider the risks of complications or side effects.

Complications can occur around the time of the operation. They include such unplanned events such as infection, too much bleeding, reaction to anesthesia, or accidental injury. Some people have increased risk of complications because of other medical conditions.

In addition, there may be side effects after the operation. For the most part, side effects can be anticipated. For example, your surgeon knows that there will be swelling and some soreness at the site of the operation.

Also, there is almost always some pain with surgery. Ask how much there will be and what the doctors and nurses will do to reduce the pain. Controlling the pain will help you be more comfortable while you recuperate and improve the results of your operation.

What will happen if I don't have the operation? What are my chances of survival without the operation? Do I need this surgery immediately? How long can the surgery be postponed, and how dangerous would waiting be?

Will the surgery be less successful if I wait? Do you use a surgical checklist prior to the operation? What are the chances of survival with the operation? What should the outcome be?

Based on what you learn about the benefits and risks of the operation, you might decide not to have it. Ask your surgeon what you would gain—or lose—by not having the operation now. Could you be in more pain? Could your condition become worse? Could the problem go away?

As a patient, be aware that beginning July 2004 surgical teams must take new steps to ensure that they are operating on the right body part and right patient. If they do not take these new steps, the Joint Commission on the Accreditation of Health-care Organizations can revoke the accreditation of hospitals or other surgical sites that do not comply with the new safety procedures. Some of these new rules include:

- The surgeon must literally sign the incision site while the patient is conscious, and cooperating if possible, with a marker that will not wash off in the operating room.
- The new rules emphasize that no mark should be placed on any site that is not being operated on. Surgeons should avoid the use of the letter "X" and should use either the doctor's initials or some other mark that is used hospitalwide. Regulators have found that an "X" can mean "operate here or not here" and writing out "not this leg" can cause problems if the "not" becomes smudged and is not readable.
- The entire operating team must halt all other work prior to the beginning of the surgery and proceed through a checklist to ensure that the right patient is on the table and that everyone—surgeons, nurses, anesthesiologists, technicians—agree what procedure is being performed and on what body part.
- If you are about to be anesthetized and have not witnessed the surgical team double-check your identity and your surgical site, for your own safety, ask them if they carried out their surgical double-check.

Where can I get a second opinion?

A second opinion from another doctor is a very good way to ensure that having the operation is the best decision for you. Many of the best insurance plans require patients to obtain a second opinion before they have certain nonemergency operations. Private insurance plans typically pay for second opinions (though not by doctors who are not in a plan's network). If your plan does not require a second opinion, you may still ask to have one. Check with your insurance company to see if it will pay for a second opinion. If your health plan won't cover a second opinion, pay for one yourself if at all possible. Also, if you use the Internet to seek second opinions, be very careful. Thousands of Web sites claim to offer opinions by qualified doctors, and it is difficult to detect quacks. If you obtain a second opinion, make sure to get your medical records from the first doctor so that the second physician does not have to repeat tests.

As already noted, to obtain the name of a specialist in your area who can give you a second opinion, ask your primary doctor or surgeon, the local medical society, a local medical school, or your health insurance company. Medicare beneficiaries may also obtain information from the US Department of Health and Human Services's Medicare hotline: call toll-free 1-800-633-4227.

What is your surgeon's experience in doing the operation? Does the surgeon regularly do this type of surgery? Did she or he do any last week? Last month? How many? With what result? What percentage of the operations were successful?

One way to lessen the risks of surgery is to choose a surgeon who has been thoroughly trained to perform the procedure and has a great deal of experience in doing it. You can ask your surgeon about his or her recent record of successes and complications with this procedure. If it is more comfortable for you, you can discuss the topic of the surgeon's qualifications with your regular or primary care doctor.

Can the surgery be performed on an outpatient basis or only in a hospital?

Most surgeons practice at one or two local hospitals. Find out where your operation will be done. Have many of the operations that you are considering have been performed in this hospital? The success rates of some operations are greater if they are performed in hospitals that do many of those same procedures. Ask your doctor about the success rate at this hospital. If the hospital has a low success rate for your kind of proposed operation, you should ask to have it at another hospital.

Until recently, most surgery was done on an inpatient basis—patients stayed in the hospital for one or more days. Today, a lot of the surgery is performed on an outpatient basis in a physician's office, a freestanding special surgical center, or a day surgery unit of a hospital. Outpatient surgery is less expensive because, among many reasons, you do not have to pay for staying in the hospital room.

Ask whether your operation will be performed in the hospital or in an outpatient setting. If your doctor recommends inpatient surgery for a procedure that is usually performed as outpatient surgery or recommends outpatient surgery that is usually done as inpatient surgery, ask why. You want to be in the right place for your operation.

If the surgery is to be performed in a surgical room of a doctor's office, ask your state medical society whether office surgery practices in your state require national accreditation. If so, ask your doctor whether his practice has been accredited. Also, you may wish to ask the following questions: Is a heart monitor used? How close is the nearest hospital? Is anesthesia equipment inspected, calibrated, and regularly maintained? Is it equipped with the latest safety devices? In LASIK eye surgery procedures, what kind of microkeratome (a corneal resection instrument—that is, a precision surgical instrument with an oscillating blade designed for creating the corneal flap in LASIK surgery) is used and how often is the microkeratome serviced? (You can check with the manufacturer for recommendations.) How many nurses work with the surgeon? Who assists? Is there a recovery room? Are emergency procedures in place? Is the surgeon trained in ACLS, Advanced-Cardiac Life Support? Who runs the operating room? Ask to see the room; is it tidy, clean, and organized? Do not be afraid to ask questions. A caring and competent surgeon will understand your need to be knowledgeable about these matters and will be willing to answer your questions.

Remember, as of the winter of 2001, the District of Columbia and forty-three states had no rules specifically regulating surgeries in a private doctor's office. Three states—Virginia, Illinois, and Missouri—had some kind of regulation. Four states — New Jersey, California, Florida, and Texas—had comprehensive laws covering surgeries and anesthesia in doctors' offices.

What kind of anesthesia will I need? What are the qualifications of the person who would administer it?

Anesthesia is used so that surgery can be performed without unnecessary pain. Your surgeon can tell you whether the operation calls for local, regional, or general anesthesia and why this form of anesthesia is recommended for your operation.

Local anesthesia numbs only part of your body for a short period of time—for example, a tooth and the surrounding gum. However, not all procedures done with local anesthesia are painless, and some people do have an allergic reaction to local anesthetic drugs. *Regional anesthesia* numbs a larger portion of your body—for example, the lower part of your body—for a few hours. In most cases, you will be awake with regional anesthesia. *General anesthesia* numbs your entire body for the entire time of the surgery. You will be unconscious if you have general anesthesia and major surgery requires it. But be aware that general anesthesia can bear some risks. After surgery under general anesthesia, your lungs are susceptible to pneumonia and your reflexes are weakened as you regain consciousness. If you vomit before they have returned to normal, you risk choking. Ask your primary care doctor and/or anesthesiologist to explain all the risks and side effects involved with anesthesia in your case. Also, ask whether you have a choice of the kind of anesthesia you will be receiving. While safety is your first consideration, you also must take into account your personal feelings. Some people are very fearful of being unconscious, while others of being awake and witnessing their own body being operated upon.

Anesthesia is usually administered by a specialized physician (anesthesiologist) or certified nurse anesthetist or a physician with credentials in anesthesia. Both are highly skilled and have been specially trained to give anesthesia. If you have decided to have an operation, ask to meet the person who will give you anesthesia. Find out what his or her qualifications are.

More specifically, before surgery the anesthesiologist should meet with you to explain what will be done and to ask some important questions about your previous medical history to increase your safety. These questions may include:

- Do you have any allergies?
- Do you have any medical problems such as cardiac or respiratory disease, sickle cell anemia, or diabetes?
- Are you taking any medication? If so, and you have difficulty remembering their names, make a list prior to visiting the anesthesiologist for his/her review.
- Have you had anesthesia in the past?
- If so, how recently? (Some anesthetic agents cannot be given again until a certain amount of time has passed.)
- Have you ever had problems receiving or recovering from anesthesia? Ask what the side effects and risks of having anesthesia are in your case.
- Have you ever had a fever or other problem after taking any kind of anesthetic?
- Have you ever had a reaction to a local anesthetic, such as a shot given at the dentist's office?
- Do you have a history of abnormal bleeding?

In what kind of hospital will the operation be performed?

Generally, the choice is between a medium-sized community hospital, a larger hospital that trains resident physicians, and a major medical center teaching hospital.

For major surgery, avoid small community hospitals. If you are trying to decide between a moderate-sized hospital (150 to 300 beds) with a good reputation and a major medical center, consider the quality of the nursing care. Community hospitals usually may show much more concern for your needs. Almost inevitably, major medical teaching centers may give less personalized care. The world-renowned surgeon there is apt to delegate much more of your preoperative and postoperative care to a less-experienced physician. Ask your family physician about the qualities of the various hospitals in which you are considering having the surgery performed.

What will the recovery period be? Will I need help at home? What kind of assistance? How will the operation affect my health and lifestyle? Are there any activities I will not be able to do after surgery?

Your surgeon can inform you how you might feel and what you will be able to do—or not do—the first few days, weeks, or months after surgery. Ask how long you will stay in the hospital. Find out what kind of supplies, equipment, and any other help you will require when you go home. Knowing what to expect can help you deal better with your recovery.

Ask when you can start regular exercise again and go back to work. You do not want to do anything that will slow down your recovery process. Lifting a ten-pound object may not seem to be "too much" seven days after your operation, but it could be. You should follow your surgeon's advice to make sure you recover as soon as possible.

How much will the operation cost? Will my insurance cover all the costs, including special tests?

Health insurance coverage for surgery can vary, and you may have to pay part of the costs. Before you have the operation, call your insurance company to find out how much of these costs it will pay and how much you will have to pay yourself. Ask what your surgeon's fee is and what it covers. Surgical fees often include several visits after the operation. You also will be billed by the hospital for inpatient or outpatient care and by the anesthesiologist and others providing care related to your operation.[20]

The answers to these questions from both your primary care physician and your surgeon will help you make the best decision that is appropriate to your situation. If you do not understand the answers, ask your doctors to explain them clearly. Patients who are well informed about their treatment tend to be more satisfied with the outcome or results of their treatment.

AMBULATORY SURGICAL CENTERS

As the healthcare industry has become more responsive to economic pressures, one kind of treatment facility that developed very quickly during the 1980s was the ambulatory surgical center. Since 1984, the number of inpatient surgeries performed has dropped by approximately two million procedures, whereas the number of ambulatory surgeries has nearly doubled. According to a 1995 survey performed by the American Hospital Association's (AHA) Society for Ambulatory Care Professionals, the decrease in inpatient procedures is due to advances in surgical techniques and the availability of new anesthetics and pharmaceuticals. According to the American Hospital Association, in 2000 there were 16.4 million surgeries performed on an outpatient basis versus 9.7 million inpatient (nearly all community hospitals, regardless of size or location, now have some sort of ambulatory facility).

One of the reasons why ambulatory surgical centers have expanded so rapidly is their ability to perform a diverse array of procedures. Another factor contributing to their rapid growth is pressure from managed care organizations and public payers for procedures to be performed in the most cost effective setting. More than twenty-five hundred types of surgical procedures are currently performed on an outpatient basis.[21]

While outpatient surgery has been performed at hospitals for many years, a facility devoted totally or principally to ambulatory surgery is a relatively new concept. Many are affiliated with hospitals, while others are freestanding independent facilities. Other outpatient sites are units in physicians' offices. Freestanding facilities—those not physically connected to a hospital—may be hospital-owned, independently owned, corporately owned, university-owned, a joint venture, or a limited partnership. These facilities may be single-specialty or multispecialty, and they may provide patients with additional nonsurgical services as well.

In addition, the ambulatory surgical facilities are evolving into new models of care. An ambulatory surgical center (ASC) may arrange with a nursing home to care for its postoperative patients. In some areas, ambulatory surgical centers contract with a hospital for the use of its recovery or sub–acute care beds, which are priced lower than acute care beds. Some states are permitting the building of dedicated recovery care centers or specialty hospitals, focused only on the care of postsurgical patients and often attached to an ambulatory surgical center.[22] However, the advantage of hospital-based units is that, if complications develop, patients can be transferred immediately to the area of the hospital that contains intensive-care units and staff who treat the critically ill. While most physicians who perform minor surgery in their offices and free-standing clinics have an agreement with a nearby hospital to allow their patients to be admitted in case of complications, the disadvantage of the situation is that the transfer could cause a dangerous loss of time in an emergency.

The first ASC was built in 1970. Now, each year more than eight million surgeries are performed in more than four thousand ASCs across the country. As already noted, one of the principal reasons for their rapid growth is costs. In fact, estimates show that surgery performed in outpatient ambulatory centers costs 60 to 70 percent less than surgery performed in inpatient facilities.[23] A study by the US Department of Health and Human Services showed that using a hospital was 73.6 percent more costly for cataract surgery and 43.8 percent higher for colonoscopies than ambulatory centers.[24] There are various reasons for these cost differences, but basically the ambulatory surgical centers do not provide the scope of work that hospitals provide, especially operating an emergency room twenty-four hours a day. In addition, hospitals must take anyone regardless of their ability to pay; most free-standing clinics do not. Because they have to shift the cost of covering the uninsured to the insured, hospitals are more expensive per operation. In addition, recovery from an ambulatory surgical center occurs at home, or in a recovery center with minimal staff; it has less capital investment and lower overhead compared with a hospital; and because an ambulatory surgical center provides only a specific and limited set of services, it does not need all the rules and procedures that an acute care hospital requires and which makes it more expensive. The primary charges of the ambulatory surgical center are for preoperative and operative activities.

The kind of operations these surgical centers perform include cataract surgery; removal of tonsils and adenoids (tonsillectomy and adenoidectomy); cystoscopy (an examination of the inside of the bladder); breast biopsy as well as dilation of the cervix and scraping the lining (curettage) of the uterus (D&C); excisions of skin lesions such as warts, small skin cancer, mole, or cyst; operations on eye muscles; breast augmentation surgery; orthopedic procedures such as setting an uncomplicated fracture; vasectomy; and face-lifts. Essentially, the centers can perform any operation that does not require prolonged general anesthesia and extensive postoperative care. Instead of staying overnight in the hospital, the patient is sent home with instructions on how to care for themselves.

"That's why I chose to have my surgery done on an outpatient basis," said Gerald. "I was in and out of the center within twenty-four hours."

"But, how did you decide on that kind of surgery?" asked Tamar. "Isn't surgery safer in a hospital? Look at all the equipment they have there." Gerald responded that it was not an overnight decision. He studied up on the centers, the quality of care they deliver, the kind of doctors they have, their experience with mortality rates, and any medical complaints about their services. He asked a lot of questions until he was satisfied with his decision. He knew that "safety" was the determining factor—that were it not safe, surgery outside the hospital would be banned.

Is Same-Day Surgery for You?

To determine your eligibility for same-day surgery, your doctor will take the following into consideration.

- Your general physical condition. Usually, but not always, same-day surgery is restricted to patients who are under sixty years of age and don't have a history of stroke or such chronic illnesses as arthritis, heart or blood vessel disease, high blood pressure, or diabetes.
- Whether you have someone to take you home after the surgery. (Driving is usually forbidden after surgery.)
- Whether there is someone to care for you after the surgery is completed and you return home.
- Whether you are considered a low risk for complications from anesthesia and postoperative bleeding. If tests or your medical history indicate a problem such as blood-clotting or vomiting from anesthesia, your doctor is in the best position to judge whether same-day surgery probably is a good idea for you.
- Whether you are the kind of patient who cannot be trusted to take your medications or who denies pain and then has to be hospitalized because you won't seek medical attention if complications develop after you go home.
- The nature of the surgical procedure. It should take normally less than one or two hours and normally there should be few complications in the three to four days following the surgery.

There are exceptions to these guidelines. An elderly person whose health is questionable may qualify for same-day surgery if there is someone capable of caring for the patient at home. Same-day surgery can also be appropriate for children and others who are afraid to stay in the hospital. That's because the patient doesn't have to be separated from the family for as long as he or she would be otherwise. Immediately before or after the operation, a child (or any anxious patient) can be comforted and reassured by parents and other family members.

What You Should Ask Ahead of Time

Before you decide to undergo elective surgery in an ambulatory surgery center, you can ask many of the same questions that have already been noted:

- Get a second opinion if you have any questions in your mind about submitting to the procedure. Ask your family doctor or surgeon if the procedure is really necessary and what the expected outcome is. In some states, insurance companies require such a second opinion.
- Ask about the facility's accreditation. Has it been approved by an accrediting organization such as the Accreditation Association for Ambulatory Health Care (AAAHC) (Tel: 1-847-853-6060 or at http://www.aaahc.org), the Joint Commission on the Accreditation of Healthcare Organizations (JCAHO) (Tel: 1-630-792-5000 or at http://www.jcaho.org), or the American Association for Accreditation of Ambulatory Surgery Facilities, Inc. (AAAASF) (Tel: 1-847-775-1985 or at http://www.aaaasf.org) or has membership in a group like the Federated Ambulatory Surgical Association (FASA) (Tel: 1-703-836-8808 or at http://www.fasa.org). These criteria are not a guarantee of quality, but they do indicate that the facility has met certain high standards. Accredited and licensed facilities in hospitals and clinics, for example, must meet stringent requirements for physician accountability, analysis of specimens, and availability of emergency equipment.
- What about the cost? Is the ambulatory surgical center Medicare approved? Your insurance company may be able to help you with this. Where private freestanding surgery centers exist, you can check the cost of a procedure by calling the center. The information may be more difficult to get from a hospital facility, because the hospital does not know in advance what tests your doctor will order or how long you will stay.
- How well trained and experienced are the center's health professionals?
- Is the center affiliated with a hospital? If not, find out how the center will deal with any emergency that could take place during your visit.
- Make the appropriate decision. Whether you decide to have surgery in a hospital or in an ambulatory surgical center, don't base your decision on the fact that you have been paying for hospital insurance for a very long time and may as well use it. Base your decision on what is the most appropriate setting and resources for the condition you wish to correct.

The Advantages of Ambulatory Surgical Centers

Seeking care in an ambulatory care facility has various advantages. These include:

- Less expense. Surgeons' fees are usually the same whether the surgery is performed on an inpatient or same-day basis. But you can save a great deal of money by not staying in a hospital.

- Convenience. Scheduling can be more flexible at an ambulatory care facility than at a facility within a hospital. Whether the center is hospital-based or private, there are less official forms and routine, resulting in delays in getting business done, because records are less detailed than those required for hospital inpatients.
- Less emotional trauma. For children and others who may be afraid of hospitals, the opportunity to be with relatives before and immediately after surgery is a decided advantage.
- Less physical discomfort. Same-day procedures are short and the effects of the anesthetics used aren't as long lasting as those used in other procedures. Because of this situation, there is usually less postsurgery discomfort than there is with longer inpatient operations.
- Insurance coverage. Most commercial insurers routinely pay for surgery in private freestanding centers. Almost all will pay for same-day surgery in hospital facilities. Blue Cross plans also pay for same-day surgery in hospital units (although not all plans have such facilities in their areas). Many Blue Cross plans also pay for same-day surgery in private freestanding centers. Ask your local Blue Cross plan whether it does so. Also, check with your local Blue Shield plan as to whether it pays for surgeon's fees if the operation is performed in a hospital or freestanding ambulatory facility. Insurance coverage for same-day surgical procedures is becoming more and more widespread. In fact, insurance companies are actively promoting same-day surgery. Also, you may wish to protect your family in another fashion. Ask your insurance broker about the availability of *short-term surgical survival insurance*, its maximum amount of coverage, its premium cost, and its terms—that is, the beneficiary of the insured receives the specified amount within thirty days as a result of the operation. This added protection may give you peace of mind regarding your family's financial health prior to any surgery.

Patient Responsibilities

If you decide you wish to have same-day surgery, you will have to assume some of the responsibilities that doctors and nurses assume in the hospital. For example, as in a hospital, you shouldn't have anything to drink or eat the night before surgery. Your family must also assume some of the responsibility for your postoperative care. Relatives must be completely briefed on the aftereffects of surgery and told what to look for. If you (or the person who will be caring for you) are unable to assume postoperative responsibilities for your care, same-day surgery should not be performed.

What Happens at Ambulatory Surgical Centers?

If you and your doctor decide that you want to have your surgery on the same day in an outpatient facility whether it be freestanding or hospital-affiliated, your physician will make an appointment that is convenient for you, the center, and your surgeon.

Some facilities will mail you literature regarding your responsibilities before the surgery and what to expect when you arrive for the procedure. The information will inform you as to what you can eat beforehand and what time you should come to the facility.

Your physician may order various tests such as x-rays, as well as an electrocardiogram to check your heart.

Upon your arrival at the center, a nurse or a physician will ask a few questions about your medical history, take a sample of your blood, and measure your blood pressure. Then you will sign a consent form authorizing the operation.

After you exchange your clothes for a gown, the anesthesiologist will again review your history, check the results of your laboratory tests, and listen to your heart and lungs.

If you fail to follow the presurgery instructions you are given, your surgery may have to be postponed. If all your tests turn out fine, you may be given medication so that you will relax until the surgeon is ready to begin the procedure.

When it is the proper time to receive your anesthetic, you will probably be given a quick-acting anesthetic that puts you to sleep immediately. After the anesthesia, you awaken rapidly and with few side effects. Some patients only require a local anesthetic.

After surgery, you will be taken to a recovery room until the surgeon or anesthesiologist decides you are ready to be discharged—under the supervision of another adult. Before you leave the facility, you will be given instructions as to exactly what you can do, or whom to call if problems arise.

Most procedures take less than four or five hours, from the beginning to the end.[25] In summary, if you really want outpatient surgery you must ask yourself the following:

- Will my insurance cover it?
- Can I save a large amount of money?
- Do I have someone willing and able to help me when I return home?
- How do I feel about hospitals? Would I feel more anxious in a hospital or does the idea of going home after surgery somehow frighten me?

In deciding upon outpatient surgery, you should know exactly how much care you will need afterward; how you will manage your personal recovery; whether you have someone to assist you or have to hire a homecare nurse through a service (your doctor can help recommend such a service); and whether you can afford homecare if your health insurance does not cover it. These also are important considerations when making your decisions.

INPATIENT SURGERY

"I'm having my surgery at St. Ann's Hospital next week and am concerned," said Charles. "It is not a serious operation, but my friend went into the hospital for minor

surgery and died on the operating table. He was only in his thirties!" Charles knew
the statistics were on his side and that most people who undergo surgery survive.
Nevertheless, he was scared.

Surgery today is far more sophisticated than years ago, and so is the knowledge and training of the surgeon. Doctors know more about postoperative care and can better inform their patients to ensure a successful recovery. Even the cost of surgery has dramatically diminished because of public and private financing. All odds are now on the side of the patient for a successful recovery. If you require inpatient surgery, there are a number of steps you can take to increase the success of your hospital stay and to reduce the costs of your hospitalization.

- Make sure you know the surgeon who is performing the operation. Check his reputation, education, experience, board certification, and the reputation of the hospital in which your operation is taking place since better hospitals tend to have better surgeons.
- Find out from your doctor exactly what hospital tests you really need prior to the operation. Ask your doctor if you have had any of these tests recently and, if so, do they need to be repeated? You can also determine whether an ordered test is really necessary by asking the following questions: What would occur if you waited and took the test only if the condition got worse? Will the test actually affect treatment? What are the chances of inconclusive or false positive results and would such results lead to more tests or treatment? In this fashion, you can reduce the costs of your hospitalization in this area and limit needless tests. Adults younger than age forty generally may need nothing more than a simple blood count and, for sexually active women, a pregnancy test. Healthy people forty years and older may need only a few additional tests such as an electrocardiogram in addition to blood tests for diabetes, liver disease, and kidney disease. Each individual is unique, so ask your doctor what tests are absolutely necessary and make sure they are done on time.
- To avoid the risk of receiving contaminated blood, you can bank your blood ahead of time if you are likely to require a blood transfusion during your operation.
- Make sure you are given your antibiotics on time—no more than two hours before surgery—since this can lessen the chance of your developing a wound infection. Also, make sure your doctor gives the necessary orders in this regard and that the nurse follows them. (And make sure the nurse checks your wound and changes the dressing regularly after the operation.)
- As already noted, get ready for anesthesia. To reduce the risk of suffering from complications of general anesthesia, do not take any food or drink that the hospital staff by mistake may offer you eight hours before surgery. If anesthesia has made you nauseous in the past, ask for antinausea medication before the operation. Weak lungs can increase the risks from anesthesia. Smokers who are older than sixty-five or who recently had a debilitating ill-

ness should ask their doctors to examine their lungs before surgery and, if necessary, teach them deep breathing exercises to make their lungs stronger. Smokers should also cease smoking for as long as possible before surgery; even stopping for as little as twenty-four hours can help.

Find out whether your surgery will be the typical open surgery, involving a large incision, a lengthy hospitalization, a significant period of recovery, and greater risk of complications, or whether it can be performed with a minimal invasive technique—laparoscopically. A laparoscope is a thin, flexible instrument equipped with a camera and tiny surgical instruments to reach the surgical site. Compared to open surgery, this is a minimal invasive procedure where the surgeons operate through "ports" or incisions so that patients experience less trauma and scarring and improved outcomes. The patient undergoing laparoscopic surgery may receive a number of benefits including:

- Smaller incisions and, as result, reduced pain and discomfort following surgery.
- Less blood loss and a decreased need for blood transfusions.
- Reduced risk of infection.
- Shorter hospital stays. Some patients who undergo outpatient minimally invasive procedures, for example, return home the same day. Ask your physician if this is also true of inpatient surgery.
- Easier recoveries. Patients can return to work and resume their normal activities more quickly, sometimes within hours or days.
- More options for older and/or sicker patients. Some open procedures are considered too risky for very frail or critically injured ill patients. Doctors, however, can often use minimally invasive procedures to address their problems effectively and safely.
- To ease postoperative pain that can delay you from becoming ambulatory sooner, thus speeding your recovery, ask your doctor if you can receive intravenous morphine after major surgery, at least at first. You might also inquire as to whether the hospital offers patient-controlled intravenous analgesia, which allows you to administer your own medication by pushing a button on a computerized pump. But be aware that many doctors and nurses are still reluctant to give morphine, the most potent painkiller, even though the chance of addiction during your hospital stay is very small. And they only give out even the weaker painkillers on an "as needed" basis, which means you get a dose only when you complain. So ask your doctor about the administration of painkillers as it applies to your particular situation.
- To avoid the risk of developing three common postoperative complications, you can take the following steps. To avoid *phlebitis*, an inflammation of leg veins, ask the nurse to help you walk and become ambulatory as quickly as possible after the surgery. If you are overweight or have varicose veins, wear

special elastic stockings. Since urinary tract infections develop because a catheter has not been removed from your body quickly enough, find out from your doctor or nurse as to whether there is any reason why you still need the catheter or whether it's there by mistake if it has not been removed forty-eight hours after your operation. To try and avoid *pneumonia*, the same breathing exercises that can make the lungs stronger before an operation can reduce the risk of pneumonia after surgery. Pneumonia can develop because the weakness and pain that follow an operation may discourage the kind of deep breathing that ordinarily helps clear the lungs of the harmful bacteria that lead to the infection.

- To avoid errors from prescription medicine while in the hospital, you can take the following steps. Check your wristband to make sure that you name is stated correctly and that it lists any drug allergies that you have. Make sure that the nurse checks your wristband each time he or she gives you any medication.

    Many drugs begin intravenously and then are changed to an oral medication. If you are receiving intravenous drugs, ask your doctor when you can begin to take oral medication instead. If you are now eating solid food and drinking fluids but are still receiving drugs intravenously, a doctor or nurse may have forgotten to institute the change.

    When you go to the hospital, bring a list of all the drugs you have been taking at home, including their dosage, so that the admitting physician can order those drugs for you. Also, find out from your doctor whether there will be any additions, deletions, or other changes in your regular drug regimen. The doctors should add that information to your drug list, including the name, purpose, dosage instructions, and, if possible, the color and shape of the new pills. (If you can't check these items yourself, ask a relative or friend to do so.) In addition, have your doctor review all your medications at least once every seventy-two hours. One other precaution: Ask your doctor to leave standing orders for medications to treat insomnia or constipation. Otherwise, you may face a long, uncomfortable wait for the appropriate order to be written and filled if you need medications for these conditions.

By being aware of these various steps, you can do much to speed up your own recovery, reduce the costs of your hospital stay, and hasten your hospital discharge.[26]

PAYING FOR SECOND SURGICAL OPINIONS

Whether you receive surgery as an inpatient or on an outpatient basis and want to determine whether your original doctor's judgment is correct, there are various ways to pay for a second surgical opinion. If you qualify for the Medicare program and are enrolled in Medicare Supplementary Medical Insurance (Part B), Medicare will pay for a second opinion just as it pays for other services. Medicare pays 80 percent of the Medicare-approved amount for a second opinion, after you have met the Part B deductible for the year. Medicare will also provide the same coverage for a third opinion if you get one. You do not have to pay the deductible and coinsurance if Medicare's Quality Improvement Organization (QIO), formerly named Peer Review Organization (PRO), requires you to get a second surgical opinion. If the second opinion required by a QIO disagrees with the first opinion, you can obtain a third opinion without having to pay for deductibles and coinsurance. Always ask whether the physician accepts assignment of your Medicare claim. Those who accept assignment agree to charge not more than the Medicare-approved amount for their services. The Medicare carrier can provide you with a list of physicians who accept assignment. Most state Medicaid programs will also pay for second opinions. The telephone number for the Medicaid agency in your state's health and/or welfare department may be obtained from your "411" directory assistance operator or from your local telephone directory listed under "State Government Offices." Medicaid payments for the second surgical opinions vary from state to state but cover their full costs in states that have approved the benefit. If you qualify and desire, Medicaid also covers third opinion consultations as well. Check with your local welfare office to determine whether your state Medicaid program offers such a benefit. But, in general, in order to obtain more details about the DHHS's second surgical opinion program you should write to Surgery, Centers for Medicare and Medicaid Services, US Department of Health and Human Services, Washington, DC 20201.

Many private health insurance companies also offer second opinion surgical benefits to their policyholders. You can contact your health insurance representatives for details. Some commercial health insurance companies cover the full cost of a second surgical opinion while others do not. Most programs are voluntary—you, the patient, make the decision to seek a second opinion. Some plans, however, require that you obtain a second surgical opinion if the medical benefits are to be paid; others reduce the benefits paid if a second opinion is not obtained. Therefore, make sure to ask your health insurance company about the extent of its second opinion coverage. Generally, *conditions for reimbursement in this second opinion surgical program among commercial health insurers depend upon three conditions.* The proposed operation must be serious enough to require more than local anesthesia; it must be for nonoccupational injuries or diseases; and it cannot be for cosmetic or normal obstetrical purposes.[27]

Remember—your personal health is involved. Make sure you get all the facts—both medical and financial—before you decide to receive elective surgery. Your physician and your health insurance company or its local agent can assist you greatly in such medical and financial matters. Use them. You and your health can and should be the beneficiary of such knowledge.

NOTES

1. William R. Barclay, "Unnecessary Surgery," *JAMA* 223, no. 4 (July 26, 1976): 387.

2. Howie Kurtz, "Unnecessary Surgery Called Cause of 10,000 Deaths," *Washington Star*, December 1978, p. A3.

3. Ibid.

4. Spencer Rich, "Medical 2nd Opinion Urged," *Washington Post*, March 14, 1985, p. A4.

5. American Academy of Ophthalmology, "Unnecessary Surgery and Related Procedures," Advisory Opinion of the Code of Ethics, February 2003.

6. Kathryn Ramage, Information Resources Coordinator, US Agency for Healthcare Research and Quality, e-mail message to author, March 21, 2005.

7. Elizabeth Morgan, e-mail message to author, March 13, 2005.

8. *VA Cooperative Studies Program: A Legacy of Achievement* (Washington, DC: US Department of Veterans Affairs, 1997), pp. 6, 9–10.

9. Mike Schwartz, "The Unkindest Cut: More Patients and Doctors Avoid Unnecessary Surgery," *Riverside (CA) Press-Enterprise*, August 15, 2003.

10. Cleveland Clinic, "Definitions of Angioplasty on the Web," http://www.Google .com-www.clevelandclinic.org/heartcenter/pub/glossary/.asp (accessed March 4, 2005).

11. Schwartz, "The Unkindest Cut: More Patients and Doctors Avoid Unnecessary Surgery."

12. *Facing Surgery: Why Not Get a Second Opinion?* (Washington, DC: US Department of Health, Education, and Welfare, September 1978).

13. "Advance Notice for Elective Surgery," *WPS Medicare Part B* (Madison: Wisconsin Physicians Service Corporation, 2004).

14. Elizabeth Morgan, e-mail to author, March 13, 2005.

15. George Crile Jr., "The Surgery Decision," *Family Health* 11, no. 5 (May 1979): 15.

16. William A. Nolen, "When Do You Need a Second Opinion?" *McCall's*, April 1979, pp. 74, 151–52.

17. "Surgery: Do You Really Need It," *Glamour*, November 1983, p. 338.

18. US Department of Health, Education, and Welfare, *Second Opinion Program*, a press background paper, September 13, 1978.

19. *Facing Surgery: Why Not Get a Second Opinion?*

20. US Department of Health and Human Services, "Be Informed: Questions to Ask Your Doctor before You Have Surgery" (Washington, DC: Agency for Healthcare Policy and Research, January 1995), pp. 2–10; Lauran Neergaard, "No, Not That Leg!! Rules Fight Surgery Errors," *Washington Senior Beacon*, July 2004, p. 6.

21. "Trends in Outpatient Surgery," *Medical Interface*, August 1995, pp. 76, 79; *Source Book of Health Insurance Data, 2002* (Washington, DC: Health Insurance Association of America, 2002), p. 119.

22. "New Models for Outpatient Surgery Centers," *OR Manager*, February 1995, p. 10.

23. Leigh G. Anderson, "Outpatient Surgery Center Accreditation," *AORN Journal* 60, no. 6 (December 1994): 959; "The History of ASCs," *About FASA* (Alexandria, VA: Federated Ambulatory Surgery Association, 2005).

24. David Segal, "Taking a Scalpel to Surgical Costs," *Washington Post*, December 30, 1995, p. C2.

25. Dan Kaercher, "Same-Day Surgery: Prescription for High Hospital Bills," *Better Homes and Gardens*, September 1980, pp. 77–78.

26. Consumer Reports, "Surviving Your Hospital Stay," *Washington Post/Health*, March 26, 1996, pp. 12, 14.

27. "Health Groups Raps Unnecessary Surgery," *Retirement Living* 18, no. 8 (August 1978): 50.

CHAPTER SEVEN

HOSPITAL CARE

INTRODUCTION

The word *hospital*, like hotel and hostel, derives from the Latin *hospes*, which can mean either "host" or "guest." The word may well have originated from the old eastern Mediterranean tradition of hospitality, which included the provision of way stations where travelers were given food, lodging, and, if necessary, nursing care. In Greece and Egypt, the sick were taken to temples where priests practiced medicine along with religion. The relationship has remained a close one. European hospitals first developed as adjuncts to monasteries or abbeys; even today, many well-respected institutions are sponsored or operated by religious orders.

Until the last hundred years or so, hospitals were not considered as temples of healing. Rampant hospital-spread infections—called, appropriately enough, "hospitalism"—made the institution more dangerous than the disease. Hospitalization was considered as a last resort for the poor and the friendless. Those in better circumstances were treated at home. However, times changed. In 1846 the use of ether as an anesthetic was introduced, expanding the variety and scope of surgical procedures. Sterile techniques were developed in the 1860s in which everything was sprayed with carbolic acid, reducing the rate of frightening infections. Florence Nightingale's work during the Crimean War marked the beginning of professional nursing, and in 1895 medical diagnosis was revolutionized by the discovery of x-rays. These developments as well as others that followed closely were centered in the hospital environment. By the beginning of the twentieth century, doctors found that they could do more for their patients inside the hospital—and the modern healthcare institution was born.

Hospitals today are multimillion-dollar institutions. The equipment necessary for their operation ranges from nearly invisible sutures to mammoth computerized body scanners. Not all hospitals are similar. The vast majority can be described as general hospitals—those which provide a variety of services, surgical and nonsurgical, for the treatment of acute medical problems. As health and hospital services have grown more complicated, specialty institutions have also developed—hospitals for women, for children, for long-term rehabilitation, and for the treatment of specific diseases.

Accreditation is one way to judge the quality of a hospital. Hospitals, general or specialty, are said to be accredited when they have met the minimum requirements of a private organization known as the Joint Commission on Accreditation of Healthcare Organizations (JCAHO). Accreditation involves periodic examinations of hospital services, facilities, and quality of care and is the generally accepted stamp of approval in the hospital field. Hospitals can also be categorized as private nonprofit, proprietary, and governmental. Private nonprofit hospitals can be very large teaching institutions or small rural treatment centers. They may be under the auspices of educational institutions, religious organizations, or groups of private citizens. Private groups also build proprietary institutions, which are operated for profit. They are generally fewer in number and smaller in size. Governmental hospitals are tax-supported institutions controlled by cities, counties, states, or the federal government. Like the private hospitals, they differ in size and quality depending upon the adequacy of their financing and their involvement in teaching programs.

Some hospitals are also schools, and these institutions are known as teaching hospitals. Four thousand years ago it was common practice in Babylon to put a sick person in his bed outside in the street. There, passersby would stop to observe his condition and advise the physician on his treatment. In today's hospitals, in what may seem like an endless stream, doctors, nurses, and other staff may question, test, probe, and discuss a medical problem with the patient. Yet, this kind of attention goes hand in hand with the most advanced medical care in the world. Since the teaching hospital is providing education for graduate physicians, such an institution is most likely to offer the highest concentration of full-time staff and specialized services. It is in teaching hospitals that advances in technology and research are first made available to patients. Such hospitals generally receive the most difficult and acute patient cases. They often act as referral centers for a broad geographic area. An "approved" teaching hospital is an institution whose residency training programs are approved by the Council on Medical Education and Hospitals of the American Medical Association.

Healthcare and hospitals can also be classified by the level of care provided—namely, primary, secondary, and tertiary. *Primary care* is generally provided by a family doctor or an outpatient clinic and in the majority of cases is the only kind of treatment necessary. It often, but not always, means hospitalization. *Secondary services* might include maternity care, an appendectomy, treatment for a broken bone, or testing for glaucoma. *Tertiary care* is the most specialized and acute medical care available. It often involves a patient with critical injuries or illness referred from a primary or secondary facility. Open-heart surgery, intensive care facilities, burn centers, kidney transplants, microsurgery—all are examples of tertiary care. As health costs spiral and medical services and facilities proliferate, health planners are looking for the most sensible ways to organize and offer these three levels of care.[1]

UNDERSTANDING YOUR HOSPITAL

Despite the fact that there were 4,915 community hospitals—that is, nonfederal, short-term, special and general hospitals—in this country during 2000, according to the American Hospital Association, and their existence spans several centuries, to many people hospitals remain an unknown and foreign environment of which they have little understanding or personal familiarity. The general director of the Beth Israel Hospital in Boston, Massachusetts, best illustrated this situation when he described a patient's view of hospital care:

> He enters the hospital anxious, if not outright scared, about the illness. He is then stripped of his clothes and given a restrictive set of rules: where he may go, what he may eat and what he must not do. In a typical day, he might have contact with admitting personnel, several shifts of floor nurses, the attending physician, radiology and laboratory physicians, operating room nurses, house staff, aides and volunteers. All the highly developed clinical procedures of modern medicine are focused on the patient. It is not surprising that this array of hospital rules, tests, instructions, and contacts holds a large potential for miscommunication.
>
> The patient may become angry because no one knows when his physician is coming, no one can reach the physician to prescribe a stronger medication, or no one knows when surgery is scheduled. Some staff members are sympathetic about his pain; others don't seem to care. Perhaps one individual was cross when the patient asked a question, and now he is scared to ask anyone anything. Or perhaps the patient is irritated over a nonclinical problem; the television doesn't work, the admitting office can't find his insurance card or whatever.[2]

Perhaps many of these problems can be avoided if the patient has a capsule view of a hospital's operation. Familiarity with the environment in which you are recuperating from an illness can do much to speed your emotional and physical healing.

A hospital is more than a building and more than a bed; it is trained people such as your physician and other medical specialists; it is an operating room; it is housekeeping and engineering services; it is meals prepared by dieticians according to your physician's orders; it is an administrator, technicians, supervisors, general duty nurses, nurse's aides, medical record librarians, and more. Other services that your hospital may provide include the following.

Basal Metabolism Apparatus

This apparatus determines the amount of energy being used by human organisms. It measures the amount of heat given off by the patient and is helpful in diagnosing a patient's condition.

Clinical Laboratory

This service helps physicians find troubles through such various laboratory procedures as sputum tests, urinalysis, blood counts, gastric analysis, bacteriological cultures, and microscopic examination of tissues.

Electrocardiograph

This instrument is essential in cardiac diagnostic work. This electronic device aids in determining the condition of your heart by providing the physician with important diagnostic information that is not available in any other way. On the other hand, an *electroencephalograph* is a machine that records and detects brainwaves and thus is useful in diagnosing various types of brain disorders.

Medical Social Service Department

Trained social workers can often ease the patient's mind of worries that might slow down recovery. Working as part of the hospital team, the social service plays an important role in modern hospital service.

Blood Bank

A blood bank is often available for transfusions if needed. This involves special refrigeration equipment and the cooperation of many people to make this lifesaving service possible.

Medical Library

A medical library provides the physician with the up-to-date experience of the entire profession—in medicine, surgery, and other specialties. A library would include recent and past journals as well as textbooks. Hospital libraries have contributed greatly to the saving of patient lives.

Pharmacy Department

The pharmacy department plays a key role in hospital service. Recent advances in antibiotic drugs and chemotherapy make the hospital pharmacy more and more important. Here a trained pharmacist can service your drug needs.

Emergency Department

This department—open twenty-four hours a day—has the equipment to treat victims of accidents and to provide facilities in case of community disasters. Depending upon local needs, there can be a very simple or an elaborate setup for handling out-patients, especially those who require medical care but have no personal physician of their own to treat them. But, be aware, changes have taken place in the emergency department. Effective November 10, 2003, the US Department of Health and Human Services relaxed rules that say hospitals have to examine and treat people who require emergency medical care regardless of their ability to pay. Under the new rules, patients might find it harder to obtain certain kinds of emergency care at some hospitals or clinics that hospitals own and operate. The new rules clarify that hospitals do not have to have specialists "on call" around the clock. Also, hospitals have greater flexibility to transfer indigent patients to other medical facilities. Under the new rules, medical facilities such as satellite offices will be exempt from providing emergency care, but they would be required to transfer emergency patients to a hospital or dial 911. Thus, the new rules narrow the definition of "hospital property" where patients are entitled to emergency care. In addition, the new rules state that the 1986 law, the Emergency Medical Treatment and Labor Act (or Emtala), which applies to all hospitals that participate in Medicare and offer emergency services, does not apply to emergency patients after a hospital has admitted them—that is, the emergency care protections end once a person is admitted to a hospital. The purpose of the 1986 law was aimed at preventing "patient dumping" by screening and treating anyone in need of emergency care regardless of health status or income. Thus, under the 1986 law, if any person—not just a Medicare beneficiary—goes to the emergency department of a hospital for treatment, the hospital has to provide a "medical screening examination." If the examination shows an emergency medical condition, the hospital has to provide treatment to stabilize the patient's condition. Alternatively, the hospital can have the patient transferred to another institution if the expected benefits outweigh the risks. Essentially, the new rules scale back regulations that specify when and where hospitals have to provide emergency services. Patients turned away or refused emergency care can still sue, but hospitals will, in many instances, have stronger defenses.

Therapeutic X-rays

Therapeutic x-rays may be available for the treatment of internal cancer and other diseases. Great advances have been made in this field—in equipment as well as in the skill and experience of the radiologist.

Physical Therapy

Physical therapy helps patients become ambulatory and use their muscles after illness or surgery. Rehabilitation by trained physical therapists speeds recovery and the return to normal living.

Sterile Supply

Sterile supply assures an ample supply of sterile dressings and equipment for patient care. This sterilization, accomplished by steam, is an important part of the daily life in hospitals.

Diagnostic X-rays

Diagnostic x-rays are important in detecting medical problems in localized areas and in planning corrective medical or surgical treatment. New x-ray equipment and techniques make this tool an invaluable aid to your physician.

Nephrology (Renal Disease)

Treats disorders of the kidneys, located on either side of the spine, that filter bodily fluids, eliminate wastes, and regulate the balance of chemicals in the blood. Artificial kidney machines (dialysis) and kidney transplants can keep alive patients with end-stage and total renal failure.

Maternity Department

This department provides the best in care for mother and child. Incubators for premature babies are usually available. Facilities for isolation, temperature control, and germ proofing are basic considerations.

Postoperative Recovery Room

This service is an effective way to give the best care to patients immediately after surgery and anesthesia. Near the operating room, specially trained nurses make use of oxygen, intravenous fluids, and various physical aids and devices if they are required. In regard to intensive care units, some hospitals systems have begun to install "enhanced intensive care technology" called eICU. It permits critical care doctors and nurses to watch dozens of patients at different hospitals at the same time via a camera and a bank of computer screens that show such items as the patients' diagnoses and progress, doctors' notes, and the patients' vital signs such as heart rate and blood pressure. Professionals watching from a distance can warn those on duty at the hospital to changes or problems through videoconferencing equipment installed at the nurses' stations. The purpose of this technology is to supplement not substitute in-person care by alerting doctors to quickly catch and respond to trouble more quickly. With this equipment doctors can monitor a patient's ventilator, intravenous medication, and anything else in his room while speaking with the patient and hospital staff members as opposed to the traditional way in which a hospital depends on nurses to notice anything wrong with a patient. Then, the nurse has to contact the doctor(s) who then must go to the ICU to check on a patient.

Occupational Therapy

This service is available in some hospitals and assists patients in becoming as independent as possible by improving their physical and/or mental functions.[3]

All these functions and services enable your hospital to assist you in recovery. To judge the scope of your own hospital's medical care, find out what services it provides. These include not only the previously mentioned programs and technology but also, depending upon the hospital, the following services as well.

Anesthesiology

Relief from pain is an exacting medical specialty called anesthesiology. Many anesthetic drugs are used. Some are injected and some are inhaled. Anesthesia may involve the entire body or portions of it. Anesthesiologists do more than suspend and restore consciousness. Before an operation, the anesthesiologist assesses a patient's mental and physical status and tailors the anesthetic accordingly. During the surgical procedure, the anesthesiologist maintains the patient's circulation and respiration and advises the surgeon on the patient's vital signs, which may dictate changes in the procedure.

Hearing and Speech

Age, heredity, disease, or exposure to hazardous noise can harm the ear. The audiology service of your hospital's hearing and speech center can provide test results that are helpful to a physician in diagnosing the cause and severity of the hearing loss. If the disability cannot be alleviated medically or surgically, the center can provide professional guidance in the selection and fitting of appropriate aids.

Cardiology

Most often, heart disease develops as fatty deposits build up in the coronary arteries, cutting off vital blood supply to the heart muscles. Blood clots can also cause similar blockages when they lodge in a vein or an artery. Sometimes damaged hearts lose their ability to beat rhythmically, and continuous monitoring is necessary to head off serious rhythmic disturbances or even cardiac arrest. Another complication, congestive heart failure, develops when damaged heart muscle fails to pump a sufficient supply of blood to vital organs of the body. The cardiology department in your hospital is trained to diagnose, treat, and prevent these disorders. Among the services your hospital may provide is a special team that responds with intensive therapy to patients suffering cardiac arrest; a receiving station for electrocardiograms via telephone from anywhere in the world; units for performing open-heart surgery; and comprehensive diagnostic services that involve monitoring the heart's electrical activity (at rest, during exercise, and over an entire twenty-four-hour period); as well as procedures that can obtain information from high-frequency sound waves or radioactive tracing.

Dermatology

Though never thicker than three-sixteenths of an inch, the skin is an intricate and vital organ, enveloping the contents of the body for protection, regulating body temperature, and acting as a receptacle for countless environmental stimuli. Dermatology treats the disorders that occur when this finely balanced system is not functioning properly. The diseases dermatologists treat include psoriasis, acne, eczema, skin cancer, and venereal disease.

Endocrinology

Lumped together, the endocrine glands weigh no more than five ounces. Yet these tiny organs—including the pituitary, thyroid, adrenals, parathyroids, ovaries, and testes—control such essential life processes as growth, maturation, and reproduction. Their power lies in the substances they secrete, called hormones. These hormones travel through the bloodstream, regulating the conversion of food into heat and energy (the thyroid); inflammation and the repair of damaged tissue (the adrenals); and the growth of bone, muscle, and other tissue (the pituitary). One major challenge to endocrinologists is helping the millions of Americans afflicted with diabetes. This disease develops through a deficiency in or resistance to insulin, a hormone made in the pancreas. Under normal conditions, this gland secretes insulin to help the body make efficient use of glucose, one of its major fuels. In diabetes this simple sugar is not well utilized and passes out of the body in urine.

Gastroenterology

Food, when swallowed, journeys nearly thirty feet through the digestive tract. The digestive tract—the esophagus, stomach, and intestines, with support of the liver, pancreas, and biliary ductal system—can be subject to disorder or disease. Gastroenterology (commonly called GI) deals with the host of specialized problems that can affect these organs. Ulcers, polyps, tumors, or bleeding of the gastrointestinal tract have been more accurately and quickly diagnosed in recent years with the advancement of endoscopy—the internal examination of hollow areas of the body. Using an instrument that can be compared to a long flexible periscope, the physician can look inside the esophagus, the stomach, and the small intestine by passing an endoscope through the patient's mouth and down the esophagus. Disorders that may not have appeared on x-rays can be detected. The endoscope can also take samples of tissue for examination and remove growths or foreign bodies with snare wires, saving the patient from a major operation. The presence of a gastroenterologist on your hospital staff can help you with these internal disorders.

Hematology

Ten pints of fluid life, the blood, circulate around the body nearly one thousand times a day performing a host of vital tasks. Blood cells carry oxygen throughout the body and pick up carbon dioxide to return to the lungs for disposal. These cells travel in a fluid base, the plasma that comprises slightly more than one-half of the blood. Though mostly water, the plasma is filled with nutrients, proteins, hormones, white cells, and platelets. White cells fight the body's invading bacteria and, when needed, additional white corpuscles can be released from the bone marrow to join the battle. The platelets work to seal off leaks at surfaces of torn blood vessels. Hematologists are medical subspecialists in the study of the blood. They ferret out clues in the blood and its manufacturing site, the bone marrow, to aid in the diagnosis of a medical problem or disease. The problems they deal with range from iron deficiencies in women and newborns to diseases of the bone marrow such as leukemia.

Infectious Diseases

Humans share our environment with an endless number of microorganisms. Viruses, bacteria, and fungi populate the air we breathe, the food we eat, the water we drink. They inhabit our mouths, our stomachs, and our skin. For the most part, these microbes coexist peacefully with us. Some are even useful, warding off harmful intruders or breaking down food substances within the body. Others, however, wreak havoc when they enter bodily systems, causing serious illness and even death. Mumps, pneumonia, food poisoning, rabies, smallpox, influenza, polio, yellow fever, tuberculosis, even the common cold—all are caused by an invasion of these microorganisms. All are classified as infectious diseases. Vaccines and antibiotics have revolutionized the field of infectious disease making minor problems out of previously dreaded infections. But these drugs have given birth to their own set of problems. Microbes, like humans, are adaptable creatures—and they have shown a disturbing tendency to develop drug-resistant varieties. Unlike the cardiologist or gastroenterologist, who deals with a particular area of the body, the infectious disease specialist must consider the patient as a biological system.

Neurology

The human brain oversees a communications network that sends and receives signals to and from every part of the anatomy. Without it, a person would feel no pain or pleasure. He would be unable to move, eat, see, or think. This network, which includes the brain, the spinal cord, and countless nerves, is known as the nervous system. Neurologists are consulted when injury or illness disrupts the complex activities these organs perform. Neurologists treat people who suffer from such diverse problems as seizures, brain tumor, multiple sclerosis, and headache. For example, because 50 percent of the brain is involved in vision, they often work with ophthalmologists in treating eye problems. They work with oncologists in dealing with complications from cancer. As hypertension (high blood pressure) increases in the community, neurologists are seeing increasing numbers of people with hypertensive cerebrovascular disease—or stroke.

Pulmonary Medicine

For most people, breathing requires no effort and is completely involuntary. For others, each breath can be a painful struggle. Pulmonary medicine works with patients whose soft spongy lung tissue has become obstructed or diseased, making a simple breath a labored ordeal. Patients with chronic bronchitis, emphysema, or lung cancer, for example, are treated by pulmonary medical specialists. In addition, these physicians can treat respiratory failure that sometimes accompanies shock, trauma, burns, surgery complications, or other medical diseases.

Rheumatology

Rheumatism is as old as history itself. The pain, inflammation, and the loss of motion characteristic of this group of diseases severely affect the quality of life of millions of Americans—at a cost to the nation of billions of dollar a year in medical expenses and lost income and services. A rheumatologist treats rheumatoid arthritis and related disorders such as gout and osteoarthritis.

Laboratories/Pathology

Another important aspect of hospital care is a department the patient rarely sees. Yet twenty-four hours per day specialists perform tests that can confirm or refute diagnoses ranging from viral pneumonia to diabetes to lead poisoning. These tests are performed in clinical laboratories—a realm of complex instruments, intricate measuring devices, and microscopes. The laboratory has many facets. The microbes that cause infectious diseases are traced and identified in the microbiology section. The blood bank provides transfusions to numerous surgery, burn, and trauma patients. The chemistry laboratory performs tests that range from sophisticated drug measurements to simple pregnancy tests. The role that laboratories assume in restoring a patient to good health is as important as any other service a hospital provides.

Nuclear Medicine

Nuclear medicine is a peacetime application of atomic technology developed in the early 1950s. A variety of diagnostic tests and measurements utilize an innovative combination of computer science and radioisotope technology to produce images or pictures on a screen—such as pictures of the brain as small amounts of a radioisotope flow through blood vessels of the cerebellum, or pictures of the lungs, kidneys, and heart showing the structure of the organs themselves as well as the flow of blood by which they function. Nuclear medicine complements such techniques as the computed axial tomography (CAT) scanner and ultrasound. Together, these methods are revolutionizing the diagnostic process.

Obstetrics/Gynecology

Women today are increasingly aware of what affects their health and their bodies—birth control, breast and cervical cancer, natural childbirth, breast-feeding, and abortion. Obstetrics is the medical specialty dealing with pregnancy, labor, delivery, and postpartum care. Gynecology involves the management of disorders of the female reproductive tract. High-risk patients can now be identified through diagnostic tools and such tests developed in decades past as ultrasonography, amniocentesis, and fetal monitoring. New diagnostic tools have opened a new world in gynecology as well. When a pap smear indicates abnormalities in the cervix, the colposcope, a magnifying instrument, can now be used to allow the gynecologist to look directly at the abnormal area. Previously, this could be analyzed only by using surgical techniques. The laparoscope allows physicians, through a tiny slit in the abdomen, to inspect the sources of pelvic pain without a major surgery and to check for an abnormally positioned fetus. Sterilization procedures have also been simplified using this revolutionary instrument.

Ophthalmology

Today the human eye is still afflicted with many of the illnesses that affected it in the past. These include cataracts, glaucoma, and retinal detachment. But the medical specialty of ophthalmology has developed therapies that can minimize their impact.

Oral Surgery

Oral surgery goes beyond the surgical removal of teeth. On an emergency basis in a hospital, an oral surgeon may be called on to close facial lacerations, repair lip injuries, and treat fractures to the wafer-thin components of the face. The services of an oral surgery department could also include the correction of facial deformities that involve the bones or jaws as well the removal of cysts and tumors from the jaws and nearby structures. For patients with joint dysfunction, whether caused by arthritis, injury, or development, oral surgery may be indicated, or the oral surgeon may instead prescribe special therapeutic exercises.

Orthopedics

The human skeleton is a balanced tower of 206 bones, ranging in size from the pisiform, a split-pea-shaped bone in the wrist, to the femur, the twenty-inch-long thighbone. In conjunction with the muscles and connective tissue, the bones give the body support, mobility, and protection for its delicate vital organs. The hospital department of orthopedic surgery provides surgical and nonsurgical care to patients with problems of the musculoskeletal system. For example, patients with rheumatoid or degenerative arthritis, joint deformities or infections, congenital problems, injury to the hands or feet, hip or back problems, and, of course, fractures, torn ligaments, and ripped tendons may be referred to the orthopedic surgery department by private physicians or by the hospital's emergency department.

Otolaryngology

Modern otolaryngology (commonly called ear, nose, and throat, or ENT) is a combination of three specialties—otology (ear), rhinology (nose), and laryngology (throat). Advances in diagnostic technology, microsurgery, and cancer therapy have considerably expanded general ENT practice to encompass maxillofacial and plastic surgery, allergy therapy, microsurgery of the ear, and tumor surgery throughout the head and neck area.

Perinatal/Neonatal Pediatrics

The department of perinatal/neonatal pediatrics becomes involved in high-risk births long before the baby arrives. Neonatologists are consulted early in pregnancies that might be unusual or high risk, and they work with obstetricians to anticipate and prevent complications. Fetal monitoring, which measures the fetal heartbeat during labor, is a routine part of every delivery.

Physical Medicine and Rehabilitation

Helping the disabled individual maximize his capabilities and build a productive life despite his limitations are the goals of rehabilitation. A rehabilitation team may include physical and occupational therapists, rehabilitation nurses, speech pathologists, recreational therapists, social workers, and vocational rehabilitation counselors. The team functions under the guidance of a physiatrist—a physician who has specialized in physical medicine and rehabilitation. The patient and family members are included as primary team members. Treatment is tailored to individual needs and abilities with an emphasis on self-help and productive living.

Psychiatry

Individuals in deep psychic stress—problem drinkers, drug abusers, or those with mental disorders—can be overwhelmed by memories. In some cases the hospital setting provides the therapeutic environment necessary for improvement and recovery. Psychiatrists rely on hospitalization when their patients become physical threats to themselves or to others, or when their condition warrants removal from a disturbing family or life situation.

Radiology

Radiology, the branch of medical science that utilizes radiant energy, has come a long way since Wilhelm Roentgen's discovery of the x-ray in 1895. Today, through research and refinement, x-rays are used for complex diagnostic studies and as therapeutic weaponry against malignancies. Some of these examinations include gastrointestinal, genitourinary, skeletal, and cardiac radiology. One development in this field is the computed axial tomographic (CAT) scanner, which combines a computer with an x-ray machine to give a three-dimensional view of the human body and often precludes the necessity of exploratory surgery. Another is the magnetic resonance imaging (MRI) scanner, which also takes three-dimensional, cross-sectional pictures of the body, but it does not emit radiation. Instead, it obtains its images by means of radio waves and magnetic fields. MRI scanning gives more precise and complete pictures of the brain for diagnosing tumors as well as other neurological problems. It is also used in other parts of the body, including the pelvis, neck, knee, and for certain cardiac conditions. A third instrument used is the PET (positive emission tomography) scan. This is a test that combines computed tomography and nuclear scanning. During a PET scan, a radioactive substance called a tracer is combined with a chemical (such as glucose, a sugar). This mixture is generally injected into a vein (usually in the arm) but on occasion may be inhaled. The tracer gives off tiny positively charged particles (positrons) that produce signals. The chemical substance and radioactive tracer chosen for the test vary according to which area of the body is being studied. A camera records the tracer's signals as it travels through the body and collects in the organs. A computer then converts the signals into three-dimensional images of the examined organ. The three-dimensional view can be produced from any angle and provides a clear view of an abnormality. Compared to CT scans and MRIs, PET scans produce less detailed pictures of an organ. A PET scan is often used to detect and evaluate cancer, of such organs as the lung or breast. It can also be used to evaluate the heart's metabolism and blood flow and examine brain function.

Surgery

Thanks to recent developments in antibiotics, monitoring and life-support devices, anesthesia, diagnostic procedures, and blood transfusions, surgeons can operate safely today on every part and system of the human body. There are many surgical subspecialties and many specialists (ophthalmologists and gynecologists, for example) who perform surgery. But when most people speak of a surgeon, they are referring to a general surgeon. General surgery, the parent of all specialties, still includes the most extensive range of procedures. Although patients with multiple injuries may be treated by several subspecialists, it is the general surgeon who usually still heads the team.

Burn Unit

You should ask whether your hospital has a burn unit. In a burn situation, all systems of the body—the heart and blood vessels, the fluid balance, the kidneys, and the lungs—are thrown off kilter. Often with electrical burns the muscles and nerves are also damaged. And with the protective skin gone, burn treatment becomes largely a race against time—a race to cover the exposed areas of the body with new skin before infection, a burn patient's worst enemy, has a chance to invade the burn site. In the first critical hours, massive amounts of intravenous fluids and blood plasma are administered to prevent shock. Later patients are placed in the Hubbard tank, a huge kidney-shaped, stainless steel tub with water heated to almost one hundred degrees Fahrenheit, just above normal body temperature. Here burns are cleansed, and the rough leathery tissue, called eschar, that forms over deeply burned areas is removed. Ointments or solutions are applied and wounds dressed. After stabilizing the patient's body functions and removing the eschar, which normally takes two to four weeks, burn unit surgeons begin the agonizingly slow process of covering the exposed areas. Skin from unburned parts of the body is shaved off in strips, stretched, and applied as a mesh over the burn site. When donors areas have healed—usually in two to three weeks—the process is continued until all burned areas have a new covering. Even then patients may require a yearlong series of plastic and reconstructive surgical procedures to rebuild facial features and restore function to hands and fingers. There are observable distinctions between different degrees of burns. First-degree burns are bright pink or splotchy red. They are superficial, similar to sunburn. Second-degree burns turn the surface layer of the skin waxy white and dry. Third-degree burns turn the surface tissue pearly white and tan. They destroy the nerve endings, so they're painless. And their damage may extend to muscle fibers, muscles, organs, or bones. Skin grafting is usually required. Fourth-degree burns cause damage to deeper structures of the body as in the case of an electrical burn.

Neurosurgery

Only since the beginning of the twentieth century has the human brain, resting snugly within the tough skin of the dura, been considered suitable territory for surgery. Today, neurosurgeons assail the brain and central nervous system to treat head injuries, aneurysms, tumors, and strokes. Neurosurgery has been one of the major beneficiaries of the present revolution in diagnostic techniques. Computed axial tomographic scanning, nuclear imaging, and blood flow studies have proven especially effective in visualizing the soft tissue of the brain. Development of the operating microscope in decades past has increased the ability of surgeons to work in the deep recesses of the brain. At the forefront of the specialty are procedures in which a radiofrequency probe is inserted into the gasserian ganglion (nerve tissue of the face) to relieve neuralgia or acute pain. The procedure is performed with the aid of x-ray equipment and avoids the hazards of more open procedures. Vascular surgery is one of the fastest growing areas of the specialty, and bypass procedures can reroute vital blood supplies around blocked areas of the brain.

Plastic Surgery

Plastic surgery came into its own during World War I when surgeons were faced with the disfiguring injuries caused by modern weapons. Taking its name not from plastic materials but from the malleable quality of human tissue, plastic surgery now involves extensive reconstruction work that restores body function as well as appearance. The results achieved by plastic surgeons are based on precise techniques and new technology: microsurgical instruments, sutures of nearly microscopic size, planning so incisions fall along natural skin lines or folds; advanced suturing techniques; and better understanding of wounds and the healing process. The specialty is generally divided into aesthetic (or cosmetic) surgery and corrective or reconstructive procedures. They often overlap—as in cases involving burn patients whose appearance and movements are affected by extensive scar tissue.

Shock/Trauma

Referred to as trauma, accidental injuries cost the nation many billions of dollars annually in terms of medical care, rehabilitation, and lost wages. Only since the late 1960s has the field of shock/trauma emerged as a distinct subspecialty using the most advanced diagnostic, resuscitative, and monitoring techniques—as well as community teamwork—in speeding accident victims (via helicopter) to regional care centers. A hospital's trauma program relies heavily on other departments—including radiology, cardiology, operating rooms, emergency department, and laboratories—for support.

Thoracic Surgery

Thoracic surgery was recognized as a separate surgical specialty in 1950. Thoracic surgeons specialize in dealing with the organs between the neck and the diaphragm —heart, lungs, esophagus, and chest wall—as well as the vascular system, the body's major veins and arteries. Their work may involve removal of tumors and aneurysms, repair of damaged organs and tissues, bypass surgery of blocked arteries, replacement of defective heart valves, and implantation of cardiac pacemakers.

Urology

Next to the brain, the kidney may well be the most complex organ in the human body. Kidneys process wastes, regulate chemical levels in the blood, and maintain the body's balance of salt and water. The urinary system and the male reproductive process are the province of the modern urologist. The field encompasses many subspecialties, including fertility and sterility, oncology, reconstructive procedures, infectious diseases, and renal (kidney) surgery. A great deal of urology is diagnostic work. Cystoscopies, in which physicians look into the bladder through a lighted tube, are one of the more common procedures. Cystoscopy has proven especially effective in diagnosing cancer at early, treatable stages and is now recommended whenever red blood cells are found in routine urinalysis.[4]

It is important to understand the character of each of the previous services, although not every hospital provides all of them. Such knowledge can contribute greatly to your physical and emotional recuperation when you are being treated by such a medical department.

STAYING OUT OF THE HOSPITAL

Before entering a hospital for treatment, there are a few steps you can take and questions you can ask that may avoid your receiving such treatment.

- The most important is to try and establish a relationship with a physician you can trust, someone who openly tells you the advantages and disadvantages of a course of treatment or hospitalization.
- If your physician advises hospitalization and it is not an emergency, find out why you are going to the hospital. Tell your physician of any network or admission requirements under your health plan.
- Ask if there are any other options to hospitalization. Perhaps, you may be able to receive care at home from a homecare or visiting nurse agency.
- If you are to be hospitalized for diagnostic tests to find out the reason for a problem or illness, ask your physician whether all or most of the tests can be performed outside the hospital or in the hospital's outpatient department. Even when there is to be a hospital stay, many hospitals now do preadmission testing on an outpatient basis.
- If an operation is recommended—basically any operation—seek a second opinion from another qualified doctor. If you are convinced surgery is required, you may be able to receive the operation without hospitalization. Many hospitals have "in and out" surgical suites where you can go home the same day. Some hospitals, and some doctors or firms, operate competent surgical centers where some operations can be performed just as well as in a hospital.[5]

By following these guidelines, it is very possible that the inevitable hospital stay that you may think is necessary may not be at all. Also, it is to your advantage, whether you enter a hospital or not, to carry on your person your own medical history, such as the names and dosages of medication you may be taking; health insurance information; the names and telephone numbers of your regular physicians; and key aspects of your medical history, such as a heart attack or kidney disease. If you are in an accident that may or may not require hospitalization, such information can be useful to the ambulance paramedics who are treating you.

IMPROVING THE QUALITY OF YOUR HOSPITAL STAY

"You know, David, it was such a surprise. I went to my primary care doctor with a bloated abdomen; he sent me to the hospital's emergency room just for an x-ray to see what might be wrong, and next thing I know I'm admitted to the hospital for ten days with the possibility of surgery within forty-eight hours of my admittance if my condition had not improved. I felt fine only a few hours before. In fact, I was so confident that nothing was wrong, I didn't even bring any clothing or other items with me for my stay. I thought I would be returning home for dinner with my family. For the next ten days, I had x-rays, intravenous feeding, an inserted tube to empty my stomach, and a whole lot of other tests and procedures. It wasn't that the staff did not try to make me feel comfortable, but the whole experience was so unexpected and unsettling with so many tests, unknown medical staff prodding and visiting, being woken up before dawn for taking temperatures and other examinations, and answering all those medical staff questions over and over again, from medical students to interns, residents and senior staff. This was my first hospital experience as a patient and, since you never know when it can happen again, I wonder what a patient can do to make his stay as pleasant as possible."

Well there are steps a patient can take to improve his hospital stay whether he enters as a planned admission or in an emergency situation. Although no one enjoys becoming sick and entering a hospital for treatment, most patients report that they are well treated when hospitalized. Part of this may be due to the computer revolution that has been occurring in hospitals. In fact, more and more hospitals have begun handling prescriptions electronically, where information technology matches most medications and doses with patients, moving a patient's records online so that caregivers—and patients—can refer to them regardless of time and place. In addition, at an increasing number of hospitals, outpatients can book future appointments by logging on to the hospital Web site. Therefore, here are a few steps you can take to improve your stay even more.

Length of Stay

Ask your doctor how long your stay will be when he suggests hospitalization. The question itself tells the doctor that you do not wish to remain in the hospital longer than necessary. If you have a choice of hospitals, ask your physician or anyone you know who works in the health field which institution they recommend and why. A physician must have admitting privileges to treat you in the hospital of your choice.

If he does not have such admitting privileges, you will have to find another physician who does.

Specialization of Hospital

Find out whether the hospital specializes in the treatment you need. Also, ask whether your doctor believes you will receive expert treatment and if the hospital has a reputation for caring. Inquire as to where else you might be treated.

Substandard Care

If you believe the hospital is providing you with substandard care, you can leave and go to another hospital. The hospital does not have the authority to keep you against your will. In most cases, you can be transported by ambulance if necessary.

Hospital Death Rate and Reputation

If you are sent to a hospital with a high death rate or a questionable reputation, ask your physician what has been done to correct them or whether enough improvements have taken place that you can stay there with confidence. If your physician tells you why there have been high rates or what the hospital has done to correct them, you can at least feel he has thought deliberately about the subject. If a doctor hesitates to answer or answers you in a way which that makes you wary, be cautious. Some doctors practice at only one hospital and may be reluctant to tell you of problems.

Physician's Experience

Ask your doctor whether he is experienced in cases like yours. Some patients require a specialist's care. Ethical physicians will tell you so. Remember, you have the right to change physicians or to request a second opinion, even when you are in a hospital.

Clinical Pathway

Ask your doctor what will be done for you in the hospital. In this fashion, you will be psychologically prepared for any hospital procedures. Ask your hospital if it has a copy of a clinical "pathway" for various medical conditions. Thus, if something does not occur in the right order, you and your family can let someone know about it. The patient clinical pathway is a guide for you to follow during your hospital stay. Each day is mapped out as to what you will be doing and who will be working with you that day. In other words, a clinical pathway is a patient-focused tool, which describes the timeframe and order of routine, predictable multidisciplinary interventions and expected patient outcomes, for a group of patients with similar needs.

Hospital Room

Think about the kind of room you would like, if available, and any other special requests. More hospitals are offering suites with additional space and conveniences for those willing to pay extra. These luxury suites are usually found in major teaching hospitals and in hospitals with wealthy patients. Some amenities may include marble bathrooms, unrestricted twenty-four-hour visitations, a refrigerator, accommodations for family members to stay the night, valet parking, concierge services, Internet access, fax machine, and flat-screen television. In regard to other special requests, you may want a special diet, such as low-salt, vegetarian, kosher, or something else. If you find that you must share a room, speak up if you find it is unacceptable or not what you were told that you would have. If your hospital allows smoking and you want a nonsmoker, tell the admitting nurse. Also, some hospitals under pressure to shorten stays and reduce medical costs are converting empty beds into what they call "subacute care" units. These units cater to patients who need more medical attention than they could get at home or in a nursing home but less care than they would receive in a traditional medical-surgical hospital setting.

Familiarity with Hospital Staff

Make sure everyone in the hospital knows who you are and that you know the names of your current doctors and nurses who are treating you. Keep a list of names if you feel it would be helpful. If you don't recognize a health provider who is treating you, ask who he or she is. Also, make sure your name on your wristband is correct and the wristband correctly lists any allergies you may have. Then make sure—when someone is about to administer a test or a medication—that you are the correct patient and that the nurse checks the band each time he or she brings you any drugs. Find out when the nursing shift change takes place, the names of the nurses who will be attending you, and don't make a lot of complicated requests because the new nurses are very busy attending to their patients. Try to make all your requests at the same time and don't be surprised if a clerk or aide answers your call because nursing situations have to be separated out from those that can be handled by others.

Medications

Be aware of the medications you should be taking and any you have been and should continue to take. If you notice a pill you do not recognize, ask, even though it may not be a mistake. Your physician may have ordered it in response to a telephone report from a nurse or a house doctor about you. You should still be informed what it is as well as its effects. It is not only proper to ask what medications you are receiving but a key to the principle of informed consent. In asking which drugs are being prescribed, you should find out when you should take them and why, and whether any are related to drugs you are allergic to. Each time the nurse brings you pills, ask what they are, and if there is a change in dosage or medication, ask why. If you have any cause for concern, ask to see your physician. Bring to the hospital a list of all the medications you have been taking at home, including the dosages, so the physician who admits you can order those drugs. Should you be taking over-the-counter drugs and vitamins or other dietary supplements, add that to the list as well. Also, ask your physician whether there will be any additions, deletions, or other changes in your usual drug regimen. If you are prescribed a new medication, tell the doctor if you are taking a similar drug for the same condition and, as already noted, what other medications or supplements you are taking. The doctor should add that information to your list, including the name, purpose, dosage instructions, and, if possible, the color and shape of any new pills. Use that list to check all drugs your nurse brings (if you don't feel well enough, have a friend or relative check for you). Therefore, get a copy of your medication administration list, which lists the drugs you are supposed to take in the hospital. If it is not accurate, say so. Take it with you if you are transferred to another part of the hospital or to a nursing home. In addition, have your doctor review all your medications at least once every seventy-two hours. One other note of precaution: Ask your doctor to leave standing orders for medication to treat insomnia or constipation. Otherwise, you may face a long, uncomfortable wait for the appropriate order to be written and filled if the need arises. One last word of caution: Many drugs are begun intravenously (IV), then changed to an oral version. If you are receiving IV drugs, ask your physician when you will start to receive pills instead. If you are eating solid foods and drinking fluids but are still receiving drugs intravenously, a doctor or nurse may have forgotten to make the change. Also, in regard to pain relief, ask your doctor if you are eligible for a patient-controlled analgesia machine. If possible, go to a hospital with a computerized drug-ordering or bar-coding system, which matches the medications patients receive with a bar code on their ID bracelets. One last word about prescribed medications, in general. Whenever a physician gives you a prescription, understand exactly what it says and whether or not you can read what he has written. Explain to the physician in your own words what the prescription states. If you cannot read it, there is a possibility that the pharmacist who is filling it cannot read it either.

Patient's Questions

If you know your doctor is going to visit you at a specific time, write down all the questions in advance that you wish to ask him. Ask what time of day and how often your doctor will visit you. You may wish to keep a notebook with you that not only records these questions but other information as well in regard to your changes in condition, changes in medication, and other aspects of your medical treatment. Be very alert when there is a change in the level of your treatment from an intensive care unit to a regular room or being transferred from a hospital to a rehabilitation facility or a nursing home. Mistakes can be made in these transitions, and you may wish to cite these in your notebook should you suspect that they have occurred.

Finally, control the number of visitors you have and do not let them tire you out by their staying too long.

Avoiding Hospital Infections

To avoid receiving any infections during your hospital stay, have someone you can rely upon make sure that you receive antibiotics before surgery. If you have a catheter in place, ask every physician who examines you how long you will need it. Catheters can cause blood and urinary tract infections if kept in for too long. Finally, observe whether hospital workers wash their hands or change gloves when examining you, inserting tubes or changing dressings. Raising the issue may lead to their practicing good hygiene if they are not already doing so because the failure of nurses and physicians to wash their hands, their improper handling of tubes and other invasive devices, and patients not being given antibiotics before surgery can lead to your receipt of hospital infections.

Consent Forms

If you are asked to sign a consent form, read it first. If you do not feel prepared to sign it, if you want to know about any possible ill effects, you have a right to say so. You have a right not to be pressured into signing by being given a form while those about to perform tests are there to do so. If you have any doubts, you have the right to postpone the test and discuss the situation with your physician. If you are about to be operated on and your left or right side or limb is mentioned on the consent form, make sure it is the correct side. Make sure of the same before you are given a general anesthetic before an operation. Also, if you have an *advance directive* (also called *a living will*) or a power of attorney, bring it with you to the hospital. A living will is a written document in which you give directions about who you want to speak for you and what kind of healthcare you want or don't want if you can't speak for yourself.

Effective April 14, 2003, some new federal regulations may ease your stay in a hospital. These are new privacy rules that give patients new power to keep their conditions secret, and they apply to friends, clergy, and family. They prevent the disclosure of information, without patient permission, for reasons unrelated to healthcare, and there will be new civil and criminal penalties for violators. In some hospitals, the rules will mean a delay in releasing information; in others, information once readily available will no longer be provided. Information will be available only if a patient agrees. If the patient is not available to say yes or no—for example, being treated for emergency care—most hospitals plan to keep the information confidential. No information—including even that the patient has been admitted to the hospital—may be released if a patient objects. Under the new rules, hospitals must inform patients if they have directories and give them the chance not to be included in them. Even if a patient should agree for a general listing, hospitals may release only limited information without a patient's specific authorization. They may disclose only where the patient is in the hospital and give a one-word condition, such as good, fair, serious, or critical. Hospitals may inform callers that a patient has died, but they cannot give the time or cause death without permission from the next of kin. The federal rules also allow hospitals to be flexible in regard to patients who have not yet had an opportunity to express a preference. Federal guidelines interpreting the regulations say the hospital may disclose information about a patient's condition if "the disclosure is in the individual's best interests as determined in the professional judgment of the provider." Despite that flexibility, most hospitals will withhold the information if they don't have a clear patient directive to release it.

Another innovation is called a *hospitalist* program. It is designed to improve, personalize, and coordinate care for patients in a hospital. In a hospitalist program, if you are admitted to a hospital as an emergency patient, you and your doctor have the opportunity to permit a hospitalist to evaluate your case and monitor your care during your hospitalization. Your regular doctor remains informed during your hospital stay. A hospitalist is a licensed physician who specializes in hospital inpatient care and becomes the doctor responsible for your care during your progress and treatment, and your physician may consult with the hospitalist or visit you if he or she is able. Many doctors can see their hospitalized patients only at certain times— usually before or after office hours. A hospitalist, however, spends the greater part of the day in the hospital and is available to answer questions, discuss treatment options, and quickly react to changes in medical data or the patient's condition. Hospitalists are on site to coordinate your tests and any needed specialty care; communicate with your regular doctor and insurance providers; plan your discharge, homecare, hospice care, or assisted-living arrangements in coordination with your doctor; and ensure that all interactions with you and your family are done in a timely and sensitive manner. The hospitalist also is knowledgeable about current medical technologies and hospital procedures. Where such programs exist, patients are pleased because the hospitalist is dedicated to their care throughout their hospital stay.

But, if your hospital does not have a hospitalist program and if you are too ill to speak up or look after yourself in a hospital, try to have a family member or a friend accompany you when you are admitted, visit you daily, and stay with you when you feel it is needed (taking into consideration that person's time as well). The family member or friend should be assertive and not be afraid to speak up on you behalf.[6]

Finally, should your child require hospitalization, there are a number of steps you can take to improve the quality of your child's hospital stay. Find out whether your hospital has a program that will tell children what they can expect during a hospital visit and will describe the specific procedures they will receive, all in words and pictures that are appropriate to their age. Also, ask the hospital whether as a parent you can be the last person the child sees before a procedure and the first person he sees when he awakens. In addition, as a parent try to find out whatever worries your child may have. If your child does not have the vocabulary to explain his fears about being treated by a doctor or being in a hospital, ask him to draw a picture of the hospital or pretend that he is the doctor and you as parent are the patient. Also, if you have an opportunity, visit the hospital ahead of time so that your child will know what the room looks like, whether there are chairs for parents and visitors who can sit with them, and where the bathrooms are. Do not surprise your children that they are going to be hospitalized, but toddlers and preschool children only need advance warning of a day or so because they lack an adult's sense of time and may worry unnecessarily for days before entering the hospital. Finally, be honest with your child. Don't tell a child that something may not happen when it usually does because the next time your child will not trust your words, and if you need help ask your doctor or nurse what is the best way you can prepare your child for a hospitalization so that he can recover as speedily and healthfully as possible and will have as pleasant a hospital stay as possible.

HOW PATIENTS CAN REDUCE THEIR HOSPITAL BILLS

Of all the medical care services provided in this nation today, hospital care is the most expensive. In fact, in 2000 hospital care ($412.2 billion) represented thirty-seven cents of every dollar spent for healthcare in this country.[7] From the 1970s to 1999 the average stay in a community hospital increased from $300 to almost $10,360.[8] The average expense of hospital care in many areas of the country in 2000 was about $2,884 per day—a 9 percent increase over 1999; in the early 1950s, it was only $15 per day.[9] Consequently, the question arises as to what the individual patient can do to control the costs of his hospital bill; fortunately, the patient has the following options available.

Medications

Try not to take more medication in a hospital than is being prescribed. Although it is not true for every single drug, inpatient hospital prescriptions tend to be higher in price than the same drug purchased on an outpatient basis at your community pharmacy. One reason is that the overhead of operating a hospital pharmacy may be higher than that of a community pharmacy as a result of the hospital pharmacy employing more technicians and administrative personnel. Another reason is that the hospital pharmacy is one of the few departments that generates income to the hospital. Thus, the price of the prescribed drug may take into consideration the costs of other departments that do not generate income to the hospital or lose money in their operations. Find out if you can bring your own medications to the hospital and save money.

Avoid Weekend Admissions of Nonemergency Care

For elective nonemergency care, try to avoid admission to a hospital on weekends. Many hospitals reduce their staffing over the weekends, and tests may not begin until the following Monday. Meanwhile, you will be charged for that weekend stay. If your physician wants you to enter a hospital on a weekend, find out whether it is absolutely necessary and whether the hospital will begin your treatment that same weekend.

Room Rates

Find out differences in price for various classes of rooms—private and semiprivate. There may be significant variations in the daily private and semiprivate rates. Also, find out whether your hospital allows you a choice of the kind of room in which you wish to recuperate such as private or semiprivate, rather than automatically assigning you a room regardless of its costs or privacy.

Diagnostic Procedures

Ask your physician how many of his diagnostic procedures and routine laboratory tests can be performed outside the hospital. Then have as many of these tests as possible carried out on an outpatient basis. Tests done outside the hospital are usually cheaper than the same tests performed in a hospital. Check with your insurance carrier as to the kinds of tests and services it covers on an outpatient basis rather than in a hospital setting. If you find that tests that have been performed outside the hospital are again being done within the hospital, tell those who are carrying out the tests that these examinations have already been done and when they were given and by whom. The federal government's Food and Drug Administration claims that up to one-half of all diagnostic x-rays made in hospitals are unwarranted. In fact, medical x-rays, regardless of origin, are the single largest source of human-made radiation to which Americans are exposed. Also, be aware that many physicians today practice "defensive medicine," which is the ordering of extensive tests and x-rays even if not needed in order to protect themselves against the possibility of medical malpractice suits as well as for the patient's care. Thus, again, find out why the testing is being done and if it is necessary, especially if the tests and procedures have already been performed outside of the hospital, particularly in the recent past. Keep a record of past examinations in your wallet for an easy reference. (The Food and Drug Administration has printed cards for this purpose.) You may also ask what are the odds that the test(s) will actually find something wrong? What would happen if you waited and took it only if the condition got worse? Will the test actually affect treatment? How likely are inconclusive or falsely positive results and would such results lead to further tests or treatment? Ask your doctor what tests he or she plans while you are in the hospital. Does the hospital that I am going to require me to accept tests you don't order? Why? Do I have alternatives? You have a right to refuse to be taken to unexpected or unexplained tests. Also, patients often spend extra time in the hospital because staff members failed to withhold food, administer an enema or laxative, or make other preparations for a scheduled test. To avoid needless delays, learn what preparations you will need and see that they are performed on time.

Becoming Ambulatory

Try to become ambulatory as quickly as you can. Early mobility means faster recovery, fewer complications, and, perhaps, an earlier hospital discharge.

Blood Donations

Donate blood to the hospital. If you require a blood transfusion, you may not have to pay for it if you have done so or if a friend or relative donates an equivalent amount of blood to the hospital. Check with your hospital about its policy on this matter.

Veterans Administration Benefits

Take advantage of Veterans Administration benefits if you qualify. Veterans Administration hospitals are located throughout the country and treat all service-connected disabilities. Veterans may also be treated for non-service-connected ailments if beds are available. Since the 1990s, the Veterans Administration has adopted a high-technology medical record–keeping system. Within this system, doctors have access on a nationwide basis to a patient's medical file from old treatment notes to the most recent tests and can be alerted as to whether a recommended test has not been performed. Such a system can improve the quality of care that is being delivered in such areas, for example, as chronic care and preventive conditions.

Hospital Billings

Ask about your hospital's operational procedures in such areas as billing and checkout time. Many hospitals begin their billing day at midnight; therefore, if you enter a hospital a few minutes before midnight or leave a few minutes after the official checkout time when a new billing day begins, you might be charged for a whole day's stay in the hospital that you never really incurred.

Rooming-in Facilities

Ask your hospital if it maintains facilities in which you can stay by rooming-in so that you can be near a loved one. Also find out what charges, if any, there are for this service. You may also want to ask whether the hospital will allow you to perform services for your loved one that a nurse might ordinarily do, thus freeing the nurse to perform other duties: perhaps you might not have to pay for these nursing-substitute tasks. Also find out if the hospital will permit you to hire a private-duty nurse as a "sitter" when a family member or friends can't be there. Your hospital or local home healthcare agency might have list of available nurses, even though health insurance rarely covers this kind of service.

Second Opinions

If you are advised by your physician to have surgery, seek a second opinion. The federal government has initiated a program for Medicare and Medicaid patients that enables Medicare patients to obtain second surgical opinions. The federal government pays 80 percent of the reasonable charge, while the Medicaid program pays the whole cost. In addition, private health insurance companies, both Blue Cross and commercial health insurance carriers, have begun to provide second surgical opinion benefits in their policies. Ask your private health insurance carrier if it provides such a program.

Homecare

If you have a choice of remaining in a hospital or being treated at home through a homecare program, investigate the advantages that the latter may afford you. This decision depends upon the nature and extent of a given illness, but homecare programs are much cheaper than hospital stays. Homecare programs are now covered under Medicare and private health insurance. Having nursing care at home is much easier on the family, offers good care, and can save you money. Although the ultimate decision rests with your doctor, you should discuss this option with him. If you are discharged from the hospital, make sure that you receive a formal plan that includes provisions for follow-up care such as visits from the physician or transfer to a nursing home or rehabilitation hospital if you are not to receive homecare. You should receive clear instructions about wound care, medications, any limitations on physical activity, dietary restrictions, and what kind of symptoms are to be expected and which are a reason for concern.

Outpatient Treatment

Try to have as many treatments performed on an ambulatory and outpatient basis as possible. Find out what kinds of outpatient services your health insurance plan covers. The principal argument for ambulatory care surgical centers, for example, is that various kinds of minor surgery or otherwise straightforward surgical procedures like tonsillectomies, biopsies, and some forms of plastic surgery can be less expensive when done on a walk-in, walk-out basis, thereby avoiding much of the administrative, lodging, food, and other costs associated with a hospital stay. Another benefit, some doctors say, is that the psychic trauma of entering a hospital is avoided. Ask your physician or local medical society about the quality of such centers if they exist in your community.

The Hill-Burton Program

If you cannot pay for hospital care, you may qualify for free or low-cost hospital services under the Hill-Burton program and the US Department of Health and

Human Services. A Hill-Burton hospital is a facility that has received funds from this federal program for construction and modernization. In return, the hospital has agreed to provide a reasonable volume of services to persons unable to pay and make their services available to all persons in the facility area. Therefore, when you enter a hospital, look for a sign in the hospital's emergency room, business office, or admissions office that says: *NOTICE—Medical Care for Those Who Cannot Afford to Pay.* Ask the admissions office for copy of the Individual Notice, which will tell you what income levels qualify for free care and what types of free care the hospital is providing. The hospital may ask for proof of your income. Also, you can ask for free care at any time, even after you have received the services. The program only covers hospital costs, not private physician bills. Once hospitals have given out a certain amount of free care each year, they can stop. You have to request these services yourself, so ask the admissions office how to apply. Hill-Burton hospitals have two working days to determine whether you are eligible for the program and must provide you with a written statement that says either you can receive free services or why you have been denied. If you have not heard from the hospital after two days, ask for a copy of the Determination for Eligibility. For more information about the program, you can contact the regional office of the US Department of Health and Human Services in Boston, New York, Philadelphia, Atlanta, Chicago, Dallas, Kansas City, Denver, San Francisco, or Seattle. You can also learn about the program by *calling toll free 1-800-638-0742 in any state except Maryland. In Maryland call 1-800-492-0359.* If you wish to file complaints about the program, you may contact the local regional office, your legal aid services, or call the previous toll-free hotline telephone numbers.

Examination of Your Hospital Bill

Examine your medical bill very carefully when you leave the hospital. But even before you are admitted to a hospital for treatment, make sure you read your master health insurance policy to find out what services your health insurance will cover during your hospital stay and what treatments and procedures as well as preexisting illnesses and experimental procedures it will not cover.

If you are a Medicare beneficiary, you can read the *Summary of Benefits* booklet that Medicare sends you each year. You may call 1-800-633-4227 or visit http://www.Medicare.gov if you have questions about such benefits or other aspects of the Medicare program. Also, make sure that the insurance carrier has your correct Social Security number and date of birth; otherwise, your hospital bill may be rejected for payment by the insurer. In addition, find out if everyone who treats you during your hospital stay participates in your insurance plan. Even if a third party such as Blue Cross, a commercial health insurance company, or a governmental medical program is paying most or all of the cost, it is important that you make sure you are not being overcharged or being charged for services that were never given. Keep a log of procedures and medications you receive during your hospital stay or have a family member or a friend do it. Also, check with the hospital's billing department ahead of time to find out what items are not included in the price of your room such as hospital gowns. Then, ask if you can bring your own to the hospital so that you won't have to pay for these items in addition to the cost of your room. If you need a cane, bring one along because medical supplies in a hospital can cost far more than those purchased outside.

Ask for an itemized bill. Don't pay bills that place charges under summarized headers like "hospital incidentals." Don't accept a bill that uses generalized words like "laboratory" or "radiology." Find out exactly what tests were given within those categories. Laboratory tests and x-rays may be ordered and later cancelled, but the charge slips have already been submitted so that you pay for tests never given. As another example, the most common billing errors involve hospital pharmacy charges for drugs. These err on the side of overcharging. Data entry errors also can cause problems. If the wrong key is pressed, a $50 charge may be recorded as a $500 charge. If you see anything on your bill that is labeled a "tray," "package," or "pack," find out its contents and make sure that no item within that package is listed separately on your bill as an additional charge—for example, syringes. Ask for a breakdown of "miscellaneous" charges on your bill. You may be billed for tissues that should be included in the daily room charge or operating room equipment that is already accounted for in the general operating room charge. If you do not examine your bill very carefully, you will pay for your hospital bills in other ways—higher health insurance premiums or higher taxes to pay the costs of public programs. Again, make sure that all services are itemized. Ask your hospital's medical records department if you can obtain a copy of your medical records and compare what's on the itemized bill with what is on your medical record. If you see something on your bill that is not on your medical record, you cannot be charged for it. "Phantom billing" is adding legitimate claim charges for services that were never performed. Some providers have been known to perform uncovered services but bill the insurers for different services that are covered. To obtain a copy of your medical record, submit to the hospital a written request, which includes your name, signature, and Social Security number as well as the date of your hospitalization and where you want the records sent. The hospital may charge you a small retrieval fee for photocopying your records.

Also, wait for an "explanation of benefits" statement from your insurer before paying any bills. Compare it with the hospital bill. Report any differences to the hospital and the insurer. You may also want to ask your insurer whether certain hospital charges should be bundled or be separate charges. Should blood tests performed in one day be combined into one charge or listed as separate charges? As another example, should the cost of surgical drapes and floor mats be included in the price of the operating room or be separated out as individual charges?

If you find that the hospital bill is wrong in any respect, report such discrepancies to the hospital's billing department and your doctor—and, if necessary, to your local Centers for Medicare and Medicaid Services (CMS) office if you are a Medicare beneficiary or consult "government" listings in the *Yellow Pages* for one of the regional CMS offices nearest you, or to your local welfare office if you are a Medicaid recipient, or to your private health insurance company. Ask the hospital or insurance carrier or both to audit the bill for errors. In a number of hospitals, ombudsmen are employed—sometimes called a patient-relations or guest-relations representative—who help you with all kinds of nonmedical problems without charge, such as finding inexpensive accommodations for visiting relatives or smoothing out a bumpy relationship with a hospital staff member. You should ask their help if the billing office cannot sufficiently explain its charges. They may be able to direct you to the appropriate people in the billing department. If you are told that the hospital does not provide itemized bills or you get the runaround, go to the hospital administrator or express your complaints in writing. Every state now requires healthcare facilities to provide itemized bills. Finally, never pay your bill before leaving the hospital and never sign a payment plan that you cannot comfortably afford. You need time to look the bill over for mistakes. For additional help, you may contact local groups like Detroit's Organization for People (1-313-640-6400), which review consumers' bills at no charge. If the billing department still won't correct the problem, no matter how much you complain, you have alternatives. You can appeal to the state consumer protection agency or to the healthcare fraud division of your state attorney general's office. Telephone numbers are listed on the National Association of Attorneys General's Web site at http://www.naag.org.

Also, remember that if you do not resolve your billing problem with the hospital billing department, many hospitals now send delinquent accounts to collection agencies in less than ninety days. An unpaid bill notation is sent to credit-reporting agencies—without your knowledge. To find out whether charges have been added to your reports, ask the three major credit-reporting agencies for a statement on your credit rating: Equifax (http://www.equifax.com; tel: 1-800-685-1111); Experian (http://experian.com; tel: 1-888-397-3742); and TransUnion (http://www.transunion.com; tel: 1-800-888-4213). There are a few states where you can receive one statement a year from each agency free of charge. If your hospital bill is listed as an unpaid account, write or contact the credit bureaus to explain that there is an ongoing dispute between you and the hospital. The bureaus must review your complaint and make the corrections.

Once you are discharged from the hospital, don't be surprised if you receive many bills that look like they are for the same services. If you examine these bills closely, you will probably see that they are for different services. Doctors who provide specialized services in a hospital generally bill independently of the hospital using an arrangement known as separate billing. Your emergency room doctor, radiologist, anesthesiologist, and pathologist generally bill separately. Most of these doctors are not paid by the hospital. They make themselves available to the hospital with the understanding that they will bill the patients they serve. As noted previously, you will also receive a bill from the hospital for the use of drugs, supplies, and services of nurses and others for whatever services your health insurance does not cover.

Also, remember that every medical procedure is assigned a number known as a CPT (code of procedural terminology). The CPT, identifying the procedure, may appear on the bill your doctor sends you. So when you get a bill after you leave the hospital, in addition to the actions outlined previously, you can take the following steps to understand your bill.

- As already noted, the first notice you will probably receive is an Explanation of Benefits (EOB) from your insurance company or a Summary of Notice from Medicare that tells you the total amount the hospital is charging, what amount of that charge your insurance company is paying, and what you owe in deductibles or copayments. Do not throw out these statements just because they may say "This is not a bill." Because if the EOB states that you owe an amount that is not what you expected to pay, you should contact the insurer to find out what wasn't covered and why. If you owe nothing, just file the EOB statement away; any overcharges must be settled between the hospital and the insurer. The next statement you will receive is a summary bill from your hospital. Compare the charges on your EOB to your hospital bill. If the charges seem excessive, as already noted, ask to see your medical records to learn if you received the care for which you are being billed. Check for common billing errors like typographical errors, incorrect dates of service, and unbundling of services, as already noted. *Unbundling* means the following: Instead of charging one single fee for an operation, some surgeons may unbundle that fee and charge you for each step that makes up the overall fee, which may include everything from visiting you in the hospital prior to an operation to the initial incision and final suturing, so that each step, when added together, amounts to a bill that is higher than just the operational fee alone. Also, watch out for duplicate or incorrect orders for medications, laboratory work, tests, or room fees. In addition, watch out for upcoding of your diagnostic medical procedure. *Upcoding* is a practice that takes a diagnostic procedure and makes it a more serious procedure at a higher cost to you and your insurer. Look at the doctor's orders for treating that diagnosis to make sure it is the same as the procedures listed on the bill. You can check codes on the Internet at http://www.cdc.gov/nchs/icd9.htm. Dates of service can be a problem because most insurers do not allow hospitals to charge for your date of discharge, although many hospitals do, but the day you are admitted to a hospital can be charged as a full day even if you were admitted late at night. Finally, should you require surgery, look at the operating room time on the anesthesia record as to when your surgery began and ended. Generally, operating room time is billed by the hour, half hour, or quarter hour. So make sure if you had surgery you were not billed for three hours when the operation only took two hours. Also, check which provider sent you the bill. Sometimes groups that provide you with services have names that resemble the hospital in which they practice.
- You also may be billed by doctors who saw you very briefly or even doctors you did not see, such as the anesthesiologist who performed medical services while you were unconscious in surgery or the pathologist who examined your tissue in a laboratory.

- Make sure the dates on the bill are the same as the dates you were hospitalized. Ask the provider's billing office about any charges that are wrongly dated or not clearly identified on the bill.
- If you are calling a hospital or a doctor's billing office about any questions having to do with your medical bill, keep a record of the people you talk with, what they say, and the dates of the calls. The telephone number of the billing office should appear on the bill.
- When paying a bill by check, make sure to write down the account number shown on the bill in order to make sure that the billing office properly credits your account.
- Also, remember that if you have excessive medical costs even after the insurer pays your bills, you can write off on your income tax filing only for that portion of your total medical expenses that exceeds 7.5 percent of your adjusted gross income.

In summary, therefore, a number of alternatives are available to the patient-consumer for reducing the costs of his hospital care: homecare programs; outpatient laboratory tests and surgery; ambulatory care centers; proper self-medication; knowledge of hospital pricing systems, billing procedures, admittance, and checkout times; knowledge of personal health insurance coverage and sources of government program aid; and careful review of your hospital bill. If these and other steps are taken, you will be able to control your hospitalization costs to some extent.

HOW PHYSICIANS CAN REDUCE YOUR HOSPITAL BILL

Your physician can also take various steps to lessen the costs of your hospital stay. In fact, the American Medical Association, in developing a *Physician's Cost Containment Checklist* for hospital care, has addressed the following questions to your physician in the hope that their answers will reduce your hospital costs:

- Are you familiar with your hospital's current admitting and discharge regulations?
- Do you try to schedule admissions and discharges in order to avoid charges for extra days or weekend stays when needed services may not be available?
- Are you aware of your hospital's policy concerning ordering combinations of diagnostic tests? Do you have the option to order tests individually?
- Do you order preadmission testing to shorten necessary hospital stays?
- Do you notify hospital administration when delayed or neglected tests or procedures necessitate a longer hospital stay for your patient?
- Do you routinely review copies of your patients' hospital bills? Do you notify administration when unnecessary duplications or procedures are ordered for your patient or when items are incorrectly billed to your patient?
- Do you and your colleagues use your hospital medical staff organization to

suggest cost-containment efforts that medical personnel and hospital administration might initiate? For example:

(1) Are charges printed on order forms for lab tests and x-rays?

(2) Has your medical staff considered including an "economic case" in its morbidity and mortality conference?

(3) Are new interns and residents at your hospital given a "cost-containment orientation" and provided with manuals detailing patient charges?

(4) Does the medical staff representative to the board of directors of the hospital encourage and endorse cost-containment efforts that are consonant with quality patient care?

- Do you initiate early discharge planning when you know one of your patients may need extended-care facility or home health services following hospitalization? (If you feel there is a shortage of these services in your community, have you communicated with your local health planning agency?)

Attention to the previous cost-containment checklist can contribute significantly to helping the physician assume an important role in achieving cost containment of the patient's hospital bills.

THE PATIENT'S BILL OF HOSPITAL RIGHTS

The community hospital performs many functions including the prevention and treatment of disease, the education of both the health professional and the patient, and, where possible, the conduct of clinical research. Historically, the hospital has been viewed as the citadel of alleviating illness, and the physician as the patient's friend has been its instrument for achieving this goal. But in recent years the medical-hospital establishment has become from some patients' viewpoint the adversary who is taking advantage of the patients' illness for personal economic gain. In order to correct these negative perceptions, many hospitals have adopted a patient's bill of rights and responsibilities that reaffirms the recognition of the patient's dignity as a human being. The following represents a Bill of Patient's Rights as revised by the American Hospital Association in 1992. Ask whether your hospital has adopted it or a similar document, for it tells you what you may expect when you are admitted to the hospital and what in turn the hospital expects of you.

Your Rights as a Patient

1. The patient has the right to considerate and respectful care.
2. The patient has the right to and is encouraged to obtain from physicians and other direct caregivers relevant, current, and understandable information concerning diagnosis, treatment, and prognosis.

   Except in emergencies, when the patient lacks decision-making capacity and the need for treatment is urgent, the patient is entitled to the opportunity to discuss and request information related to the specific procedures and/or treatments, the risks involved, the possible length of recuperation, and medically reasonable alternatives and their accompanying risks and benefits.

Patients have the right to know the identity of physicians, nurses, and others involved in their care, as well as students, residents, or other trainees. The patient also has the right to know the immediate and long-term financial implications of treatment choices, insofar as they are known.

3. The patient has the right to make decisions about the plan of care prior to and during the course of treatment and to refuse a recommended treatment or plan of care to the extent permitted by law and hospital policy and to be informed of the medical consequences of this action. In case of such refusal, the patient is entitled to other appropriate care and services that the hospital provides or a transfer to another hospital. The hospital should notify patients of any policy that might affect patient choice within the institution.

4. The patient has the right to have an advance directive (such as a living will, healthcare proxy, or durable power of attorney for healthcare) concerning treatment or designating a surrogate decision maker with the expectation that the hospital will honor the intent of that directive to the extent permitted by law and hospital policy. (Give copies to your doctor, family, and care team. If you and your family need assistance in making difficult decisions, counselors, chaplains, and others are available at the hospital to help.)

   Healthcare institutions must advise patients of their rights under state law and hospital policy to make informed medical choices, ask if the patient has an advance directive, and include that information in patient records. The patient has the right to timely information about hospital policy that may limit its ability to implement fully a legally valid advance directive.

5. The patient has the right to every consideration of privacy. Case discussion, consultation, examination, and treatment should be conducted so as to protect each patient's privacy.

6. The patient has the right to expect that all communications and records pertaining to his/her care will be treated as confidential by the hospital, except in cases such as suspected abuse and public health hazards when reporting is permitted or required by law. The patient has the right to expect that the hospital will emphasize the confidentiality of this information when it releases it to any other parties entitled to review information in these records. (You should receive a Notice of Privacy Practices that describes the way your hospital uses, discloses, and safeguards patient information and that explains how you can obtain a copy of the information from the hospital's records about your care.)

7. The patient has the right to review the records pertaining to his/her medical

care and to have the information explained or interpreted as necessary, except when restricted by law.

8. The patient has the right to expect that, within its capacity and policies, a hospital will make reasonable response to the request of a patient for appropriate and medically indicated care and services. The hospital must provide evaluation, service, and/or referral as indicated by the urgency of the case. When medically appropriate and legally permissible, or when a patient has so requested, a patient may be transferred to another facility. The institution to which the patient is to be transferred must first have accepted the patient to transfer. The patient must also have the benefit of complete information and explanation concerning the need for, risks, benefits, and alternatives to such a transfer.

9. The patient has the right to ask and be informed of the existence of business relationships among the hospital, educational institutions, other healthcare providers, or payers that may influence the patient's treatment and care.

10. The patient has the right to consent to or decline to participate in proposed research studies or human experimentation affecting care and treatment or requiring direct patient involvement, and to have those studies fully explained prior to consent. A patient who declines to participate in research or experimentation is entitled to the most effective care that the hospital can otherwise provide.

11. The patient has the right to expect reasonable continuity of care when appropriate and to be informed by physicians and other caregivers of available and realistic patient care options when hospital care is no longer applicable.

12. The patient has the right to be informed of hospital policies and practices that relate to patient care, treatment, and responsibilities. The patient has the right to be informed of available sources for resolving disputes, grievances, and conflicts, such as ethics committees, patient representatives, or other mechanisms available in the institution. The patient has the right to be informed of the hospital's charges for services and available payment methods.[10]

While the previous enumeration of patient's rights and responsibilities is intended as a statement of the ideals of a hospital and its patients, the declaration does not presume to be a complete representation of mutual rights and responsibilities. For example, as a patient, you are also entitled to request that a person of your own sex be present during an examination; to decline a visit from anyone you do not wish to see; and to be transferred to another room if the behavior of someone else in the room disturbs you. In fact, a patient's bill of rights can be so important that Herbert S. Denenberg, former Pennsylvania insurance commissioner, developed a set of patient hospital rights while in that office. Some are included in the previous statements, while others are listed as follows:

- The public has the right to good quality care and high professional standards that are continuously monitored and reviewed, including frank disclosure to the patient when it is discovered that poor quality care has been delivered or when there has been medical or hospital malpractice.
- The public has a right to economical care and to hospital management that operates efficiently and eliminates waste, such as unnecessary services and duplicative and unsafe facilities.
- The public has a right to have its voice heard in the management, control, and planning of hospitals; in the case of community hospitals it should be assured of a board of directors that represents a broad cross-section of the community.
- The public has a right to full information about the finances and activities of the hospital.
- The patient has a right to a redress of grievances in a reasonably efficient and timely fashion.
- The patient and public have the right to full disclosure of any hospital relationships that pose an immediate or potential conflict of interest such as when a physician has an interest in or owns a for-profit hospital or outside laboratories, nursing homes, or health facilities to which he sends his patients.
- The patient has a right to continuity of care, including timely response to his needs and appropriate transfer to other facilities.
- The public has a right to expect a hospital to behave as a consumer advocate rather than as a workshop for doctors and hospital officials. The hospital should provide leadership in improving healthcare in the community.[11]

Whether or not you agree with these principles of patients' rights and responsibilities in a hospital, they do present a framework of what you should expect and what is expected of you as a patient. Knowing these rights and responsibilities should answer many questions, thus allowing you to recuperate with a greater ease of mind and leave the hospital more quickly. Ask whether hospitals in your community have a patient's bill of rights and whether you could obtain a copy.

HOW TO JUDGE THE QUALITY OF A HOSPITAL

Thus far, we have discussed the kinds of services and medical departments a hospital may provide and contain, the kinds of measures you as a consumer can take to reduce your personal hospital bill, and the rights and responsibilities you have when you are admitted to such an institution. While the establishment of patients' rights is one barometer of a hospital's quality in terms of patient care, there are other measures available by which to judge its standing versus that of other hospitals in your community.

"Michael, why do you have so much faith in the quality of the hospital to which you're being admitted and how do you know it has the ability to treat your illness

successfully? My wife and I don't have much experience with hospitals except for the times when our children, Yael and Talya, were born there."

"Well, Barry, the whole health field has changed since those days. Do you realize that the Internet didn't even exist at that time. Today, you can go online and look up various 'report cards' about different hospitals and the quality of care they deliver. Even Medicare, for which I still do not qualify, has a place on its Web site that compares hospitals in this country. Have you ever heard of the Joint Commission on the Accreditation of Healthcare Organizations? Well, this group examines various aspects of a hospital's operations, and if the hospital passes its examination, the Joint Commission will give the hospital its accreditation. That is another good sign you should look for. Also, check on the quality of the hospital's staff, if you can, before you get sick. There are certain benchmarks you should be looking for in this regard as well."

"Michael, this is great advice. I plan to look into these various areas in more detail."

Hospital Accreditation

Regardless of your physician's hospital affiliation, if there is more than one institution in your community, you can have confidence that any hospital which has accreditation has voluntarily met high standards of patient care and is continually trying to offer the best health services possible. A Certificate of Accreditation is granted a hospital if it has met the standards established by the Joint Commission on Accreditation of Healthcare Organizations, which represents the American College of Physicians, the American College of Surgeons, the American Hospital Association, the American Medical Association, the American Dental Association, and the public. The following are among the criteria by which the Joint Commission judges the quality of a hospital prior to awarding or denying accreditation:

- a safe and sound physical plant
- good facilities and equipment
- special services such as pharmacy and dietary
- a competent and qualified medical staff
- a responsible governing body
- trained nursing staff and adequate personnel
- a medical library
- trained administration
- good medical records
- a review of the hospital's medical cases and their medical outcomes[12]

Beginning in January 2003, the Joint Commission on the Accreditation of Healthcare Organizations announced that its hospital inspectors will look at eleven mandatory patient safety standards to reduce medical errors. The standards are the organization's first detailing of specifications for patient safety. They list six goals:

- improving the accuracy of patient identification
- improving effectiveness of communication between caregivers
- improving safety of potentially lethal medication
- eliminating wrong-site surgeries
- improving the safety of using infusion pumps to administer intravenous medication
- improving the effectiveness of audible alarms signaling when a patient is in distress

In more specific terms, some of these standards include:

- demanding better methods of correctly identifying patients when giving blood tests or medication;
- doctors and nurses using at least two methods of identifying a patient when taking blood samples or administering medication and verbally conducting a final verification process to confirm the correct patient and procedure;
- making sure concentrated solutions like potentially deadly medications—such as potassium chloride used to treat kidney disease and other conditions—are stored in hospital pharmacies, not patient care units, because they require careful dilutions and measurements and can be fatal if given at full-strength;
- checking to be sure intravenous infusion pumps have a device that prevents too much medication from flowing freely into a patient's blood stream; and
- verifying that hospitals make sure alarms such as those on heart monitors really work and not sound when there is no emergency allowing some hospital workers to ignore them when there is real crisis.

The Joint Commission on the Accreditation of Healthcare Organizations has stated that many of these rules are already at hospitals nationwide, but the rules are not always followed.

As already noted, this accreditation is done on a voluntary basis. There is no legal requirement that a hospital or any other kind of healthcare facility seek it. Thus, it speaks well of such a facility if it asks for and obtains accreditation. The Joint Commission on the Accreditation of Healthcare Organizations also operates similar programs of accreditation for long-term care facilities, adult psychiatric facilities, children's and adolescent's psychiatric facilities, drug-abuse treatment programs, alcoholism treatment programs, community mental health services, homecare agencies, ambulatory healthcare organizations, and services for mentally retarded and other developmentally disabled persons.

In addition to reviewing the previous facets for hospital administration when determining whether or not a hospital should be accredited, the Joint Commission survey team examines other aspects of hospital care. They verify the ownership of the hospital to determine who is ultimately responsible for the facility's performance. The team checks the bylaws of the hospital, and then decides whether the medical staff follows the bylaws. They inquire into the way hospital privileges are granted and delineated. The hospital survey team studies the hospital's provisions for evaluating its own performance and its procedures for self-evaluation, as well as the medical outcomes of these methods—doing the right things right. Thus, the accreditation process is not only a standards-based snapshot of a hospital but also has become, in part, a continuous motion picture that includes performance measures or medical outcomes in a program called ORYX that the board of commissioners of the Joint Commission approved in January 1997 as part of the accreditation process for hospital and long-term care facilities. The quality of medical care rendered can be judged in various ways, such as by the completeness of the patient's medical charts, the frequency with which the mortality review committees meet, and the details covered in these meetings. The survey team examines the records of peer-review committees, organized to determine inconsistencies and deficiencies in the management of patients and to guard against the abuse of hospital privileges, as well as the records of staff utilization committees, which determine whether available bed space is being used efficiently.

Quality of Hospital Services

In examining each service and department, the survey team evaluates the hospital's documented evidence that it is conforming to the Joint Commission standards for accreditation. The evaluation not only includes functional safety and sanitation, infection control, laboratories, and radiology services but also anesthesia services, physical medicine, medical social services, emergency services, hospital-based homecare, pathology services, nuclear medicine services, respiratory services, outpatient services, and special care units.

When the survey team finishes its on-site review, it sends its findings and recommendations to the Joint Commission Hospital Accreditation program. After an overall review, the report and its recommendations are sent to the accreditation committee of the board of commissioners, which may give the hospital one of three ratings: accreditation with commendation for those institutions with the highest scores; accreditation for those institutions in "substantial compliance" with JCAHO standards; or a conditional accreditation, for organizations with serious deficiencies, which then must file a plan of correction and undergo a follow-up survey within six months to become fully accredited or receive no accreditation. Hospitals receiving accreditation usually display their certificate in the lobby. But if you are not sure whether your hospital is accredited, you can find out from the hospital administrator or by writing to the Office of Public Information, Joint Commission on the Accreditation of Healthcare Organizations, One Renaissance Boulevard, Oakbrook, IL 60181.

The Joint Commission on the Accreditation of Healthcare Organizations has also given the consumer an opportunity to participate in the accreditation process. Individuals and representatives of interested groups can now request a hearing before the on-site surveying team. The testimony is taken into account by both the survey team and the Joint Commission when the accreditation is evaluated and made. According to the Joint Commission policies ratified in August 1972, a hospital is required to reveal the date of the impending survey and is expected to post a notice in a public place on the premises at least four weeks prior to the visit. The hospital and the Joint Commission survey team must hold a public information interview, if requested in writing, at the time of the survey.

If, as a consumer, you are not satisfied with the quality of an accredited hospital, there is still another source available to which you can voice your grievance. Under the 1972 Amendments of the Social Security Law, the US Department of Health and Human Services is required to investigate any "substantial allegation" that a hospital receiving funds under Medicare is not complying with prescribed standards of safety and health. If an investigation reveals that a hospital is actually violating federal standards, Medicare funds may be withheld from the institution. A consumer who wishes to make a "substantial allegation" should first become familiar with the Medicare standards—copies of which may be found at your local Centers for Medicare and Medicaid Services office—and then address the specific complaint to the Director of the Bureau of Health Insurance, Centers for Medicare and Medicaid Services, US Department of Health and Human Services, 7500 Security Blvd, Baltimore, MD 21244-1850.

If there is more than one hospital in the community, it is possible that your physician has several institutional affiliations. If he does not have especially strong feelings about admitting you to a particular institution for a special reason (as in the case where open-heart surgery is needed and only one hospital in the community has such a unit), then there are other ways to judge a hospital's quality, accreditation, and cost.

Quality of Hospital Staff

Another yardstick by which you can judge a hospital is whether or not the hospital has a formal program for training medical personnel—that is, is it a teaching hospital or is it affiliated with a medical school? If a hospital has such an affiliation, it has more sources of revenue as well as a wider range of medical skills and diagnostic and treatment sources not normally available to community hospitals, which are supported entirely by taxes and patient charges. Teaching hospitals with medical affiliations are likely to have available, as needed, the services of qualified family doctors and specialists in all fields; they often have full-time staff physicians in charge of key departments; and they attract many of the best young physicians who want residency training in specialties. Such an environment is likely to bring out the best in medical practice among physicians. If your hospital is not affiliated with a medical school or one approved for residency training, you should next consider a hospital that trains house staff and nurses. A hospital that has a nursing school or is approved for training by the AMA Council on Medical Education is preferable to one without such a program.[13] Other aspects of the quality of the hospital's medical staff include:

- What percentage of the staff physicians are board certified? Nationally, about 65 percent of all physicians are board certified. At a good hospital in a large urban center, that figure may reach 80 percent or more. Smaller, more rural communities typically have fewer certified physicians.
- Are doctors available in most specialties and subspecialties? The more serious the ailment or the more complex the operation, the greater the need to have a full range of physicians on hand who can treat any unexpected problems.
- Do the major clinical departments have full-time chiefs? Full-time status allows chiefs to spend more of their time overseeing the department. It also reduces their dependence on referrals from other doctors in the department, leaving them freer to discipline the doctors when that becomes necessary.
- What percentage of the nurses are RNs? Registered nurses have substantially more training than the other principle type, licensed practical nurses (LPNs). About 70 percent of the nurses in the average hospital are RNs.
- How many patients does each RN care for? Ideally, there should be one RN for every one or two patients in an intensive-care unit and for every six patients or so in most other areas of the hospital.

Hospitals that cultivate a progressive philosophy that is strongly concerned with satisfying the patient tend to do the following:

- use primary nursing, in which nurses are assigned to particular patients rather than particular tasks (such as examining patients or giving medications)
- offer self-administered pain medication
- employ a full-time patient advocate and provide full information on patients' rights
- employ social workers who counsel patients or who help them obtain various rehabilitative, social, or financial services
- have a hospice program for dying patients and encourage the use of living wills
- have a birthing center, allow a woman to deliver and recuperate in the same room, and employ midwives
- operate community outreach programs such as support groups for breast cancer or diabetes patients
- have reasonable, flexible visiting hours
- allow friends and relatives to bring food to patients who are not on a special diet, or have kitchens where those patients can prepare their own food[14]

As far as selecting a hospital according to its daily costs is concerned, one way to compare an institution's daily costs is to call and survey all hospitals in your community. In addition, if your state has a state hospital cost commission such as those in Maryland and Massachusetts, this or another health regulatory agency might be able to direct you toward a lower-cost hospital. But the problem with this approach is that the hospital you select in this manner may not have granted to your physician its privileges of practicing in the institution, so you will have to select another doctor. Also, the chances are that the hospital with the lowest daily rate is a municipal one. You may not have the same regard for municipal hospitals as you do for private voluntary community hospitals—even though you may have superb facilities and staff in government-supported hospitals, especially those affiliated with medical schools. But again, since individual municipal hospitals vary from each other in regard to physical and medical care quality, you should check into those in your community to determine their medical status. In addition, do not equate size with quality—depending upon your illness and the kind of medical attention you will require, a smaller hospital may provide you with less hurried and more personal care, which is difficult to measure in terms of monetary and psychological cost.[15] The real worth of a hospital lies in the capacities and abilities of its attending staff as well as in the adequacy and competency of such basic ancillary services as the pathology lab, the chemistry department, and the radiology section. Remember, your physician will make a diagnosis and formulate therapy on the basis of their reports. The reliability of these reports determines the real value of the hospital and the ultimate outcome of your treatment.

Report Cards

One of the newest innovations in judging the quality of hospital care is report cards. This effort to judge the quality of hospital care is so new that there is no standardization in writing these reports or agreement on the contents of care they should measure and include. They are beginning to be available nationally, by state, and locally. But, be aware of their shortcomings. First, these report cards are not available in all parts of the country. Second, hospitals do not routinely measure the coordination of care among various providers, error rates, the sufficiency of pain relief, or functional outcomes of medical treatments.

National

There are at least four national report cards published by various organizations. These include *U.S. News & World Report*, which publishes an annual survey of *America's Best Hospitals*. The Consumers' Checkbook publishes a *Guide to Hospitals*. Health Grades, Inc. publishes *Hospital Report Cards*, and the Joint Commission on the Accreditation of Healthcare Organizations publishes *Quality Check*. In more specific terms:

- *America's Best Hospitals* ranks fifty hospitals in each of seventeen specialty areas. The listing is based on mortality rates, available technology and services, nursing staff levels, and a physician survey. The reader may access the list by Web site (http://www.usnews.com) or telephone (1-800-436-6520). It is searchable on the Web site by hospital location or specialty area. It is also available on the newsstands at the magazine price since it is a *U.S. News & World Report* publication; it is free on the Web site.

- *Guide to Hospitals* examines forty-five hundred hospitals. Mortality rates for ten common medical conditions, two kinds of surgery, and adverse-outcome rates for seven kinds of surgery are all compared to national averages. Those who subscribe to Consumers' Checkbook may visit this information free online. For others there is a price for the print copy. The Web site is http://www.checkbook.org and the telephone number is 1-800-213-7283.
- *Hospital Reports Cards* rates more than five thousand hospitals based on volume and mortality rates for more than twenty-five common procedures and diagnoses. Obstetric data are available for some states, including Cesarean rates, volume, and complication rates. The Web site is http://www.healthgrades.com. While free for limited use, the site does sell comprehensive reports on individual hospitals.
- *Quality Check*, published by the Joint Commission on the Accreditation of Healthcare Organizations, does not contain disease-specific or volume information. Rather, it presents the results of the most recent reviews by the Joint Commission. Scores for hospitals, services, and systems are compared with national results. It is free and may be viewed on the Web at http://www.jcaho.com.

Selected States

In addition to national information, as of the winter of 2003, report cards are also available for selected states. These include California, Florida, Illinois, Iowa, Maryland, Massachusetts, New Jersey, New York, Pennsylvania, Virginia, Washington, and Wisconsin. The following is one such report:

- *Healthcare Choices*. While not including any outcome information regarding medical treatment, this report card does contain volume information for specific states on high-risk cancer and cardiac surgeries. This site, which is free, also links to individual state hospital-report sites. The Web site address for this report card is http://www.healthcarechoices.org.
- *Individual states have their own Web sites to check up on hospitals.*
  - ▼ California (http://www.oshpd.state.ca.us)
  - ▼ Maryland (http://hospitalguide.mhcc.state.md.us)
  - ▼ New Jersey (http://www.state.nj.us/health)
  - ▼ New York State (http://www.health.state.ny.us/nysdoh/healthinfo/index .htm or http://hospitals.nyhealth.gov/)
  - ▼ Pennsylvania (http://www.phc4.org)
  - ▼ Texas (http://www.dshs.state.tx.us)
  - ▼ Virginia (http://www.vhi.org)
  - ▼ South-Central Wisconsin (http://www.qualitycounts.org)

Selected Cites and Regions

In addition to national and statewide report cards, there are also report cards available for selected cities and regions. These include Atlanta, Buffalo, Cleveland, Indianapolis, and southeast Michigan. The following is one such report card: *Hospital Profile Consumer Guide* is published by a consortium of major employers, labor unions, and consumer groups. This report contains hospital-specific quality, volume, and patient-satisfaction information for a variety of conditions and procedures, depending on the geographic locale. Quality measures are not the same for each, depending upon the desired outcome. This Web site is free and can be reached at http://www.hospitalprofiles.org.

Medicare's Hospital Compare

Medicare has a Web site, http://www.hospitalcompare.hhs.gov, that provides you with information on how well the hospitals in your area care for all their adult patients with certain medical conditions. For certain basic measurements this information will allow you to compare the quality of care hospitals provide, not only in terms of comparing the hospital of your choice to other hospitals in your state but also to other hospitals in the country. You will see some of the *recommended care* that an adult should receive if being treated for *a heart attack, heart failure, or pneumonia*. The Web site has quality measures on how often hospitals provide some of the recommended care for adults with these conditions to obtain the best results for most patients. The hospitals have agreed to submit these data. This information helps you, your healthcare provider, family, and friends compare the quality of care provided in acute-care hospitals (general hospitals) and critical-access hospitals (small, remote hospitals) that agree to submit data on the quality of certain services they provide for certain conditions. As of 2005 quality information was not available on this Web site for children's, psychiatric, rehabilitation, or long-term care hospitals because they generally do not treat adult patients for heart attack, heart failure, or pneumonia. To find out information about a hospital in your or other areas of the country, you can enter on the Web site the hospital's name, address (state, county, city, zip code), telephone number, and other important information. Hospital Compare was created through the efforts of the Centers for Medicare and Medicaid Services (CMS) of the US Department of Health and Human Services as well organizations of the Health Quality Alliance: Improving Care through Information (HQA), which is a public-private collaborative project established in December 2002 to promote reporting on hospital quality of care. The Health Quality Alliance represents hospitals, doctors, employers, accrediting organizations, other federal agencies, and the public. The information on the Web site can be used by any adult needing hospital care.

   In the *New England Journal of Medicine* (July 21, 2005) the HQA reported on its findings of examining ten quality measures in the treatment of Medicare patients for congestive heart failure, heart attacks, and pneumonia. The study included 3,558 hospitals and found that hospitals which treated a high number of patients outscored those who treated fewer patients on almost every measure. Teaching hospitals did better than nonteaching hospitals in treating congestive heart failure— with 85 percent and 81 percent, respectively—in performing all the recommended steps. On the other hand, the teaching hospitals were 2 percent higher in treating heart attacks than nonteaching hospitals, while nonteaching hospitals were higher by the same amount than teaching hospitals in treating pneumonia. In addition, nonprofit hospitals were about 1 to 2 percent better than for-profit hospitals in treating pneumonia, congestive heart failure, and heart attacks.[16]

In addition, in July 2002 the Joint Commission on the Accreditation of Healthcare Organizations implemented standardized performance measures that were designed to follow the performance of accredited hospitals and encourage improvement in the quality of care. On July 21, 2005, the JCAHO published in the *New England Journal of Medicine* the findings of a study it conducted between 2002 and 2004 on how well 3,087 hospitals followed its guidelines in treating congestive heart failure, heart attacks, and pneumonia. Some of the indicators used included asking patients to stop smoking, administering aspirin to heart attack victims, quickly prescribing antibiotics to patients with pneumonia, and examining how well the heart's principal pumping chamber was working in heart failure patients. The analysis revealed a significant improvement in the performance of US hospitals on fifteen of eighteen measures, and no measure showed a significant deterioration. The size of improvement ranged from 3 to 33 percent over eight quarters studied from July 2002 to June 2004. The JCAHO concluded that, over the two-year study period, it observed consistent improvement in measures reflecting the process of care for acute myocardial infarction, heart failure, and pneumonia.[17]

Ownership Status

Finally, you may wish to think about the ownership status of the hospital in deciding which kind you wish to enter. Of course, you can only be admitted to those hospitals in which your doctor has privileges to practice, but your physician might have privileges in the three kinds of hospitals with different ownership status. These include the voluntary nonprofit community hospital, the privately owned proprietary hospital, and the hospital sponsored by the government—municipal, county, state, or federal. It should be noted at this point that ownership status, whether it be a nonprofit voluntary community hospital or a profit-making proprietary institution, does not reflect the quality of medical care delivered. A proprietary hospital can provide excellent medical care while a nonprofit voluntary hospital may deliver poor care. As far as government-sponsored hospitals are concerned, they may differ from these two kinds of facilities in that they may not possess their luxury or their number of private rooms. The degree and excellence of care a hospital delivers does not depend on its ownership status; as a consumer, you should judge the hospitals on their own merits as healthcare institutions. A nonprofit community hospital, for example, operates under religious or other voluntary auspices. Ultimate responsibility for all the hospital's operations remains with a board of trustees, who generally represent the community's business and professional people. The hospital is managed by a paid administrator, whether he is a layman educated in hospital administration or a new physician. When a doctor disagrees with hospital policy, the view of the board, acting through the administrator, takes precedence. On the other hand, public hospitals are supported by public funds, and services may be lowered when public budgets are reduced. Publicly funded hospitals share a common mission—provision of medical services to the poor. But nonindigent patients may also be admitted to public hospitals, in which case they would be billed at standard rates.

In terms of internal operations, one important element distinguishes public, for-profit, and nonprofit hospitals. In the best of voluntary hospitals, there are strict provisions for the inspection, evaluation, and control of the medical activities of affiliated physicians. Government-sponsored hospitals also tend to have rigid standards. This might not always be the situation in regard to proprietary hospitals, although a proprietary hospital might have a certificate of accreditation from the Joint Commission on Accreditation of Healthcare Organizations. But proprietary hospitals, with notable exceptions, tend to concentrate on illnesses that can be treated relatively simply, without the elaborate equipment or highly specialized technical staff that you might find in a university-affiliated teaching hospital. Statistically, proprietary hospitals have less than their proportional share of blood banks, electrocephalographic services, medical libraries, postoperative recovery rooms, radioactive isotope departments, therapeutic x-ray services, and open-heart surgical units. Rather, they stress surgical operations that require a minimum of operating room personnel and equipment—appendectomies, voluntary abortions, and tonsillectomies, for example. But again, each hospital is dissimilar; look into the facilities and the nature of the procedures offered by the proprietary hospital.

Thus, a proprietary hospital may not have the facilities or health personnel you need for some serious illnesses; on the other hand, for hospitalization calling for routine obstetrical care or bed rest, traction, and analgesics for a back disorder, a patient may do just as well medically and, perhaps, even better financially in an accredited proprietary hospital than in a more expensive accredited nonprofit voluntary institution. Proprietary hospitals may have lower daily charges than nonprofit community hospitals because of reduced operating costs and better management efficiency since they operate on the profit motive and seek to achieve such efficiencies. Despite their profit motive and need to pay taxes (from which voluntary hospitals are exempt) proprietary hospitals, by offering fewer medical services, can sometimes achieve savings in capital expenditures and staff expenses.[18] Of course, it is recognized that some geographic areas may not have a hospital, or only maintain one hospital, which may or may not be accredited. Where you have a choice, look at the various features of a hospital's operation, as already discussed. If you have any questions concerning your local hospital, ask your physician, local county medical society, or state hospital association.

Today's hospital has its problems of rising costs and staffing as a result of many rapid technological innovations taking place in American medicine. It tries to give you every advantage of the new methods of diagnosis and treatment that medical science discovers while providing you with friendly and personal care. But the principal goal of hospital care is and has always been the same—to restore your health and prolong your life.

NOTES

1. "What Is a Hospital?" *Centerscope* (Washington, DC: Washington Hospital Center, Fall/Winter 1977), p. 4.

2. *Controlling Hospital Liability: A Systems Approach* (Chicago: American Hospital Association and Maryland Hospital Education Institute, 1976), p. 23.

3. *What Everyone Should Know about Hospitals* (Springfield: Illinois Department of Public Health, Statewide Health Coordinating Council, 1978), pp. 6–10; Robert Pear, "Emergency Rooms Get Eased Rules on Patient Care," *New York Times*, September 3, 2003; and Ceci Connolly, "Hospital Rules Change Faulted," *Washington Post*, September 4, 2003, p. A2.

4. "What Is a Hospital?" pp. 7–40.

5. Victor Cohn, "Surviving the Hospital," *Washington Post/Health*, April 17, 1985, p. 11.

6. Ibid., pp. 10–11.

7. *Source Book of Health Insurance Data, 2002* (Washington, DC: Health Insurance Association of America, 2002), p. 90.

8. Ibid., p. 91.

9. Ibid.

10. *A Patient's Bill of Rights* (Chicago, IL: American Hospital Association, 1992).

11. Herbert S. Denenberg, *The Shopper's Guide to Citizens' Hospital Rights* (Washington, DC: Consumer News, Inc., 1974), pp. 112–13.

12. *What Everyone Should Know about Hospitals*, p. 11.

13. *The Medicine Show* (Mount Vernon, NY: Consumers Union, 1976), pp. 341–42.

14. Consumer Reports on Health, "Surviving Your Hospital Stay," *Washington Post/Health*, March 26, 1996, p. 15.

15. Sylvia Porter, *The Money Book* (New York: Avon Books, 1976), pp. 258–59.

16. Ashish K. Jha et al.,"Care in U.S. Hospitals—The Hospital Quality Alliance Program," *New England Journal of Medicine* 353, no. 3 (July 21, 2005): 265–74.

17. Scott C. Williams et al., "Quality of Care in U.S. Hospitals as Reflected by Standardized Measures, 2002–2004," *New England Journal of Medicine* 353, no. 3 (July 21, 2005): 255–64.

18. *The Medicine Show*, pp. 341–44.

CHAPTER EIGHT

NURSING HOME CARE

INTRODUCTION

Within recent years, especially since 1965 when the Social Security Act was amended to include both Title XVIII (Medicare) and Title XIX (Medicaid), nursing homes have assumed an ever-increasing role within our society for delivering healthcare services. This role stems from our desire to use skilled nursing homes both as institutions for providing long-term care and as extended care facilities for providing post–acute short-term hospital care in order to reduce, in part, the costs of hospitalization. Thus, the nursing home has become an integral and important part of our healthcare delivery system. As the number of individuals who seek services in nursing homes increases in the future, the healthcare role these facilities presently assume will continue to grow and flourish.

In 1997 there were seventeen thousand nursing home facilities in the United States. They had 1.8 million beds and housed 1.6 million patients. Thirteen percent of the nursing home facilities were hospital based. Medicaid paid 68 percent of nursing home costs; Medicare, 8 percent; and private pay, 23 percent. However, nursing home care is not only for the elderly. Persons with AIDS require nursing home care sometime during the progression of their disease, and special nursing facilities devoted to the care of AIDS patients have developed since the early 1990s.[1] There are also more than a million children in this country with severe chronic illnesses, some of whom require nursing care in a facility or at home.[2] Some of these children may have birth defects or may be retarded or dependent upon machines. Often, for these families, the only recourse is to institutionalize the child—at great cost and heavy emotional sacrifice—or to become "poor" enough to qualify for Medicaid to pay for homecare. A major federal program for children with special health needs is known as Title V of the Social Security Act. However, it provides limited services.[3]

384

In fiscal 2001 Americans spent an estimated $99 billion for nursing home care; that is, about one out of every seven dollars spent in that year for national healthcare ($1.4 trillion). This increasing demand for nursing home care has led to the development of a giant new industry. In addition, the demand for this care is growing at such a rate that it threatens to overwhelm such public medical care programs as Medicaid.[4]

In 1999 about seven million men and women over the age of sixty-five were estimated to need long-term care. By 2020 twelve million older Americans will need long-term care. According to the US Government Accountability Office (GAO), estimates suggest that the future number of disabled elderly who cannot perform basic activities of daily living without assistance may as much as double from 2000 through 2040, resulting in a large increase in demand for long-term care services, especially as the estimated 76 million baby boomers born between 1946 and 1964 become elderly. Most will be cared for at home; family members and friends are the sole caregivers for 70 percent of elderly people. But a study by the US Department of Heath and Human Services indicates that people who are sixty-five years of age face at least a 40 percent risk in their lifetime of going into a nursing home. About 10 percent of the people will stay there five years or longer, with the risk much higher for women than men.[5] The American population is growing older, and the group over age eighty-five is now the fastest-growing segment. Today, the elderly, numbering more than thirty-five million people, represent almost 13 percent of the population. It is predicted that by 2030 this number will double to seventy million persons and about one in five Americans, or 20 percent, will be sixty-five years of age or older.[6] The chances of entering a nursing home, and staying there for a long period, increases with age. In fact, statistics demonstrate that, at any given time, 22 percent of those age eighty-five and older are in nursing homes ands adults age eighty-five and older are the fastest-growing segment of the population with expected growth from four million as of 2001 to twenty million by 2050. Because women generally outlive men by several years, they confront a 50 percent greater likelihood than men of entering a nursing home after age sixty-five.[7]

Whereas once the old and the sick cared for themselves as best they could, or moved in with their children, or were sent to old-age homes for custodial care, there are now nursing home companies all over the country whose principal purpose is to care for the elderly in our society. Increasing age increases the chances of functional limitations. One-third of elderly women age seventy-five and older are functionally dependent and in need of considerable assistance, while another study revealed that 9 percent of people age sixty-five through sixty-nine required day-to-day assistance, including help with bathing, dressing, and eating, compared with 50 percent of those age eighty-five and older.[8]

As in other areas of the healthcare field, fraud and scandal still plague the nursing home industry. Yet there are also nursing homes in which fraud and substandard care do not exist and the elderly can receive the kind of care they require for such illnesses as arthritis, diabetes, cancer, stroke, and heart disease.

The cost of nursing home care can be a financial burden. During 2001, as a national average, a year in a nursing home was estimated to cost $54,900. By 2003 the average national cost of nursing homes was almost $58,000 a year. In some regions of the country, it can easily cost twice that amount. Even homecare can be expensive. Bringing an aide into your home just three times a week—to help with dressing, bathing, preparing meals, and similar household chores—could easily cost $1,000 per month, or $12,000 per year. When the cost of skilled help, such as physical therapists, is added, these expenses can be much greater. By 2004 in-home assistance averaged $18 per hour, or $37,000 per year for forty hours a week.[9] Fortunately, some assistance is available to help individuals pay for part of their nursing home care. This includes public programs such as Medicare and Medicaid and private health insurance plans. Of the estimated $92.2 billion spent for nursing home care in 2000, federal and state governments paid about $55.9 billion (more than one-half the costs); the remainder was paid out of pocket by the patients or their families, private health insurance, or other private sources.[10] Thus, it is very important to become knowledgeable about nursing homes, because at some point in time either you or someone in your family may have to enter a skilled nursing facility. As people live longer, skilled nursing homes can fill a special need caring for people who need health supervision and daily attention but do not require a full range of hospital services. Skilled nursing homes treat young and old alike, even though most nursing home residents are senior citizens. These facilities also treat convalescents recuperating from hospital treatment as well as those who are chronically ill and require the kind of close nursing supervision not available in their family homes. Learning about skilled nursing homes will help you find the kind of facility you want when the time arrives for such a decision.[11] This chapter will discuss the variety of nursing homes available for your needs, the programs available to help you pay for such care, and the kinds of questions you should ask before selecting such a residence for a loved one.

SERVICES AVAILABLE IN NURSING HOMES

Essentially, nursing homes offer three basic kinds of services, as described here:

- *Nursing Care*
     Certain nursing procedures require the professional skills of a registered or a licensed practical nurse. These include administration of medications, injections, catheterizations, and similar procedures ordered by the attending physician. Posthospital stroke, heart, or orthopedic care is available with related services such as physical therapy, occupational therapy, dental services, dietary consultation, laboratory and x-ray services, and a pharmaceutical dispensary.
- *Personal Care*
     This care embraces such services as walking, getting in and out of bed,

bathing, dressing and eating, and the preparation of special diets as prescribed by a physician.
* *Residential Services*

    These services involve general supervision and a protective environment, including room and board as well as a planned program for the social and spiritual needs of the residents.[12]

CLASSIFICATION OF NURSING HOMES

The three basic categories of care described above can be found in a variety of facilities. Your individual personal needs will determine which kind you want. The following facilities provide these different levels of assistance:

* *Skilled Nursing Facilities (SNFs)*

    These nursing homes provide continuous nursing service on a twenty-four-hour basis for convalescent patients. Registered nurses, licensed practical nurses, and nurse's aides provide services prescribed by the patient's physician. Emphasis is placed on medical nursing care with restorative, physical, occupational, and other therapies provided. This kind of facility is eligible to participate in both Medicare and Medicaid.
* *Intermediate Care Facilities (ICFs)*

    These facilities provide regular medical, nursing, social, and rehabilitative services in addition to room and board for individuals who are not capable of fully independent living. Intermediate care facilities are for residents who require less intensive nursing care than that provided by skilled nursing homes. This kind of facility may elect to be recognized for the Medicaid program. Skilled nursing facilities and intermediate care facilities that choose to participate in Medicare and Medicaid must meet the National Fire Protection Association's Life Safety Code.
* *Residential Care Facilities*

    These facilities provide safe, hygienic, sheltered living to individuals who are capable of functioning in an independent manner. The residential care facility stresses the *social* needs of the resident, rather than the *medical* needs provided by skilled nursing facilities and intermediate care facilities. Residents are provided dietary and housekeeping services, medical monitoring, and social, recreational, and spiritual opportunities.
* *Adult Daycare Facilities*

    These facilities provide nursing and nutritional services and medical monitoring in a clean and comfortable nonresidential environment. Adult daycare affords the older person an opportunity for making his or her own decisions, while allowing the long-term care facility the opportunity to participate actively in community affairs.

- *Mental Healthcare Facilities*

    As governments reduce their support for public mental healthcare facilities, a growing number of patients are entering alternative long-term care facilities for comprehensive psychosocial services with therapeutic intervention and remedial education in a homelike setting. Long-term care facilities have begun to fill this social and healthcare need.

- *Childcare Facilities*

    These facilities meet the long-term needs of chronically ill children. A close staff/parent/child relationship must be formed to guide the ill or impeded child toward normal development. Specialized nursing, social, and educational services are provided under medical supervision in close concert with all members of the family.[13]

After you and your physician discuss the kind of nursing home service you want, obtain a list of those that serve your community. Your physician and social worker will be familiar with such facilities. Other sources of information and referral include your state nursing home association, your local Social Security agency, your local medical society, your community welfare agency, or your state health and welfare departments, as well as the yellow pages of your local telephone directory. Your friends or neighbors are also good sources of advice if they are acquainted with someone in a nearby nursing home. Your church and synagogue can also give you the names of nursing care facilities. By telephoning the homes in the initial list, you usually can narrow the field to two or three that offer the services and the location you seek. Plan to visit each of these homes. Talk with administrators and tour the facilities.

Many qualified nursing homes participate in two voluntary standards programs. One is conducted by the Commission for Accreditation of Rehabilitation Facilities, which might include nursing homes. The other is the accreditation program of the Joint Commission on Accreditation of Healthcare Organizations. Their certification is based upon on-site surveys of the facility's operations to determine whether they are in substantial compliance with the standards of the Joint Commission. Find out whether your nursing home has been reviewed by both the state and the national associations for accreditation and what were the results of their reviews.

DEFINITION OF A SKILLED NURSING HOME

"Elaine, I think the time has come to think about putting Mother into a nursing home. We both work and Mom now requires 'round-the-clock care each and every day, and we simply can't provide it anymore."

"John, Mom will never agree to go into a nursing home. We all have read all those terrible stories about what goes on in those places."

"But, Elaine, it's always the bad news that makes the headlines. You never hear about the good nursing homes in this country and there are many of those, too."

"But, how do we go about checking out these facilities to decide if they are good or bad. We don't know anything about nursing homes or the care they provide. We don't even know what to look for or even the kind of questions we should be asking if we walked into a nursing home today."

"Well, Elaine, I know if I was just walking into one, I would like to know who is operating the nursing home, the kind of patient care they deliver, what kind of physical environment the patients live in and how safe is the home itself. How many times have we heard about nursing home fires where not all the patients are sufficiently ambulatory and get out in time."

"John, these are good points you are raising. I am sure that there must be some kind of checklist available that tells persons what to ask and look for when deciding upon a nursing home."

There are many ways to judge quality of care. But in order to do so, you need a set of standards against which to judge each nursing home you visit. One of the best standards available at the moment is the Medicare program, which offers, among other benefits, nursing home coverage to elderly persons who qualify for it. In examining any skilled nursing facility, find out whether, as a minimum, it adheres to the following Medicare standards in its daily operation. If it does not, it is likely that Medicare did not certify the facility—in which case be careful. Find out whether the nursing home has other qualities you desire. To be certified under the Medicare program a skilled nursing home must meet the following standards:

- *Licensure*

   A skilled nursing home must be licensed in accordance with state and federal laws, including all applicable laws relating to staff, licensing and registration, fire, safety, and communicable diseases, as well as other standards required by various state and local laws. Write to the state government nursing home licensure agency, which may be either in your state health or welfare department, to obtain a copy of its licensure standards.

- *Physician Services*

   A skilled nursing home must have a medical plan designed by a doctor. Furthermore, doctors must always be on call for routine medical examinations as well as for emergencies.

- *Governing Body and Written Policies*

   A skilled nursing home must have a governing body legally responsible for policies and the appointment of a qualified administrator, as well as written policies established in consultation with and periodically reviewed by a professional group that includes a physician and a registered nurse.

- *Utilization Review Plan*

   A skilled nursing home must have a utilization review plan in which a committee of medical people regularly review and evaluate the entire medical program—policies, admissions, treatment, and case histories—to determine whether Medicare coverage should be continued.

• *Physician's Recommendation*

Skilled nursing home care can be covered by Medicare only if the patient is admitted on a physician's recommendation. Each patient must be under the regular care of a physician.

• *Twenty-four-Hour Nursing Care Services*

A skilled nursing home must have twenty-four-hour nursing care services. There must be enough nurses on duty at all times, including at least one registered nurse employed full time. There must be a registered nurse or a licensed practical nurse in charge of each tour of duty who knows about such things as medications, special feeding methods, and skin care. There must also be a continuing in-service educational program for all nursing personnel.

• *Hospital Transfer*

A skilled nursing home must have an agreement with one or more Medicare-participating hospitals for transferring patients when such transfers are medically determined by the patient's physician.

• *Drugs*

A skilled nursing home must have appropriate methods for obtaining and dispensing drugs and biologicals according to accepted professional standards. Emergency drugs must be available and stored in an appropriate manner.

• *Medical Records*

A skilled nursing home must maintain a separate and confidential clinical record for each patient, including individual care plans and case histories.

• *Rehabilitation Services*

A skilled nursing home must provide skilled rehabilitation services in such areas of posthospital care as speech, hearing, and physical therapy to help the patient maintain and improve his functional abilities.

• *Social Services*

A skilled nursing home may provide for the patient's medically related social needs (by its own staff or by arrangement with the local welfare department) but is not required to do so.

• *Other Medical Services*

A skilled nursing home must have arrangements for obtaining required clinical, laboratory, x-ray, and other diagnostic services such as those provided by dentists.

• *Food*

A skilled nursing home must serve adequate food to meet the dietary needs of patients. A qualified person must prepare food in compliance with all sanitary and safety codes. Therapeutic diets, as prescribed by a doctor, must be given and meals must be served three times a day.

- *Activities*

    A skilled nursing home should encourage self-care—that is, the patient's return to normal life in the community through social, religious, and recreational activities and by visits with relatives and friends.

- *Building and Maintenance*

    A skilled nursing home must be constructed, equipped, and maintained to insure a safe, functional, sanitary, and comfortable environment for patients. Fire rules must be posted.

- *Infection Control*

    A skilled nursing facility must have an infection control system under the supervision of a committee composed of members from all staff departments of the facility.

- *Institutional Plan*

    A skilled nursing home should have an institutional plan that is available to the public and includes such information as its personnel policies and its operating budget.

- *Staff Education*

    A skilled nursing home should have ongoing programs to keep all personnel informed of new methods in patient care.

- *Admission Policies*

    A skilled nursing home should have admission policies that do not discriminate against race, color, creed, or national origin.

- *Emergency Plans*

    A skilled nursing home must have emergency plans for evacuation and must regularly hold fire drills involving staff and patients.[14]

Although the previous enumeration centered on the standards that skilled nursing homes must meet under government medical care programs, be careful as to the kind of facility you choose—be it skilled, intermediate, or residential care. If Medicare and Medicaid payments are involved, make sure that the facility has been given its proper designation—skilled nursing facility (SNF) for Medicare or Medicaid or intermediate care facility (ICF) for Medicaid eligibility—and confirm that the home participates in these programs. As your physician will advise you, you do not need a higher quality of services than the situation requires. Choosing a nursing home according to your individual needs will not only hold down your health costs but also will allow others who are in greater need of more services to obtain them. Tour a nursing home several times at different times of the day, and make notes about what you observe. Do not forget, many nursing homes have waiting lists. Also, remember that you will rarely find the nursing home's services clearly defined in the name of the facility. For this reason, it is important to use the previous enumeration of standards as a checklist against which to judge the quality as well as the range of services a nursing home offers. In addition to voluntary accreditation certificates noted earlier, there are several other certificates and licenses a nursing home should have and display so you will know that it has met all the laws set by federal, state, and local governments:

- *Current State Nursing Home License*
  Licensing periods and facilities standards vary from state to state. Check with your state health and/or welfare department to determine whether the nursing home in which you have a selection interest has a current license to operate. Beware of temporary or provisional licenses.
- *Current Administrator License*
  This license is required of all administrators and is subject to periodic renewal (usually every one to two years).
- *Current Fire Safety Certificate*
  Issued by the National Fire Protection Association, the certificate indicates that the facility has met fire safety standards as set forth by the Fire Safety Code.
- *Periodic Nursing Home Inspections*
  Inspections are carried out by an independent state agency certifying that all state requirements have been met. Find out from your state health and/or welfare agency which agency makes these inspections in your state. Ask about their findings, and even recommendations, about the quality of the nursing home in which you are interested. In the fall of 2002, a federal district court in Washington, DC, upheld the government's right to inspect, cite, and sanction nursing homes that jeopardize their residents' health and safety. The judicial decision reaffirms the power of the enforcement system that has been established to protect nursing home patients. It is law that the state inspection report (CMS-2567) be posted conspicuously at the nursing home. Look for it. If it is not posted, this fact should raise suspicions about the quality of the facility. You should also review several inspection reports from several years to determine how consistent the nursing home's record is. In addition, look at complaint files and lawsuits that can also reveal the quality of care that a nursing home provides.

The previous licenses and certificates are required in each state. If they are not on display, find out whether the nursing home has obtained these various seals of state approval. Ask to see them for your own peace of mind, safety, and well-being. The American Health Care Association recommends that consumers not use a nursing home that does not have a current state operating license or whose administrator is not currently licensed by the state.

The most important element in selecting a nursing home is the condition of the prospective patient. An older patient has different needs than a younger one. A bedridden patient has different needs than an ambulatory one. Remember, you cannot change the patient or resident to fit the home—you must pick the home to fit the patient. If possible, look into nursing homes long before your relative needs one.

Once your relative becomes a resident, get involved in the initial care plan and attend monthly care plan meetings. To help your loved one obtain the best care, it is helpful for the nursing home staff to know about that person. You may want to share such information as the new resident's interests or hobbies; personality and ability to cope with problems; work history and educational level; cultural and religious background; values and beliefs; routines and habits; likes and dislike; important relationships (past and present); how the person may be consoled if upset; the individual's losses, disappointments, or successes; his family of origin, and where he was born and lived; and other kinds of information that will enable the staff to understand your loved one and provide the kind of care he needs. Speak up when the care you find is poor or even mediocre. Praise the staff when the care is good. Although no checklist or guide is a foolproof guarantee against selecting the wrong nursing home for your needs, your chances of making a mistake can be considerably lessened if you obtain the following information. For this reason, I have divided the operation of nursing homes into four broad categories: administrative management, patient care, environmental health, and fire safety/construction standards.

ADMINISTRATIVE MANAGEMENT

One of the most important aspects of a nursing home's operations is the administrative management policies it adopts and adheres to in its daily activities. These policies ultimately have a direct influence on the patient's well-being. For example, an administrator's training and education can determine how well he is able to understand and meet the medical, social, and psychological requirements of his patients. The kind of residents with whom the patient associates is determined by the admission policies of the facility. The adequacy of the food service and housekeeping operation has a direct impact on the patient's nutritional health as well as on the kind of physical environment in which the patient resides. Consequently, in examining the administrative aspects of any nursing home you are considering, you will need the following the information:

Administrator's Qualifications

- What kind of education does the nursing home administrator have? Is it just a high school education, or college, or graduate school? What is his field of training—social work, gerontology, sociology, psychology, business administration, law, or other fields?
- When the administrator is absent, who assumes the responsibility for the nursing home's operation? How competent is this individual and what is his or her background, training, and education for this field and position? When absent from the facility, can the administrator be easily reached? On weekends? In emergencies?

- Does the administrator participate in extracurricular or continuing-education programs to keep up-to-date on knowledge related to his position?
- Does the administrator have preemployment as well as annual physical examinations to protect his own health as well as that of the patients?
- What is the minimum age at which an individual can serve as an administrator? Do you consider this age too young for the patient's safety and well-being?
- Is the administrator courteous and helpful? Does he know the patients by name? Does the nursing home administrator make himself readily available to patients and visitors alike or answer questions, hear complaints, or discuss problems? If you find that the state survey's results are poor or there are areas of the nursing home that you find troublesome, will the administrator be receptive to your questions and answer them in a manner that you find informative and acceptable?
- What kind of ownership does the administrator work for? A corporation or a nonprofit or religious group? Ask the administrator whether the nursing home has been accredited by the Joint Commission on the Accreditation of Healthcare Organizations? Has it ever applied for accreditation?
- Does the administrator post addresses and telephone numbers of the nearest state nursing home ombudsman and state and local agencies responsible for nursing home regulations and benefits in a prominent patient/resident activity area as well as provide this information upon request?

Personnel Policies

- Does the nursing home require preemployment physicals and x-rays as well as annual physical and x-ray examinations of all its personnel so as to protect them and nursing home patients from illness, especially communicable disease?
- Does the nursing home maintain current employee records, including the records of all employee illnesses and accidents occurring while employees are on duty?
- Does the nursing home maintain an in-service training program for its personnel?
- Does the nursing home maintain written job descriptions for each employee's position so that each employee knows what is expected in terms of contributing to a healthful environment for the patients?

Residency Policies

- Does the nursing home permit patient visiting hours? Are these visiting hours on a daily, weekly, or monthly basis? What hours of the day are set aside for visiting a patient? Are visiting hours flexible during the day or are they fixed or limited—such as an hour per day or, for example, between 7:00 PM and 9:00 PM? Do the visiting hours accommodate residents and relatives?

- Does the nursing home allow patients to attend religious services if they wish and are able to do so? Does it allow religious observances to be a matter of choice?
- Does the nursing home grant privacy in receiving and sending a patient's mail? Does the resident have freedom and privacy to attend to personal needs?
- Is there a resident council in the nursing home? How often does the council meet? Is it on a regular or infrequent basis? How are complaints from patients and residents handled? Has the nursing home established a procedure that includes the designation of a staff member who is responsible for handling the recommendations and maintaining a record of comments, recommendations, and steps taken by the facility to address the issues raised?
- Does the nursing home provide social and recreational activities suited to the needs and interests of the patients as an important adjunct to an active treatment program? Are individual patient preferences respected? Are they group or individual activities or both? Does the nursing home encourage self-care and resumption of normal activities by the patient? Do all patients have opportunities to socialize? Do the residents look happy?
- Can a patient veto experimental research as in regard to drugs, treatments, and other matters? Does the nursing home provide the resident this protection if the patient did not sign an informed and written consent?
- Does the resident have the right to see anyone except the attending physician and facility nursing staff for medical purposes?
- Does the resident have the right to obtain knowledge of all medical tests and medications through his/her attending physician or physician-designated staff member?
- Does the nursing home provide residents and their families with discharge planning services?
- Can married couples share a room unless medically contraindicated and documented by the attending physician on their medical records? Does the nursing home separate nonmarried male and female patients?
- Does the nursing home allow residents the opportunity to meet privately at any time with individuals of their choice in a manner that does not interfere with the equal rights of fellow patients?
- Are residents prohibited from smoking in their rooms?
- If the nursing home accepts children, does it separate the older patients from the children, or family groups or children thereof?
- Does the nursing home maintain a record of a patient's personal possessions? Does the nursing home provide residents with individual storage space for their private use?
- What is the minimum age for entering the nursing home as a patient?
- Are private rooms available? Is the resident allowed to bring his or her own furniture? Are the nursing home patients permitted to decorate their own bedrooms? Wear their own clothes? Do the rooms look personal or institutional?
- Does the nursing home have a patient's bill of rights? In 1999 the US Supreme Court reinforced disability rights laws, ruling that if a disabled person prefers

to live in the community and care services would cost the same or less than a nursing home, restricting him to an institution is isolating and discriminatory, with the result that older Americans have begun to use these disability laws in suits to rejoin the community. Are the rights clearly posted? Does the home observe civil rights regulations, including the right to privacy and to be secure from unreasonable governmental search or seizure of his/her person, papers, or effects; the right to vote and not to be deprived of life, liberty, or property without due process of the law; and the right to enter into contractual relationships, including marriage and divorce, and execute legal instruments such as wills? May a resident communicate with anyone without censorship? Can patients and relatives discuss complaints and voice grievances without fear of reprisal as guaranteed by the Nursing Home Reform Act of 1987?

- Can patients manage their own finances if capable or obtain an accounting of their funds if not? What provisions are there to handle funds of patients who are unable to handle money themselves? How are residents' personal cash and valuable possessions protected? Do residents get receipts and regular reports?
- Are residents, visitors, and nursing home volunteers pleased with the facility? Ask their opinion about how the facility treats them as well as what life is like within the facility.
- Do staff members respond quickly to patient calls for assistance? Is the staff neat, clean, and well groomed?
- Do patients find that staff members have an interest in and affection for them? Is the staff courteous and respectful or angry and intimidating? Do they find time to talk with patients and make them feel at home? Are the patients spoken to as adults or as children? Do you see staff members on the floor actually helping residents, or are they all gathered around the nursing station, or are they nowhere in sight? Does the staff honor a resident's privacy? Does the staff knock before entering a resident's room?
- Do patients find that the nursing home is warm, pleasant, and cheerful? Do you have similar feelings? How do the residents look? Are they out of bed, dressed, clean, chatting among themselves and staff, or are they slumped in wheelchairs? Is there a general level of chatter as in a normal household? Or is there noise blaring from the TV and cries of help or "nurse"? Is there a sense of fellowship among the residents? Be cautious about the facility if the nursing home administrator does not allow you to talk freely with patients and staff.

Patient Transfer Arrangements

- Does the nursing home transfer or discharge patients without first notifying the patient's next of kin or sponsor? Does the nursing home transfer or discharge the patient arbitrarily? According to the Nursing Home Reform Act of 1987, nursing homes must give notification to a resident prior to an impending discharge or transfer plan.

- Does the nursing home have in effect patient transfer agreements or arrangements with other institutions such as hospitals when the need arises? Is emergency transportation readily available?
- Will it be necessary for a resident to move if the resident needs more or less care in the future?
- Are the residents, family, and, where applicable, guardian informed at admission of the reasons for which patients may be involuntarily transferred or discharged by the facility, including nonpayment of charges for their stay and services (except as prohibited by Medicare and Medicaid regulations); the physical, mental, and/or medical welfare of the patient or that of other patients; and medical reasons that include the reclassification of the level of care by the attending physician or a government agency that is responsible for determining the placement of patients for Medicare/Medicaid eligibility.

Food Service Regulations

- Does the nursing home allow animals in the food service area? Many states prohibit this situation for the patients' health and safety?
- Is the nursing home's milk and ice supply sanitary?
- Does the meat, poultry, or meat products used by the nursing home come from state or federally inspected and approved sources?
- Do the food handlers have hand-washing facilities in the nursing home?
- Do food service personnel wear clean washable garments and hair nets or clean caps?
- Does the nursing home employ, or has it a record of employing, persons with symptoms of communicable or infectious disease?
- Is a professional dietician responsible for the nursing home's food service? If not, does it have the consultation services of a professional dietician or other person with suitable training? Does a dietician plan menus for patients on special diets?
- Does the nursing home prepare and serve therapeutic diets as prescribed by the attending physician?
- Does the nursing home follow dishwashing procedures as outlined in the state's nursing home licensure manual? You can obtain a copy of this manual from the nursing home agency of your state health and/or welfare department.
- Does the nursing home follow and provide the minimum daily food allowances enumerated in its state licensure manual (for those states that have such regulations) or the dietary allowances of such organizations as the Food and Nutrition Board of the National Research Council of the National Academy of Sciences, Washington, DC—dietary allowances that are adjusted for age, sex, and activity?
- Does the nursing home have sanitary refrigeration for perishable food? Is food needing refrigeration left standing out on counters? Is waste properly disposed of?

- Are personal patient likes and dislikes in regard to food taken into consideration?
- Is there a variety of food served from meal to meal? Does the food look appetizing and is there enough of it? Does the food from the kitchen smell good? Is the food tasty? Eat a meal if you can. If not, ask residents how the food is. Are they eating it? Are fresh fruits and vegetables served?
- Are meals served at convenient hours? Are at least three meals served each day? Are meals served at normal hours?
- Does the nursing home allow sufficient time for eating meals?
- Are nutritious between-meal and bedtime snacks available to patients?
- Is food delivered to patients who are unable or unwilling to eat in the dining room?
- Does the nursing home provide help with eating when such assistance is needed? Do they get this help promptly? Does there appear to be enough staff to help those who cannot feed themselves? Be aware that as of October 26, 2003, the US Department of Health and Human Services permits nursing homes to hire less trained, lower-paid workers to feed residents who cannot feed themselves. Until that October date, this task was performed only by licensed nurses, certified aides, and other care providers. The feeding assistants are not required to pass a competency test as required in the instance of aides, and they can feed residents without direct supervision from nurses or aides. The feeding assistants are only required to receive eight hours of training—far less than the seventy-five hours the nurse's aides must complete. Critics of this new rule state that the new rule may raise the risk of choking and other problems among the residents.
- Is food served at the proper temperature? Are warm dishes served warm and cold dishes served cold? Are warm dishes served in covered plates? Are patients served food on regular dishes with silverware, or must they eat from paper plates with plastic utensils?
- Are the food preparation, dishwashing, and garbage areas separated? Is the kitchen clean—the floors, the stove, and the refrigerator?
- Do the meals match the posted menus? Do the residents seem to be enjoying themselves? Can residents have visitors join them at mealtime? Is there a charge? Meals become very important to nursing home residents. Ask to have a meal with them.

Admission Policies

- If the patient has private insurance, does the nursing home inform the patient upon admission as to how much the insurance policy covers in terms of basic care and how much the patient may have to pay out of pocket?
- Does the nursing home admit Medicaid patients?
- Does the nursing home admit narcotic addicts?
- Does the nursing home admit alcoholics?

- Does the nursing home admit mentally ill patients who are dangerous to themselves and others? If so, are the mentally disturbed allowed to mingle with the rest of the patients? If not, where do the mentally disturbed reside in the nursing home? Does their place of residence ensure and protect the safety of the other residents? According the Nursing Home Reform Act of 1987, each state must have a screening program to determine whether the admission of mentally ill or retarded persons is appropriate, or whether they could be cared for somewhere else if they do not need nursing facility care.
- Does the nursing home admit maternity patients?
- Does the nursing home admit acutely ill patients who require the kind of medical or surgical care that is more than just first aid? What facilities are available in the nursing home for treating such acutely ill patients?

Housekeeping Services

- Does the nursing home provide sanitary laundry and linen service? How is laundry handled? Is it ironed? Is there an extra charge for this service? How often are the bed and table linens changed?
- Is the nursing home free from insects and rodents? Does the home use an extermination service? How often do they visit?
- Are the furniture, towels, and bedding clean?

Transportation

- Does the nursing home provide transportation for residents?
- Is the home located on a bus route for the convenience of residents and visitors?

Lifecare Contracts

- Does the nursing home offer a lifecare contract? Lifecare contracts are legal agreements that, when entered into without competent legal advice, objective financial analysis, and a complete medical evaluation of an individual's life expectancy, are fraught with many pitfalls for the unwary patient. For example, lifecare contracts can be noncancellable—if a resident does not like the nursing home and wants to move elsewhere, he cannot rely upon getting back the balance of the money given to the nursing home for the purposes of lifecare. Lifecare contracts may not always cover skilled nursing care—if a patient needs the kind of long-term care that is not available under the contract, he may never receive the service. Finally, a lifecare contract may deprive both the resident and the nursing home of the welfare benefits to which the resident would otherwise be entitled. However, it should be noted that there is a possibility that patient's contract might provide that a deposit be made by the resident to the nursing home from which monthly payments to the facility are drawn; when the deposit is exhausted, the resident might be able to apply for welfare payments, with the nursing home agreeing to keep the resident at the welfare rate. Consequently, before signing a lifecare contract with a nursing home explore all of its ramifications.

Selecting a nursing home that will provide loving and high-quality care for a loved one can be a very difficult task. The answers to previous questions directly affect the emotional and physical well-being of the patient. We are living in an era in which healthcare is becoming quite complex in terms of the delivery of such services, in the development of new techniques for patient care, and in the complexities of financing the delivery of care through third-party mechanisms. Consequently, it is important to know the educational backgrounds of administrators, and their ability to understand and deliver the quality of services sought in nursing homes should be questioned when you are selecting such a facility.

Another area you should examine is the facility's admission policies. A relatively small number of facilities are exclusively devoted to the care and treatment of narcotics addicts, mentally ill patients, alcoholics, acutely ill patients, and maternity patients. It can, however, be a very unhealthy experience, emotionally or psychologically, to institutionalize the aforementioned patients in the same facility with those afflicted with heart disease or arthritis. Make sure that the admission policies of a nursing home meet your particular needs for the care of a loved one. Even if the nursing home is equipped with such installations as a laboratory, treatment rooms, and therapy rooms, make sure it has the staff to perform the specialized functions required.

Food preparation is another important aspect of the nursing home's operation. This is extremely important because testimony before the Senate Special Committee on Aging in 1997 indicated that thousands of American nursing home residents are suffering needlessly from preventable malnutrition and that inadequate staffing, poor care, and lax enforcement of federal nursing home regulations are making the problem worse. Many factors can contribute to this problem, including the patient having one or more conditions that interfere with eating such as missing teeth, gum diseases, dementia, pain, tremors, difficulty in swallowing, or an appetite diminished by illness, depression, or drug side effects. Other causes of malnutrition can be linked to management factors such as inattention to personal food preferences, a lack of ethnic food for minorities, institutional rules about what and when people can eat, and unappetizing pureed food for those with no teeth or dentures. Therefore, ask whether the state authorities check samples of the food, drink, or other substances for wholesomeness. For purposes of food cleanliness, make sure that the food service personnel have to wear clean garments and hairnets or caps. Also, make sure that sanitary conditions are maintained in the storage and preparation of food. Ask to see the facility's food preparation facilities. Find out from your state or local health authority whether they have inspection reports on file that you may examine in regard to any food or other violations of health or safety standards in the nursing home. Ask the administrator if he would be willing to show you the reports of state or local government inspections.

In judging the quality of the administrative procedures, look at such house-keeping measures as insect/rodent control and the frequency of laundry/linen changes, on the one hand, and the nursing facility's policies, on the other hand, regarding patient transfer arrangements with other institutions—and whether the nursing home consults with or obtains permission from appropriate persons prior to making the transfer arrangements. Each affects the patient's health.

Finally, look at the setting. It is important to consider whether the patient prefers a country or an urban location since this choice may affect his attitude toward a nursing home stay. You should try to ease the patient's transition to the facility by being with him or her on admission day and staying a few hours to get the patient settled in. Try to visit as often as possible and ask friends to make similar visits. Be willing to provide the patient with as much affection and concern as you would if he or she were able to be at home.

One last word of caution. After you find a facility you feel is suitable for your loved one, you may find that it has no vacancies at the moment. Place your name on a waiting list and check interim alternatives such as daycare, nightcare, home health agencies, and other community resources that meet your immediate needs; also con-tact your local social service agency and hospitals to determine whether they pro-vide services that will help your relative or friend. In this fashion, your loved one will continue to receive assistance until a nursing home vacancy occurs.

PATIENT CARE STANDARDS

Another area of great concern to the patient relates to the quality of patient care that a nursing home can render. As of 1996, reports of abuse and neglect in the nursing home industry were widespread, according to state officials and advocates for the country's nursing home residents.[15] In 1986 a US Senate Special Committee on Aging issued the results of a two-year study in which it stated that more than one-third of the nation's skilled nursing homes fail to meet basic federal health and safety standards, and many "resemble 19th-century asylums more than modern healthcare facilities." Senator John Heinz wrote in the report's preface, "We've allowed bed, board and abuse to replace the medical and rehabilitative care the law demands."[16] About four decades earlier, in 1960, another US Senate Subcommittee stated, in part, that "every troubled son or daughter, anxious to find a good nursing home for a mother or father, is dismayed and often shocked by the inadequacy, the hopeless-ness, inherent in most nursing homes. Those who have wandered from home to home seeking decent facilities, a therapeutic environment and a life restoring force pulsing through its system too often have given up in frustration. Or with no other solution feasible or possible, they may consign a parent or troubled relative to an inadequate nursing home, but with a troubled conscience and feelings of guilt. . . . It is this lack of medical care and restorative service in the great majority of homes, labeled nursing homes, which is the number one problem in the nursing home field."[17] These various public and private reports summarize the feelings of many people today who seek nursing home care for a loved one. While there are many fine nursing homes in this country, there are others that are not so good. Therefore, when considering a nursing home for a loved one, don't settle for a single visit. After visiting the nursing home the first time, visit it again several times at different times of the day, such as on the weekend or in the evening when many nursing homes reduce their staff, and make notes about what you observe. Make sure you are completely satisfied with what you have found. Consequently, when examining the issue of patient care in a nursing home today, be sure to ask many questions, including those relating to physician services, physical therapy, restorative care, laboratory/diagnostic activities, dental care, social service, nursing care, utilization review procedures, grooming services, medical records, and pharmaceutical services.

Physician Services

- Will the patient be under the personal medical supervision of a physician licensed by the state? Does the nursing home have an advisory physician or medical director who accepts the responsibility for the medical guidance of patient care within the facility? How much time does he or she spend at the nursing home?
- Does the patient want the service of a private family physician? Is the resident's physician willing to visit the home? Is the nursing home convenient for the patient's personal doctor? Is the nursing home close to a hospital with which the family physician is associated? Is a private physician allowed to attend to the resident? The Nursing Home Reform Act of 1987 guarantees patients a choice of physicians. If a private physician is used, can he or she visit the patient at least every thirty or sixty days as required or even more frequently if needed? Are there regular reports or contacts by the nursing home with the resident's own doctor?
- Does the nursing home have a physician available for emergencies? How often does the nursing home's own physician visit the facility—on a daily, weekly, or monthly basis? Does the nursing home have psychiatric and psychological services available?
- Does the nursing home require that the patient have a physical examination prior to or upon admission to the facility?
- Does the nursing home require annual physical examinations of the patient?
- Is the patient or family allowed to be involved in his plans for treatment? Does the nursing home maintain a plan of patient treatment as required by the Nursing Home Reform Act of 1987? Is the treatment plan reviewed on a regular basis? Is there any evidence of bedsores among patients, indicating that patients are not turned regularly? Do patients get exercise? To assess the res-

idents' health status, nursing homes must fill out a federal form called a minimum data set.

- Are chemical (drugs to control behavior through ingestion or injection of prescribed medication) or physical restraints (to prevent the resident from moving around freely) used on patients only upon physicians' orders? (Some drugs prescribed to control agitation and anxiety can cause the elderly to lose their equilibrium and fall, while some frail elderly patients seriously injure themselves by trying to climb over bed rails that are supposed to prevent falls.) If so, for how long and with what means—torn sheets, leather straps, adult high chairs, or other means? To determine possible abuse in the use of restraints that the Nursing Home Reform Act of 1987 is supposed to curtail, look for redness, bruising, blanching, or welts. Do the restraints cause pain in wrists, waist, chest, or feet? Is there squirming in an attempt to become comfortable? Does the resident bend forward trying to loosen the restraints or rock back and forth? If you suspect any kind of abuse of an elderly patient or want information on the subject, you can visit http://www.safetyforum.com and click on "Nursing Home Abuse Action Group," make a toll-free telephone call to the Association for the Protection of the Elderly at 1-800-569-7345, or go online to http://www.nhadvocates.org, which lists not-for-profit independent citizen advocacy groups throughout the country that are not affiliated with the nursing home industry or federal or state governments and that are concerned with improving the quality of life of nursing home patients.
- Does the nursing home have arrangements with various medical specialists such as those concerned with eye care? What do these services cost in addition to basic charges?
- Can x-rays and cardiograms be done in the nursing homes?
- Do the patients appear alert unless very ill?

Physical Therapy

- Does the nursing home provide physical therapy, if ordered by a physician, under the direction of a qualified full-time physical therapist?

Restorative Services

- Does the nursing home provide restorative services if ordered by a physician? (These may include physical, occupational, or speech therapy as well as podiatry.) Are there specialists in various therapies readily available when needed? What do these services cost in addition to basic charges? Is oxygen available in the nursing home? Does the nursing home have resuscitation facilities available or must it call upon a rescue squad when these services are needed?

Laboratory Services

- Does the nursing home provide laboratory/diagnostic services if ordered by a physician?

Dental Services

- Does the nursing home have arrangements for dental services as required by the Nursing Home Reform Act of 1987?
- Is a dentist available for consultation or emergencies?
- Does the nursing home provide dental examinations of the patient upon admission if ordered by the physician?
- Does the nursing home provide annual dental examinations of patients?

Social Services

- Is a social worker available to help residents and families? Do the social services meet the medically related needs of the patient if the need exists? What kind of social services are provided? Does the nursing home have a social services director? Are there any other counseling services available?

Nursing Services

- Who is in charge of nursing services—a registered or a licensed practical nurse? A registered nurse has a higher level of skills and training. In a skilled nursing home, is a registered nurse in charge or the director of nursing services? Is there a registered nurse (RN) or a licensed practical nurse (LPN) on the floor? Is at least one registered nurse or licensed practical nurse on duty day and night? Is a registered nurse on duty during the day seven days a week?
- What is the ratio of nurses and aides to patients? A ratio of three to one would be considered very good. Since the aides are in most frequent contact with patients, inquire about their training programs, ongoing training, and performance evaluations. In regard to aides themselves, an ideal ratio is one aide to eight residents; more often it is one aide to ten or twelve residents. This ratio often drops at night. Are there enough nurses on hand at all hours? The Nursing Home Reform Act of 1987 established minimum training standards for aides in nursing homes that receive Medicare and Medicaid money and required states to keep registries of aides who passed the required test. A nursing home must check its state's registry before hiring, but there is no national registry, so some aides move to other states and get certificates there if they did something illegal.
- Is there an in-service training program for nurses in the facility?

- Does the nursing home use the services of geriatric nurse practitioners? These are individuals who have received advanced education, most often at the master's level, in the nursing care of the elderly and disabled persons. In addition to advanced nursing education, they also learn the basic elements of medical diagnosis and the management of common problems affecting the elderly.
- How much nursing care per day is provided to patients?
- Does the nursing home have a nursing care or treatment order plan for the patients?
- What kind of patient hygiene is provided? What constitutes these services?
- What is the minimum age of persons allowed to nurse in the facility?
- Do nursing personnel also perform nonnursing duties?
- Can the nurses start intravenous fluids if the patient becomes dehydrated? Can they insert nasogastric tubes and draw blood?

Utilization Review Committees

- Does the nursing home have a utilization review committee?
- What are the duties of the utilization review committee?

Grooming Services

- Is assistance provided in bathing if necessary? Are the residents clean? Do patients have some degree of privacy? Are doors closed or screens installed when patients are given baths? What provisions does the home have for assisting patients out of bathtubs or whirlpools? Are there machines for this or does the home rely on its maintenance man to help lift heavy patients into or out of a bathtub?
- Are barbers and beauticians available for men and women? Are the residents well groomed? Residents may reach out to you. Take their hands. Are they clean, with well-lubricated skin and trimmed nails, or are their hands sticky or dry, with ragged nails?
- Does the nursing home staff encourage a neat appearance and give help when needed? Are patients dressed in clothes that are neat and clean or are they wearing hospital dressing gowns? Can they wear clothes of their own choice? Do they wear stockings, shoes, or slippers?

Medical Records

- Is confidentiality of medical records assured? Are medical records available only to authorized personnel such as those having licensing responsibility for the nursing home?
- Are medical records removable from the nursing home only upon court order?

- How many years after a patient's discharge does the nursing home keep his or her records?
- Does the nursing home maintain the following kinds of records for patient care?
  - ▼ admission record
  - ▼ admission physical examination record
  - ▼ physician order record
  - ▼ physician progress notes
  - ▼ nursing notes
  - ▼ medication record
  - ▼ physician visit record
  - ▼ patient accident/incident record
  - ▼ utilization review plan
  - ▼ death record
  - ▼ discharge record
  - ▼ dental service record
  - ▼ laboratory report record
  - ▼ x-ray record
  - ▼ specialist's consultation record

Pharmaceutical Services

- Are pharmaceuticals only dispensed on the order of the attending physician or dentist?
- Are medications stored in a locked cabinet?
- Are medications that are poorly labeled or damaged returned to the pharmacy for disposal or relabeling?
- Does the medication label include the patient's name, pharmacy, prescriber, date, directions, dosage unit, and prescription number?
- Does the patient have the freedom to purchase medicines outside the home?
- If a medication is prescribed for a specific patient, does the nursing home allow it to be administered to another?
- Is the patient's medication stored and kept in the original container unless otherwise authorized by a physician?
- Can a prescription order be renewed without a physician's permission? If so, why? Under what conditions?
- Does a qualified pharmacist maintain and monitor a record of each resident's drug therapy?
- Is there an excessive use of drugs and tranquilizers? Many listless and drowsy patients may be an indication.
- Does the nursing home keep poisons and medications "for external use only" in a locked cabinet and separated from other medications?
- After the expiration date, is the prescription medicine removed from use? If not, why?

- Are medicines requiring refrigeration kept in a refrigerator?
- If a patient should be discharged or die, is the unused portion of his medication destroyed by the nursing home? If not, what happens to it?
- Can nurses package or repackage, bottle or label, in whole or in part, any medication?
- Does the nursing home prohibit unlabeled medications or medications with illegible labels?
- Does the nursing home have automatic stop orders for dispensing medication after a given time has passed, unless otherwise authorized by a physician?
- Does the nursing home make an inventory of narcotics that is signed and recorded by the nurse in charge, and on what basis—daily, weekly, monthly?
- Does the nursing home maintain a record of the use of narcotics by the patient?
- Are unused narcotics destroyed according to state/federal government regulations?
- Does the nursing home maintain first aid supplies?
- Does the nursing home maintain a pharmacy whose operation permit is approved by the state board of pharmacy? Does the nursing home have a room for storing drugs and other pharmaceutical items?
- Is a state-licensed pharmacist in charge of the pharmacy?
- If the nursing home has no pharmacy on the premises, then does it have contractual services with a pharmacy outside the facility? Does the pharmacy deliver drugs promptly?
- Are residents allowed to choose their own pharmacist?
- Can prescribed medication only be dispensed by a licensed pharmacist/pharmacy?
- Does the nursing home keep an emergency drug kit on the premises? Is the kit kept in a locked box? Are narcotic drugs kept in the emergency drug kit? Does a pharmacist or physician inspect the drug kit to account for and replace used drugs? Can emergency medications in the kit be used only on the orders of a physician or a dentist? If not, who else had the authority to order their use? When medication is used from the kit, does a pharmacist replace the medications and is the kit resealed? If not, why? Are emergency medications issued only in the name of the patient?

In examining the patient care services of a nursing home, try to determine whether the nursing care facility provides just minimal basic services or provides care beyond this level. Basic minimal services may include a patient having a physician to care for him, an emergency physician available to the facility, a registered or licensed practical nurse in charge, medications only administered upon a physician's order, and medications kept in a locked cabinet. Care beyond these minimal services may include the provision of physical therapy; dental, social, and laboratory services; maintenance of an emergency medication kit; and the existence of in-service nursing training programs and nurses' procedure manuals. Find out how much more extra services, supplies, and medications will cost.

Other criteria by which to judge the quality of patient care a nursing home renders are the minimum time intervals that pass between physician visits to a patient and whether annual physical examinations are given to a patient. Ask your physician what his policy is in this regard. Also, find out whether the nursing home has an advisory group of physicians, or an advisory physician, that accepts the responsibility for the medical guidance of patient care. In addition, find out whether the nursing home has a utilization review committee. Extended care facilities certified under federal law must maintain such bodies. Such a committee might review such conditions as overuse or underuse of services, proper use of consultation, and whether or not required nursing and related care is initiated and carried out.

Another way to judge whether the nursing care facility provides certain patient services is by the absence or presence of medical records. The nursing home should, for example, maintain dental consultation and laboratory/x-ray records. It should have physician visitation records to check up on the date and number of visits a physician makes to a patient. It should keep physician progress notes which the physician fills out when visiting a patient. If these records are absent and not kept by the nursing home, it is very likely that such services are not provided. If you desire such services for a loved one, you should probably avoid such a nursing care facility. It is the patient who will ultimately suffer—many patients do not have their own physician, and the doctor who is called in an emergency must work against a serious handicap if the patient's medical history is not available.

Another area to examine in selecting a nursing home is its policy regarding the administration, disposal, and inventory control of narcotics and drugs. Check with your local or state health department to find out whether it has had reports of drug abuse in regard to the facility you are considering. Find out whether a nursing home keeps an emergency medication kit or even a first aid kit. The charge nurse or someone of similar authority should make an inventory of narcotics on a daily basis, which she records and signs, so that the facility's narcotics will not be abused and improperly administered. The nursing home should prevent drug abuse by not allowing a prescription order to be renewed without a physician's permission and by prohibiting the administration of one patient's medication to another. Without these prohibitions, a problem is created whereby a patient can receive a continuous dosage of medication at a level and at a time of treatment when it is no longer needed. The nursing home should be concerned about the age and potency of the patient's medication by requiring that poorly labeled medication containers be returned to the pharmacy for disposal or relabeling and by requiring that the medication be removed from use after its expiration date. The registered or licensed practical nurse should have the responsibility for supervising the administration of a drug. If not, the possibility exists that individuals of a lesser skill or knowledge or training may be supervising such activities. Unless such individuals have the rudimentary knowledge of the characteristics of the drugs for which they are responsible, dire consequences may befall the patient upon the receipt of such a drug. The nursing home should make sure that all the information that a state requires be placed on the label. Find out from your state health agency what information it requires and check it against the nursing home's policy. Also, make sure that the nursing home takes appropriate safeguards with the correctly labeled medication by safely storing and keeping it in its original container unless otherwise authorized by the patient's physician. Make sure that the nursing home keeps poisons and medications marked "for external use only" in a locked cabinet and separated from other medications. These are some of the ways of determining the policies the nursing home has adopted to prevent drug abuse in its facility. To make sure of its compliance, obtain from the nursing home licensure agency of your state/welfare department its licensure requirements, in which the state's standards for pharmaceutical and other services are listed. Also, write to the state pharmacy board for its nursing home requirements so that you can probe into the subject matter in more depth and ask the kind of questions that matter most to you about the facility's patient care policies.

Medicare's Nursing Home Compare

There is another mechanism available to consumers to judge the quality of a nursing home. In November 2002 the Centers for Medicare and Medicaid Services established a new feature on Medicare's Nursing Home Compare Web site (http://www.medicare.gov/nhcompare/home.asp) that provides quality indicators on nearly seventeen thousand nursing homes in the United States. For each nursing home, Medicare has established as many as fifteen long-term performance categories that show the percentage of long-term residents in physical restraints, with weight loss, and with the inability to perform basic daily tasks. Other categories show the percentage of patients with bedsores, pain, urinary tract infection, worsening of ability to move in or around their room, most of their time spent in bed or a chair, catheter inserted and left in bladder, depression or anxiety, and bowel or bladder problems. Some of the short-stay measures (three) include patients with delirium, moderate to severe pain, and pressure sores. But some words of caution: The measures do not address quality-of-life issues such as activities for patients in the nursing home, its overall environment, or the quality of its staff—all important issues in good nursing home care. Also, as another example, there are no comparative numbers on staffing levels—a category considered crucial in determining quality in a nursing home. If you do not have access to a computer or the Internet, you may telephone Medicare at 1-800-633-4227 for information. Be aware that the nursing home is responsible for reporting its own quality indicators—for example, the percentage of patients in pain. But the nursing home may not have sufficient staff to identify all of those patients in pain. Also, the General Accounting Office (GAO), now renamed the Government Accountability Office, that performs studies for the US Congress has stated that 17 percent of the nursing homes listed online had four or more positive indicators and no highly negative scores—all apparently good homes. Yet all those homes, the GAO stated, had been cited by state authorities for practices that physically harmed the patient. So be careful. The data at this site is just one more tool to use in selecting a nursing home for a loved one, but it is no substitute for visiting the facility and talking with staff and families of the residents and asking the questions that are listed in this chapter. Also, be aware that the government has a system called the Scope and Severity Index, which rates the seriousness of a violation of federal minimum standards for patient care. For each violation, a state inspector determines the harm to a resident and how widespread the problem is within a nursing home. Each violation is assigned a letter grade A to L. A is the least serious. Ask the state if these results are available to you in a report so that you can determine the quality of care that the nursing home delivers.

ENVIRONMENTAL HEALTH

A third important aspect of nursing home administration is related to the issue of whether or not a favorable environment exists in the facility for the physical and emotional well-being of the patient. In its certification requirements for extended care facilities, the US Department of Health and Human Services recognizes this fact by requiring extended care facilities to be equipped and maintained to provide an environment that is functional, sanitary, and comfortable. The presence or absence of recreation areas, dining rooms, adequate bedroom furnishings, special care, and physical examination rooms as well as safe and sanitary electrical-mechanical systems can enhance or detract from the functional aspects of the facility's operation—also, they can affect the spirit, attitude, and, ultimately, the basic health of the patients themselves. One innovative approach for improving the environment of nursing homes is the "Eden Alternative" promulgated by the Eastern Idaho Special Services Area (EISSA) VI Agency on Aging, Idaho Falls, ID (1-800-632-4813). The "Eden Alternative" transforms nursing homes into lush, lively human habitats. Gardens, animals, birds, and children bring life and involvement to settings once associated with death and infirmity. So ask for a tour of the home. Walk around on your own. Chat with some of the residents and friends and relatives of residents. Do you like what you see? Does the nursing home's atmosphere seem welcoming? Are things attractive, comfortable, well lit, and clean—as clean as you wish it to be? Consequently, in examining the environment of a nursing home look at the following areas.

Lobby

- Is the atmosphere welcoming? Is there a lounge? Is it being used by the patients?
- Is the furniture attractive and comfortable? Are plants and flowers present?
- Are there wall decorations, as well as a bulletin board activities schedule?
- Are certificates and licenses of the nursing home on display?

Patient's Bedroom

- Does each bedroom have an attendant/nurse call system by each bed? Is there easy access to each bed? Does the bedroom open onto a hallway? Is a public telephone available for the residents' use? Does the bedroom have a window to the outside?
- What kinds of furnishings are in each bedroom? Do they meet the requirements of the patient? Is there a reading light and a comfortable chair, as well as adequate drawer and closet space for a patient's personal possessions? Is there a possibility for individual decorations or preferences?
- Are there screens or draperies for privacy in multipatient bedrooms? Is there fresh drinking water beside each bed?
- Does the nursing home allow more than four patients in each bedroom? How does the patient feel about sharing his bedroom with others? Would he or she be compatible with the roommates? Does the resident have any input into the assignment of roommates?
- Is the bedroom designed to accommodate wheelchairs? Is there at least one comfortable chair for each patient?

Special Care Room

- Is there an isolation room with a bed and a bathroom available within the facility to provide for the special care of patients who develop a contagious or an acute illness while in the facility and for patients who are in the terminal phase of illness?

Physical Examination Room

- Is there a special room provided for the examination and/or treatment of the patient?

Nurses' Station

- Is there a nursing station in the facility? In a multifloor nursing home, is there one on each floor?
- What is the maximum number of beds serviced by the nurses' station? From thirty-five to fifty beds is average in some states.
- How far away is the nurses' station from the most remote room served? About 100 to 120 feet is average in some states.

Utility Room

- Is there a utility room in the facility?

Recreation/Dining Area

- Is there a living room in the nursing home? Is it comfortably furnished?
- Is there a dining room in the nursing home? Are patients allowed to eat in their rooms or must they eat all meals in a dining room? Is it attractive and inviting? Are there comfortable chairs and tables? Are small tables used rather than mess-hall-type tables? Is it easy to move around in? Are the tables convenient for those in wheelchairs? Is the dining room separated from the food preparation area?
- Is there recreation space in the facility? What activities are available, how are they utilized, and are patients satisfied with them? Is there an activities director? Are there volunteers who visit the home and provide entertainment and instruction in such areas as arts and crafts? Is there anything for patients to do other than watch television? If there is equipment available such as games, easels, and other material, do the residents use it? Does the nursing home have an organized program of activities as required by the Nursing Home Reform Act of 1987? Do the patients have a choice in activities and are they allowed a voice in planning them? Does the nursing home have a varied program of recreational, cultural, and intellectual activities for its residents? Does the staff assist the residents in getting from their rooms to activities? Are there outside trips and excursions? Does the staff speak to the residents about activities and where the residents are being taken? Are residents encouraged to participate in community activities outside the nursing home (health permitting)? Are interesting sounding daily schedules posted and given to residents? Are those posted activities actually taking place? Are activities provided each day? Are some activities scheduled in the home on weekends? Is warmth reflected in the nursing home's operations through parties and remembrances of birthdays and anniversaries? Are there group as well as individual activities? Are residents encouraged but not forced to participate? Are the lounges or sitting rooms and common areas used, pleasant, and comfortable? In good weather, can residents sit or walk outdoors?
- Is there an area that provides privacy for meeting visitors and making telephone calls?

Sanitation

- Is the nursing home as clean as your personal standards wish it to be? Is the facility free of unpleasant odors? Are incontinent patients given prompt attention?
- Is the sewage disposal, water supply, and refuse/garbage disposal sanitary? Check with your local health department to learn whether they have on file any violations by the nursing home in this regard.
- Are the lavatory/bathroom facilities clean? Are they convenient to the bed-

rooms? Are they accessible to handicapped residents? Are the lavatory/bathroom areas wide enough for wheelchairs and easy for a wheelchair patient to use? Do they contain any nurse call bells? Are there handgrips on or near toilets? Do the bathtubs and showers have nonslip surfaces and handgrips? Does each bathroom contain a sink, a toilet, and a shower?

* Does the nursing home have an incinerator?
* How is the heating and ventilating system? Are the rooms kept at a comfortable temperature and well ventilated? Is the nursing home air-conditioned?

Grounds

* Can residents get fresh air?
* Are there ramps for the handicapped?
* Is there outdoor furniture for the residents to use?
* Is the atmosphere pleasing to the patient? Are there outdoor patios with shade? Are there hazardous objects in areas where patients may walk?

Geographic Location

* Is the nursing home conveniently located near family and friends for visits?

In examining the physical layout of a nursing home, the presence of an isolation unit for acutely ill or terminally ill patients, an examination/treatment room, and a nurses' station within the facility very greatly influence the quality of care rendered. For example, special care isolation rooms can protect a facility's residents from those who have dangerous communicable diseases or can provide privacy for those in the last moments of their lives; examination/treatment rooms afford the patient the dignity of privacy when he is so engaged. It is also important to know how many patients are allowed in a multipatient bedroom. Many states recommend four, some even six. This knowledge is very pertinent when you realize that the physical and emotional well-being of any patient can be impaired if he or she is subject to overcrowded conditions. Also, some nursing home operators may not be concerned as to whether or not a patient resides under desirable conditions. The lack of the aforementioned units in a facility can continue the impairment of a patient's physical status; the lack of recreational areas for patient social activities and the lack of dining facilities that allow the patient to leave a possibly overcrowded bedroom to enjoy nourishment can be an emotional setback. By determining the kind of environmental health a nursing home will provide for a loved one, you will have another basis on which to judge whether the facility you are considering can meet the complex demands of patient care today and tomorrow without using yesterday's techniques and equipment.

FIRE SAFETY AND CONSTRUCTION

A fourth important aspect of nursing home administration pertains to the patient's physical safety, which, in turn, results from both the protective fire measures a facility adopts and the physical construction of the facility. All too often public attention is focused on the nursing home field for the wrong reasons; an example is when fire or other disaster strikes a facility with the ensuing loss of human life, sometimes owing to the fact that improper measures were taken initially to protect the facility's residents. Thus, both fire safety and construction are interrelated in the sense that the quality and extent of construction can determine the spread or magnitude of a fire or other disaster. Therefore, in examining a nursing home, be sure to ask the following questions.

Fire Safety

- Does the nursing home meet the National Fire Codes of the National Fire Protection Association?
- Does the nursing home meet federal and/or state fire standards?
- Does the nursing home have smoke detectors?
- Is there a written emergency evacuation plan with floor plans posted throughout the facility?
- If the nursing home is higher than one story, are there adequate fire escapes? What are they made of and are they operable?
- Does the nursing home have frequent fire drills involving both the staff and the patients?
- Are exits clearly marked and unobstructed?
- Are exit doors unlocked on the outside? Are they unlocked from the inside?
- Are doors to the stairway kept closed?
- Does the nursing home designate areas where smoking is restricted?
- Are exits clearly marked and signs illuminated?
- Does the nursing home have a fire alarm and sprinkler system? Are they in good operating condition?
- Is there a fire extinguisher in the facility and is it easily accessible in time of need?
- What about electric wiring? Are bare wires exposed?
- How is the nursing home constructed—brick, wood, or other materials? Was it built originally as a nursing home or was it converted? Were any additions made to the original facility? If so, do they have heat, electricity, and adequate fire protection? How old is the nursing home?
- If there is carpeting on the floor, what is the flame spread rate? A facility without sprinklers and with carpeting should have its carpet certified as having a flame spread rating of 75 or less on the American Society of Testing and Materials E-84 Tunnel Test.

- Does the nursing home have a telephone?
- Does the nursing home store flammable liquids and gases in proper storage facilities? Check with the local health department to learn if the nursing home has been cited for any violations of this safety precaution.
- Does the nursing home require that combustible, decorative, and acoustical material be flame resistant?

Construction

- Are hallways, corridors, stairways, and landings unobstructed? Are the halls roomy? Are there ramps for the handicapped?
- Does the facility have emergency lighting?
- How good is the nursing home's security?
- Is the heating plant (boiler/furnace room) enclosed as protection in the event of explosions?
- Are there warning signs posted around freshly waxed floors?
- Are chairs sturdy and not easily tipped?
- Are interior stairwells enclosed? Do the stairways have handrails? Do the stairways have illumination?
- Are the corridors free of hazards? Do the corridors have illumination and handrails on both sides? Are the corridors wide enough for two wheelchairs to pass with ease?
- Are there any signs of plaster falling from walls or water damage indicating roof leaks? Is the facility freshly painted? Are the walls and floors in good repair?
- Are there windows that open in each room?

In examining the fire safety and construction standards of a nursing home, you should be aware of the implications of the previous questions. If a nursing home does not maintain a written fire evacuation plan, the patient may be placed in a very precarious position when his very condition—many times a bedridden one—depends upon the training and sure judgment of another individual. If, in addition, fire drill records are not kept, who is to judge whether such drills take place and decide that the personnel of any given facility in the event of fire or other disaster can act effectively to protect the safety of the patients? Without fire alarms and a telephone, a nursing facility lacks the quickest means of communication in order to notify the proper authorities. Also, the nursing home would lack in the absence of a sprinkler system and fire extinguishers the equipment to eradicate or control the fire until the proper assistance arrives. Unless it has flame-resistant combustible, decorative, and acoustical material, enclosure of the heating plant, and smoking restrictions within given areas of the facility, the nursing home exposes itself to the dangers of conflagration. In such an event, it is important that passageways and stairways contain handrails to assist the residents who need such support. Do not select a nursing home that has not been inspected and cleared for safety during the past year.

Each of the four broad areas just discussed, individually and collectively, has great relevance to the physical and emotional well-being, as well as the safety, of a loved one. No question is too trivial if you feel the answer is important for your peace of mind and that of the prospective patient. The care of the elderly requires much patience and the intangible factor of innate kindness. A warm, pleasant, and cheerful atmosphere within the facility can contribute much to a loved one's attitude toward his stay in the nursing home and to the maintenance of his health.

THE PATIENT'S BILL OF NURSING HOME RIGHTS

In addition to the previous questions, there is another criterion by which to judge the quality of the nursing home—namely, its adherence to a patient's bill of rights, which many hospitals observe today. On October 3, 1974, the US Department of Health, Education, and Welfare (now the Department of Health and Human Services) published regulations in the government's *Federal Register* that set forth a bill of rights for nursing home patients. It is important for you and your loved one to become aware of each of these principles. When considering placing a loved one in a nursing home, try to determine whether these rights have been preserved for those patients already in the facility. If you place a relative in such a facility, make sure that these rights are not compromised in any way. The bill of rights which follows requires that each patient admitted to a facility:

1. Is fully informed, as evidenced by the patient's written acknowledgement, prior to or at the time of admission and during stay, of these rights and of all rules and regulations governing patient conduct and responsibilities;
2. Is fully informed, prior to or at the time of admission and during stay, of services available in the facility, and of related charges including any charges for services not covered under titles XVIII (Medicare) or XIX (Medicaid) of the Social Security Act, or not covered by the facility's basic per diem rate;
3. Is fully informed, by a physician, of his medical condition unless medically contraindicated (as documented by a physician, in his medical report), and is afforded the opportunity to participate in the planning of his medical treatment and to refuse to participate in experimental research;
4. Is transferred or discharged only for medical reasons, or for his welfare or that of other patients, or for nonpayment for his stay (except as prohibited by titles XVIII or XIX of the Social Security Act), and is given reasonable advance notice to ensure orderly transfer or discharge, and such actions are documented in his medical record;
5. Is encouraged and assisted, throughout his period of stay, to exercise his rights as a patient and as a citizen, and to this end may voice grievances and recommend changes in policies and services to facility staff and/or to out-

side representatives of his choice, free from restraint, interference, coercion, discrimination, or reprisal;

6. May manage his personal financial affairs, or is given at least a quarterly accounting of financial transactions made on his behalf should the facility accept his written delegation of this responsibility to the facility for any period of time in conformance with state law;

7. Is free from mental and physical abuse, and free from chemical and (except in emergencies) physical restraints except as authorized in writing by a physician for a specified and limited period of time, or when necessary to protect the patient from injury to himself and others;

8. Is assured confidential treatment of his personal and medical records, and may approve or refuse their release to any individual outside the facility, except in case of his transfer to another healthcare institution, or as required by law or third-party contract;

9. Is treated with consideration, respect and full recognition of his dignity and individuality, including privacy in treatment and in care for his personal needs;

10. Is not required to perform services for the facility that are not included for therapeutic purposes in his plan of care;

11. May associate and communicate privately with persons of his choice, and send and receive his personal mail unopened, unless medically contraindicated (as documented by his physician in his medical record);

12. May meet with, and participate in, activities of social, religious, and community groups at his discretion, unless medically contraindicated (as documented by his physician in his medical record);

13. May retain and use his personal clothing and possessions as space permits, unless to do so would infringe upon rights of other patients, and unless medically contraindicated (as documented by his physician in his medical record); and

14. If married, is assured privacy for visits by his/her spouse; if both are in-patients in the facility, they are permitted to share a room, unless medically contraindicated (as documented by the attending physician in the medical record).

In addition to the patient's bill of rights, make sure that the nursing home also respects a patient's civil rights. Find out whether the bill of rights is posted anywhere in the facility. The patient's bill of rights enunciates many of the principles toward which some of the previous questions address themselves; the fact that a nursing home has adopted such criteria for its own mode of operation speaks positively about the facility you are considering. The more you can learn about a nursing home's operation, the easier will be your eventual decision about placing a loved one in it. Tour the facility during the mornings, afternoons, evenings, and all meal times. Call ahead for appointments. Be thorough.

LONG-TERM CARE INSURANCE

"Edith, I think the time has come to think about the remaining years ahead. Medicare is a great program but unfortunately does not cover long-term care if one or both of us has to go into a nursing home for an extended period of time or perhaps require other kinds of long-term services. Given our economic circumstances, we certainly do not qualify for Medicaid that also covers nursing home care."

"Bill, what do you suggest?"

"I think it's time to look into long-term care insurance. It pays for such basic benefits like nursing facility care and home and community-based care. You can even obtain supplemental benefits like durable medical equipment coverage and other benefits. Plus, these policies give you a choice of increasing your coverage to keep pace with rising medical costs by paying a higher premium But they also give you the choice of not doing so and keeping your premium at whatever price level you are paying when the option to increase the premium is offered."

"Bill, I think this is a great idea to protect our economic security so let's do it."

While no one can predict what kind of care will be needed in the future or how much it will cost, it's very appropriate to know whether you should protect yourself against long-term care expenses through insurance. Who needs protection? People with assets of $100,000 to $1 million (not counting your home) who want to save it for their heirs. If you have more than $1 million, you can afford to pay your long-term care bills out of pocket. Under $100,000 look to Medicaid, which picks up the bill when your money runs out.[18] The kind of protection you require the most is against the catastrophic costs of long-term care. And the diseases for which most long-term care insurance claims are filed include Alzheimer's and other types of dementia followed by complications resulting from stroke, fractures from falls, and heart disease. So before purchasing such insurance, you might want to discuss with your doctor your family history and your risk for any of these illnesses. Also, remember that the vast majority of plans are "tax qualified." This means that some or all of your premium charges, up to specified limit based on age, may be tax deductible and, more important, any benefits you receive won't be taxed. In addition, expenses not reimbursed for qualified long-term care services will be tax deductible under the medical expense deduction of the Internal Revenue Code, to the extent that all deductible medical care expenses exceed 7.5 percent of your adjusted gross income. Many elderly are attracted to home healthcare insurance, hoping that it will keep them out of the nursing home. But if you become disabled so that you need home health payments such as becoming bedbound, are wandering, or are too weak to dress, you are not likely to remain at home for long. Therefore, buy long-term nursing home care first, then add a home health rider if you can afford it.[19] The principle under which long-term care insurance operates is similar to other forms of insurance. You pay a known premium that offsets the risks of much greater personal out-of-pocket expenses. Although long-term care insurance is relatively new, more than one hundred companies now sell this kind of coverage.

Several types of policies are being sold. But most are *indemnity* policies. This means they pay a fixed dollar amount for each day you receive specified care either in a nursing home or at home. No policy is guaranteed to cover all expenses. Policyholders usually have a choice of indemnity amounts, ranging from $40 to more than $200 a day for nursing home care, that is geared to whatever the current average daily costs may be. The daily benefit for at-home care is usually half the benefit of nursing home care. Note, though, that you are actually responsible for your actual nursing home or homecare costs. Try to insure for the amount of the daily nursing home cost that exceeds your discretionary income from pension, Social Security, and so on. If your income is $30 per day and the nursing home costs $100, insure for $70. Because the per-day benefit you buy today may not be sufficient to cover higher costs after a number of years, most policies now include an *inflation adjustment* feature. In any policies, for example, the initial benefit amount will increase automatically each year at a specified rate (such as 5 percent) compounded over the life of the policy. Some life insurance policies offer long-term care benefits. Under these "accelerated" or "living benefit" provisions, a portion of the life insurance benefit is paid to the policyholder instead of to the beneficiary at the policyholder's death. Some companies make these benefits available to all policyholders; others offer them to people buying new policies.

In terms of cost, as of 1995 individual policies without an inflation adjustment feature ranged in cost from about $350 per year to more than $3,800. *Inflation adjustments* can add from 30 to 90 percent to your premium, depending on the option you choose, but can keep benefits in line with rising costs.[20] However, the actual premium you will pay depends on many factors, including your age, level of benefits, and the length of time you are willing to wait until the benefits begin. Premiums generally don't increase with age but remain the same each year (unless they are increased for all policyholders at once). The younger you are when you first purchase a policy, the lower your annual premium will be. The premium is also directly influenced by the amount of the daily benefit and how long the benefits will be paid. For example, a policy that pays $100 a day for six years of nursing home care costs more than a policy that pays $50 a week for three years. So-called *elimination or deductible periods* refer to the number of days you must be in residence at a nursing home or the number of homecare visits you must receive before policy benefits begin. Most policies offer a choice of a deductible ranging from zero to one hundred days. A twenty-day elimination period, as an example, means that your policy will begin paying benefits on the twenty-first day. The longer the elimination or deductible period, the lower the premium. Therefore, you can lower your own expenses for long-term care coverage by purchasing a policy at a young age and by choosing carefully both the level of benefits and the deductible benefits. *An industry rule of thumb is to spend no more than 7 percent of your annual income on long-term care insurance.* And ask about spousal and family discounts. Some companies also give price breaks to very healthy individuals. Also, find out whether your premiums can be paid automatically from your bank account, so the policy won't lapse if you become ill or become forgetful. Ask about a *third-party notice*. If your coverage is about to end because you forgot to pay a premium, you need this notice so a warning goes to someone you can trust. In making your choices, remember that while 45 percent of nursing home stays last three months or less, more than one-third last one year or longer. The average length of a claim on long-term care insurance policies is about two years. According to the National Association of Insurance Commissioners, if you eliminate nursing home visits lasting less than three months, only one-third of the population will spend time in a care facility.

In terms of coverage, new policies no longer require that you stay in a hospital before paying nursing home benefits. Newer policies no longer require a certain period of nursing home care before paying for home healthcare services. Most long-term care policies will begin to pay benefits either when the need is shown by the inability to perform a specific number of personal functions or activities of daily living (ADLs), such as bathing, dressing, or eating, or when care is needed because of cognitive impairment, or when care is medically necessary and prescribed by the patient's physician.

Today's policies pay for skilled, intermediate, and custodial care in state-licensed nursing homes. Long-term care policies also usually cover homecare services such as skilled or nonskilled nursing care, physical therapy, homemakers, and home health aides provided by state-licensed and/or Medicare-certified home health agencies. Many policies also cover adult daycare and other care in the community, alternate care, and respite care for the caregiver.

If your policy includes alternate care, this kind of benefit refers to nonconventional care and services developed by a physician that can serve as an alternative to more costly nursing home care. Benefits may be available for special medical care and treatments, different sites of care, or medically necessary modifications to the insured's home, like building ramps for wheelchairs or modifications to a kitchen or bathroom. A healthcare professional develops the alternate plan of care, the insured or insurer may initiate the plan, and the insurer approves it. Note that the benefit amount will reduce the maximum or lifetime benefit available for later confinement in a long-term care facility and that most policies limit the expenses covered under this benefit (i.e., 60 percent of the lifetime maximum limit). Finally, Alzheimer's disease and other organic cognitive disabilities, leading causes for nursing home admissions, are generally covered under long-term care policies.

All long-term care policies have *limitations and exclusions*, but their nature varies from policy to policy. For example, some mental and nervous disorders are often not covered, while alcoholism and drug abuse are usually not covered, along with care that is needed as a result of an act of war or an intentionally self-inflicted wound. Most policies will pay for whatever level of care you require. A few mandate a certain period of nursing home care before you become eligible for homecare. Generally, the fewer the restrictions, the more useful the policy.

Despite some move to uniformity—basically all policies now cover Alzheimer's disease, as noted, and no longer require a hospital stay before paying nursing home benefits—different policies have different options. If you are in reasonably good health and can take care of yourself, and if you are between the ages of fifty and eighty-four, you can probably buy long-term care insurance. Most companies do not sell individual policies to people under age fifty and over age eighty-four. These age limitations apply only to your age at the time of purchase, not at the time you use the benefits.

Long-term care policies generally limit benefits to a maximum dollar amount or a maximum number of days and often have separate benefit limits for nursing home care and home healthcare within the same policy. For example, a policy may offer five years of nursing home coverage (many policies now offer lifetime nursing home coverage) and two years of home health coverage. *Generally, companies define a policy's maximum benefit period in two ways. Under one definition, a policy may offer a one-time maximum benefit period.* A policy with five years of nursing home coverage, issued by a company using this definition, would pay just once in a policyholder's lifetime. *Other policies offer a maximum benefit period for each period of confinement.* Under this second definition, a policy with a five-year maximum benefit period would cover more than one nursing home stay lasting up to five years each if the days were separated by six months or more.[21] Virtually all long-term care policies sold to individuals are *guaranteed renewable*; they cannot be canceled as long as you pay your premiums on time and as long as you told the truth about your health on the application. Premiums can be increased, however, if they are increased for an entire group of policyholders. The renewability provision, usually found on the first page of a policy, specifies under what conditions the policy can be canceled and when the premiums may increase.

Find out whether the policy has a *nonforfeiture benefits provision*. This benefit returns to the policyholders some of their payments if they stop their coverage. The most common types of nonforfeiture benefits offered today are "return of premium" or "reduced paid-up." With a "return of premium" benefit, the policyholder receives cash, usually a percentage of the total amount of the premiums paid to date, after a lapse or death. With a "reduced paid-up" benefit, the long-term care coverage continues but the daily payment amount is reduced as specified in the policy. A nonforfeiture benefit can easily add 20 to 100 percent to a policy's cost.

The *waiver of premium provision* permits you to stop paying premiums during the time you are receiving benefits. Read the policy carefully to determine whether there any restrictions in regard to this provision, such as a requirement to be in a nursing home for any length of time (ninety days is a typical requirement) before premiums are waived.

Your medical history is important because the information you provide on your application is used by the insurance company in determining your eligibility for coverage. The application must be accurate and complete. If it is not, the insurance company may be within its rights to deny coverage when you file a claim.

Remember, new long-term care insurance policies may have more favorable provisions than older policies. Newer policies, as already noted, generally do not have requirements for prior hospital stays or for prior levels of care. But if you do change, provisions for specified periods of time will have to start again. So you should never change policies before making certain that the new policy is really an improvement over the policy you already have. And you should never get rid of the old policy before making certain that the new policy is in force.

Do not forget, insurance policies are legal contracts. Read and compare the policies you are considering before you purchase one, and make sure you understand all the provisions. Read the policy itself before purchasing it rather than just relying upon marketing or sales literature. Discuss the policies you are considering with people whose opinions you value such as your doctor, your children, or an informed friend or relative. Also, ask about the insurance company's financial rating and for a summary of each policy's benefits or an outline of coverage. (Ratings result from an analysis of a company's financial records.) To find out about an insurance company's ratings and their meaning, the National Association of Insurance Commissioners recommends among different services:

- *A. M. Best* (http://www.AMBest.com)
- *Fitch Ratings*, tel: 1-800-893-4824 (http://www.fitchratings.com)
- *Moody's Investors Services*, tel: 1-212-553-0377 (http://www.moodys.com)
- *Standard & Poor's Insurance Rating Services*, tel: 1-212-438-2400 (http://www.standardandpoors.com)
- *Weiss Ratings*, tel:1-800-289-9222 (http://www.weissratings.com)

Also, a wise choice may be to look at a company's size and its experience with long-term care insurance and other insurance. And remember, even after you buy a policy, if you determine that it doesn't meet your needs, you generally have thirty days to return the policy to get your money back. This is called the *free look*.

Don't give in to high-pressure sales talks. And don't be afraid to ask your insurance agent to explain anything that you do not understand. If you are not satisfied with an agent's answers, ask for someone who you may contact in the company itself. Call your state insurance department if you are not satisfied with the answers you obtain from an agent or another company representative.

Information is available from the Area Agency on Aging. For your local office, call 1-800-677-1116. Also, check with your local Better Business Bureau. Additional information about healthcare coverage and long-term care is available from:

- American Health Care Association (1201 L St. NW, Washington, DC 20005; tel: 1-202-842-4444; Web site: http://www.ahca.org)
- National Association of Insurance Commissioners (2301 McGee St., Suite 800, Kansas City, MO 64108-2662; tel: 1-816-842-3600; Web site: http://www.naic.org)
- The National Council on the Aging (United Seniors Health Council Program,

300 D St. SW, Suite 801,Washington, DC 20024; tel: 1-202-479-1200; Web site: http://www.ncoa.org)

In summary, according to the National Association of Insurance Commissioners, consumers should look for the following standards in a long-term care policy:

- At least a year of nursing home or home healthcare coverage, including intermediate and custodial care. Nursing home or home healthcare benefits should not be limited primarily to skilled care.
- Coverage for Alzheimer's disease if the policyholder develops the disease after buying the policy.
- An inflation protection option. The policy should offer a choice among:
    - ▼ automatically increasing the initial benefit level on an annual basis;
    - ▼ a guaranteed right to increase benefit levels periodically without providing evidence of insurability; and
    - ▼ covering a specific percentage of actual or reasonable charges.
- An "outline of coverage" that systematically describes the policy's benefits, limitations, and exclusions, and also allow you to compare it with others.
- A long-term care insurance shopper's guide that helps you decide whether long-term care insurance is appropriate to you.
- A guarantee that the policy cannot be canceled, nonrenewed, or otherwise terminated because you become older or suffer deterioration in physical or mental health.
- The right to return the policy within thirty days after you have purchased the policy (if for any reasons you do not want it) and to receive a premium refund.
- No requirements that policyholders:
    - ▼ first be hospitalized in order to receive nursing home benefits or home healthcare benefits;
    - ▼ first receive skilled nursing home care before receiving intermediate or custodial care nursing home care; or
    - ▼ first receive nursing home care before receiving benefits for home healthcare.[22]

The United Seniors Health Cooperative also has its own recommendations. The cooperative was renamed the United Seniors Health Council after its merger as a program with the National Council on the Aging on January 4, 2002, a consumer advisory group in Washington, DC, that is concerned with the quality and cost of healthcare. The United Seniors advises buying long-term insurance only if

- annual income exceeds $30,000 per person in your household
- assets exceed $75,000 per person
- you could still pay the premiums if they rise 20 or 30 percent
- paying the premiums doesn't crowd out other items out of your budget

If you decide to purchase a long-term care policy, United Seniors states it should have the following features, some of which have been recommended by other insurance groups:

- Coverage of all levels of care—skilled, custodial, and intermediate. And prior hospitalization should not be a requirement for obtaining benefits.
- Flexibility. It should cover various forms of care, including adult daycare, respite care, and home healthcare.
- Inflation protection. If you are seventy-five or younger, you should get a policy with benefits that rise at a 5 percent compound annual rate, even though it will add to your cost.
- Reasonable eligibility benefits. Policies usually require certain impairments before paying benefits. You must show such circumstances as medical necessity, cognitive impairment, problems with activities of daily living, and the like. United Seniors recommends policies that treat these impairments separately rather than requiring several combined to obtain benefits.

Purchasing long-term care insurance poses many perplexing questions to which you might not have the answer at the time you are considering purchasing it. For example, what are your chances of ever being admitted to a nursing home? If you went, how long would you have to stay? If you became sick, could you stay at home and have a relative care for you? Would you be better off taking the insurance premiums you pay annually and depositing the money in an investment account? And how do you know when you might need a nursing home or another kind of long-term care? You might need it next month or next year or never at all. United Seniors also recommends that you should review the companies with which you might want to do business. You may be using this product many years after you buy it, so you want a company that will still be there. Stay with large, well-known companies and review their ratings. (Look for an industry rating of A or A+ or better) A. M. Best (a commercial service that assigns large insurers a rating based on their financial strength) and Standard & Poor's, as already noted, are among the companies that evaluate insurers for financial soundness, and their publications are usually available in public libraries. You don't want a company whose business profile indicates that it can go out of business. Also, don't buy the policy just based on the company ratings. Look at policy price and benefits.

Most important of all, United Seniors recommends that you ask yourself whether long-term insurance is an appropriate and suitable product for you. This means examining and judging your financial and medical conditions and your family situation. Look at how much you could afford on your own, allowing for inflation, and look for a policy that will fill the gap. If you can afford to pay your own way or are likely to qualify for Medicaid, you may not need private insurance. People who may be able to rely on family members for some help should make flexibility a major priority in their policy. They can't be sure at this point how much help the family will be, so they want a policy that is likely to pay for benefits under a variety of care arrangements. Single persons with no dependents probably need less flexibility because they will probably go into assisted living or a nursing home if they need care.[23]

Of course, there are some risks in this kind of insurance just as there are in other kinds. *If you are dealing with an insurance agent in buying a long-term care policy, here are a few key questions you might ask your insurance agent about policies that may interest you:*

- What are the provisions for custodial and homecare benefits? What are the benefit amounts? How many home visits are allowed and what type of institution or home health organization may provide such services? Do such facilities exist in your area?
- Will the policy pay benefits even if you are paid under another policy?
- What optional coverages are available—for example, an inflation rider on daily benefit amounts? What does such an option—or any other you might want—add to the basic premium?
- What happens if you fail to pay your premium—or pay it late? Typically (but not always), there is a "grace period" for late payment of premiums, ranging from seven to thirty-one days during which you are fully covered. After that, your policy may be canceled.
- As already noted, does the policy cover Alzheimer's disease and other organic nervous/mental disorders? These are among the longest-term, costliest conditions for which older people are institutionalized today.
- What is the maximum lifetime benefit in dollars?
- What is the maximum time you can collect benefits for one confinement— two years?—four years—six years—no limit?[24]

In addition to asking the previous questions, *you can avoid being ripped off by an insurance salesman by being aware of the following points*:

- Beware of a salesperson's exaggeration of benefits. You have to understand the benefits of the policy. Ask the agent to leave a sample policy with you so you can read it. If you are not in a position to do that, ask a relative to help you—or show the policy to a lawyer. This will cost some legal fees, but since you are paying thousands of dollars in premiums for the policy over the course of your life, the lawyer's fee may be well worthwhile.
- Agents can use scare tactics to sell policies, emphasizing the costs of nursing home care and the benefits Medicare doesn't cover. Become familiar with the Medicare program and your own financial situation. Don't let any agent scare or pressure you into buying a policy immediately.
- Agents may be evasive about the policy's premium increases—but increases probably can and will happen. Many policies guarantee a certain premium for the first three years, but after that, it can rise substantially. Take this into con-

sideration when you purchase a policy. If you are having problems paying for the policy now, there's a real chance you won't be able to pay for the policy in the future. And even if the policy is guaranteed renewable, that will not help you if you cannot afford the premiums.

- Agents may sometimes tell consumers to fudge or even lie on their applications, a process called "clean sheeting." These statements can involve the person's health, age, or the conditions under which they live (alone or not). However, if the company finds out that the application was not true, it can revoke the policy and refund the premiums—years after the application was filed and just when the consumer needs the policy's coverage. Don't let an agent tell you that accuracy on an application isn't important—it's very important.

- Agents may not discuss specifically the obstacles you may have to overcome before the company will pay a claim—"gatekeepers" in the language of the industry. A letter from your doctor is usually not enough to begin policy payments or keep them coming. Many companies require that the plan of care be approved by a long-term coordinator who is either named by the insurer or must be approved by the insurer. Also, insurers often reserve the right to have the doctor examine you and reexamine you periodically afterward to determine whether you still qualify. As already noted, most insurance companies use trigger clauses called activities of daily living (or ADLs). Examples include bathing, dressing, and eating. Typically, policies pay if you cannot do two or more activities of daily living. Other obstacles for activating the long-term insurance may include a requirement that you be hospitalized first (although this is becoming less common), that the facility be licensed and/or have certain staffing levels, and that the facility have a minimum number of residents.

- Finally, agents have financial incentives to sell new policies and may therefore want to replace your old policy with a new one. Up to 80 percent of the first-year premiums may be a commission but much less in subsequent years. So if you already have a policy, be sure any new policy is truly better before you change.[25]

So be vigilant and read your policy very carefully before purchasing it. Because long-term care insurance contracts can be complex, you may want to have someone who is knowledgeable about such contracts look at it before signing up such as an attorney who specializes in eldercare law, insurance law, or estate planning. Your local bar association can refer you to such an attorney or you can check with the National Academy of Elder Law Attorneys (http://www.naela.org) for a list of attorneys. Members of the American Association of Retired Persons (AARP) can obtain a free thirty-minute consultation through the Legal Services Network (1-888-687-2277; or online at http://www.aarp.org/lsn). For general information about long-term care insurance consult the AARP site (http://www.aarp.org). If you need more time than thirty minutes, you can still get a discount off the attorney's hourly rate. Also, in the summer of 2003 millions of federal and postal workers and all government retirees, as well as retired military personnel, became eligible to purchase long-term care insurance through the federal government. Also eligible are their immediate families, including their adult children, current spouses, parents, parents-in-law, and stepparents. For more information on the federal program, you may call 1-800-582-3337 (or 1-800-843-3557, TDD, for the hearing impaired) or you may go to the Web site, http://www.ltcfeds.com. By following the previous guidelines, you should be able to understand and purchase the kind of long-term care policy that is best suited to your personal needs, again taking into consideration such key components as dollar-per-day benefits, duration of coverage, and whether or not the policy is inflation protected (i.e., making sure your daily allowance is keeping up with the dollar's real value).

PUBLIC PROGRAMS TO FINANCE NURSING HOME CARE

There are many other ways to finance nursing home care. Aside from long-term care insurance, these might include Social Security payments, your own funds, assets in escrow or as an endowment, assistance from the local welfare department, or assistance from private organizations such as veterans' groups, trade unions, fraternal organizations, or, as already noted, private health insurance plans. Many health insurance carriers provide nursing home coverage. Be sure to check with your insurance agent and/or group insurer to determine the kind of benefits he or she offers. But remember, neither Medicare nor private Medicare supplement insurance nor the hospitalization health insurance you may have through you employer or on your own (except for specific long-term care insurance) will pay for long-term care. Medicare supplement insurance (often called Medigap or Medsupp) is private insurance that helps covers some of the gaps in Medicare coverage. Those gaps are hospital deductibles, doctors' deductibles, and coinsurance payments or what Medicare considers excess physician charges—but they are not long-term care.

Almost one-third of all nursing home costs are paid out of pocket by individuals and their families. Medicare also pays for some skilled at-home care but only for short-term unstable conditions and not for the ongoing assistance that many elderly people require. As already noted, Medicaid pays most of the balance of the nation's long-term care bill—more than half of all nursing home expenses—either immediately, for people meeting federal poverty guidelines, or after nursing home residents "spend down" their own savings and become eligible. Many people who begin paying for nursing home care from their own their funds soon discover that their savings are not sufficient to cover lengthy stays. If they become impoverished after entering a nursing home, they turn to Medicaid to pay their bills. Using Medicaid once meant impoverishing the spouse who remained at home as well as the spouse in the nursing home. Recent changes in the law, however, permit the at-home spouse to keep a specified level of assets and income.[26]

Thus far, we have reviewed the kinds of questions you should ask in choosing a nursing home. However, to control costs for this care to the extent that may be possible, as your doctor would probably advise, you do not need a higher quantity of services than your personal situation requires. *Also, when meeting nursing home administrators, discuss the financial situation in detail. Recognize that the more services needed, the greater the financial burden. Get the facts straight regarding basic charges and additional costs for extras. Make sure to get all financial agreements in writing and keep a copy of the final arrangements. Before signing any papers you may wish to ask questions pertaining to the following areas:*

- Is the home certified to participate in the Medicare and/or Medicaid programs?
- Is a deposit required? When a patient's private funds are gone, is the deposit returned?
- Does the nursing home require you as a Medicaid-eligible person to make contributions, donations, or gifts as a condition of admission or continued stay in the home? If so, this action is illegal. Regardless of your paying status, be it as a public or a private paying patient, check with your lawyer or ombudsman in this regard.
- Does the contract require a resident to continue paying privately, even if personal resources are exhausted and he or she becomes eligible for Medicaid? These contracts, called "duration of stay" contracts, require payment at a certain rate for a designated period and have been ruled illegal by attorneys general in some states. If the contract contains clauses such as "waivers" of responsibility for lost possessions or injury, or requests "blanket" approval for certain treatments, these are not legal and check with a lawyer or ombudsman about such conditions.
- Do the residents' assets remain in his or her control or that of his or her family? How are cash and assets that are entrusted to the home protected? Is a receipt given to the resident? Are withdrawals noted by signed receipt so that the resident can keep abreast of his account?
- Are the agreed date of admission and the degree of care to be furnished set forth in the written agreement? Does the contract between the resident and the home clearly state discharge and transfer conditions?
- Prior to or at admission does the nursing home furnish the resident, family, or guardian, where applicable, a statement of the facility's current charges, including information about daily or monthly charges? Are all the services covered in the basic daily charge? If not, is a list of specific services and their fees not covered in the basic rate available? (Some homes have cost schedules covering linen, personal laundry, haircuts, shampoos, dental care, and other services.) Are many of the services the patient needs included in the basic charge?
- Are the patients, where customary or as specified by federal or state requirements, billed monthly with copies of the bill being given to the patient, family, or, where applicable, guardian? Does the bill show the amount due for the daily or monthly charges and a list of all other charges as set forth in the facility's

policy statement? How are charges handled for doctor visits, prescription drugs, and supplies such as wheelchairs, lotions, tissues, and other items?

- Does the facility announce through the issuance of written notices to all residents/patients at least thirty days before the changes become effective any changes in the facility's daily or monthly rates? Does the statement specify the facility's policies regarding what may be purchased outside the facility and the standards that those items or services must meet, such as appropriate labeling and availability of drugs? Does the facility also provide, if appropriate, a list of incidental or commonly used products with accompanying prices if purchased from the facility, along with a suggested supply for customary usage when bought outside the facility?
- Do the estimated monthly costs (including extra charges) compare favorably with the costs of other homes?
- Will the nursing home keep patients when they apply for Medicaid?
- Will the patient or resident and/or his family receive a refund of any advance payments if he or she leaves the facility or dies? At the time of transfer, discharge, or death, is the individual's account settled within thirty days (whenever possible) with refunds promptly and courteously given to the individual, guardian, or estate as is appropriately established by law?

While we have briefly mentioned many sources of assistance to finance nursing home care, there are two major government programs for which most of the elderly qualify and which do much to defray their personal nursing home expenses. These plans are Medicaid and Medicare. You should be knowledgeable about the kinds of nursing home care available and the conditions under which Medicaid and Medicare will pay the costs and to what extent.

Medicaid is a federal-state government grant-sharing program that is designed to meet the cost of financing medical care for the poor and the medically needy—persons who do not qualify for welfare but still cannot pay for medical care. States design their Medicaid programs within broad federal guidelines. Thus, Medicaid programs will vary from state to state. The Medicaid program uses the same definition of a skilled nursing home to which it will make payments under certain conditions that Medicare uses. The US government sets the standards for services, safety, and sanitation. States must obey the federal guidelines for inspection and certification of nursing homes receiving reimbursement under Medicaid and Medicare. Medicaid will pay for skilled nursing care in a facility where such round-the-clock services are available. A physician must approve this type of care for an applicant to be eligible for this aspect of Medicaid. (For data on your state regulations, ask your state or local welfare office.) On the other hand, unlike Medicare, the Medicaid program also pays for care in intermediate care facilities, which were described previously. The intermediate care facility caters to those who need some health services in addition to nursing supervision along with assistance in eating, dressing, walking, and other similar essentials. For those patients who qualify for both Medicare and

Medicaid, the Medicaid program may pick up charges after your one hundred days of skilled nursing home care under Medicare are used up. Thus, if you are a Medicaid recipient and eligible for payment, seek a nursing home certified for intermediate care or skilled nursing care by the federal government. Such a selection will do much to help alleviate your personal costs for such long-term care.

In addition, in 1988 Congress enacted spousal impoverishment reforms in the Medicaid program that allow a spouse who remains in the community when the other spouse is in a nursing care facility to keep one-half of the couple's assets up to a maximum of $76,000, in addition to the family home and car. In some states, the healthy spouse can keep $76,000, even if it represents more than one-half of the couple's savings. This so-called protected amount is subject to annual increases to keep pace with inflation. While most government Medicaid offices tell applicants for nursing home care that they must "spend down" their assets until there is only $2,000 (varies by state) remaining to qualify for nursing home care benefits, this is true only for individuals but does not take into account special provisions for married couples when one spouse remains at home.[27] Medicaid allows individuals to reduce their assets in various ways such as paying off their debts, prepaying their burial expenses, modernizing their home, or purchasing an automobile. Find out from your state Medicaid program which assets are applicable in your jurisdiction. In addition, some states are looking at a combination of Medicaid and private insurance as a way of keeping public costs down while allowing individuals to protect some of their assets. Under this partnership, the person who needs care is allowed to keep assets equal to the amount paid out by insurance and still qualify for Medicaid. As of 1996, New York, Connecticut, Indiana, and California had such programs. Find out whether your state has established such a program under Medicaid. On February 8, 2006, President Bush signed into law the Deficit Reduction Act of 2005 (Public Law 109-171) part of which is designed to prevent wealthy senior citizens from qualifying for Medicaid by transferring money to their children so that the seniors appear poor and thus have Medicaid pay for their nursing home costs. As already noted, only seniors with $2,000 or less in assets, excluding a house or a car, can qualify for Medicaid. (Married couples are permitted more resources.) In addition, they had to prove under the former law that, in the previous three years, they had not tried to defraud Medicaid by giving away assets. The new law in 2006 extends the previous three-year restriction to five years and limits the value of the excluded house to $500,000. However, each state has the option of raising that equity ceiling to $750,000. Gifts to a spouse or a disabled child are permitted. If seniors have transferred the money improperly, they are not permitted to be covered by Medicaid for months or years, depending upon how much they transferred. The new rules strengthen that penalty. You should check with the Medicaid program in your state or with a lawyer experienced in this aspect of the law to find out how the new law affects you should you find yourself in the position of needing Medicaid to pay for your nursing home care and have transferred assets to others in the previous five years.[28]

As far as original Medicare is concerned, it consists of two parts. Part A is the hospital insurance program that helps pay the cost of care in a skilled nursing home; Part B is a voluntary medical insurance program that, for a monthly premium, pays for physician and surgeon services, including those provided in a skilled nursing home, as well as home health services, outpatient hospital services, and other medical and health services such as surgical dressings, rental and purchase of medical equipment, outpatient physical therapy, outpatient maintenance dialysis (kidney) treatments, and certain colostomy care supplies. The other two parts, Part C, Medicare Advantage (managed care), and Part D, the prescription drug program, were not part of the original Medicare program, which became operational in the 1960s.

While the hospital insurance program (Part A) of Medicare does not cover physician services while you are in a skilled nursing home, it does pay for up to one hundred days of care in each benefit period while you are in such a facility. A benefit period begins the first day you receive covered services in a hospital. It ends after you have been out of a hospital or skilled nursing facility for sixty consecutive days (including the day of discharge). The hospital insurance program under Medicare pays for all covered services for the first twenty days while you are in nursing home and, as of 2006, all but $119 per day for up to eighty more days if *all* of the following four conditions are met:

- You have been in a hospital for at least three consecutive days (not counting the day of discharge) before you transfer to a skilled nursing facility.
- You are transferred to the skilled nursing facility because you require care for a condition that was treated in the hospital.
- You are admitted to the facility within a short time (usually thirty days) after you leave the hospital. If you leave a skilled nursing facility and are readmitted within thirty days, Medicare will cover you without your having to return to the hospital for a new three-day stay. In some instances, you may exceed the thirty-day criterion if for some reason you are discharged from the hospital but still cannot undergo treatment within thirty days because of the nature of your condition.
- A doctor certifies that you need, and you actually receive, skilled nursing or skilled rehabilitation services on a daily basis.

Medicare's hospital insurance program *pays* for the following major services when you are in a skilled nursing home:

- a semiprivate room (2 to 4 beds)
- all your meals, including special diets
- regular nursing services
- rehabilitation services, such as physical, occupational, and speech therapy
- drugs furnished by the facility during your stay
- medical supplies such as splints and casts
- use of appliances such as a wheelchair

Medicare's hospital insurance program (Part A) *cannot pay* for the following services when you are in a skilled nursing home:

- personal convenience items you request such as a television, a radio, or a telephone in your room
- private-duty nursing by skilled nurses and medical social workers
- any charges above the hospital's semiprivate room rate, unless you need a private room for medical reasons
- the first three pints of blood you receive in a *benefit period*. If you need blood while you are an inpatient of a hospital or a skilled nursing home, the hospital insurance program under Medicare pays the full cost of the blood starting with the fourth pint in a *benefit period*. If you are covered by a blood donor plan, it can replace the first three pints of blood for you. Or, you can arrange to have someone donate blood for you. A hospital or other facility may not charge you when you arrange for the replacement of the first three pints of blood for which Medicare does not pay. Also, under the medical insurance program (Part B) of Medicare, the medical insurance pays, after you pay the annual deductible, 80 percent of the reasonable charges for blood starting with the fourth pint in a *calendar year*. Medical insurance does not pay for the first three pints in each calendar year.

Finally, it should be noted that certain services are not covered under either the hospital insurance program (Part A) or the voluntary medical insurance program (Part B) of Medicare. These include:

- Custodial care (help with bathing, dressing, toileting, and eating) for personal needs that do not require professional skills and training.
- Routine physical examinations and tests directly related to such examinations.
- Eyeglasses and related eye examinations. But, effective July 1, 1981, optometrists' services to patients with the condition of aphakia (absence of the natural lens of the eye) is covered under Medicare.
- Routine dental care. But effective July 1, 1981, Medicare covers services performed by dentists *if* those same services are presently covered when performed by a physician. Medicare also covers hospitalization for noncovered dental services where the severity of the procedure or the condition warrants hospitalization.
- Hearing aids and related examinations for prescribing, fitting, or changing hearing aids.
- Dentures.
- Orthopedic shoes.
- Private-duty nurses.
- Personal services in your hospital or nursing home such as a television, a telephone, and other services already noted.

- The first three pints of blood or packed red cells: per benefit period (under hospital insurance) or per calendar year (under medical insurance).
- Acupuncture treatments and cosmetic surgery.
- Drugs *are covered* under the hospital insurance plan (Part A) if furnished to a patient in a hospital or a skilled nursing home; drugs are *not covered* under the medical insurance plan (Part B) unless *administered* as part of a physician's professional services and which *cannot be self-administered.* But beginning January 1, 2006, prescription drugs are covered under Part D of the Medicare program.
- Immunizations (except for pneumococcal vaccine, effective July 1, 1981) for which Medicare will not pay unless required because of an injury or an immediate risk of infection.
- Supportive devices and routine foot care except, beginning in 1981, for plantar wart treatment (warts on feet).

Remember, many nursing homes provide only room and board with *limited* medical services and are not considered skilled nursing homes. Even though this care is important and is needed by many people, there is no reimbursement from Medicare for intermediate care.

When Medicare and Medicaid are involved, the US government sets the standards for services, safety, and sanitation of skilled nursing homes, as we have already discussed. States must obey the federal guidelines for inspection and certification of nursing homes receiving reimbursement under Medicare or Medicaid. All other nursing homes come under state inspection and approval standards.

The federal government frequently revises its own rules and standards under Medicare. Make certain that the nursing home you select conforms with current rules. Do not forget that many homes are certified as both skilled nursing homes and as intermediate care facilities and, therefore, are eligible for Medicare and Medicaid payments. Finding and selecting a nursing home that meets your particular needs may not be an easy emotional or financial experience. By being aware of various sources of financial aid available from both public and private agencies as well as the kinds of questions you should ask when inspecting a nursing home yourself, you can ease—for both yourself and a loved one—the transition, whether entering the facility for long-term or short-term convalescent care.

WHERE TO TAKE NURSING HOME COMPLAINTS

In our discussion we have reviewed a variety of areas of a nursing home's operation including its costs, administration, patient care, environmental health, safety, and construction. Needless to say, just as an individual may have many questions to ask, he also may have many complaints—whether he is a resident in such a facility or a friend or a relative. In order to have you complaints heard, there are a variety of sources to which you can bring your grievances for hopefully corrective action. These include:

- The head nurse on unit, who may be called the charge nurse.
- The director of nursing.
- The nursing home administrator.
- The facility's residents' council.
- Your local Social Security district office, which functions as a clearinghouse for complaints about all nursing homes, whether or not they receive government funds.
- The American Health Care Association (1201 L Street NW, Washington, DC 20005), if the home is a member. Its Web site is http://www.ahca.org.
- The American Association of Homes and Services for the Aging (2519 Connecticut Ave. NW, Washington, DC), if the home is a member. Its Web site is http://www.aahsa.org.
- The National Citizens' Coalition for Nursing Home Reform (1828 L St. NW, Washington, DC 20036). Its Web site is http://www.nursinghomeaction.com.
- The American College of Health Care Administrators (300 North Lee St. Alexandria, VA 22314), if the administrator is a member. Its Web site is http://www.achca.org.
- The patient's caseworker or the county welfare office, if the patient is covered by Medicaid.
- The state Medicaid agency, if the home is certified by that program.
- The state health department and state nursing home licensing authority (which may be located in the state health or welfare department).
- The nursing home ombudsman, if such an office has been established in your community or in your state Office of Aging. The federal Older Americans Act requires each state to have an ombudsman program to serve as an advocate for residents of nursing homes, board and care homes, and assisted living facilities. For the telephone number of your state or local long-term care ombudsman program, telephone 1-800-677-1116 or visit http://www.aoa.dhhs.gov. The ombudsman may have a directory of facilities in your area and information about problems particular facilities may be having, including your own.
- Your congressmen and senators (address congressmen at the US House of Representatives, Washington, DC 20515; senators at US Senate, Washington, DC 20510).
- Your state and locally elected representatives, including members of your state house and city council.
- The Joint Commission on Accreditation of Healthcare Organizations (One Renaissance Boulevard, Oakbrook Terrace, IL 60181), if the nursing home has received accreditation from this organization). Its Web site is http://www.jcaho.org.

- Your local Better Business Bureau and Chamber of Commerce.
- Your local hospital association and medical society.
- A reputable lawyer or legal society.

All these sources of assistance exist to help you with your nursing home problems. You should take advantage of them. Remember, those nursing home administrators who operate homes of quality will welcome your opinions. Your stay, treatment, and physical well-being—or your loved one's—will ultimately be affected.

NOTES

1. *Source Book of Health Insurance Data* (Washington, DC: Health Insurance Association of America, 1995), p. 121; "Nursing Home Care," *Vital and Health Statistics*, (Hyattsville, MD: National Center for Health Statistics, November 7, 2000), series 13, no. 147.

2. Nancy L. Ross, "The Long-Term Care-Care Tangle," *Washington Post*, January 31, 1989, p. D5.

3. John F. Wasik, "Can You Afford to Take Care of a Loved One," *Parade*, December 16, 1990, pp. 14–15.

4. *Health, United States, 2003, with Chartbook on Trends in the Health of Americans* (Hyattsville, MD: National Center for Health Statistics, September 2003), p. 309 (table 115).

5. *Guide to Long-Term Care Insurance, 1999* (Washington, DC: Health Insurance Association of America, 1999), pp. 4–5; "GAO Issues Report on LTC Financing" (Washington, DC: US Government Accountability Office, April 2005), pp. 2, 4.

6. "65+," *Washington Post/Health*, July 23, 1996, p. 7; Mary Beth Franklin, "Elder Law: Saving Your Life Savings," *Washington Post/Health*, July 23, 1996, p. 16; and US Department of Health and Human Services, *CDC Fact Book 2000/2001* (Atlanta, GA: Centers for Disease Control, September 2000), p. 53.

7. *Guide to Long-Term Care Insurance, 1999*, p. 5; *Fact Sheet: The American Geriatrics Society (AGS)* (New York: American Geriatrics Society, 2001).

8. "65+," p. 7.

9. *Guide to Long-Term Care Insurance* (Washington, DC: Health Insurance Association of America, 1996), p. 3; "Nursing Home Costs Top $80,000 a Year," *Silicon Valley/San Jose Business Journal*, March 4, 2002; "2003 GE (General Electric) Nursing Home Cost of Care Survey," conducted by Evans Research, July 31, 2003, as cited in long-term care insurance material sent to author, January 2005, from General Electric Capital Insurance Company; and "Be Prepared for Long-Term Care," Cox News Service, March 15, 2004.

10. *Source Book of Health Insurance Data, 2002* (Washington, DC: Health Insurance Association of America, 2002), p. 98 (table 5.1).

11. *What Everyone Should Know about Skilled Nursing Homes* (Springfield: Illinois Department of Public Health, State Health Coordinating Council, 1977), pp. 2–3.

12. *Thinking about a Nursing Home?* (Washington, DC: American Health Care Association, 1979), pp. 2–3.

13. Ibid., pp. 3–5.

14. *What Everyone Should Know about Skilled Nursing Homes*, pp. 5–10.

15. "Nursing Homes in Area, Nationwide Plagued by Reports of Abuse," *Washington Post*, October 13, 1996, pp. B1, B6.

16. "Third of U.S. Nursing Homes Faulted on Care," *Washington Post*, May 21, 1986, p. A15.

17. *The Condition of the American Nursing Home: A Study* (Washington, DC: US Senate Subcommittee on the Problems of the Aged and Aging of the Committee on Labor and Public Welfare, 1960), pp. 1–2.

18. Jane Bryant Quinn, "Long-Term Health Care: An Insurance Checklist," *Washington Post*, May 24, 1992, p. H3.

19. Ibid.; Russell Wild, "Someone to Watch Over Me," *AARP* 1 (January/February 2003): 27–28.

20. *Guide to Long-Term Care Insurance, 1996*, p. 5.

21. Ibid., p. 9.

22. Ibid., pp. 13–14.

23. Albert Crenshaw, "Long-Term Care Is Hot Topic in Insurance," *Washington Post/Health*, June 18, 1996, p. 10.

24. Esther Peterson, *Choice Time: Thinking Ahead on Long-Term Care* (Hartford, CT: Aetna Life Insurance and Annuity Company, undated), pp. 20–21.

25. Albert Crenshaw, "Long-Term Policies: Beware of False Promises," *Washington Post*, June 30, 1991, p. H3.

26. *Guide to Long-Term Care Insurance, 1996*, pp. 3–4.

27. Mary Beth Franklin, "Elder Law Saving Your Life Savings," pp. 17–18.

28. Crenshaw, "Long-Term Care Is Hot Topic in Insurance," p. 10; Alice Dembner, "Medicaid Proposal Could Hurt Seniors," *Boston Globe*, January 30, 2006 (Your Life section); Jonathan Weisman, "Budget Cuts Pass by Slim Margin," *Washington Post*, February 2, 2006, pp. A1, A7; and Joe Barton, "House Approves Medicaid Reform, Digital TV," US House of Representatives, Committee on Energy and Commerce, December 19, 2005.

CHAPTER NINE

HOME HEALTHCARE AND HOSPICE CARE

INTRODUCTION

One of the oldest forms of healthcare services in existence today is home healthcare programs, yet they represent one of the "newest" solutions to rising hospital costs and escalating health insurance premiums. Even though home healthcare agencies have operated for decades, federal and state government funds for long-term care have been geared to nursing home care—with little or no support for in-home care programs. Yet, various estimates indicate that many hospital and nursing home patients could be cared for in their own homes. The benefits of homecare are not only financial but also emotional and psychological. The advantages to a patient who obtains peace of mind through his convalescence at home, upon his physician's recommendation, rather than in an institution, cannot be measured. Home healthcare agencies provide a wide range of services to the public. As a partial listing, these include blood tests, home kidney dialysis, medical social services, and skilled nursing care, as well as intravenous, inhalation, physical, and occupational therapy. Also, some agencies provide a wide range of personnel, including nurses, social workers, and speech, physical, and occupational therapists, as well as home health aides who attend to housekeeping, marketing, and personal patient needs such as bathing and hair washing. Other agencies are more specialized.

In 2000 about 70 percent of home health patients (70.5 percent) were sixty-five years of age and over, and almost 22 percent of home health patients (21.9 percent) were eighty-five years of age and over. Two-thirds of home health patients were women.[1] Among home health patients in 2000, almost 48 percent (47.5 percent) of the admission diagnoses were composed of the following five conditions: diseases of the heart (10.9 percent), diseases of the musculoskeletal system and connective tissue (9.8 percent), diabetes (7.8 percent), cerebrovascular diseases (7.3 percent), malignant neoplasms (4.9 percent), and respiratory diseases (6.8 percent).[2] But babies born with severe birth defects, persons with multiple sclerosis, young mothers injured in automobile accidents, and children in traction are all eligible for treatment at home. In some communities, hospital discharge planning teams, which might include a public health nurse, suggest when patients might go home and recommend the care the patients will need when they get there. However, homecare is not just for the sick and the elderly. It can be for anyone—individuals and families who may have a variety of health and social problems, aside from short- or long-term illness, such as an injury, mental disorders and retardation, alcoholism, and physical or social handicaps, among others. In most places, however, it is the responsibility of the patient or his family to investigate the possibility and availability of homecare and then ask his physician to order it. Good care at home often can prevent or delay the patient's need to enter a nursing home and spare the family the ordeal of visiting the patient in an institution, running the household, and holding down several jobs at the same time.[3]

BASIC SERVICES

Homecare is not just a single service but rather a wide variety with a common goal: to preserve the home and to improve the quality of life by providing help in the home. These services include the following:

- *Social Services* to identify and overcome specific problems within the home, supervise services, and coordinate homecare with other community programs. These services involve:
  - ▼ medical care
  - ▼ nutrition services
  - ▼ skilled nursing (giving drugs and other prescribed treatments) therapy for specific problems: speech therapy, respiratory therapy (breathing), physical therapy (movement), occupational therapy (managing household or work tasks)
  - ▼ personal care (bathing, dressing, eating, taking temperatures, changing dressings, helping with exercises)
- *Homemaking Services* to improve or maintain the home, including:
  - ▼ environmental care (light housekeeping, doing the laundry, food shopping, planning, and preparing meals)
  - ▼ teaching home management (budgeting, home safety) and parenting (childcare skills and family relations)
- *Supplemental Services* to improve the quality of life.
- *Pastoral Counseling* to give comfort and advice to individuals and families, especially the seriously ill.
- *Chore Services* to help with or do heavy-duty household tasks and to maintain safety in the home, including:
  - ▼ minor home repairs (step, rail, or electrical repair)

> ▼ heavy cleaning (outside window washing and cleaning attics or basements)
> ▼ yard tasks (lawn cutting or snow removal)

- *Meal-on-Wheels* to deliver nutritious meals to the homes of those unable to prepare or obtain their own meals.
- *Friendly Visiting* to provide regular visits, at least once a week, to the homebound who are lonely for companionship. Visitors talk, write letters, read, or often just listen.
- *Telephone Reassurance* to link the homebound to the community via a seven-day-a-week call system. Telephone reassurance lessens loneliness, depression, and fears common to those living alone and assists in emergency situations.
- *Transportation and Escort Services* to help those needing assistance to get out of the home. Minibuses, cars, or public systems may be used as transportation to medical or community services. Escorts provide physical assistance, support, or protection needed to encourage the elderly and the disabled to venture into the community. Often these two services work hand in hand.
- *Equipment Services and Loan Closets* to provide needed healthcare equipment such as hospital beds or wheelchairs. Equipment services rent or sell equipment; loan closets lend healthcare devices as needed at little or no cost.

Steve worried about his elderly parents. He knew the time had come to bring help into the house. His father could not take care of himself like before, and his mother could not juggle the household chores and still take care of his father. He discussed the dilemma with his brother Mitchell, suggesting that homecare might alleviate their mother's pressure. "It could be difficult for them to accept this change in their lives," said Steve. "Mom and Dad are two independent people who have always taken care of each other and their family. Still, I think it's time, while they still have the energy to care for each other." Mitchell had no argument. He knew they qualified for Medicare even though Medicaid, other public programs, and private insurance provide coverage. "Well, it's better than a nursing home," agreed Mitchell. "The folks at least will be in their home surroundings, and with friends and relatives who can visit anytime without official visiting hours. It's important they maintain a quality of life." The brothers agreed to look into homecare agencies and the services provided. Steve knew about Medicare's Internet Web site, a valuable resource for comparing the quality of homecare agencies around the country.

A plan for homecare and the specific services needed, how often, and for what period of time they are needed can be designed to match individual needs. Could homecare assist you or someone you know? The following questions may help you decide:

- Are you having trouble caring for yourself, your home, or your family because of age, health, or social problems?

- Are you able to provide adequate care but feel angry, frustrated, or exhausted at the end of each day? Are family relationships breaking down as a result?
- Are you homebound, living alone, and feeling depressed, fearful, or lonely?
- Are you in a hospital or about to go home without a satisfactory plan for your care following your release?
- Are you missing workdays to care for a family member?[4]

If the answer is "yes" to any of these questions, homecare could make an important difference in your life.

ADVANTAGES OF HOMECARE

In area after area where home health programs have been developed, organizations that have developed and offered these programs to the public have achieved financial savings. In a Connecticut homecare program, a Blue Cross plan study of 991 patients showed a total reduction of 8,919 days (an average of nine days per case) and money savings of $801,511. And in Philadelphia, in just two years, another long-standing plan saved an average of 12 days per patient and shaved $2.5 million from hospital bills, or an average of $869 per case.[5] The potential savings that homecare programs can achieve in reducing unnecessary hospital stays, health insurance premiums, and individual costs, perhaps, have no limit as our population, especially the elderly, grows in future years. Because such chronic illnesses as diabetes, hypertension, arteriosclerotic heart disease, cerebral-vascular disorders, arthritis, neurological problems, malignancies, and other long-term partially disabling illnesses are prevalent and can be treated at home, the immense good that homecare programs can render society is inestimable.

AVAILABILITY OF HOMECARE

The US Department of Health and Human Services has certified many agencies to provide home healthcare services under the Medicare program. This certification means that the agency meets the minimum federal standards and qualifications in order to receive Medicare reimbursements. However, there are many home health agencies that are not so certified. This failure to meet Medicare certification does not necessarily mean that the agency is providing poor services. Rather, the agency might only wish to provide services to non-Medicare patients and not get involved in the federal government program.

The services that home health agencies provide vary widely. Some of the more sophisticated agencies deliver services similar to those of hospitals. These might include nurses with advanced training in chemotherapy, social workers, speech pathologists, occupational therapists, and pediatric nurse practitioners, as well as specialists in nutritional therapy or in caring for surgical patients. Some agencies are able to set up traction in a patient's home; others provide medical supplies or equipment and intravenous drug therapy as well as arrange transportation to the hospital or doctor's office for periodic treatments or follow-up examinations. However, most agencies are not so elaborate in regard to their services. Most have only three or four nurses, a few home health aides, and usually a physical therapist.

Just like hospital and physician care, the quality of home healthcare can vary. Screening and supervision of workers may be slipshod, and a number of abuses have been reported to Medicare officials. *Therefore, before engaging the services of a home health agency, there are several questions you should ask to assess its quality to the extent that is possible*:

- How long has the agency been in business? New agencies may be good ones, and old agencies may be poor, but fly-by-night services are growing in number. Does the agency have any literature that explains its services, eligibility requirements, fees, and funding sources, as well as a patient's bill of rights that details the rights and responsibilities of the agency, patient, and caregivers alike? Ask the agency to explain what your insurance covers and what will be out of pocket. Also, does the agency publish an annual report and other kinds of information about itself?
- What are the agency's hours? Can you obtain help every day, seven days a week, or just five days a week? What about nights and weekends or emergencies? Night or weekend care may be vital but in some cases a superior agency may provide only daytime services, while an inferior agency may offer round-the-clock care. What steps does the agency have in place to handle emergencies, as on nights and weekends? Make sure about the availability of the agency's services to meet your personal needs.
- How soon can the agency begin helping you? Most agencies can at least make an assessment visit and often start services within forty-eight to seventy-two hours, often sooner; more time may be needed for complex or high-tech care. If an agency can't respond to a simple request within three business days, seek another agency.
- Is the home health service certified by Medicare? To determine the quality of a Medicare-certified agency, you can review its Medicare Survey Report. For assistance in receiving this report, contact you state health department or health insurance counseling program, which offers free information specifically about Medicare home health benefits. These offices can direct you to the state's Medicare hot line for information about the quality of services that Medicare-certified home health agencies and hospices provide in your area. Also, find out whether the agency is approved to receive Medicare and Medicaid payments? How much does the agency charge? Will the agency tell you what your private health insurance—or Medicare or other programs—covers? Does the agency help with the insurance billing?

- What are the qualifications of its staff members? What are their credentials, experience, and references? Are they bonded? Does the agency perform staff background checks?
- Does the agency have written statements outlining its services, eligibility, cost, and payment procedures; employees' descriptions; malpractice and liability insurance? Does the agency protect its workers with written personnel policies, basic benefits, a wage scale for each position, and malpractice insurance? Does the agency have a board of directors or advisory committee representative of the community? Is a list of those persons available? How does the agency ensure patient confidentiality?
- If only limited services are available, what assistance can be provided to obtain other homecare services as needed, such as home-delivered meals? Will the agency arrange extra support services such as meals-on-wheels? Also, does the agency offer personal services such as bathing or dressing and other support services such as laundry or help with shopping?
- Can the agency provide you with references from professionals, such as hospital or community agency social workers, doctors, and discharge planners, and other patients, and their family members, who have used this agency? A good agency will provide references upon request. Also check with the Better Business Bureau, the local Consumer Bureau, or your state attorney general's office for information about their experience with the agency. Some of the questions you may ask when seeking references include: How frequently do you refer patients to this agency? Do you have a contractual relationship with this agency? If so, do you require that the agency meet special standards for quality of care? Is a list of these standards available to the public? Do you have any opinions that you received from the patients who used this agency, either informally or through an official survey, that are available to the public? Ask the agency whether it knows of any patients who required treatment similar to your own or your loved one's. If so, can the agency help you contact these persons?
- Is the home health agency a member of the National Association for Home Care and Hospice?
- Is the home health agency certified or licensed by the state? Have any complaints against the agency been filed with the state licensing body? Does the agency issue an annual report and make it available to the community?
- Is the home healthcare agency accredited by organizations dedicated to promoting excellence in homecare? If so, it means the home health agency passed careful review of all services and practices as well as met basic standards of quality, which these organizations developed. For example, the Joint Commission on the Accreditation of Healthcare Organizations accredits hospitals whose review includes homecare services (tel: 1-630-792-5000); the National League for Nursing and the American Public Health Association (tel: 1-202-777-2472) jointly accredit community nursing services such as

visiting nurse associations and home health agencies; and the National Home Caring Council accredits programs that provide homemaker–home health services such as reviewing the screening, training, and supervision of aides. You may also want to contact Accreditation Commission for Home Care, Inc. (tel: 1-919-873-8609; the Community Health Accreditation Program (tel: 1-800-669-1656); and Homecare University, part of the National Association for Home Care and Hospice (tel: 1-202-547-3576).

- What is the agency's ratio of professional staff to aides? If one professional nurse is responsible for two hundred aides, supervision will be spotty at best.
- Is the agency's plan of care carefully and professionally developed with you and your family and your doctor (good agencies will work with the doctor as a matter of routine, and just because an agency asks for your doctor's telephone number does not mean this will happen)? Or is the plan of care based solely on your own view of the home situation and request for services? Seek a professional evaluation before contracting with the agency. *Look for these clues as reflective of quality*:
    - ▼ The evaluation is performed by an experienced registered nurse or social worker, not an agency clerk. Ask what it includes.
    - ▼ The evaluation is done in the home, not on the telephone.
    - ▼ The evaluation determines what you can do for yourself.
    - ▼ The evaluation includes consultation with the family physician and/or other professionals already providing you with health and social services; and, if you agree, consults other members of your family.
- Once developed, is the plan of care written out? Are copies of the plan given to workers in the home? Ask for a copy of the plan for yourself whether you are the patient or his or her family. Make sure that it lists specific duties, work hours/days, names, and telephone numbers of the supervisor in charge. When agency personnel report to the home, ask if they have seen the plan of care. If necessary, provide a copy and discuss duties. Has the home health aide been instructed in regard to the duties and any special tasks included in the plan of care? Do the caregivers update the plan as changes in care occur? Does the agency take time to educate family members on the care being administered to the patient?
- If you are dealing with an agency, are references required by the agency and on file? If you cannot learn about the references, ask how many references the agency requires. Any agency should require several (two or more).
- Are homemaker–home health aides who are not required to be licensed or certified adequately trained? Has the aide received at least sixty hours of training? Does the aide receive continuous in-service education? Has the aide been instructed as to the duties and any special tasks included in the plan of care? Will the same aide or nurse or therapist continue with you to ensure continuity and quality of care? Are homemaker–home health aides who are not required to be licensed or certified adequately supervised? Is supervision pro-

vided in the home? How often? How soon? This is difficult to learn. Judge the agency's answer. Any supervisor other than a registered nurse or a social worker should have at least a four-year college degree in an area related to homecare such as home economics. When home health services (personal care and/or basic home nursing) are needed, the supervisor should always be a registered nurse. Is the supervisor a registered nurse or a social worker? If not, who will provide supervision? What are his or her qualifications? How often does the supervisor visit the home? Keep track of the supervisor's contacts to ensure that proper supervision is being provided. Telephone supervision alone is not acceptable. At a minimum an in-home visit should be made at least every three months. The first in-home visit by the supervisor should take place before or at least within the first two weeks of service. Between in-home visits a supervisor should be available by telephone to the family and to the homecare personnel at all times while on assignment.

- How available is the supervisor? What arrangements are made for emergency situations? Ask the supervisor for specific times and days when he or she is available. Then check the system by calling on those days. If the supervisor is not available, who else can the patient and his or her family members call with questions or complaints? How does the agency follow up and resolve such problems?
- What is the patient load of the home health agency?
- Does the home health agency have professional staff education programs?[6]

The answers to these questions will enable you to determine the agency's ability to serve your needs as you perceive them as well as the quality of those professionals who are delivering that care.

In addition to the previous questions, another tool has become available to Medicare recipients to help them judge the quality of care a home health agency provides. Now available on Medicare's Web site (http://www.Medicare.gov), "Home Health Compare" provides quality-of-care information about homecare agencies throughout the country. These measures offer information about patients' physical and mental health and whether their ability to perform basic daily activities is maintained or improved. The quality-of-care measures are grouped into four categories and include:

- four measures related to improvement in getting around;
- four measures related to meeting the patients' activities of daily living;
- two measures related to patient medical emergencies; and
- one measure related to improvement in mental health.

The quality measures are based on data collected about home health patients whose care is covered by Medicare or Medicaid and provided by a Medicare-certified home health agency. To reduce the chance that a home health agency that serves sicker, older, or frailer patients looks worse in the quality measures, the quality measures are risk adjusted. This means that some of the percentages have been changed to account for the fact that the agencies treat sicker patients. In more specific terms, the Web site informs you of the following quality-of-care measures:

- percentage of patients who get better at walking or moving around
- percentage of patients who get better at getting in and out of bed
- percentage of patients who get better at getting to and from the toilet
- percentage of patients who have less pain when moving around
- percentage of patients who get better at bathing (improvement in ability); percentage of patients who stayed the same or don't get worse at bathing measures maintaining (stabilizing) ability
- percentage of patients who get better at taking their medicines correctly (by mouth)
- percentage of patients who get better at getting dressed
- percentage of patients who had to be admitted to the hospital
- percentage of patients who need urgent, unplanned medical care
- percentage of patients who are confused less often

By looking at these various quality-of-care measures for a home health agency, in addition to asking the questions already cited about the agency and its operations, these various tools can help you make the kind of decisions as to what agency will best meet your personal health needs. *Again, to access the comparative information, you can log onto the Medicare consumer Web site, http://www.Medicare.gov, and click "Home Health Compare." Once on the site, you can search for home health-care information by state, county, zip code, or name of agency. Consumers may also obtain the information via Medicare's twenty-four-hour hotline at 1-800-MEDICARE (tel: 1-800-633-4227).*

DEFINITIONS OF BONDED, LICENSED, AND CERTIFIED HEALTH PERSONNEL

As already noted, certain terminology is employed in regard to homecare personnel. These include their being bonded, licensed, and certified.

Bonded Personnel, like bonded agencies, have some protection or "insurance" against consumer claims. So if a consumer has a problem with a bonded employee—for example, personal property damage—and takes court action and wins, the bond can pay for the damages. The term "bonded" does not mean that employees are qualified to provide safe and satisfactory care.

Be aware that when agencies use the term "bonded" this almost always refers to the agency and claims against it, not their employee. Although agencies could bond employees, few do so because of the expense involved. It is rare for individual employees to bond themselves.

Licensed Health Personnel pass a state test. Once passed, the state department of health or education issues a license that permits them to work. Every state licenses doctors, dentists, registered nurses (RN), licensed practical nurses (LPN), and physical therapists. Some states license social workers; dental hygienists; occupational, speech, and respiratory therapists; and laboratory personnel. Homemaker–home health aides are not generally licensed by states.

Certified Health Personnel must meet the specific standards set by the national organization representing their profession. For example, the American Dietetic Association represents and certifies dieticians. The standards usually require passing a national test and/or providing proof of work experience. Social workers and therapists are among health personnel who are generally certified. Homemaker–home health aides are not certified by a national organization.

State licensure and certification help protect the public against unqualified health personnel working in homecare, health facilities, and private practice. But standards vary from state to state, and in all cases your best defense is to screen carefully and supervise workers yourself—or rely upon a good homecare agency.[7]

HOW TO FIND HOMECARE AGENCY SERVICES

The most common form of homecare assistance in many communities is an informal system of friends, family, or individually hired help who make their living by performing work in the home, including childcare, home nursing, homemaking, or chore work. However, more and more assistance is provided through a variety of agencies, public and private.

"Steve," asked Mitchell, " in looking for a homecare agency, what exactly are we looking for? This whole field is new to me. I know, in general, what homecare programs do. How and where do we get started in looking and exactly what kind of organization provides it?"

In looking for agencies that provide homecare services, there are a variety of sources you can use. You can find their names and addresses from your physician, the public health department of your community or state, which can refer you to Medicare/Medicaid-certified home health agencies, your state or local welfare department, a hospital social service department, or the visiting nurse association in your community. Homecare agencies may be listed in the yellow pages of your telephone directory under "Nursing," "Nursing Services," "Homemaker–Home Health Aide Agencies," "Home Healthcare," "Social Service Organizations," or "Home Health Services." In the white pages, look for Meals-on-Wheels (home-delivered meals); Homemaker–Home Health Aide Services; Visiting Nurse Associations; Family Service Agencies; Catholic Charities; Jewish Family Services or other religiously related agencies; or local offices of the American Red Cross or the United Way (sometimes called United Fund or Community Chest). Your place of religious worship may also be able to help you find homecare providers. You may also wish to check your telephone books in "Information and Referral (I&R) Service or System," "Community Service," "Action Lines," "Hot Line," "CONTACT," "HELP," or ask your local phone operator for assistance. Your community's Information and Referral Service can connect people to a variety of health, social, and consumer services and is often sponsored by city or county offices such as social service departments or community organizations such as the United Way. In addition, there may be Area Agencies on Aging in your community that sponsor homecare and other community programs to assist those age sixty and older to remain independent. Although they are established for services to older citizens, they will often help people of any age trying to find community homecare. The Eldercare Locator, financed by the US Administration on Aging, also may be able to provide information about services available in your area. (Telephone 1-800-677-1116, toll free, or visit http://www.aoa.dhhs.gov on the Internet.) The American Association of Retired Persons (AARP) also may provide information to its members. Write to AARP, Department P, 601 E St. NW Washington, DC 20049 or visit http://www.aarp.org on the Internet. If you need homecare services related to a specific problem such as cancer, blindness, mental retardation, or other illnesses, contact the appropriate community voluntary health agency such as the local office of the American Cancer Society. Most agencies have "patient services" divisions that may assist you in locating services. Finally, don't overlook city, county, or state officials. Call the mayor's office, the board of supervisors, state senators, or your congressional representative.[8] The following are common home health agencies.

Voluntary Tax-Exempt Agencies

Voluntary agencies are locally funded, community-based, and usually operated by a volunteer board of interested citizens. Like the public health services, the agencies, concerned with a broad base of clients, usually offer a sliding scale of fees and are good sources for information and referral. Most of the voluntary agencies are visiting nurse associations.

Public Health Services

About one-half of the Medicare-certified home health agencies are government sponsored, usually under the support of a city or county health department. Most charge for services but arrange reduced rates or free care for those who cannot pay. Some may restrict services to the poor or the elderly, but most serve a broad-base clientele. Even if public health departments do not provide direct homecare, they usually can refer callers to agencies that do.

Hospital-Based Agencies

A small number of hospitals operate home health agencies. Many of the clinical services available in the hospital are provided, such as laboratory work and physical therapy. Nearly all restrict themselves to providing follow-up care for patients released from the hospital. Find out whether your community hospital provides homecare services.

Proprietary Agencies

A number of profit-making organizations offer home health services in cities throughout the United States. Not all proprietary agencies are eligible for Medicare reimbursement. You should ask your agency whether you qualify for Medicare benefits. It is more common, but not universal, that private insurance plans reimburse proprietary agencies. While proprietary agencies do offer skilled services, many agencies emphasize nonskilled care, such as homemakers, companions, and home health aides.

Private Nonprofit Agencies

These are usually small organizations owned by families or individuals who technically earn a salary, rather than take a profit. This arrangement makes such agencies eligible for Medicare reimbursement, regardless of state licensing procedures, and Medicare patients constitute a high percentage of their clients. The majority of private nonprofit agencies operate in urban areas where there are large numbers of elderly individuals.

Employment Agencies and Nurses' Registries

For a fee, these agencies refer and place health personnel in your home. You assume responsibility as an employer. In general, employment agencies and nurses' registries provide a referral system that helps you find and employ individuals willing to work in your home; but they do not supervise them once they have been placed. Thus, an agency concerned with good quality of care—whether profit making, nonprofit, or governmental—and which supervises its employees, provides additional services that are not available to you otherwise.[9]

In looking for a home healthcare agency, call the various organizations previously listed, explain the kind of health problems for which you seek their assistance, and choose the agency that seems most likely to answer your personal needs. A good agency carefully evaluates the home situation and works with you to develop a plan of service that matches your health, social, and financial needs. This is very important. A good agency will only provide services that you require. For example, it will not provide round-the-clock services when a few hours a day is all that is necessary. It would not provide assistance for tasks you would and could do yourself. This can help you keep or regain your independence and help lessen costs to you. A good homecare agency supervises all personnel coming into the home, including the volunteers, so problems are prevented or corrected as soon as possible if they happen.

HOMECARE PERSONNEL

There is a wide variety of personnel who provide homecare services. These include the following major categories:

- *Physicians* (doctors of medicine and osteopathy) may prescribe homecare for their patients. They outline specific health or other services that are needed and the level of care. Sometimes doctors provide medical care at home.
- *Social Workers* provide counseling and find and coordinate resources and supervise homecare services.
- *Registered Dieticians* or nutritionists plan special diets to speed recovery from illness or injury or to manage health conditions such as high blood pressure or diabetes.
- *Speech Therapists* help those with communications problems, such as learning to speak after a stroke.
- *Respiratory Therapists* help patients with breathing difficulties so that their lung function is restored or kept at its highest possible level.
- *Physical Therapists* use exercise, heat, light, water, or other methods to treat patients with problems of movement.
- *Occupational Therapists* teach people how to manage daily activities at home and/or work despite physical or mental disabilities; for example, carrying out housekeeping from a wheelchair.
- *Nurses*: registered nurses (RNs) provide skilled nursing care and licensed practical (vocational) nurses (LPNs) also provide nursing care.
  - ▼ Registered nurses are more highly skilled and educated than LPNs. RNs are best prepared to manage the critical needs of patients who may require complex treatment. The RNs often act as homecare supervisors. RNs with public health education may be employed to coordinate agency services with other health and social services available in the community.
  - ▼ Licensed practical nurses have less education in nursing than RNs. LPNs are equipped to take care of patients with simpler nursing needs who usually require more routine treatment and care.
- *Homemaker–Home Health Aides* may provide one or more services: homemaking services (environmental care and home management), personal care, childcare, and others. Job titles for the aide often vary depending upon local practice and specific duties in the home. For example, when employed primarily to perform household duties, aides may be known as "homemakers,"

"housekeepers," or "home helps." When they carry out personal care services, they may be called "nursing assistants," health aides," "home health aides," or "attendants." Because the aide's job usually involves health and safety, a good agency provides aides who have at least sixty hours of training as recommended by the National Home Caring Council. Training should cover personal care, basic home nursing, working with people, food and nutrition, home safety and management, budgeting, childcare, and family relations. Ongoing training should be provided to keep skills up-to-date. Nurse's aide training and experience are not considered a good substitute. In hospitals, supervisors are available as soon as the need arises. In a home an aide must be trained so as to work with little immediate supervision. He or she must know how to "make do" with what is at hand and know what to do in an emergency.

Certified homecare aides and personal care aides, who provide similar services, will visit your home for as little as four hours or up to twenty-four hours a day to provide assistance with personal hygiene, toileting, light housekeeping, shopping, and meal preparation. They also offer companionship. However, you must pay the costs of such aides yourself because Medicare, Medicaid, and private insurance usually do not cover the services of personal care aides when the physician does not order such care. Thus, this is the kind of care you can receive without a physician's order. Your aide's supervisor, who should be a registered nurse, should visit your home to make sure your needs are being met. Together, you write the assignments you wish the aides to complete. The nurse supervisor should return to your home at intervals of no more than sixty days and should help you maintain your health by evaluating your general physical condition as well as your home's environment for safety. The supervisor should also be accessible at any time for your questions and concerns.

If you decide to hire a home health aide on your own, whether you locate the person through a newspaper advertisement, a friend, or a relative, make sure the candidates give you character and personal references as well as information about their work performance. Be thorough in asking the candidates about their work and personal history, obtaining their names and addresses, Social Security numbers, information about past work experience, at least three professional references (with names and telephone numbers of their past supervisors), and five personal references. Be sure to call these references and interview them as well to make sure the candidates have told the truth. You can also contact investigative agencies that are listed in the yellow pages of your telephone directory to perform a criminal check on the candidates. You will pay a fee for this service, but it is worth the money if it prevents someone with a criminal history from working in your home. Remember that federal law also requires that private employers withhold Social Security monies from the income of home workers who are paid more than a minimal amount. Also be sure that you have sufficient insurance to cover the claims of workers who may injure themselves on your property. In addition, tell your friends and relatives that you have hired a home healthcare aide and ask them to visit you unannounced so that they can witness how you and your home health aide are doing. In case of any emergency, tell the home health aide which friends, relatives, or neighbors the home health aide should contact.

Also, if you are hiring a home health aide on your own, think about employing a case manager to watch over the delivery of care. A case manager is a professional, usually a nurse or a social worker, who will thoroughly review your needs and coordinate your services. To learn the names of qualified case managers in your local area, contact the National Association of Professional Geriatric Care Managers in Tucson, Arizona, at 1-520-881-8008 or click on its Web site at http://www.caremanager.org. Telephone the suggested care managers and interview them about their professional work experience and fees. Always prepare a checklist of duties you wish the home health aide to perform. It is important to pay home health aides fairly for their services, reward them for the way they work, and treat them as professionals. Do not allow the home health aide to perform duties related to your personal estate or valuables, including handling your mail, signing checks, visiting the bank, reviewing insurance information, or similar duties. If you require a money manager to oversee your financial affairs, you can hire such a person who will help you with check writing and banking activities and can watch over your income and expenses. Before hiring anyone, ask about the individual's fees. To find the names of a qualified manager, you can telephone the American Association of Daily Money Managers at 1-301-593-5462 or go to its Web site at http://www.aadmm.com.

- *Volunteers* assist with supplementary services such as friendly visiting, telephone reassurance, meals-on-wheels, transportation, and escort services
- *Chore Workers* perform or assist with chore services: home repair, heavy cleaning, or yard work.[10]

In addition to the previous personnel, others may also provide homecare services. These include the clergy, laboratory technicians, and others.

HOW TO PREVENT PROBLEMS

"Steve, the idea of homecare is great, but we're going to have a big problem with Mom and Dad. They may not trust strangers in their home. How can we assure them it is safe and make certain they are comfortable with strangers who are now part of their family life? You know that elderly people are notoriously forgetful. Mom refers to these episodes as her 'senior moments.' She could be resentful, thinking the homemaker had stolen some missing object rather than considering the possibility that she herself may have misplaced it. We can't be with them all the time to monitor."

Mitchell's concern was well taken. Whether you use a home health agency or hire help yourself, there are certain steps you can take to avoid problems and improve services in the home.

- *Discuss security in detail.* Anyone entering your home should have proper identification. Always ask for receipts for any monies received or purchases made. Most good agencies have a system for this. Store large sums of cash, jewelry, or other valuables in a safe place—if possible, in a bank.
- *Treat homecare workers with respect.* Once again, remember they are there to help and are not servants. Make their jobs easier by letting them know in advance how you like things done. Whenever possible, they will try to comply with your requests. For example, if an article of clothing wears out, it would be helpful for the head caregiver to receive money from the supervising parent (or child) instead of the caregiver buying it and getting reimbursed.
- *Discuss confidentiality when dealing with an agency.* Responsible agencies will not give out any information about those receiving care without their written permission. When care is not for yourself, find out what arrangements must be made so you are kept informed.
- *Involve those for whom homecare is sought as much as possible, even if they are very young or very old.* Let them know someone will be coming to the house and what will be done. If possible, be there yourself the first day services begin and stop in periodically.
- *Keep important telephone numbers handy.* Make sure homecare workers know how to reach you, the doctor, and the local fire and police stations. Provide backup names and telephone numbers of relatives, neighbors, or friends who should be contacted when you cannot be reached.[11]

HOW TO EVALUATE SERVICES

Even when you carefully select an agency or an employee, problems can occur once services begin. When care is not for you, but for young children or someone living alone, be extra cautious for signs of trouble:

- *Poor Work Habits.* Is the worker frequently late or absent? Does he or she leave early or do just enough to get by?
- *Indifferent Care.* Does the worker provide rough care? Fail to respond to reasonable requests? Act in a rude or discourteous manner?
- *Untrustworthy Behavior.* Is money or personal property missing that is not misplaced and otherwise cannot be accounted for?
- *Poor Home Environment.* Is appearance of house clean and orderly? Is food improperly stored? Are garbage and trash not attended to? Are toilets, bedpans, or bathtubs dirty?

- *Poor Personal Care*. Does the person being cared for appear clean? Smartly dressed? Is clothing improper for weather or living conditions? Are there unexplained or unusual marks, cuts, or bruises? Are bed sores developing or getting worse? Are there signs of unhappiness, fear, or depression? Are the person's eyes bright? Is there eye contact?

If the answer to any of these questions is "yes," problems exist—usually with the worker. However, unhappiness, fear, or depression may mean that the mental or physical health of the person receiving care is declining or there is a worsening of social factors in the home.

HOW TO HANDLE PROBLEMS

If you suspect problems in the homecare or they have already happened, do not delay. Take action immediately before the situation worsens.

- *If the problems do not appear too serious*, you may wish to discuss them first with the worker.
- *If a serious situation exists*, call and discuss the problem with the agency supervisor, not the homecare worker. Put your complaint in writing as well. Keep a copy of your letter. Do not wait long to see results. If the situation does not improve in one to two weeks (depending upon the nature of the problem), complain again. Consider changing agencies.
- *Contact the police first*, in cases of clear-cut theft, fraud, physical or mental abuse, or suspected child abuse. Don't hesitate to exercise this basic consumer right to protect yourself and others.

Finally, if problems cannot be resolved to your satisfaction, you can and should take other consumer action.

- *Make your complaints a matter of public record*. Contact the appropriate agencies such as the city, county, or state consumer affairs or protection offices, or get in touch with the state attorney general. If your community has a Better Business Bureau, register your dissatisfaction there. If the homecare workers or agencies at fault are licensed or certified, or if an agency is accredited, notify the organization in charge. In addition, you can notify the homecare provider's chief supervisor or administrator, the state health department, or the Medicare hot line. If you suspect fraud, no matter how slight the fraud may appear, you should report these activities to your state department of health. In the case of the delivery of Medicare home healthcare services, contact the Office of Inspector General hot line, tel: 800-HHS-TIPs (1-800-447-8477).
- *Find out where the agency gets its financial support and complain there*. If

public funds such as Medicare and Medicaid are involved, complain to your elected federal, state, county, or city officials as well as to the state agencies in charge. As public advocates they may be more receptive to consumer charges.

Though complaints can usually be made with a telephone call, it is usually more effective to write. Be specific in your charges. Support the charges where possible with proof that problems exist—for example, with written complaints you have made already to an agency. Keep a record of all complaints made, the office or party contacted, the date contacted, and any follow-up.

Your action will not always solve your problems, but it will help. It will fore-warn other consumers and alert key public and private officials and organizations. Licenses, certification, and accreditation can be revoked for unsafe care and unethical practices.

COST OF HOMECARE SERVICES

As far as fees and visit charges are concerned, most homecare agencies charge for professional services by visit. Bringing an aide into your home just three times a week (2 to 3 hours per visit) to help with dressing, bathing, preparing meals, and similar household chores can cost $1,000 per month or $12,000 per year. In 2004 the national average cost for homecare provided by a home health aide was $18 per hour, or $37,000 per year for a 40 hour week of help, but expect to pay more in or near cities, less in rural areas. Add in costs of skilled help such as physical therapists and these costs can be greater. In comparison, nursing home care during 2001 as a national average cost more than $54,900 per year and by 2003 almost $58,000, and much more than this amount in some regions of the country.[12] An official home health agency is an organization sponsored by a unit of the government such as a city or county, while nonofficial agencies are all nongovernmental home health organizations whether they operate on a profit or nonprofit basis. Proprietary agencies may charge a little less per hour than public agencies. A minimum stay of two to four hours is often required by proprietary agencies (thus sometimes raising the cost per visit), although this is subject to negotiation. Therefore, when you engage the services of a home healthcare agency, ask what its fees and minimum-stay policies are in advance. Some services such as meals-on-wheels, friendly visiting, and telephone reassurance usually operate at little or no cost because of volunteer help. The same may be true in some cities where transportation and escort services operate as community services. You will be able to assess these various costs for yourself. Remember, fees rise with inflation. *In assessing the costs of homecare or homemaker–home health aide services, ask the following questions*:

- Does the agency provide written statements explaining all the costs and payment plan options associated with homecare? What are the hourly fees? Are there minimum hours or days per week required? Are there a minimum amount of services you must pay for? Generally, you can expect to pay more when additional services are needed; service periods are long and/or frequent; and services are provided by highly trained personnel. For example, per-hour charges for registered nurses are usually more than licensed practical nurses, whose fees are usually more than homemaker–home health aide service.

- Does the agency set a sliding scale based on the ability to pay?
- Who pays for the employee's Social Security or other insurance? Are there any additional costs such as travel? For supervision or home evaluation? Medical supplies such as dressings? (Most quality agencies include supervision and evaluation in their fees.)
- How does the agency handle payment and billing? Make sure you obtain all financial arrangements—costs, payment procedures, and billings—in writing. Read the agreement carefully before signing. Be sure to keep a copy.[13]

By asking the proper questions, you can do much to control the costs of your home healthcare expenses.

HOW TO FINANCE HOME HEALTHCARE SERVICES

In determining whether you can afford homecare services, you should know that there are a variety of private and public sources available to help you pay for such care. These sources include Medicare, Medicaid, other public programs, private health insurance, and health maintenance organizations (HMOs), as well as charitable funds. However, it should be noted that government and private assistance may not be sufficient to pay for all your homecare services. Some of the funding is too limited in the types of services covered; as a result, a patient sometimes can pay more out of his own pocket when he stays at home than if he were hospitalized and an insurance plan paid for the hospital stay. Moreover, some people who could be cared for at home must enter an institution or give up the homecare because they cannot meet all the third party's (insurance or government assistance program) requirements for payment. Consequently, if you need homecare, the following sources may help you pay for it. But find out in advance what restrictions home health agencies may impose in order to receive their services. Then you will know what kind of financial burden you may have to assume in deciding whether you can afford to receive care at home.

Medicaid

All states and the District of Columbia are required to provide Medicaid payments for three home health services: nursing, home health aides, and medical supplies and equipment. At the option of the states, Medicaid may also provide other services such as physical therapy, occupational therapy, and speech and hearing services.

Find out from your local or state public assistance or welfare department, your local department of social services, or your local Social Security office whether Medicaid in your state pays for these additional services.

Blue Cross

Many Blue Cross plans provide some form of home health benefits. A majority no longer require prior hospitalization. If you have Blue Cross coverage, find out from your plan or insurance agent whether this waiver applies to you. Many plans also pay for comprehensive homecare services: drugs, medical-surgical supplies, transportation, nutritional guidance, counseling, social service, and rental of equipment are covered in addition to visits by medical professionals. Homemaking services are usually not covered.

Private Insurance

Many Americans who have major medical insurance may have homecare benefits included in their insurance coverage plan. Except for prior hospitalization and coverage of prescription drugs, the restrictions of the insurance coverage are similar to those of the Medicare program. Many private insurance programs require the patient to pay a deductible and a percentage (usually 20 percent) of any charges beyond the deductible. Except in some states where home healthcare coverage is mandatory, private hospitalization plans probably will not cover homecare. Check your policy carefully or contact the private insurer. In some cases, homecare services will not be listed specifically in the policy, but they may be covered under "miscellaneous" or "other" clauses.

Federal Programs

Aside from Medicaid and Medicare, for persons who qualify there may be other federal program funds available for home health services. Homemaker services may be provided to needy persons under Title XX of the Social Security Act. Where these programs are available, they are usually administered by the local welfare agency. Money for homecare for the elderly is available on a limited basis under an Administration on Aging program or Older Americans Act; check with your local agency or state Agency on Aging. Disabled persons may qualify for home health services under the Developmentally Disabled Assistance Act. An agency that deals with rehabilitation of the handicapped may be able to help.

Health Maintenance Organizations

A federal qualified health maintenance organization is required by law to provide home health services to its members. Others may include some aspects of homecare in their consumer health plans.

Charitable Funds

Nonprofit home health agencies such as visiting nurse associations often receive United Way funds to help offset the costs of homecare when the patients cannot pay the full cost of service.[14]

Special Insurance

Special insurance such as worker's compensation, disability, home liability or care insurance may cover homecare services under specified conditions—for example, if care is needed as a result of an injury at home or work or in a car.

Department of Veterans Affairs

This federal agency provides homecare benefits for military-related illnesses or injury.

While the aforementioned sources should be examined as ways to finance home health services, one major source of assistance that is readily available to millions of elderly citizens in this country is the federal government's Medicare program. Because of the importance of the Medicare program to the elderly and the fact that most homecare program patients are elderly, the following discussion presents in more detail the homecare benefits in the Medicare program.

HOME HEALTHCARE AND MEDICARE

Given a choice, most elderly people would rather remain at home when they are sick rather than go to a nursing home or a hospital. Home healthcare is not only more comfortable but also can cost less than institutional care. Some illnesses, of course, may make homecare impossible. According to the federal government's General Accounting Office (now named the General Accountability Office), however, until the patient becomes greatly impaired and needs more extensive care, being treated at home is the preferred option to institutional care.[15]

During calendar year 1999, about 2.7 million Medicare enrollees received over 113 million home health visits. Total program charges were almost $11.4 billion of which payments of $7.9 billion were made. In contrast, a decade earlier, in 1988, 1.6 million Medicare enrollees received 37.7 million visits for whom total program charges were almost $2.5 billion, of which $1.9 billion in program payments were made. This growth was basically the result of the 1988–1989 liberalization and standardization of coverage for home healthcare services, which, in turn, spurred a substantial increase in the number of home health agencies certified by Medicare. Between 1989 and 1999, the number of agencies increased by almost 40 percent (from 5,676 to 7,857).[16]

Under Medicare home healthcare was originally conceived as a means to facilitate earlier hospital discharge; that is, it was to be a transitional relationship following hospitalization. In fact, before 1980, Medicare regulations stipulated that only beneficiaries who had been hospitalized could receive home health services. In 1980 this requirement was removed and home healthcare began to be used more broadly. Toward the end of the decade, the Medicare manual for home health agencies was revised in response to litigation. Two changes were critical: first, coverage could no longer be denied solely because a patient had chronic disease; and second, a physician's prescription of home health services could no longer be rejected unless objective clinical evidence contradicted the order. In the 1990s these changes laid the foundation for the rapid growth of home healthcare under Medicare, which is used primarily to provide long-term care.[17]

It is the physician who decides whether or not the patient's medical needs can be met at home. But the suitability of the home must be examined not only in terms of its physical layout but also in terms of the ability and willingness of the family members to provide what help is needed. For example, are the home and the neighborhood quiet? Must the patient climb any stairs? Will the patient have his or her own room? Are bathroom facilities easily accessible? Will the house accommodate a walker or a wheelchair?

While few homes meet all these conditions, suitable arrangements can often be made to adapt to the patient's needs. The family also has to be considered. Having a patient at home may mean changes in your lifestyle. Therefore, make sure that the nature of the patient's condition would respond to homecare rather than requiring the security and appropriateness of round-the-clock institutional care. A patient who is extremely nervous, demanding, or crotchety could make matters worse for the family at home.

On the other hand, home healthcare is so important because it gives you more freedom as a patient:

- You can sleep as late as you wish.
- You can eat what you crave and when you want.
- You can dress as you desire.
- You can sleep in your own bed, wearing your selection of clothes.
- You can keep your home at any temperature you want.
- You can visit with your friends as often as you please in addition to being with your family.
- You can enjoy more privacy in your own home with your own family.
- Your family can often assist you with rehabilitation therapy.
- You do not have to worry as much about your family when they are right there.
- You may feel like doing more yourself so as not to inconvenience your family.
- You can still receive the individual attention you need from nurses, technicians, and other professionals.

- You can receive a "lift" from going from hospital to home. Such progress can make you feel better.
- You open up a hospital bed for someone else who needs hospital care.
- Your care at home is less expensive than in a hospital or a skilled nursing facility.[18]

Given the advantage of receiving homecare services, the question arises as to how an individual qualifies for them under Medicare. The following requirements must be met:

- You must be sixty-five years or older or have been entitled to Social Security disability benefits for twenty-four consecutive months.
- You must be under a physician's care.
- Your physician must certify that you need specified home health services which can be provided by a home health agency participating in the Medicare program.

The Medicare program provides homecare services under its hospital insurance program (Part A) and its voluntary medical insurance program (Part B). Coverage under the hospital insurance to which all Social Security beneficiaries are automatically entitled pays the reasonable cost of unlimited home health visits during a benefit period. A benefit period begins with the first day you receive covered inpatient services in a hospital. It ends when you have been out of the hospital or the skilled nursing facility for sixty consecutive days (including the day of discharge). There is no limit to the number of benefit periods a person may have. The payment for the home health visits may be made for a non-calendar year (365 days) after the start of each benefit period. Therefore, you qualify for home health visits under the hospital insurance (Part A) of Medicare if you meet the following conditions:

- You are in a Medicare program–participating hospital. Effective July 1, 1981, the three-day prior hospitalization requirement qualifying for homecare visits under Part A was eliminated by the Omnibus Budget Reconciliation Act of 1980 (Public Law 96-499). In other words, you can qualify directly for homecare under Part A of Medicare without first being hospitalized.
- Your home health plan is set up by a physician within fourteen days after you leave the hospital or the skilled nursing home if you need such services before receiving home care.
- Your homecare program is for further treatment of a condition for which you received treatment in the hospital or the skilled nursing facility if you required such prior care or you can receive homecare directly without first being hospitalized. You are confined to your home.
- Your condition is such that you need skilled nursing care on an intermittent basis or physical or speech therapy.

In addition to the home health benefits of the hospital insurance plan (Part A), additional home health benefits are available under the medical insurance plan (Part B) of Medicare for which you can sign up on a voluntary basis. The home health services under the supplementary medical insurance program are without limit within a calendar year. *The benefit period provision does not apply in the Part B program* as it does in Part A and, also like Part A, *no prior stay in a hospital or a skilled nursing home is required in the Part B program of Medicare before these home health benefits become effective.* Consequently, you can become eligible for home health benefits under the supplementary insurance program (Part B) of Medicare if the following conditions are met:

- If you have voluntarily signed up for this insurance, it will pay 100 percent of the reasonable costs of the covered services.
- You are confined to your home.
- A doctor orders and reviews periodically the plan for home healthcare.
- Your condition is such that you will need skilled nursing care on an intermittent basis or physical therapy or speech therapy. If you qualify for any of these home health benefits, your eligibility for home health services may be extended solely on the basis of your continuing need for occupational therapy.

Homecare services provided under the Medicare program are carried out by home health agencies that qualify for participating in the Medicare program. Such agencies have policies established and supervised by physicians and registered nurses, are licensed under state and local laws, and are approved for participation in the Medicare program. They keep clinical records of all patients and carry out the orders of the patients' physicians. In addition, services may be performed outside of your home if they require special equipment that cannot be brought to your home. The following services are paid for by Medicare and are provided by a home health agency:

- *Professional Skilled Nursing Care (part-time)*
  A registered nurse carries out the physician's plan of treatment. The nurse reports your progress to your physician and instructs you and your family regarding your care.
- *Practical Nursing Care*
  Under the supervision of a registered nurse, licensed practical nurses perform such services as giving you simple treatments and keeping records.
- *Physical Therapy Services*
  Under a physician's orders, qualified physical therapists may treat you to relieve pain and restore muscles by such services as exercise, massage, heat lamps, and baths. Also, physical therapists may instruct you on how to use braces, crutches, wheelchairs, and canes. They arrange for equipment and teach your family how to help you.

In addition, under the supplementary medical insurance (Part B) program of Medicare, you are entitled to outpatient physical therapy services under the supervision of hospitals, approved clinics, rehabilitation centers, and local public health agencies.

- *Speech Therapy Services*

    Your physician's plan may include speech therapy provided by qualified specialists if you need this help because of a speech disorder.

- *Occupational Therapy Services*

    Your physician's plan may also include the services of a specialist in occupational therapy to guide you in creative and self-care activities and to instruct you in ways to help you.

- *Medical Social Services*

    Qualified medical social services may be part of your physician's plan to help the team understand the social and emotional problems or personal difficulties related to your health and recovery.

- *Home Health Aide Services*

    Part-time services of home health aides provide needed care for patients under physician's orders and under the supervision of a nurse or therapists, including assistance with such personal needs as bathing, personal grooming, exercises, and grooming.

- *Medical Supplies*

    Includes such supplies as surgical dressings, oxygen, gauze, cotton, rubbing alcohol, and intravenous fluids. However, medical supplies do not include drugs or biologicals.

- *Medical Appliances*

    This includes the use of such appliances as wheelchairs, crutches, hospital beds, oxygen tents, trapeze bars, and air pressure mattresses as prescribed by your physician.

- *Physician Services*

    Physician services are covered if you signed up voluntarily for the supplementary medical insurance (Part B) of the Medicare program.[19]

However, although many services are covered under Medicare's home health services program, many are not. *Medicare does not cover the following home health services:*

- full-time nursing care
- drugs and biologicals
- personal comfort items
- general housekeeping services
- meals-on-wheels (meals delivered to your home)
- ambulance or special transportation to and from your home when you receive covered services on an outpatient basis

In seeking homecare services, you can find out whether a home health agency is Medicare approved by asking your local Social Security agency, your physician, or the home health agency itself. If you qualify for the hospital insurance program (Part A) under Medicare and voluntarily purchase the supplementary medical insurance (Part B) of Medicare, you will not have to decide whether to receive your home health benefits under the hospital insurance (Part A) or the medical insurance (Part B) program. If you meet the hospitalization requirements of Part A, you will *automatically* come under the hospital insurance plan and its home health benefits. If you do not meet Medicare's hospitalization requirements, your home health benefits will *automatically* come under the medical insurance plan, *if you have purchased this insurance.* After you receive your home health visits, you do not have to pay the home health agency directly and then collect the cost of the service from Medicare. Rather, the home health agency will collect from Medicare directly. And if you are living in a rest home, you are still eligible for home health benefits because the rest home is your place of residence. In addition, the home health agency provides services for the treatment of mental illness if you meet all the qualifications for receiving home healthcare under Medicare.

Consequently, Medicare can assist people age sixty-five years or over, or people who have been entitled to Social Security disability benefits for twenty-four consecutive months, with the best in skilled nursing care and other therapeutic services in their own homes through the coordinated planning, evaluation, and follow-up efforts of the professional health team of the physician, hospital, and home health agency. Finally, make sure that you always carry your Medicare card with you. It has your personal claim number and shows what benefits you are entitled to. If you lose your card, notify your Social Security office and they will help you get another. Your Medicare card, whether it enables you to receive homecare or other kinds of health services, is one mechanism that enables you to have as healthful a life as possible.

COMMUNITY ASSISTANCE OUTSIDE OF MEDICARE

While for-profit and nonprofit homecare agencies, whether they are Medicare certified or not, provide a great deal of the homecare services in this country, there are other means of receiving care at home that are available within your own community. These may be private-like assisted living facilities or public federal government programs or other public programs operated by your state or local government. The following are the kinds of organizations and programs that may be available within your community and can provide care within a homelike setting. *The Eldercare Locator of the US Administration on Aging can help you find necessary and convenient services that serve the elderly in your community. Its telephone number is 1-800-677-1116.*

Board-and-Care Homes

Board-and-care homes are group living arrangements designed to meet the needs of people who cannot live independently but also do not need nursing home care. These homes offer a broader range of services than independent living choices. Most provide assistance with some of the activities of daily living, including eating, walking, bathing, and toileting. In some instances, private long-term care insurance and medical assistance programs will help pay for this kind of arrangement. Remember that many of these homes do not receive payment from Medicare and Medicaid and are not closely monitored.

Continuing Care Retirement Communities (CCRCs)

Continuing care retirement communities are housing communities that provide different levels of care, based on the requirements of a resident, ranging from independent living apartments to skilled nursing care in an affiliated nursing home, which may be on or off campus. The independent living arrangement may be set up as a cooperative, a condominium, or a rental arrangement. These communities are usually restricted to persons over a specific age. Residents move from one care setting to another depending upon their needs but continue to remain part of their continuing care retirement community. Make sure you check the record and quality of the CCRC's nursing home. Your CCRC contract will require that you use it. Many CCRCs require a large payment prior to admission and also charge monthly fees, which cover a resident's fee for housing, social activities, meals, services, and nursing care. For these reasons, many CCRCs may be too expensive for older people whose incomes are not in the higher brackets. However, if you can afford a CCRC, you have the freedom to enjoy your own home and daily chores as well as have a variety of clubs, groups, and organizations to serve your interests and needs.

Dementia Care Facilities

These multiunit developments are licensed by the state as adult homes. Their physical layouts, programmatic goals, staffing, and care plans are designed to address the needs of people with Alzheimer's disease or other dementia conditions.

Assisted Living Communities

Assisted living communities offer personal services, twenty-four-hour supervision and assistance, along with activities and health-related services. Medicare does not cover the cost of assisted living, which means the resident or the family must pay for this living arrangement themselves. In addition, assisted living does not necessarily provide the medical and nursing care available in a nursing home. Unlike skilled nursing homes, there are no federal regulations or even a single term that defines all assisted living facilities. Each state defines and regulates assisted living differently. Assisted living is designed to minimize the need to move; meet an individual's needs and preferences; maximize an individual's dignity, privacy, independence, choice, and safety; and encourage family and community involvement. More than a million persons live in more than thirty-six thousand licensed facilities generally considered assisted living operations, which do not include skilled nursing homes. While many of these homes are small and house only a few residents, others are far larger. The more amenities a facility offers, the higher the cost. There are many questions you may ask before moving into an assisted living facility, but one of the services you should ask about is its provision of healthcare. The following questions may help you determine the nature and quality of services an assisted living community provides:

- Does the assisted living community perform a preliminary assessment of the kinds of services a resident requires? Are family members or appropriate healthcare professionals participating in the assessment?
- Does the community establish a service plan for each new resident member? The service plan should include specifics about the services to be provided, their frequency, and the period of time over which the services will be delivered. The service plan should be updated as the resident's needs change. Ask if you can see a sample service plan.
- Does the organization coordinate healthcare services for your loved one?
- Who provides the direct care? What training/certification do the caregivers have? What are the trainer's qualifications? Is there a physician on staff who visits regularly and is on call the remainder of the time? If they wish, can residents keep their own doctors? Is there a pharmacy service? A medical room? What are the community's policies in regard to treating medical emergencies?
- Are health-related services and trained staff available should the resident need them? How much does it cost? How many staff persons are there for each shift or time of day? What are their responsibilities? What other duties do the staff members have during these hours? Are they trained in the techniques and care of mentally confused residents and are there specific areas and/or units within the community that are designed to provide specialized care and programs for those who are cognitively impaired?
- For how many residents is each direct staff person responsible? What is the ratio of staff to residents on all shifts? This ratio is an indication of how fast they can help residents who need assistance.
- Is there a nurse? Is the nurse licensed? What are the nurse's responsibilities and hours? Nurses available twenty-four hours per day? Who is responsible when the nurse is not on duty?
- Who provides the medications? If not the nurse, how are staff trained and supervised? Is medication management provided?
- What health services are available at the community: wound care, hospice,

pharmacy services, laboratory work, medical room, capability for x-rays, physical therapy, social work, podiatrist, dentistry, physiotherapy, and others? If the resident has chronic hypertension (high blood pressure), will the person's blood pressure be taken and recorded on a regular basis? Also, is there convalescent care (during acute illness or recovery from surgery)? If so, how extensive and at what cost? What happens if the resident requires additional services such as nursing care? Can additional services be purchased on a longer-term basis? What does the home provide and what can outside agencies provide?

- As the resident's requirements change, what guidelines will be used to determine whether he or she will be able to continue living in the community?
- Does the community provide twenty-four-hour supervision or is assistance available if a resident needs it?
- For what reasons may a resident be discharged? How does the facility help you if you need to be discharged?
- Has the Joint Commission of Healthcare Organizations that also accredits hospitals and other health organizations accredited the assisted living community? Communities voluntarily seek accreditation through the Joint Commission as evidence of their commitment to delivering quality healthcare. Also, communities can receive special recognition for Health Services Coordination.

There are a number of nonhealth questions you should ask about in terms of the community's operations. How much is its monthly fee? Can it change and what does the fee include? Must you sign an admission contract and does it explain in detail the various services you will receive such as room and board, housekeeping, personal care (such as help with bathing, dressing, and eating), and supervision? Is it twenty-four-hour supervision? Does the community offer choices in regard to single or double occupancies? Does the community provide any written description of its services and fees? Does the contract spell out the responsibilities of the resident and the home and can the resident change the contract? Also, find out what happens if you no longer have any funds? Is there any financial help available and are there any agencies that can help you? Will the community try to assist you to maintain your autonomy and independence?

In case of a power failure or a natural disaster, ask if the community has an emergency plan in place to deal with it. Can you see a copy? You have to know that in case of some kind of emergency the community can still provide services to its residents.

Ask about your rights and responsibilities as a resident? Does the community have a copy of such information that it can give you? Also, does the community have a quality improvement program? Is their a mechanism in place that allows the resident to file his complaints with the community?

Has the community established a family council that allows the families of residents to interact and discuss the care their family members are receiving? Does the community's management welcome any suggestions from the family council, families, or residents or does it oppose the existence of such a council?

What about the community's menu? Three meals a day? Does the community prepare a variety of foods and meet an individual's food preferences and needs? Can it provide special diets that are medically required? Can you bring food into the community from the outside? Can food be brought to a resident's room if the person feels too ill to come to the dining room? Can residents cook within their residencies if they wish?

In terms of meeting the spiritual, mental, physical, psychological, and emotional needs of its residents, does the community provide transportation to outside community activities like shopping or social events as well as have social/recreational activities within the community as well? Do these activities satisfy the residents' needs and interests? Opportunities to attend religious services? Does the community have a homelike atmosphere, encouraging friendships among residents, reaching out to less sociable residents? Is it easy to get around the facility if a resident uses a walker, a wheelchair, or requires the use of handrails?

For a complete list of questions regarding assisted living communities, contact the Consumer Consortium on Assisted Living at 1-703-533-8121 or visit the organization's Web site at http://www.ccal.org. Other organizations providing information in regard to assisted living facilities include:

- *The American Association of Homes and Services for the Aging (AAHSA)*
  National organization of not-for-profit nursing homes, continuing retirement communities, assisted living facilities, senior housing facilities, and community service organizations. The AAHSA can help you find AAHSA-affiliated assisted living residencies in your community. Telephone: 1-202-783-2242. Web site: http://www.aahsa.org.
- *The Assisted Living Federation of America (ALFA)*
  A national organization of for-profit and not-for-profit providers of assisted living, continuing care retirement, independence living, and other forms of housing and services. Telephone: 1-703-691-8100. Web site: http://www.alfa.org.
- *The National Center for Assisted Living (NCAL)*
  Assisted living branch of the American Healthcare Association, a national organization representing long-term care providers. Telephone: 1-202-842-4444. Web site: http://www.ncal.org.
- *The Long Term Community Coalition (LTCC) (Former Nursing Home Community Coalition)*
  Devoted to improving care for the elderly and disabled and publishes booklets on assisted living facilities. Telephone: 1-212-385-0355. Web sites: http://www.assisted-living411.org; http://www.ltccc.org; and http://www.nursinghome411.org.

These various organizations can help you with any questions you may have in regard to assisted living communities.

Program of All-Inclusive Care for the Elderly (PACE)

PACE is unique. It is an optional—not mandatory—benefit under Medicare and Medicaid that concentrates totally on older people who are frail enough to meet their state's standards for nursing home care. It features comprehensive medical and social services that can be provided at an adult day health center, home, and/or inpatient facilities. For most patients, the comprehensive service package allows them to continue living in their own home while receiving services, rather than be admitted to an institution. A team of doctors, nurses, and other health professionals including physical, occupational, and recreational therapists, social workers, and dieticians assess the patient's needs, develop care plans, and provide all services, which are integrated into a complete health plan. Other members on the team include personal care attendants and drivers. Generally, the PACE team has daily contact with its enrollees. This enables team members to detect slight changes in the enrollee's condition, and they can react quickly to changing medical, functional, and psychosocial problems.

Enrollment in PACE is voluntary, but an enrollee must be at least fifty-five years of age; live in a PACE service area; be screened by a team of doctors, nurses, and other health professionals; and sign and agree to the terms of the enrollment agreement.

The PACE service package must include all Medicare and Medicaid services provided by that state. At a minimum, there are at least sixteen services that a PACE organization must provide, including social work, drugs, and nursing facility care. Minimum services that a PACE center must provide include:

- primary care services
- social services
- restorative therapies
- personal care and supportive services
- nutritional counseling
- recreational therapy
- meals

When an enrollee is receiving adult daycare services, these services also include meals and transportation. Services are available twenty-four hours a day, 7 days a week, 365 days a year. Generally, these services are delivered in an adult day health setting, but they may include in-home and other referral services that enrollees may require. This includes such services as medical specialists, laboratory and other diagnostic services, and hospital and nursing home care.

The PACE organization receives a fixed monthly payment per enrollee from Medicare and Medicaid. The amounts are the same during the contract year, regardless of the services an enrollee may need. Persons enrolled in PACE may have to pay a monthly premium, depending upon their eligibility for Medicare and Medicaid.

PACE is only available in states that have decided to offer PACE under Medicaid. As of February 2006, PACE sites were available in California, Colorado, Florida, Kansas, Maryland, Massachusetts, Michigan, Missouri, New York, Ohio, Oregon, Pennsylvania, Rhode Island, South Carolina, Tennessee, Texas, Washington, and Wisconsin. To find a PACE site in the previous states and its contact telephone number and address, go the Web site at http://www.cms.hhs.gov/pace.

Expanded In-Home Services for the Elderly Program (EISEP) and Community Services for the Elderly

These programs are available, for example, in New York State. You should check with your county Office of Aging to see whether they are available in your own community.

These state-supported programs provide supportive services to older persons in their own homes/apartments, including case management, homemaking, housekeeping, and other services. Home services, like meals-on-wheels and friendly visiting, and shopper services are found in most communities. These programs are available to older persons whose income level exceeds Medicaid eligibility levels, and charges are assessed on a sliding scale basis.

Long-Term Home Healthcare (LTHHC) Program

Available in New York State, this program, operating under a specific federal Medicaid waiver, may also be available in your community. Contact your county's Office of Aging, Department of Social Services, or Health Department to find out.

As an alternative to long-term care in an institution, this program provides nursing home services and other care to disabled and chronically ill persons in their homes and apartments. Individuals are eligible for the LTHHC program if the assessment shows that they are eligible for nursing home care but choose to be maintained at home and if the services required will cost no more than a specified percentage of what those same services would cost if provided in a nursing home.

Personal Care and Home Health Aide Services

In addition to telephone book listings, you may also contact your County Public Health Department and your County Department of Social Services about these listings.

Services are available to older persons in their own homes or apartments, including housekeeping, personal care, and home health aide services. Services are available to seniors and families on a private-pay basis in New York State or to those who are eligible for Medicaid reimbursement if income eligibility limits are met. While these requirements relate to New York State, find out if they also pertain to your own community as well.

Social HMOs (SHMOs)

The social HMO (SHMO) was developed in the 1980s as a new approach to improve care for frail Medicare beneficiaries in the community. Combining managed care and expanded home- and community-based care services, social HMOs now enroll a broad range of Medicare beneficiaries. The extra services are targeted to those who are at greatest risk of being admitted to a nursing home or those who have significant healthcare needs. Basically, social HMOs are a special kind of health plan that provides the full range of Medicare benefits offered by standard Medicare HMOs, in addition to chronic care/extended care services that include the following: care coordination, prescription drugs, chronic care benefits covering short-term nursing care, and a full range of home- and community-based services such as respite care, adult daycare, homemaker and personal care services, and medical transportation. Other services that may be provided include eyeglasses, hearing aids, and dental benefits. However, there are only four such SHMOs in the country. In general, social HMOs do not charge HMO enrollees premiums if they have both Medicare and Medicaid. They usually charge premiums to enrollees who only have Medicare. Three (the first generation) are located in Portland, Oregon (Kaiser Permanente); Long Beach, California (Senior Care Action Network, known as SCAN); and Brooklyn, New York (Elderplan). The remaining one, Health Plan of Nevada, is in Las Vegas/Reno, Nevada (second generation).

In brief, each of the plans has the following criteria:

- *Kaiser Permanente, Portland, Oregon*

   The enrollee must be at least sixty-five years or older, must have Part A and Part B of Medicare, must continue to pay the Medicare Part B premium, and must live in Kaiser Permanente's Social Managed Care Plan service area. The enrollee *cannot* have end-stage renal disease or reside in an institutional setting. In order to obtain the long-term care benefit, an expanded care resource coordinator will visit you at home to determine if you qualify for nursing home certification based on criteria established by the state of Oregon's Senior and Disabled Services. These criteria may include needing daily continuing assistance from another person with one of the following activities of daily living: walking or transferring indoors, eating, managing medications, controlling difficult or dangerous behavior, controlling your bowels or bladder, or the need for protection and supervision because of confusion or frailty.

- *Senior Care Action Network (SCAN), Long Beach, California.*

   The enrollee must be sixty-five years of age or older, must have Medicare Part A and Part B, must continue to pay Medicare's Part B premium, and must live in SCAN's service area. The enrollee *cannot* have end-state renal disease. In addition, in order to receive extended home care services, members must have a Nursing Home Certificate which indicates that the members' informal support system, such as a family member or a caregiver, is not enough to keep the member out of a nursing home.

- *Elderplan, Brooklyn, New York*

    The enrollee must be sixty-five years of age or older, must have Medicare Part A and Part B, must continue to pay the Medicare Part B premium, and must live in the Elderplan's service area. The enrollee *cannot* have end-stage renal disease. In order to receive chronic care benefits, the enrollee must meet the state's nursing home certificate criteria.

- *Health Plan of Nevada, Las Vegas, Nevada*

    The enrollee must be at least sixty-five years of age, or may be under sixty-five, if disabled. The enrollee must have Medicare Part A and Part B, must continue to pay Medicare's Part B premium, and must live in Health Plan of Nevada's service area. The enrollee cannot have end-stage renal disease. For the long-term care benefit, the beneficiary must meet certain criteria based on established medical, psychological, functional, and social criteria.

Each plan has different requirements for premiums. All plans have copayments for certain services. To find out more information about SHMOs, you can go to the Medicare Web site, http://www.Medicare.gov/nursing/alternatives/shmo.asp.

Area Agencies on Aging

On July 14, 1965, President Lyndon B. Johnson signed into law the Older Americans Act (OAA). In addition to establishing the US Administration on Aging, the OAA established a network, headed by the US Administration on Aging, comprised of State Units on Aging, Area Agencies on Aging, tribal organizations, local service providers, and volunteers. The OAA authorized grants to states for community planning and services programs, as well as for research, demonstration, and training projects in the field of aging. Later amendments to the act added grants to Area Agencies on Aging for local needs certification, planning and funding of services, including but not limited to nutrition programs in the community as well as for those who are homebound; programs which serve Native American elders; services aimed at low-income minority elders, health promotion, and disease prevention activities; in-home services of frail elders; and those services which protect the rights of older persons such as the long-term care ombudsman program.

On November 13, 2000, the Older Americans Act Amendments of 2000 were signed into law (Public Law 106-501), extending the act's programs through fiscal year 2005. The law created a new program, the National Family Caregiver Support Program, whose purpose is to aid the many thousands of family members who are struggling to care for older loved ones who are ill or have disabilities. Under this program, state agencies on aging work with Area Agencies on Aging and community and service provider organizations to provide support services, including information and assistance to caregivers, counseling, support groups and respite care, and other home- and community-based services to families caring for their older members. The National Family Caregiver Support Program also recognizes the needs of grandparents who are caregivers of grandchildren and other older individuals who are relative caregivers of children who are eighteen and older. Telephone 1-800-861-8111 to learn about and contact this program.

The following provides an overview of the range of supporting services available to older residents in their communities through the OAA and other federal, state, and local programs.

- *Senior Transportation Services*—make it possible for individuals who do not drive or whose physical condition prohibits them from using public transportation to obtain rides for essential trips like medical appointments, business errands, shopping, and senior activities. Door-to-door transportation is available in many communities.
- *Outreach*—identifies homebound or isolated persons in need of services. Once they are identified, they are aided in receiving necessary services.
- *Information and Referral Assistance Programs*—assist older persons, their families, and community agencies who need information but do not know where to turn. Many state Agencies on Aging have toll-free statewide 800 numbers that assist with linking older persons with appropriate services. Anyone regardless of age may telephone the Area Agency on Aging for information on services and resources available in the community to individuals sixty and older.
- *Escort*—provides support for older people with limited mobility to obtain needed services. Escort service is often provided by volunteers. It might mean picking up an individual at his home, accompanying him to a doctor's appointment, or spending the afternoon together running errands.
- *Case Management*—services aimed at providing a single access point in the community to reduce the distance an individual must go to initiate entry into the service system. Drawing upon a variety of resources, the case manager meets with the individual, assesses his or her needs, and develops a service plan to meet those needs. Once the service is initiated, a case manager can provide follow-up to assure that needed services are being provided.
- *Home Healthcare*
- *Home-Delivered Meals*
- *Nutrition Education*
- *Homemaker and Chore Services*
- *Respite Care*—provision of short-term relief (respite) to families caring for their frail elders offers tremendous potential for maintaining dependent persons in the least restrictive environment. Respite services encompass traditional home-based care, as well as adult day health, skilled nursing, home health aides, and short-term institutional care. Respite can vary in time from part of a day to several weeks.

- *Friendly Visitors and Telephone Reassurance*—programs, which have different names in different communities, that provide regular personal or telephone contact for older persons who are homebound or telephone contact for older persons who are homebound or live alone.
- *In-Home Services*—includes a wide range of supporting offered services to individuals who are homebound because of illness, functional limitations in activities of daily living, or disability. Their availability often is credited for permitting people to remain in the community.

For further information on the services listed here as well as senior centers, housing services, energy assistance, physical fitness, and other programs /services, contact your local Area Agency on Aging using the Eldercare Locator of the US Administration on Aging, which can help you find necessary and convenient services that serve the elderly in your community. The Eldercare Locator telephone number is 1-800-677-1116.

Medicaid Waivers

Medicaid, a public assistance program financed by federal, state, and local governments, is available in all states as well as the District of Columbia, Puerto Rico, and the Virgin Islands. As a minimum, all Medicaid programs offer a variety of benefits for the elderly, including inpatient hospital care, outpatient hospital care, skilled nursing facility services for persons over age twenty-one, and home health services for persons eligible for skilled nursing services. Also, in many states Medicaid pays for such additional services of interest to the elderly as dental care, prescribed drugs, intermediate care facility services, optometrist services and eyeglasses, clinic services, hearing aids and prosthetic devices, as well as diagnostic screening and rehabilitative services. Check with your local welfare department whether these additional services are available in your jurisdiction's Medicaid program.

As authorized under section 1915C of the Social Security Act, Medicaid has waiver programs. This section of the Social Security Act gives states greater flexibility to serve individuals with substantial long-term care needs at home or in the community rather than in an institution. Under this section the federal government can "waive" certain Medicaid rules. This allows a state to choose a portion of the population in Medicaid to receive specialized services not available to all Medicaid recipients. For example, in New York State and Connecticut waivers have been granted for providing services and treating persons with traumatic brain injury, while in New York State waivers have been granted for providing services and treating persons with mental retardation or other developmental disabilities such as autism, cerebral palsy, epilepsy, mental retardation, and/or other neurological impairments. The waivers allow Medicaid funds to be used to allow persons with disabilities to choose to live at home or reside in other living arrangements of their choice with the type and degree of support needed to increase independence in their home and community rather than being required to live in a nursing home, intermediate care facility, or other institution in order to receive Medicaid benefits. You should check with your local or state welfare department to determine whether the medical condition you have can be covered by Medicaid, if you are eligible, or whether waivers have been granted to your state Medicaid program through which you can receive treatment for your condition

Veterans Administration Home Healthcare

Home healthcare is skilled home care provided by the VA and contract agencies to veterans who are homebound with chronic diseases and includes nursing, physical/occupational therapy, and social services. There are several kinds of home healthcare offered to eligible veterans. These include:

- homemakers for shopping, cleaning, or meal preparations
- home health aides for help with bathing and dressing
- nursing assistants for bathing
- nurses to help you with your medications and dressing changes
- physical therapists to help you with strength and mobility exercises
- occupational therapists to help you relearn activities like eating, dressing, and the like
- speech therapists to help you with relearning to speak following surgery or a stroke

If you and your VA provider agree that you need these or other services, depending upon your eligibility, the VA may pay for the care. To find out what may be available, speak with your VA healthcare provider or your VA social worker.

Nursing and Rehabilitation Centers

These centers provide care to individuals who need specialized care on a regular basis but do not need to be hospitalized. Care is administered under the direction of a physician. Each resident is charged a basic daily rate for the fundamental services that he or she receives as well as additional charges for any supplemental services.

Licensed Homecare Service Agencies (LHCSAs)

These agencies provide homecare services including a level of nursing care, various therapies, home health aides, and personal care aides to clients who pay privately, have private insurance coverage, or are covered through a variety of government payers. Many also deliver services under contract with local departments of social services or other service authorizing agents. For example, in New York State services through Medicaid Personal Care and Private Duty Nursing Programs are delivered in this manner. Licensed agencies may also subcontract with other homecare providers to deliver services to beneficiaries as they do in New York State. These agencies may offer a full range of services from skilled to paraprofessional or may choose to focus on the delivery of one service or population, such as high-technology pediatrics or aides to seniors.

Adult Daycare and Adult Day Healthcare (ADHC)

This is a service for frail, physically or cognitively impaired seniors such as those with Alzheimer's disease and their caregivers. The inclusion of the word "health" in the kind of daycare a center provides should indicate that it also provides elements of healthcare and the purpose of the center is not just for socialization and taking care of seniors. The designation of Adult Day Healthcare (ADHC) in many states refers to those centers that the state has licensed to deliver health and medical-related care services, similar to what a state-licensed nursing home or a state-licensed assisted living facility might provide. In most states a senior or adult daycare center that is not designated as adult day healthcare will not be licensed to include, or have available on site, psychological evaluations, licensed social workers, administration of medications, assistance with bathing and hair washing, dressing of wounds, and assistance with feeding. If Medicaid covers adult day healthcare as a benefit, it will not also reimburse adult daycare. Most states require a licensing process for adult day healthcare and a state licensing process that must be approved for Medicare reimbursement and/or Medicaid reimbursement.

Medicare does not cover daycare costs, but in a licensed medical or Alzheimer's environment Medicaid may pay all the costs if the senior qualifies financially. Some daycare centers offer need-based scholarships. Private medical insurance policies sometimes pay a part of the daycare costs when registered, licensed medical personnel are involved in the provision of the care. Long-term care insurance policies can cover daycare as well.

In deciding upon an adult day center, the National Adult Day Services Association's *NADSA Guide to Selecting an Adult Day Center* and others recommend that you should first find out what kind of services are important to the elderly person:

- Is the environment safe and secure?
- Any social activities?
- Is social isolation and the mental decline that accompanies it prevented?
- Help with eating, walking, toileting, medicines?
- Are there physical, speech, occupational group therapies?
- Is the person's health monitored—blood pressure, food or liquid intakes, weight?
- Are nutritious meals, snacks, or special diets provided?
- Exercise?
- Does the center provide mental stimulation?
- Is there personal care—bathing, shampoos, shaving?
- Does the center improve or maintain an elderly person's level of independence?

- Does the center help cognitively and physically impaired adults maintain or improve their level of functioning?

For the families of those with dementia or Alzheimer's disease, adult daycare centers offer:

- assistance with care
- relief from care
- reassurance
- short- or long-term care
- services at affordable prices
- transportation to and from the facility

There are various sources available to locate such an adult day center in your community. You can ask your family physician, who can also advise you under what circumstances you may wish to place a person with Alzheimer's disease in an adult day center. These centers can be listed in the yellow pages of your telephone directory under such classifications as "Adult Daycare," "Aging Services," and "Senior Citizen Services." You can telephone the Eldercare Locator of the US Administration on Aging at 1-800-677-1116. The Eldercare Locator can direct you to the Area Agency on Aging in your community, which can help you find such a center. Local social services or health departments can also inform you of adult daycare centers in your community. There are also local senior centers and mental health centers.

Once you find such a center, ask it to send you a flier or brochure, eligibility standards, a monthly activity calendar, a monthly menu, and application procedures. When you receive the material, the National Adult Day Services Association suggests you review it for the following information:

- Who is the owner or sponsoring agency?
- How many years has it operated?
- Is it licensed or certified? (if required by your state)
- What are its hours of operation?
- What days is the center open?
- Is there transportation to and from the facility?
- What does the center cost—hourly or daily fees, other charges, financial assistance?
- What kind of conditions does the center accept—such as memory loss, limited mobility, incontinence?
- What are the staff's credentials?
- What is the ratio of staff members per participant?
- What kind of activities does the center provide? Is there a variety and choice of individual and group activities like trips, if appropriate for an elderly person's profile
- Is there menu-appeal, balance?

If you find one or more centers that interest you, you should then make an appointment for a visit. Again, the National Adult Day Services Association and others recommend that you take note of the following observations:

- Did the center make you feel welcome?
- Did someone try to find out what you personally wanted and needed?
- Did anyone explain clearly the nature of services and activities the center provides?
- Did you get any information about the center's staffing, costs, program procedures, and what responsibilities they expect from the caregiver?
- Did you find the center appearance to be a clean, pleasant, and odor free?
- Were the building and rooms accessible for wheelchairs?
- Was the furniture firm and comfortable? Do the chairs have arms? Are there lounges for relaxation?
- Does the center have a quiet location for conferences?
- Is there a location where sick persons can be separated from other attendees?
- Were the staff and attendees cheerful?
- Do volunteers help?
- Do attendees contribute to the planning of the center's activities or are they allowed to make other suggestions?
- Are persons with Alzheimer's disease treated with respect?

The previous questions should be of value in helping you judge which center best satisfies your requirements. Do not forget to check references or ask several persons who have used the center for their opinions about the facility. Use the center for a few days, recognizing that the transition from home to a center for a loved one may not be free of troubles in terms of adjusting to the new routine and environment. If there are any problems, ask the center's staff for their ideas so as to make the transition easier for a loved one or a friend. The staff is familiar with the problems of caregiving and the various resources in the community to make it easier. Remember, the purpose of these centers is to provide assistance to families and/or caregivers who have a care recipient who cannot be left alone during the day. Daycare centers are generally open five days a week, and some may even have extended evening and weekend hours. If the elderly person in your life requires more care than this, it may be time to consider residential care or twenty-four-hour in-home care.

For more information about adult day services you should contact:

- National Adult Day Services Association, Inc.
  2519 Connecticut Avenue, NW
  Washington, DC 20008
  Tel: 1-800-558-5301 (toll free) or 1-202-508-1205
  Web site: http://www.nadsa.org

- Alzheimer's Association, Inc.
  225 North Michigan Ave., 17th floor.
  Chicago, IL 60601
  Tel: 1-800-272-3900 (toll free)
  Web site: http://www.alz.org
- Eldercare Locator
  US Office of Administration on Aging
  Washington, DC 20201
  Tel: 1-800-677-1116 (toll free)
  Web site: http://www.eldercare.gov

A PATIENT'S BILL OF HOMECARE RIGHTS

As a consumer, the National Home Caring Council developed on your behalf from the American Hospital Association's "Patient's Bill of Rights" the following bill of rights that you should expect as a homecare patient. You have the right

1. To receive considerate and respectful care in your home at all times;
2. To participate in the development of your plan of care, including an explanation of any services proposed, and of alternative services that may be available in the community;
3. To receive complete and written information on your plan of care including the name of the supervisor responsible for your services;
4. To refuse medical treatment or other services provided by law and to be informed of the possible results of your actions;
5. To privacy and confidentiality about your health, social, and financial circumstances, and what takes place in your home;
6. To know that all communications and records will be treated confidentially;
7. To expect that all homecare personnel within the limits set by the plan will respond in good faith to your requests for assistance in the home;
8. To receive information on an agency's policies and procedures including information on costs, qualifications of personnel, and supervision;
9. To homecare as long as needed and available;
10. To examine all bills for service regardless of whether they are paid for out of pocket or through other sources of payment;
11. To receive nursing supervision of the paraprofessional if medically related personal care is needed.[20]

When you are receiving home healthcare services, make sure that your rights as a homecare patient are respected.

BACKGROUND OF HOSPICE CARE

One form of care that can be delivered at home, in a nursing home, in a hospital, or in any other kind of inpatient facility is a relatively recent addition to the US health-care system insofar as the services it provides, the illnesses it treats, and its methods of financing. Its name—hospice care. The focus of the hospice movement is so basic that it is unthinkable for most people—namely, our death. Yet, the hospice movement suggests a way to make comfortable, for lack of a better word, that final event with a sensitivity which combats the dread. Hospice care represents an approach to providing a more humane context for the dying and for their families. In the words of advocates of the system, "The hospice groups now springing up around the country are responding to one of the deepest needs in all of us, the need to feel that when our time comes to die, we will be able to do so in conditions which reduce the physical suffering and spiritual anguish to a minimum."[21] Therefore, because hospice care has become an important alternative treatment within our healthcare system, it is important to understand its nature and purpose.

The idea of hospice care began when a group of Catholic widows established a hospice in Lyon, France, in 1842 for young women with incurable disease and inoperable cancer. In the mid-1800s, the Irish Sisters of Charity established a hospice for the dying in Dublin, Ireland. The genesis of today's hospice care movement began in England in 1967 when Dame Cicely Saunders founded St. Christopher's Hospice in London to provide care for terminally ill patients. This hospice has served as a model for a movement that has spread to northern Europe and the United States. In 1974 the first hospice in this country was opened in New Haven, Connecticut.[22] As of January 1, 2001, the National Hospice and Palliative Care Organization (NHPCO) had knowledge of 3,139 operational or planned hospices programs in all fifty states and the District of Columbia, Puerto Rico, and Guam. The NHPCO estimated that hospices admitted 700,000 patients in 1999, an increase from 540,000 patients in 1998. The hospice organization further estimated that 600,000 Americans died while receiving hospice care in 1999 (or 29 percent of all Americans who died in that year). By 2002 it is estimated that US hospice programs had served 885,000 persons.[23]

The word *hospice* had its origin in medieval times and means a way station where a traveler on a difficult journey could find rest, food, and medical care. Today, hospice represents a concept of healthcare for the terminally ill. The theory is based primarily on the relief of pain so that the dying patient may make fuller use of the final stages of his life. Thus, a hospice is not necessarily as much a physical place as it is a concept. Although some hospices may provide care in discrete units of hospitals or other freestanding facilities, it is the *nature* of the services and the underlying philosophy rather than the setting which distinguishes a hospice program from other approaches to terminal care treatment.

At present, hospices care for about one out of every three cancer and AIDS patient deaths in America. Thus, hospices now care for over half of all Americans who die from cancer, as well as a growing number of patients with other chronic, life-threatening illnesses, such as end-stage renal disease and heart or lung disease.[24] America's hospices were also leaders in caring for terminally ill patients with HIV/AIDS. Admission to hospice programs is usually limited to terminal cancer patients, although some groups admit other kinds of patients as well. It is up to the individual program to determine its admission policies. Usually, prior to admission, patients have been diagnosed as having a very short life expectancy as measured in weeks or months. In 1999 the average length of stay (ALOS) for all patients admitted to a hospice program of care was forty-eight days.[25] Some groups require that the patient reside in the county where the hospice program exists and in some instances a certain distance from the project. However, the program's present emphasis on terminally ill cancer patients is quite significant for demonstrating the potential of hospice care. Thus, the hospice program's promise of bringing some measure of physical, spiritual, and financial relief to millions of Americans in the last stages of their human existence is inestimable. Beyond direct service to patients and families, many hospice programs also offer services to the community as a whole. These activities range from support groups and memorial services to educational programs, individual and family counseling, crisis counseling, and specific children's programs.

Hospice care is the grassroots answer to the usual way this country handles the dying. Many terminally ill patients with chronic degenerative diseases remain for long periods of time on life-sustaining machines and potent drugs that sometimes do little or nothing to change the outcome of their illness, while their medical bill (often paid in part by government or by private health insurance or both) rises and rises. Hospice care, on the other hand, provides psychological help, among other services, to the terminally ill as well as to their families, sometimes for as long as a year after the patient has died. Thus, hospice teaches family members how to care for patients, how to administer medications, how to prepare tasty but nutritious foods, and other practical things. Hospice also educates the family regarding the progression of the illness so that no one will be surprised by new developments. Family care, as already noted, continues through the bereavement period. Every family, following the death of a patient, may receive a visit from the nurse who carried the primary responsibility for the patient, as well as periodic telephone calls. If the family needs additional help in coping with their loved one's death during that difficult period, a volunteer bereavement team may assume a continuing role for as long as its help is needed. But the first function of hospice care is nursing care that allows the patient to remain at home as long as possible. A 1992 nationwide Gallup poll commissioned by the National Hospice Organization revealed that, given six months to live, nine out of ten (87 percent) of those surveyed would choose to be cared for and die in their own or a family member's home. Care is less expensive in the home setting or in a hospice than it would be in a hospital. Although there is no nationwide standard on what the cost of caring for a hospice patient is, the closest determination is Medicare per diem rates (daily–all inclusive), which in 2000 were about $101 per day for homecare and $453 per day for general inpatient care. A study commissioned by the National Hospice Organization and released in 1995 demonstrated that for every dollar Medicare spent on hospice care, it saved $1.52 in Medicare Part A and Part B. In addition, the 1995 study also showed that in the last year of life, hospice patients incurred $2,737 less in costs than those not on the Medicare Hospice Benefit. These savings totaled $3,192 in the last month of life, as hospice homecare days often substituted for expensive hospitalizations.[26]

In today's healthcare system, healthcare institutions are oriented toward curative care and rehabilitation of the patient. Routine medical procedures, visiting hours, meals, even the physical environment itself are all designed with the acutely ill patient in mind. Thus, the terminally ill patient, with special emotional and physical needs, may suffer a sense of isolation and frustration if he feels that the physician and his staff have a feeling of helplessness in treating him. Consequently, hospice groups believe that their support and assistance can have a positive and beneficial influence on the patient in the final stages of his life. As already noted, the hospice organization is prepared to step in with medical help and emotional support during the patient's illness and during the bereavement period that follows.

CHARACTER OF HOSPICE CARE SERVICES

"Verna, I just don't want to die in a cold impersonal institution surrounded by strangers and hearing calls for doctors and nurses over the hospital intercom system. I prefer home-cooked meals, and I don't want to dress in institutional gowns. I don't want to worry about somebody coming to visit, visiting hours, and all the other emotional discomforts of hospitals, nursing homes, or some other institution. I want to die in my own bed, in the warmth of my own home, surrounded by the love of my family and friends. I want to look out of my own window and into my own garden and the familiar neighborhood."

Like Anthony, millions of people share these feelings—be they young, middle aged, or elderly. Hospice care is the answer.

Hospice care is provided in several basic ways. One of the first things hospice will do is contact the patient's physician to make sure he or she agrees that hospice care is appropriate for this patient at this time. (Hospices have medical staff available to help patients who have no physician.) The patient will be asked to sign consent and insurance forms. These are similar to the forms patients sign when they enter a hospital. The so-called hospice election form says that the patient understands that the care is palliative (that is, aimed at pain relief and symptom control) rather than curative. It also outlines the services available. The form Medicare patients sign also tells how choosing Medicare hospice benefits affects other Medicare coverage for terminal illness. If the conditions are right, a patient may be kept at home, where the hospice team sets up a schedule of care and works with the family to carry out the program. In fact, more than 90 percent of hospice care hours are provided in the patients' homes, thus substituting for more expensive multiple hospitalizations.[27] If the patient's needs are too demanding upon the family or too specialized for homecare, the patient may be shifted to an inpatient facility of the hospice, if one is available. Or the patient may go directly to an inpatient facility such as the section of a hospital or a nursing home that has been set aside for this purpose. As of 1999, approximately 44 percent of hospices were independent community-based organizations; 33 percent were divisions of hospitals; 17 percent were divisions of home health agencies; and 4 percent were divisions of nursing homes or under other auspices. In addition, as of 1995, 77 percent of hospice patients died in their own personal residence; 19 percent died in an institutional facility like a hospital or a nursing home; and 4 percent died in other settings.[28] No matter what the physical arrangements may be, patients receiving hospice care are encouraged to wear their own clothes, not institutional garments, and to bring with them their favorite possessions—plants, photographs, perhaps even a pet. One sign of a well-operated hospice is the availability of a comfortable meeting room where the family can talk privately with the patient day or night.[29] If the patient's condition improves and the disease seems to be in remission, patients can be discharged from hospice and return to aggressive therapy or go on about their daily lives. If a discharged patient should later need to return to hospice care, Medicare and most private insurance will allow additional coverage for this purpose.

The provision of hospice care involves individuals possessing a wide range of disciplines and skills, some of whom alleviate physical pain while the others try to help the patient and his family with spiritual, relational, and financial pain. Depending upon the organization, the hospice staff may include physicians, psychologists, nurses (registered nurses, licensed practical nurses, nurse's aides, or visiting nurses), nutritionists, pharmacists, occupational and physical therapists, social workers, home health aides, clergy, administrative personnel, and volunteers. Individuals who volunteer to serve in the hospice program may perform a variety of duties such as reading to patients, providing automobile transportation, staying with patients while family members leave the house, and assisting family members with chores.

GOALS OF THE HOSPICE PROGRAM

"Hope," said Ann, "our doctor just informed me that Peter's cancer has progressed and now it is terminal. He has less than four months to live. I don't know what to do. After all these years together, I cannot put Peter in a nursing home for his remaining days. I want him home with me, but the children live far away. At my age and in my health, I worry about caring for someone who is slowly dying."

Ann was reassured that no longer would she need to worry. Hospice provides the level of care that she is seeking. Hospice will provide Peter and Ann with all the assistance they need from doctors to social workers. Peter can remain at home during his final days with Ann at his side. Medicare will cover everything needed. The program cannot extend Peter's life, but it will enhance the quality of life during his final days. The hospice team will make certain that he is as comfortable as possible, emotionally and physically. The patient's comfort and peace of mind is the ultimate goal.

Hospice is dedicated to the individual needs of each patient. Such comfort comes about through the regular control of pain and the management of symptoms, that is, nausea and shortness of breath, that are associated with terminal illness. To ease the dying process, the hospice program focuses on the following:

- to help the patient to live as fully as possible;
- to provide support for the entire family as the unit of care;
- to make it possible for the patient to remain at home as long as homecare is appropriate;
- to supplement rather than duplicate existing services; and
- to keep expenses down.[30]

As already noted, hospice care emphasizes what doctors call palliative treatment. In addition to emotional, social, and spiritual comfort, this means that medications are administered mainly to relieve stressing symptoms and to ease pain and not to prolong the irreversible. If a patient's condition so requires, medication is administered on a regular basis before the patient feels the need. The source of what the patient interprets as pain must often be found and help provided to meet each symptom. The aim is to find the point at which discomfort ceases but before the sedation begins. Thus, pain is something to be prevented and controlled. "At least, at the time of passing, there will be no pain," is the wish of many. Hospice workers state that the doses of narcotics are always concentrated downward to get the minimal effective dose to alleviate pain without making the patients into drugged zombies. By contrast, in standard medical practice medication is used not to control pain but to subdue it after its strikes. This standard approach to pain can often be excruciating for the terminally ill patient—both physically and emotionally. For any patient, the expectation of pain can cause great anxiety. For the terminally ill patient, that fear—of devastating, inescapable pain—can intensify the actual experience of physical pain. Thus, to reverse this situation, hospice care employs the concept of symptom control in treating the dying patient. On the other hand, a person in hospice care doesn't give up all access to medical technology: about one-half of US hospice programs admit patients requiring "high-tech" therapies, and almost all will consider such patients on a case-by-case basis. Hospice patients, of course, have the right to change their minds and be admitted to a hospital for high-tech treatment.

Most terminal care now occurs in general hospitals, nursing homes, or other facilities where the environment—institutional regulations, procedures, personnel, and costs—may not only be inappropriate for the dying patient but even counterproductive.[31] The needs of the terminal patient—comfort, communicating with family and friends, sharing his feelings, loving and receiving love from others, freedom from pain, and reasonable healthcare costs—are among the major purposes of the hospice movement. The attitude of the hospice movement toward dying makes it possible for staff, patient, family, and friends to deal with the greatest crisis that any of us will ever face as something that can be managed, something that can be eased.

JUDGING THE QUALITY OF A HOSPICE PROGRAM

"Helen," said Ted, "I have been thinking of getting my father into a hospice program. I have a general idea what these program do, like providing dignity and peace to the terminally ill. Although I know the program provides many kinds of professional help to the family in need, how do I judge the quality of care my father will receive? I know his days numbered. How do I check out hospices in our area, and what should I expect them to deliver in the quality of their services? I know that Medicare pays for hospice care. Do other public programs and private insurance plans cover hospice care?"

Ted learned that operational guidelines have been established to ensure American citizens extended benefits for hospice care and private healthcare programs. Regulations and operating standards governing hospice care vary widely from place to place; they are nonexistent in some communities and are just getting started in others.

As of 1999, forty-four states had hospice licensure laws defining requirements for operating as a hospice program. However, some jurisdictions may regulate hospices under existing statues relating to the licensure of other healthcare agencies like homecare, nursing homes, or hospitals. Consequently, it is important to remember that there is more to hospice than just a name. Admitting a terminally ill patient to a section set aside as "hospice" in a hospital or a nursing home is no automatic guarantee of specialized care. Here are the principal characteristics of a hospice qualified to carry out its mission:

- If possible, the dying patient should be cared for at home. And the homecare part should consist of managing the pain and symptoms; instructing the family in basic nursing care, including diet, medicine, and exercises; and offering a system of emotional support until death and through bereavement. The program should include an arrangement for inpatient care in a special facility of the hospice if attending to the patient at home becomes impractical.
- Hospice services should be available twenty-four hours a day, seven days a week, under the supervision of a licensed physician in cooperation with a family member designated to be in charge. Besides doctors, basic hospice teams should include nurses, mental health specialists, therapists, social workers, chaplains, and volunteers.
- The program should emphasize preserving the quality of the patient's life till

the end without resorting to heroic efforts to maintain it artificially. This does not eliminate surgery, chemical treatments, or x-rays if the goal is mainly to relieve pain. The hospice arrangement also encourages the use of certain painkilling drugs that are sometimes withheld in hospitals as a result of institutional policy.

- Admission and care should be permitted regardless of age or ability to pay and only if the attending physician and designated family members give their informed consent and participate actively.[32]

In June 1978 the American Medical Association approved a resolution declaring its endorsement of the hospice movement "to enable the terminally ill to die in surroundings more homelike and more congenial than the usual hospital environment."[33] Since that period, the number of hospice programs has grown rapidly in this country. Hospice care has become more accepted within the healthcare field and among the ranks of health professionals generally—despite its nontraditional focus on palliative treatment rather than cure, its regard for the dying patient and his family as unit of care, and its emphasis on emotional, social, and spiritual needs as well as physical ones. The previous as well as the following guidelines should be of great assistance in judging the quality of a hospice unit.

NATIONAL HOSPICE ORGANIZATION RECOMMENDED STANDARDS OF A HOSPICE PROGRAM OF CARE, 1979

1. Appropriate therapy is the goal of hospice care.
2. Palliative care is the most appropriate form of care when cure is no longer possible.
3. The goal of palliative care is the prevention of distress from chronic signs and symptoms.
4. Admission to a hospice program of care is dependent on patient and family needs and their expressed request for care.
5. Hospice care consists of a blending of professional and nonprofessional services.
6. Hospice care considers all aspects of the lives of patients and their families as valid areas of therapeutic concern.
7. Hospice care is respectful of all patient and family belief systems, and will employ resources to meet the personal philosophic, moral, and religious needs of patients and their families.
8. Hospice care provides continuity of care.
9. A hospice care program considers the patient and the family together as the unit of care.
10. The patient's family is considered to be a central part of the hospice care team.

11. Hospice care programs seek to identify, coordinate, and supervise persons who can give care to patients who do not have a family member available to take on the responsibility of giving care.
12. Hospice care for the family continues into the bereavement period.
13. Hospice care is available twenty-four hours a day, seven days a week.
14. Hospice care is provided by an interdisciplinary team.
15. Hospice programs will have structured and informal means of providing support to staff.
16. Hospice programs will be in compliance with the Standards of the National Hospice Organization and the applicable laws and regulations governing the organization and delivery of care to patients and families.
17. The services of the hospice program are coordinated under a central administration.
18. The optimal control of distressful symptoms is an essential part of a hospice program requiring medical, nursing, and other services of the interdisciplinary team.
19. The hospice team will have:
    a. a medical director on staff.
    b. physicians on staff.
    c. a working relationship with the patient's physician.
20. Based on the patient's needs and preferences as determining factors in the setting and location for care, a hospice program provides inpatient care and care in the home setting.
21. Education, training, and evaluation of hospice services is an ongoing activity of a hospice program.
22. Accurate and current records are kept on all patients.[34]

FINANCING HOSPICE CARE

Financial coverage for hospice care has become widespread since the program began in the United States in the 1970s. More than 75 percent of hospices are either Medicare certified or pending certification. To receive Medicare certification, a hospice program must provide the following:

- twenty-four-hour staffing
- medical and nursing care
- home health services
- access to patient care
- social work services
- counseling, including bereavement counseling
- medications, medical supplies, and durable medical equipment
- physical, occupational, and speech therapy

In 1999 Medicare spent about $2.5 billion of its budget on hospice services, or $5,324 per person served. Twenty-eight percent of all Medicare costs goes toward the care of people in their last year of life, regardless of the site of medical service; almost 50 percent of those costs is expended in the last two months of life. Hospice care is also covered under Medicaid in forty-three states plus the District of Columbia. Coverage for hospice care is also provided to more than 80 percent of employees in medium and large business. Eighty-two percent of managed care plans offer hospice services. In addition, most private insurance plans include a hospice benefit as does the former federal CHAMPUS program (the Civilian Health and Medical Program of the Uniformed Services), now called TRICARE.[35] Thus, coverage for hospice care services is available to millions of beneficiaries in both the public and the private sectors of our society. As of 2000, 73 percent of all hospice patients received their care under Medicare (65 percent) and Medicaid (8 percent). In addition, according the National Hospice and Palliative Care Organization, 12 percent had private insurance coverage, 4 percent were indigent, and 10 percent had "other" coverage to pay for hospice care. Also, hospices will assist families lacking insurance to explore other options for coverage. And most hospices will provide for anyone who cannot pay, using money raised from the community or other donations. This situation is in stark contrast to the period when the hospice movement began in the 1970s and one of its major problems was getting reimbursed from such third parties as Blue Cross, commercial insurance companies, Medicare and Medicaid, as well as other private and public programs that cover and pay for the healthcare expenses of the American public.

Reimbursement from any general health insurance policy for hospice care is complicated by the fact that hospice care involves inpatient confinement, outpatient services, and home healthcare. Some insurance policies do not cover psychological counseling or bereavement support to the family but do pay for services provided in the home by doctors, speech and physical therapists, registered nurses, and social workers. The same services on an inpatient basis in a facility lacking legal credentials may not be covered, according to the commercial health insurance industry, which has studied the hospice concept. On the other hand, they may be covered if a hospice occupies part of a nursing home that is officially qualified to offer skilled nursing care. Such is the basic problem of hospice care insofar as receiving insurance coverage for these services. Some of the hospice services, such as skilled care in a nursing home or homecare coverage by Medicare, Medicaid, and private insurance plans, are already part of official programs that are hospice oriented, while other services may not be.

Most private insurance plans presently reimburse patients for hospice care. Some unions have made hospice care a collective bargaining goal. Check whether your union or insurance company presently covers or plans to cover hospice care— even if only for experimental or demonstration purposes—and the conditions under which you might qualify for such coverage if you desire it. Blue Cross and Blue Shield plans as well as commercial insurance companies are independent entities. As such, each decides the question of hospice reimbursement for both inpatient and homecare services.

In some areas, commercial insurers and Blue Cross provide more liberal coverage of hospice services than do Medicare and Medicaid. Since many hospice patients are both elderly and low income, this presents a problem. As a result, those who are under sixty-five years of age and have a low income may receive more comprehensive coverage from their private health insurance carrier for the care they receive from the same hospice than those who are more than sixty-five years of age, in the same category, and covered by Medicare and Medicaid. But there are various sources of public assistance available to the elderly for some hospice care services. To place into proper context the public assistance you may and may not expect to receive for hospice services, let us briefly examine the general framework of hospice care.

Each hospice determines the range of services it provides. Although a given hospice may not provide all these services, the hospice concept includes the following types of care: inpatient skilled nursing care in a nursing home or hospital; physician services; homecare, including nursing and personal services; physical, speech, and occupational therapy; pain relief treatment; emotional support services; and spiritual support.

Given these services, hospices face the following problems. Prior to 1982, Medicare and Medicaid did not recognize a hospice as a specific category of health provider eligible for program reimbursement. However, if the hospice could be certified by Medicare, for example, under another classification—such as a qualified home health agency—the hospice could receive Medicare reimbursement for those home health services that are eligible for Medicare payments. Remember, we have already noted that both hospice- and non-hospice-oriented organizations provide some hospice services. Coverage of such services under Medicare and Medicaid as skilled nursing care in a nursing home or homecare were part of these programs long before the hospice movement began. Thus, the hospice as a Medicare-certified home health agency is able to receive Medicare payments that partly cover the expenses of home health aides, physical therapists, visiting nurses, and social workers. In addition, the hospice may also receive payment through Medicaid, Blue Cross, and private insurance companies, all of which may be required by state law, as in Connecticut, to include home healthcare in insurance coverage. As of 1995, hospice care revenues broke down as follows: Medicare, 74 percent; private insurance, 12 percent; Medicaid, 7 percent; and other (e.g., donations, grants, private pay), 7 percent.[36] On the other hand, Medicare regulations do not cover services unique to the hospice movement alone, such as travel between home and institution as the patient's condition permits. Rather, if the patient is traveling to a skilled nursing home, the Medicare regulations require that admission to a skilled nursing home be preceded by a three-day stay in the hospital.

For those who are elderly or have low incomes or both, there are four government programs that can help pay for some of the hospice services you may require.

Medicare

This program provides two basic types of protection:

- Hospital insurance benefits under Part A (generally financed by special Social Security taxes) cover inpatient hospital services and post-hospital care in skilled nursing facilities and patients' homes.
- Supplementary medical insurance benefits under Part B, a voluntary program financed by premiums of enrollees and general federal contributions, cover physician services and many other medical services, including outpatient hospital and home health services.

Anyone who is covered by Part A of Medicare is eligible for the hospice care under Medicare. The Medicare hospice benefit pays for care related to terminal illnesses when all three of the following conditions are met:

1. The patient's physician and hospice medical director certify that a patient is terminally ill (a life expectancy of six months or less).
2. The patient chooses to receive care from a hospice instead of standard Medicare benefits for curative treatment of his or her terminal condition.
3. Care is provided by a hospice program certified by Medicare.

Under this benefit a patient may be asked to pay:

- 5 percent of the cost of outpatient drugs or $5 for each prescription, whichever is less
- 5 percent of the Medicare rate for respite care.

Medicare covers many services under hospice care, including:

- nursing services on an intermittent basis.
- physician services.
- drugs, including outpatient drugs for pain relief and symptom management.
- physical therapy, occupational therapy, and speech therapy pathology.
- home health aide and homemaker services.
- medical supplies and appliances.
- short-term inpatient care, including respite care.
- medical social services.
- psychological counseling, including bereavement counseling.

Medicare pays covered costs for:

- two ninety-day periods.

- one additional thirty-day period.
- an unlimited extension, if the patient is recertified as terminally ill.

Remember, under Medicare if a patient is recertified as needing hospice care, the benefit can be extended indefinitely, and a hospital cannot discharge a person without good cause. If private insurance is paying for hospice care, the coverage for extended periods varies. Some plans define a dollar limit, while others follow the Medicare rules. If you are paying for hospice care yourself, the admission criteria and other policies and procedures of the hospice govern the situation.

As already noted, under Medicare the patient may stop hospice care at any time and return to cure-oriented care. Any remaining days in a benefit period are forfeited once the hospice care is stopped.

On the other hand, the Medicare hospice benefit does not pay for treatments or services unrelated to the terminal illness. Any attending physician charges would continue to be reimbursed in part through Medicare Part B coverage. However, the standard Medicare benefit program still helps pay covered costs necessary to treat an unrelated condition.

Medicaid

As of 1995, Medicaid covered hospice care in thirty-six states plus the District of Columbia. Medicaid is a grant-in-aid program in which the federal government and state governments share the costs of providing medical services to those who qualify for welfare programs and to the medically needy—those whose incomes are too high to qualify for welfare programs but who still cannot afford to pay for medical care. Medicaid is administered by the state under federal regulation. States with Medicaid programs must provide inpatient and outpatient hospital, skilled nursing facility, physician, laboratory and x-ray, home health, family planning, and preventive care. States can also choose to cover any other medical or remedial services recognized under state law and approved by the US Department of Health and Human Services. The specific scope and limitations on hospital, nursing homes, home health, and other medical services covered under Medicaid varies from state to state.

Older Americans Act of 1965

The Older Americans Act of 1965, as amended, authorizes projects to help elderly Americans maintain a dignified and, to as great an extent as possible, independent lifestyle. Generally, persons age sixty and over are eligible for services under the Older Americans Act. Many of the projects contain home health components and other health-related features, including visiting nurses, home health services for homebound elderly, homemaker services, health education, immunization and screening programs, home repairs, and home-delivered meals. Another part of the Older Americans Act is designed to improve the well-being of older persons through nutrition and social service programs. Meals and supportive services are provided in congregate settings as well as in the home.

Social Service Programs

A variety of social services, including home-based services, can be covered and funded from state programs established under Title XX of the Social Security Act, commonly known as the Social Services program. The US Department of Health and Human Services is responsible for this program. The home-based services can include homemaker, home health aide, home management, and personal care. Although the covered services under Title XX vary from state to state, at least one home-assisted service is included in each state program. Welfare and other low-income persons are eligible for these services.[37]

PUBLIC PROGRAM COVERAGE OF HOSPICE-RELATED SERVICES

In more specific terms, the previous programs as of 1995 made or restricted payments under the following conditions for the ensuing services included in hospice care:

- *Physician Services*
  Both Medicare and Medicaid pay for physician services. No problems should arise in a hospice receiving payment for these services under Medicare. Make sure that your state Medicaid program does not severely restrict the number of physician visits allowed.
- *Physical and Occupational Therapy*
  Medicare pays for these services if prescribed by a physician. Find out if your state Medicaid program covers these services. Many states do pay for such services.
- *Homemaker Services*
  In addition to the hospice benefit under Medicare, both the Social Service and the Older Americans Act programs allow homemaker services to be covered. Many states and aging agencies do cover these services.
- *Emotional Support Services*
  Although federal law has no specific restrictions on mental health benefits under Medicaid, except for those in institutions, most states provide only limited mental health benefits. Also, if mental health benefits are provided under a state's Social Service program or an agency's Older Americans Act program, they are usually quite limited. Medicare does cover medical social services under its hospice benefit. Generally under Medicare, medical social services are defined as those services necessary to assist the patient and his family in adjusting to social and emotional problems related to the patient's

health problem. Medicare requires that the services be provided by a qualified psychiatrist or medical social worker.

• *Home Healthcare Services*

Medicare, Medicaid, Social Services, and Older Americans Act programs all provide home healthcare services. Potential problems in obtaining Medicare payments for hospice home health services arise because of several Medicare requirements. One requirement is that the patient must be home-bound; that is, unable to leave home except for infrequent or brief absences to obtain services in another setting. Many terminal cancer patients, who represent the vast majority of hospice patients, remain ambulatory and thus are not homebound until the very last days of their lives. Unless the homebound requirement is eliminated, many hospice home health visits could not be covered by Medicare.

Another requirement that could pose problems is that services provided by a nurse during a home health visit must involve skilled nursing care before a Medicare payment can be made. In other words, at least one service that meets the definition of skilled nursing care under Medicare must be provided. In hospice care, many home health visits are for observation. Medicare does not routinely cover such but can if certain conditions, such as a probability of a change in the patient's condition, are met. Also, personal care services provided by home health aides are not covered unless they are provided in connection with skilled nursing care under an approved plan of care. Many home health aide visits under hospice care may not meet these skilled nursing care requirements.

Under Medicaid and Social Service programs, states are allowed great latitude in designing their home healthcare programs. The same is substantially true under the Older Americans Act. Thus, the requirements for and limitations on reimbursement under these programs vary from state to state and from area to area. Some use Medicare requirements and limitations, while others are either more or less restrictive.

• *Inpatient Care*

Both Medicare and Medicaid cover inpatient hospital and skilled nursing facility services. Medicaid also covers intermediate care facility services. If the inpatient care provided by a hospice meets the definition applicable to these levels of care under these programs' guidelines, then Medicare and Medicaid would pay for such services up to a beneficiary's maximum benefits. The main question that could arise concerning coverage of inpatient hospital services for hospice patients is whether it is necessary for the patient to receive the service in a hospital. For Medicare, an inpatient hospital is defined as a facility primarily engaged in providing to inpatients—by or under the supervision of a physician—diagnostic, therapeutic, and/or rehabilitative services for medical diagnosis, treatment, care, or rehabilitation of injured, disabled, or sick persons. To be covered as inpatient hospital services, it is required that the services be medically necessary and that it is necessary that the services be provided in a hospital and not at a lower level of care. Medicaid uses the same definition. Of course, if the service could be provided adequately at a lower level than hospital care it should be.

For Medicare and Medicaid, the definition of a skilled nursing facility is the same: a facility engaged primarily in providing skilled nursing care and related services or rehabilitation services to injured, disabled, or sick persons on a daily basis. Again, in order to be covered by Medicare and Medicaid, it must be necessary to provide the services in the skilled nursing facility. Assuming the necessity requirement is met (and for Medicare the three-day prior hospitalization requirement before being allowed to enter a skilled nursing home), hospices should be able to obtain Medicare and Medicaid reimbursement for the skilled nursing facility services they provide. In fact, Medicare presumes that a patient is eligible for skilled nursing care for a period of thirty days after discharge from the hospital with a diagnosis of terminal cancer. A potential problem with Medicare coverage is the requirement that a person be hospitalized for three consecutive days before admission to the skilled nursing home. Some potential hospice patients may not meet this requirement.

Normally, hospice patients in intermediate care facilities would meet coverage requirements if eligible for Medicaid. Intermediate care facilities under Medicaid are health-related inpatient care and services provided to treat individuals who do not require the degree of care and treatment that a hospital or a skilled nursing facility is designed to provide. Because of these individuals' mental or physical condition, they require care and services (above the level of room and board) that can be made available to them only through institutional facilities.[38]

Consequently, in seeking hospice care, learn as much as you can as to what aspects of care are covered or not covered under the various programs you may be using to receive and pay for such services.

FINDING HOSPICE CARE SERVICES

The sponsorship of hospice care services in this country seems to vary widely. Many are hospital based, but some are independent corporations. There appears to be little formal sponsorship by churches, although virtually all programs have a spiritual dimension and most include clergy on either the paid or the volunteer staff. Church organizations and individual members of the clergy have also been instrumental in developing some hospices and in raising funds under the auspices of a hospital or other sponsoring body. These hospices serve a broad community and do not require patients to adhere to any particular set of beliefs. Consequently, in order to find out whether or not a hospice organization exists in your community, you can check with your physician; the local Blue Cross and Blue Shield plan or other local insurance company; your church or synagogue; the hospital administrator(s) in your community or the hospital's social services department; the visiting nurse association in your community; your local public health or welfare department; your state hospice organization; your local Social Security office; and the county medical society. Since hospice care includes care at home, homecare agencies may be listed in the yellow pages of your telephone directory under "Nursing" or "Home Health Services." *Or you may call the National Hospice and Palliative Care Organization Help line (1-800-658-8898) or visit its Web site at http://www.nhpco.org.*

QUESTIONS TO ASK WHEN SEEKING HOSPICE CARE

As far as the costs of hospice care services are concerned, check with the National Hospice and Palliative Care Organization, 1700 Diagonal Rd., Alexandria, VA 22314; Children's Hospice International, 901 North Pitt St., Alexandria, VA 22314; Hospice Education Institute, P.O. Box 98, Machiasport, ME 04655; and Compassionate Friends, P.O. Box 3696, Oak Brook, IL 60522. But it appears that a combination of hospice home and inpatient care may be less expensive than care of the same duration in the traditional acute care hospital or skilled nursing facility. In seeking a hospice facility, and remember that hospices do not require federal government certification to operate, there are some questions you may wish to ask:

- Has Medicare certified the program for hospice care?
- Has the Joint Commission on the Accreditation of Healthcare Organizations (JCAHO) certified the program? A seal of approval by the JCAHO or Medicare means that the hospice has met national standards established for quality care in medical direction, nursing, social work for both patient and family, and bereavement counseling for at least one year after the patient's death. There is no current mandatory nationwide accreditation or "seal of approval." Certification by Medicare and the JCAHO is voluntary.
- What are the hospice's hospital affiliations? Does the hospice have a satisfactory inpatient arrangement for patients who become too ill to be cared for in the home?
- Does your state license hospice services?
- What are the criteria for enrolling?
- What services does the hospice offer?
- Where are services offered?
- Does the hospice staff sound caring and competent or do they use a lot of language that make you believe that the program may be very bureaucratic?
- What are the procedures for assuring twenty-four-hour access to staff such as nurses for advice and in-home emergency assistance?

- How are professional staff and volunteers chosen and trained? Does the hospice have an active volunteer program? Volunteers provide needed companionship, reassurance, and hands-on assistance to both the patient and members of the family providing care.
- Who handles the paperwork for Medicare, insurance, and hospital billing?
- How are hospice's services arranged and paid for?
- What are the payment alternatives?
- What is the protocol for managing pain? Is it a good pain-management program?
- What role does the family physician have?
- Is the hospice willing to work cooperatively with the patient's family physician?
- How are families involved in care?
- Will the hospice work with you and your family? How?
- What are the arrangements for residential care, if and when it is needed?

You may also want to contact the hospice and find a family who would be willing to share their hospice experiences with you.

The best time to learn about hospice care is *before* a life-threatening illness occurs. Ideally, everyone should make their views about the end of life known before any illness strikes. They should also take a few simple steps to ensure that their wishes are followed if and when a crisis does occur. This involves drawing up

- a *living will* of written instructions to make known what you want done if, for example, you are gravely ill and the only way you can be kept alive is by artificial means.
- a *durable power of attorney*, which authorizes a person of your choosing (usually a spouse or a close relative) to make decisions for you if you become unable to do for yourself.

Because every state has different laws, it is best to consult a lawyer about these documents. In these documents, you may want to indicate that if you ever become terminally ill, your preference is to receive hospice care.[39]

CONCLUSION

Until now, many Americans faced with a diagnosis of terminal illness have been told that there is nothing more that professional health personnel can do. As a result of this situation, too many patients have been forced to live out the final days of their lives experiencing pain and other symptoms. Their families do not know how to deal with a loved one who is dying—they try to pamper him or her or act differently rather than promoting living as long as possible. Such patients are even shunned by their friends, to whom they are reminders of their own mortality. The result has been that many patients have died without anything resembling a sense of fulfillment.

Hospice care is trying alleviate these traumas to the extent it is possible. The concept suggests changes in family lifestyle to accommodate dying members, as long as homecare is possible. Hospice is hard at work helping people young and old to live as fully and completely as possible during whatever time they have left by emphasizing the fullness and quality of life, rather than death. Only time will determine whether it succeeds in its goals of changing our attitudes toward the dying process as it becomes an integral part of our health system.

NOTES

1. US Department of Health and Human Services, *Health United States, 2003 with Chartbook on Trends on Health of Americans* (Hyattsville, MD: National Center for Health Statistics, 2003), p. 268 (table 87).

2. Ibid.

3. Michael Scott and Barbara Mantz, "A Guide to Home Healthcare," *Better Homes and Gardens*, September 1978, p. 71.

4. *All about Home Care: A Consumer's Guide* (New York: National Homecaring Council, 1982), pp. 2–4.

5. Sylvia Porter, "Home Care Plans Cut Expenses of Illnesses," *Washington Star*, May 17, 1978.

6. Scott and Mantz, "A Guide to Home Care," p. 74.

7. *All about Home Care: A Consumer's Guide*, pp. 12–13.

8. Ibid., pp 9–10.

9. Scott and Mantz, "A Guide to Home Care," p. 78.

10. *All about Home Care: A Consumer's Guide*, pp. 7–8, 11; Anne Harrod, "How to Find a Qualified Home Health Aide," *Washington Senior Beacon*, June 2005, p. B15 (Housing Option)

11. Ibid., pp. 21–22.

12. *Guide to Long-Term Care* (Washington, DC: Health Insurance Association of America, 1999), p. 5; "Nursing Home Costs Top $80,000 a Year," *Silicon Valley/San Jose Business Journal*, March 4, 2002; "Home Care Agencies Understanding Your Options," *FYI*, October 2004, p. 14 (AARP Healthcare Options); "Be Prepared for Long-Term Care," Cox News Service, March 15, 2004; and "2003 GE (General Electric) Financial Nursing Home Cost of Care Survey," conducted by Evans Research, July 31, 2003, as cited in material sent to author from General Electric Capital Assurance Company, January 2005.

13. *All about Home Care: A Consumer's Guide*, p. 20.

14. Scott and Mantz, " A Guide to Home Care," p. 74.

15. Martha Hewson, "McCall's Family Lobby—Right Now," *McCall's*, February 1979, p. 54.

16. "Medicare and Medicaid Statistical Supplement, 2001," *Healthcare Financing Review* (Washington, DC: Centers for Medicare and Medicaid Services, 2002), pp. 217 (table 50) and 218 (table 51).

17. Ibid.

18. *You and Your Home Care* (Springfield: Illinois Department of Health, Statewide Health Coordinating Council, 1978), pp. 4–5.

19. Ibid., pp. 9, 12–15.

20. *All about Home Care: A Consumer's Guide*, p. 25; *Helping You Choose Quality Assisted Living* (Oak Brook Terrace, IL: Joint Commission on the Accreditation of Healthcare Organizations, 2005); "Questions to Ask Assisted Living Facilities," *Washington Senior Beacon*, June 2004, p. B9; Margaret Stafford, "Assisted Living in a Home-Like Environment," *Washington Post*, May 2, 2004, p. A9; *NADSA Guide to Selecting an Adult Day Center* (Washington, DC: National Adult Day Services Association, revised 1997).

21. "The Hospice Movement," *Washington Star*, October 23, 1978.

22. Matthew L. Wald, "Hospices Give Help for Dying Patients," *New York Times*, April 22, 1979.

23. *Hospice Fact Sheet* (Alexandria, VA: National Hospice and Palliative Care Organization, January 1, 2001); "Going Home," *AARP* 3 (January/February 2005): 61.

24. *Hospice Fact Sheet* (Arlington, VA: National Hospice Organization, October 10, 1995).

25. *Hospice Fact Sheet*, January 1, 2001.

26. Ibid.

27. Ibid.

28. Ibid.

29. "A Better Way to Care for the Dying," *Changing Times* 33, no. 4 (April 1979): 22.

30. John W. Abbott, "Hospice," *Aging* (November/December 1979): 38.

31. US Department of Health, Education, and Welfare," Hospice Programs," *Program Information Letter* (Washington, DC: Health Resources Administration, May 29, 1979), p. 1.

32. "A Better Way to Care for the Dying," p. 22.

33. "Hospice Leaders Hear Encouraging Reports from HEW Officials," *AMA News,* October 28, 1978, p. 2.

34. M. Caroline Martin and Gerald R. Brink, "Setting Up an In-Hospital Hospice," *Hospital Forum* (January/February 1980): 17. More detailed information is available in *Standards of a Hospice Program of Care* (Arlington, VA: National Hospice Organization, 1979). The National Hospice Organization is now located in Alexandria VA as the National Hospice and Palliative Care Organization.

35. *Hospice Fact Sheet*, January 1, 2001; "Medicare and Medicaid Statistical Supplement, 2001," in *Healthcare Financing Review* (Washington, DC: Centers for Medicare and Medicaid Services, 2002), p. 224 (table 54).

36. Ibid.

37. US General Accounting Office, *Hospice Care—A Growing Concept in the United States* (Washington, DC: March 6, 1979), pp. 1–4.

38. Ibid., pp. 23–27

39. *Hospice: A Special Kind of Caring (*Arlington, VA: National Hospice Organization, 1993), p. 2.

CHAPTER TEN

PRESCRIPTION DRUGS

INTRODUCTION

During the past five decades, a vast variety of lifesaving, life-lengthening, and health-protecting drugs have been developed to improve the lives and reduce the physical and emotional suffering of all Americans. The development of the "miracle" drugs—namely, the sulfa drugs and the antibiotics, as well as oral contraceptives, oral antidiabetic agents, hypertensive drugs, the tranquilizers and sedatives, psychopharmaceuticals, corticosteroids, and polio, measles, mumps, and rubella vaccines—attests to these advances. The producers of these substances—both prescription and nonprescription drugs—number hundreds of firms and constitute a large, rapidly growing, and important segment of this country's economy.

The predecessor of our present drug industry first appeared in America as early as 1748 when the concept of apothecary shops was imported from Europe. This country's first manufacturing pharmaceutical laboratory was opened shortly thereafter to furnish medicines to George Washington's army in 1778. Still later, during the Civil War, pharmaceutical houses increased in number and expanded vigorously. The distribution of drugs soon became nationwide in scope.

The first major crisis to challenge this growing industry came during World War I, when it became obvious that the United States was almost totally dependent upon Germany for many of the new and potent synthetics developed by German drug manufacturers. The war halted the importation of these materials, and American physicians could not obtain drugs essential for their practice. Accordingly, American firms plunged into the task of synthetic production. Until World War II these companies introduced relatively few innovations and provided only modest support for original research in this field. But after Pearl Harbor the drug industry underwent explosive growth in which many of the previously listed drugs were developed, and today the industry leads all nations in research, development, production, and distribution. The postwar period witnessed the solid establishment of the philosophy that enough research and development, properly directed, would provide the key to finding new and better drugs, with full implications for both the therapeutic and the economic benefits to be gained therefrom.

The climate for prescription drug making continues to evolve. The influence of government programs has dramatically affected the drug industry and the consumer-patient who has become actively involved in bringing about changes in drug product selection. Since 1955, compared to earlier years, fewer new products have been approved by the government for marketing. Since 1963 those that are marketed must pass more rigorous animal and human tests. Medicare-Medicaid programs and healthcare reform initiatives have created the distinct possibility that an increasingly large share of the future drug market will be partially supported by taxes. This became more relevant when President Bush signed into law Medicare's new prescription drug benefit program in December 2003.

The marketing of prescription drugs is unique. It is focused basically on a small, homogenous target group of practicing physicians and is even narrower when aimed only at specialists. The circumstance is unusual. The physician who selects and orders a drug product is not the consumer who pays for it, and the consumer has little or no voice in the selection—a marketing situation almost unparalleled in other consumer industries. Furthermore, once the producer has established the value of his product and his own integrity and reputation in the mind of the doctor, he not only has a firm grip on the market for his present products but also an entrée for future products as well. But manufacturer identification is a double-edged sword. The doctor can deny the drug manufacturer a part of the market if a product is disappointing; the doctor's dissatisfaction also may extend to other products. This possibility has increased within recent years as a result of the establishment of new government drug programs and the repeal of state antisubstitution drug laws, which give the consumer greater participation in selecting quality prescription medicine at prices he or she can afford. Beginning in the 1990s, some prescription drug advertisements began to be aimed at consumers through television and other media formats such as celebrity personnel stating the advantages of the hair restoration drug, Rogaine, or how they reach for Tagamet when they feel their ulcer acting up. Whether or not the advertising of prescription medicines to the public will increase in volume in the ensuing years remains to be seen, but barriers to the promotion of prescription drugs to the public have been breeched. Consumer advertising could play a far larger role in stimulating dialogue between patients and physicians in regard to their medication regimens than in the past, and such advertising appears to be an issue that is going to become more important over the next decades, not less.

Although this country has had a pharmaceutical industry for many years, many questions and much confusion still plague the consumer in understanding the subject of prescription medicines—a knowledge so essential for maintaining his personal health. For example, some of these questions include the following:

- What is the difference between a generic and a brand-name drug and why are the prices so different?
- What is the best way to achieve the most effective results from prescription drugs?
- How can prescription drugs be purchased economically?
- What are drug anti-substitution statutes and how can their repeal save the consumer money?
- What should you ask your doctor when he gives you a prescription?
- What should you tell your doctor before he prescribes medication for you?

These and other subjects will be examined in this chapter and hopefully will enable you to purchase and utilize quality drug products in a manner beneficial to your physical and financial health.

BRAND-NAME VERSUS GENERIC DRUGS: CUTTING YOUR DRUG BILL

"Jim, are generic drugs really that good? I know they are cheaper than the brand-name drugs I see on television, but if they are as good as brand-name products, why do they cost less?" Are drug companies skimping on their ingredients? I'll be the first to admit that I know nothing about drugs—brand name or generic—except what I see advertised on television, but I also want a quality drug when I am sick and not a drug that isn't. I just wish I understood a little more about both kinds of drugs and how the government ensures the quality of both. It sure would put my mind at ease whichever kind my doctor prescribes, and if it's generic, saving some money won't hurt either."

One of the major questions that arises in the consumer's mind when the subject of prescription medicine is discussed concerns the definition and quality differences of brand-name versus generic drugs and why their prices are so different. To answer this question, it is first necessary to discuss some very basic scientific principles.

Every drug is identified by three names—chemical, generic, and brand:

- A drug's chemical name is descriptive of its chemical structure, based on rules of standard chemical nomenclature.
- Drugs also have a shorter, more simple, established or official or generic name. It may or may not be an abbreviated form of its chemical name. It is the name most commonly used in scientific literature, by which many pharmacists and physicians learn about a particular drug during professional schooling and training.
- The brand name is the name the company gives its product to distinguish the medicine from competitive products, which may be identical insofar as active ingredients are concerned.

As an illustration, a five-grain acetylsalicylic acid tablet (chemical name), more commonly known as an aspirin (generic name) tablet, actually represents a kind or class of drug universally prescribed and used for the relief of aches and pains. Currently, aspirin is marketed under several brand names such as Bayer and St. Joseph, and they all have the same molecular entity. When the quality of brand-name drugs versus generic drugs is debated, at least two important scientific issues are raised: their chemically equivalency and their therapeutical equivalency. Drugs are said to be chemical equivalent if they contain the same active ingredients and are identical in strength, dosage form, and route of administration, and meet existing physico-chemical standards in the official compendia. But they may differ in characteristics such as color, taste, shape, packaging, expiration time, and, within certain limits, labeling. Drugs are said to be therapeutically equivalent when they are chemically equivalent and when administered in the same amounts, they will provide the same biological or physiocological availability as measured by such criteria as their rate of absorption into the bloodstream. This absorption rate can be affected by differences among the same product in terms of particle size and the methods used in their formulation, as well as in their granulation and tablet compression pressure. Yet, each product contains the same chemical equivalents from a dosage standpoint.

The brand name is used to advertise a drug to the medical profession, although the generic name must appear in advertising and labeling in letters at least half as large as those of the brand name. It is a popular misconception that brand-name drugs are produced only by large, well-known firms, while generics are made by small, unknown companies. However, a small drug company can put a brand name on its product just as a large company can sell a drug under its generic name. And many large drug firms distribute, under their brand names, products that have been manufactured, packaged, and labeled by firms that make generic drugs. Some manufacturers may make a drug and sell it under both a trade name and a generic name. In other instances, large firms may make the final dosage form from drugs purchased in bulk from other companies. In view of these manufacturing activities, consumers have raised various questions regarding the prescription of brand name versus generic drugs.

Are generic drugs as good as brand-name products?

While some drug authorities claim that chemically identical prescription drugs are not necessarily therapeutically equivalent—that is, they may not have the same curative effects—Dr. Donald F. Kennedy, former commissioner of the Food and Drug Administration (FDA) during the Carter administration, has testified in Congress that "we find no evidence of widespread differences between the products of large and small firms or between brand-name or generic drugs."[1]

Why are generic drugs cheaper than brand-name products?

All drugs have a generic name. If the Food and Drug Administration gives permission to the manufacturer of a newly discovered drug to market that drug and the product is patented, that manufacturer has the sole right to sell the drug until the patent expires. Under the present drug patent law, manufacturers are granted patents that give them exclusive marketing rights on a new drug for up to twenty years from the date a drug patent is filed, as opposed to the date on which the patent is issued and during which time no one else can copy this formula. These patents are listed in the Food and Drug Administration's "Orange Book" registry. In some instances, a patent holder may give other firms the right, usually in return for payment of a royalty, to make and sell the patented drug. While the drug is under patent protection, its manufacturer will set a price that will allow it to recoup its research, production, and marketing costs. However, once the patent has expired, other firms may manufacture and sell the drug. Since the original manufacturer's research information is now known to other firms and the generic manufacturers do not have to invent the drug, it is cheaper for the latter to make the drug and sell it under its generic name or in some cases different brand names. This is why there is such a price difference between generic and brand-name drugs. Because the generic drug must be identical to the original, the FDA approval process is much simpler and less costly. The FDA does not require the generic drug sponsor to repeat costly animal and clinical research on ingredients or dosage forms already approved for safety and effectiveness. Rather, companies simply submit an abbreviated new drug application to the FDA for approval.

How does the Food and Drug Administration (FDA) assure that the prescription drugs I am using are of proper quality?

The Food and Drug Administration's responsibility to regulate prescription drugs includes assuring the safety and effectiveness of drugs for their claimed uses before approving them; requiring complete labeling (directed to physicians) of all drugs; and the provision of drug information to physicians and others in the health profession. In February 2005 the Food and Drug Administration announced the creation of a new independent Drug Safety Oversight Board to monitor FDA-approved medications once they are on the market and keep physicians and patients up-to-date with emerging information on their risks and benefits through such methods as postings on the Internet.

The Food, Drug, and Cosmetic Act of 1938 required that drugs be proved safe before they could be marketed. In 1962 the law was amended to require that drugs be proved effective, as well as safe, before being marketed. The FDA conducted an extensive review of all prescription drugs marketed between 1938 and 1962 to determine whether they are effective by modern standards. As a result of this review, thousands of prescription drugs have been removed from the market or have had their formulation or labeling improved.

Not only must each drug meet FDA requirements but so must each drug plant.

All firms, large and small, must register with the FDA; all are subject to periodic inspection; and all must follow the FDA's Good Manufacturing Practice regulations (GMPs), which touch upon every aspect of making drugs, from building maintenance to quality control. These regulations apply to all producers and are intended to assure that all drugs meet the same standards of safety, strength, purity, and effectiveness. Other FDA standards provide further assurance of drug equivalence.

Another assurance of quality stems from the FDA's monitoring programs. The FDA periodically collects samples of all drug products, both generic and brand name, from manufacturers and from the marketplace to test them for purity and strength. When trouble is found or suspected, the drug company is notified immediately. Faulty products are removed from the market. Batch testing and certification are required by law for insulin and for biological products such as vaccines and serums, as well as for antibiotics. When the FDA discovers particular problems with a drug, it may require that each batch of that drug be tested before it can be released for sale.

How can the repeal of state antisubstitution drug laws lower my personal drug bill?

Beginning in the 1970s states began to repeal laws that prohibited pharmacists from dispensing any version of a drug product other than that specifically prescribed by a doctor. Under such laws, for example, if a doctor prescribed a certain brand of tetracycline, a pharmacist could not substitute generic tetracycline or even another brand, although they might cost less and are the chemical twin of the prescribed brand. Find out from your state pharmaceutical association or physician whether the law has been repealed in your state; if so, does it require that any cost savings achieved by substitution of a less costly equivalent drug for a brand-name product be passed onto you as a consumer? Many such antisubstitution laws, upon repeal, have such a requirement. Upon the repeal of these laws, some states permit the pharmacist to choose a substitute product unless the prescriber forbids it, while other states require a prescription form with two signature lines on which the prescriber must indicate approval or disapproval of substitution.

Therefore, the next time you obtain a prescription from your physician, you should ask whether he knows of a generic drug product that can achieve the same medical therapy as the brand-name product being prescribed and what the difference is in price. If there is such a generic drug product available, find out whether your state allows for its substitution and whether your physician will recommend such a change. In this manner, you will able to save money on your prescription drug bills.

What are the drug management companies and how may they save me money?

In this new era of managed benefits, one of the relatively newest innovations within the pharmaceutical industry are drug management companies—also known as pharmacy benefit managers, or PBMs, which act essentially as middlemen between health plans and drug manufacturers. These drug management companies originally just processed claims for insurance companies. Today, PBMs operate mail-order pharmacies that grant members significant discounts over standard retail pharmacies. PBMs also contract with large employers to provide drugs at discount prices to insurance-covered employees through networks of retail pharmacies that promise savings to patients if they buy drugs at participating stores. The drugstores are reimbursed by the management companies. These management companies draft lists of drugs approved for coverage based on assessments of their cost and effectiveness. Thus, pharmacy benefit managers administer drug plans and organize the purchasing, dispensing, and reimbursement of medicines for health insurers or other large purchasers of healthcare such as employers and unions.

The process works as follows:

- An employer issues a request for a proposal to manage its prescription benefit program for its employees.
- Prescription benefit managers submit proposals in response. Employers assume that the chosen manager can contract with pharmacies to reimburse the pharmacies based on a formula for each prescription dispensed. The drugstore is paid an amount equal to the employee copayment plus the average wholesale price of the drug minus a negotiated percentage discount.
- Beneficiaries can go to any pharmacy participating in the program, present their drug card, and pay a copayment to obtain the prescription.
- At the end of every two weeks, the benefits manager pays the pharmacy for the prescriptions it dispensed.[2]

If your company has such a plan, you as an employee may be able to save a great deal of money by enrolling in this program. Be aware that the movement to fill prescriptions for many chronic conditions through the mail is growing rapidly. For example, Blue Cross and Blue Shield informed federal retirees in 1996 that they could fill prescriptions for medicine used routinely for chronic conditions at a drugstore and pay 20 percent of the cost or could order the drugs from a mail-order pharmacy and pay nothing. Providers of mail-order drugs use large processing centers across the country that, automated with state-of-the art computers, store information about each patient and dispense prescriptions based on that patient's insurance coverage, medical needs, and the frequency with which the person tends to use a drug. Cost savings, analysts say, come from bulk purchasing. In addition, card plans are intended to save money by requiring employees to use specific pharmacies, which have agreed to offer discounts. Also, according to analysts, insurers are more aggressively asking that doctors in some instances change prescriptions to less expensive generic brands or to similar brand-name counterparts. Some doctors have criticized this "switching strategy" used by some mail-order pharmacies, saying it can lead to inappropriate substitutions that in some instances can cause adverse patient reactions. Mail-order companies say they can often change to a generic brand without calling a doctor but that they must receive a doctor's approval before switching to similar, but not identical, substitutes. Doing anything less, they say, could make them legally responsible if the substitute led to a bad reaction. So if you use mail-order pharmacies, be aware of their advantages and disadvantages compared to your local drugstore in terms of filling your prescription. Only you can decide which source is best in terms of costs, monitoring your use of drugs and possible drug interactions, ease of getting a prescription filled, and other elements that constitute quality pharmaceutical services. In addition, some businesses are opening their own pharmacies for their employees where they work. Some advocates think it is a win-win situation if companies can buy drugs at steep discounts and find it cheaper to operate a pharmacy than to reimburse employees for the medicines they buy at other drugstores.

What is the federal government's Maximum Allowable Cost (MAC) Drug Program and how may it save me money?

In August 1976 the US Department of Health and Human Services' new drug program, named Maximum Allowable Cost (MAC), became effective. The program places a price ceiling on prescription drugs at the lowest price for which that drug is widely and consistently available; for drugs whose patents have expired, which are produced by more than one company, and which are covered by Medicare, Medicaid, and Maternal and Child Health programs. Although MAC applies to the three programs, government savings were expected to come almost exclusively from Medicaid because as of 1976 Medicare did not as yet cover out-of-hospital drugs and most hospitals enforce their own cost controls on inpatient drugs. However, as already noted, as of January 1, 2006 Medicare began to offer coverage for out-of-hospital prescription drugs.

Under this MAC drug program, the US Department of Health and Human Services (HHS) sends lists of drug comparisons to physicians and pharmacists in order to encourage them to reduce patient drug costs. Before a limit on drug payments is proposed, the Food and Drug Administration will study the drug to make sure there is no quality or therapeutic equivalency problems. Under HHS regulations, manufacturers of generic drugs with known variations must match the effectiveness of the standard drug or withdraw their drug from the market. Should the price of a drug product, for which a MAC limit has been established, rise or fall in the marketplace owing to an increase or decrease in its supply, then, after appropriate review by HHS, the MAC limit can be adjusted upward or downward as the circumstances warrant.

As a consumer, if you qualify for Medicaid, Medicare, and Maternal and Child Health programs and if these programs pay for drugs, the government may pay the entire cost of the drug your physician prescribes. Or you may pay the difference between the Maximum Allowable Cost the government pays and the remaining cost the pharmacist charges you. To find out whether any of your prescription drugs qualify for this Maximum Allowable Cost drug program, ask your physician or pharmacist or write to the Centers for Medicare and Medicaid Services, US Department of Health and Human Services, Washington, DC 20201, to learn which drugs they have approved for payment under the program.

In view of the Food and Drug Administration's assurances that there are no differences between generic and brand-name drugs, why don't physicians write more generic prescriptions?

There is no single answer to this question. Some physicians may feel more confidence in the products of familiar drug companies. Others may not be aware of the difference in price between a brand-name drug and its generic equivalent, or they may not know that a generic version of particular drug is available. Another factor that plays an important role in influencing a physician's prescribing practices is the promotional activities of drug manufacturers. One form of promotion is advertising in medical journals. Another is personal visits from representatives, called "detail men," who talk up their company's products and leave samples and literature with the physicians they call on. A third channel of promotion is a publication called the *Physician's Desk Reference*, which is made available without charge to physicians and pharmacists. Drug companies pay to have essential information included in this valuable reference work. Those that do not pay do not have their products listed.

Patients who are concerned about their health dollars should ask their physicians to prescribe and their pharmacist to dispense generic drugs when they are available.[3]

Every consumer should realize that all medicines, brand name or generic, carry a risk. Along with the benefits, they also have a potential for harm. Undesirable side effects can occur. Any decision to use drugs must take into account the benefits versus the risks. Therefore, make sure to follow your physician's advice very carefully—do not take more medication than your doctor advises or use it in ways he/she does not recommend.

WHAT TO TELL AND ASK YOUR DOCTOR ABOUT PRESCRIPTION DRUGS

"Paula, do you now how many doctors I see now and all the drugs they prescribe. That doesn't include all the other drugs I take that are not prescribed like aspirin, cough medicine, antidiarrheal medicine, and others that I can buy over-the-counter without a prescription. What worries me is that despite taking all these medications, especially the ones prescribed for my illnesses, I still do not always feel well. I don't know if these drugs are helping or harming me?"

"Well, do you tell all your doctors all the drugs you are taking, both prescription and over-the-counter? What do they say when you ask them questions about these drugs?"

"Paula, how can I ask any questions? I don't know anything about any of these drugs to even know what to ask? If my doctor prescribes the drug, I just assume he knows what he is prescribing and why. He's the expert. He's the doctor. I'm not."

"June, I think you ought to make a complete list of all the drugs you are taking from all the doctors and show all of them the list because it is possible that you may have forgotten some of the drugs you are taking and didn't tell them. They will know whether or not some are interacting with each other to cause you problems. Remember, June, even a drug you buy without a prescription is still a drug. Any drugs can affect your personal health. Read the labels of the drugs. You can avoid a lot of trouble by being knowledgeable about them."

Physicians prescribe the drugs they believe are needed to diagnose or treat your particular problems. But your health is at stake, and there are many things you need to know and do to help your doctor make the right decisions and to make sure the prescribed medicines work the way your doctor intended.

You can buy some drugs "over-the-counter." They usually are intended to relieve symptoms or treat minor ills. For maximum benefit and safety in the use of these drugs, you should follow the directions on their labels whether the drug is over-the-counter or a drug prescribed by your doctor.

Important Elements on a Drug Label

- active ingredients
- uses
- warnings
- directions
- other information
- inactive ingredients

The labeling section called *active ingredients* lists the chemical compound in the medicine that works with your body to bring relief to your symptoms. It can always be found as the first item on the label. Make sure it agrees with your doctor's instructions. Also, check the drug label section named *uses*, also sometimes referred to as *indications*. This section tells you the only symptoms the medicine is approved to treat, and you can make sure this is the correct medicine for your condition. Additional information about the product such as how to store the medicine will be listed in the *other information* section. The final section is called *inactive ingredients*. An inactive ingredient is a chemical compound that has no effect on your body. Preservatives, items that bind the pill together, and food colors are listed here. By the fall of 2005, the Food and Drug Administration had not only placed the previous newly revised labeling on over-the-counter nonprescription medications but also, on January 18, 2006, announced a new prescription-drug safety format for the inserts that are found inside prescription drug packages—the first revised design of these inserts since 1975. The format requires that the prescription-drug information for new and recently approved products meet specific graphical requirements and includes the reorganization of critical information so that physicians can find the information they need quickly and to allow physicians to have more meaningful discussions with their patients concerning the medications they are prescribing. Some of the most significant changes include:

- a new section called *highlights* to provide immediate access to the most important prescribing information about benefits and risks
- a *table of contents* for easy reference to detailed safety and efficacy information
- the date of initial product approval, making it easier to determine how long a product has been on the market
- a toll-free number and Internet reporting information for suspected adverse events to encourage more widespread reporting of suspected side effects

You might first see the information, commonly called the package insert, if your doctor gives you a free sample of the drug to begin your prescription. If not, the package insert should be inside the box you receive at the pharmacy. If the pills come in a bottle and the pharmacy only gives you a leaflet of simplified information, which is often written by a separate company, ask for the genuine labeling. The Food and Drug Administration does not regulate the leaflets, and you could be missing important safety information. However, regardless of the nature of the labeling, be it official or not, always make sure you discuss the side effects and safety of the medication with your physician. When taking over-the-counter medications, the following steps should be taken:

- Always read the drug's label, even if it is a brand-name drug you have purchased before, because the ingredients and dosage instructions can change.
- Ask the pharmacist which over-the-counter drug is best for your symptoms and risk factors, including age and other medical conditions.
- Make sure you understand the drug's dose and how many days in a row it is safe to take before consulting a physician. Avoid taking over-the-counter drugs longer or in higher doses than the label recommends (unless your doctor approves). If your symptoms continue, see a doctor.
- Tell your doctor or pharmacist all the prescription and over-the-counter drugs you are taking, in addition to dietary supplements or herbs. Some can be fatal if taken together.
- If the pharmacist is too busy to give you immediate advice, ask if you can make an appointment to see him. Change drugstores if the pharmacist cannot make time.

Log on to the following Web site to learn more about over-the-counter medications, and drugs in general: http://www.bemedwise.org.

In addition to over-the-counter medication, other drugs can be obtained only with a physician's prescription. Because these drugs usually are prescribed for the treatment of specific diseases and are generally more powerful than over-the-counter medicines, they should be taken only on the advice of and under the supervision of a physician. If you do not know the difference between an over-the-counter drug and a prescription medicine, look for the legend on the drug's label. *Any drug that does not have the legend "Caution: Federal law prohibits dispensing without prescription" on the label can probably be sold over-the-counter without a doctor's prescription.* Therefore, when you purchase medication, read all the labels carefully. Also, when a physician prescribes medication for you, there is important information he should know. *Be sure to tell your doctor if you:*

- Are being treated for a different condition by another doctor.
- Require a smaller-than-usual dose of a given drug because you are over sixty-five years of age. Ask your physician if it is appropriate in your age situation.
- Have had allergic reactions such as rashes, headaches, or dizziness to drugs or foods you have taken in the past.
- Are taking other medicines, including over-the-counter drugs and such special-category drugs as birth control pills or insulin, so the doctor will not prescribe a drug that will interact with another medicine and cause unwanted side effects. When visiting your doctor, bring a written list of your allergies and the medicines to which you've had a negative reaction or that you cannot take and the reasons why. If you see more than one doctor, share that list at each visit. This will help you avoid unnecessary and risky drug combinations. Also, review each of the medications you are taking with your primary doctor at least once a year. This is a good opportunity to eliminate medications that are no longer necessary.
- Are taking vitamins, herbal products, or mineral supplements. Vitamins are substances that regulate all the chemical reactions in the body and make sure they go the proper speed. Without them, bodily functions are impaired, and the result can be disease—even death. To obtain the necessary vitamins, you should eat such foods as potatoes, tomatoes, meat, and eggs, or you may wish to take a multivitamin tablet that is sold at drugstores. Also, while taking vitamins, drink at least a quart of water a day to help wash the vitamins through your kidneys and prevent kidney stones. Don't expect instant results from taking vitamins. It is not like taking a drug—you won't find improvements instantly. You'll feel better for taking vitamins, but changes may take a month. While you cannot be allergic to the vitamin itself, you could be allergic to its coating or additives. For example, some people cannot tolerate the yeast that Vitamin B is grown in and they develop a rash. Or you might find yourself allergic to wheat germ oil, the base for some Vitamin E. This could result in such reactions as feeling the rush of blood through the veins and arteries of your neck. If you do experience any reactions when taking vitamins, contact you doctor for assistance.

- Are undergoing or have undergone diagnostic procedures, such as x-rays, under the supervision of another physician.
- Use alcohol or tobacco.
- Are pregnant or breastfeeding.
- Have liver or kidney disease or any other special medical condition (such as diabetes).
- Are on a special diet.[4]

In addition to telling your doctor about your health status, there is also information you should obtain. By asking your doctor for advice about the medication, you are, in effect, creating a safety system for yourself. If your doctor is personally dispensing the medication and discusses its purpose with you, your physician can see if he/she has misread the drug name, dispensed it from the wrong container, mistyped a label, or dispensed the wrong dosage. If your doctor is not dispensing the medication, but is having the medication filled through a pharmacist, there is still a great deal you should know about it. *Be sure to ask your doctor:*

- *Is the medicine necessary?* Many people have the mistaken idea that they must receive a prescription every time they visit a doctor. But medicine is not the answer to every health problem, and drugs should be taken only when needed.
- *What is the name of the medicine, both the brand and the generic (scientific) names? Is a generic version available?* Write it down so you will not forget. If you can't write everything down while you are still with the doctor, sit down in the waiting room and finish up while the information is still fresh in your mind.
- *Why am I taking it? What does the medicine look like?*
- *Is there any written information available about the drug? What is the drug's strength? Might my ethnicity affect the dosage strength? What do I do if I miss a dose?*
- *What results are expected from taking the medicine? Make the pain go away? Get to the cause of the pain? Reduce fever? Lower blood pressure? Cure infection? How soon should I expect results?*
- *What unwanted side effects might occur (such as sleepiness, swelling, nausea)? Which should be reported to the doctor and when? What should I do if they occur? How can I manage mild side effects so I can keep taking the medication?* If you change from a brand-name drug to a generic, report any different reactions or side effects to you doctor. Also, read about the side effects in the information you receive at the pharmacy. Reread it every time you refill the prescription because the information may have changed or you might have new questions. Also, keep a record of any side effects you might have had between doctor or pharmacy visits. Write down the date and what your healthcare provider told you to do in regard to them. Discuss what you have written with your doctor during the next visit.

- *Are there other medicines, vitamins, minerals, herbs, and dietary supplements I should not take while taking this medicine?* Some drugs cause reactions when taken with other drugs, prescription and nonprescription.
- *Are there any particular drinks or foods I should avoid while taking the medication? Will the medication, for example, interact with alcohol, tobacco, caffeine, juices, or milk?*

   Some antibiotics, for example, will not work if you drink or eat milk products. Alcoholic beverages should not be used when some drugs are taken. Alcohol is a depressant, and even a small amount can increase the depressant effect of such drugs as antihistamines. A chemical in grapefruit juice can lessen the body's capability to metabolize any one of more than two hundred medications, including cholesterol-lowering statins, sleeping pills, and antianxiety agents.

- *How and when should I take the medicine? Is there a best time to take it? If you are told to take it "three times a day," does that mean morning, noon, and night? Should you take it before meals, with meals, or after meals? If "every six hours," does that mean when you are awake, or should you get up during the night to take the medicine exactly every six hours? Should you take it on an empty stomach?* If your container says "take with food," that means your medication should be taken while you are eating or perhaps a few minutes after. If your container states that the medication be taken on an "empty stomach," then it means that food will interfere with the amount of drug your body takes up. You may not receive the full effect of your medication if you fail to take it on an empty stomach. The stomach is considered empty about one hour before a meal or two hours after. Since food affects the amount of acid in the stomach, it can affect how much of a drug is absorbed from the stomach into the bloodstream. Food can also hinder the onset of a drug's action as well as protect the esophagus and stomach from the irritating nature of many medicines.
- *How long should I continue to take it? Should I take the medicine until it is all gone, or just until I feel better? What do I do if I feel better before finishing the entire dosage you are prescribing for me?* Some medicines must be taken for long periods to cure the disease. If you stop the medication too early, even when you feel better, the symptoms and disease may return.
- *How long will it take before the medication is likely to work; and how long should you wait to report to your doctor if you see no benefits or change in your symptoms?*
- *Are there any precautions you should take while on the medication, such as not driving or operating machinery?*
- *Can your prescription be refilled?* For some drugs your doctor may indicate one, two, or even three refills. For others it may be important for the doctor to see you before additional medication is prescribed. Some drugs that have the potential for abuse are "controlled" under federal law, which places limits on the number of refills.

- *How should you store your medicine?* Some medicines should be kept cool and dry; some must be refrigerated; others must be protected from the light. Remember the bathroom where you have the medicine cabinet and kitchen tend to be the moistest part of the house and that moisture can degrade the effectiveness of the medications. Your physician or pharmacist can tell you the best way to store your medicine to ensure that it does not lose its effectiveness. Also, make sure that you store your own medication and that of loved one separately. Make sure you keep the medications out of sight and reach of grandchildren, as well as your loved one if he/she has memory problems. If you require medication during the day and are away from home, be very wary of putting a small supply of tablets in a fancy pillbox even though it is more convenient. The tablets may break apart, in which case you might not receive the correct dose. Or they could react with the metal. Or in some cases, such as nitroglycerin, they can be absorbed by plastics. Instead, explain your problem to the pharmacist; perhaps, he can put your medication in small containers.

- *Does the medicine come in another form if you have trouble taking tablets or capsules?*

  Your physician or pharmacist will know this. Be sure to ask. Your doctor's permission will be needed to change the prescription. Some tablets can be crushed and easily mixed with food or water; others should not be broken up because they are coated to prevent the drug from being absorbed too rapidly or from irritating the stomach. Your pharmacist can tell you whether a particular tablet can be crushed and, if so, what liquid can be mixed with it. When taking liquid medication, do not use a kitchen spoon to measure the dose. Household teaspoons can hold between 3 ml and 7 ml (milliliter); a "prescription teaspoon" refers to 5 ml. Either measure the dosage in the cup or dropper that accompanies the medication or ask the pharmacist for a measuring device.

- *What is the impact of drugs and smoking?* Women on birth control pills who smoke have an increased risk of heart attack, stroke, and other circulatory diseases.

  Nicotine and other tobacco constituents speed up the metabolism of theophylline, an asthma drug, and pentazocine, a painkiller, and to a lesser extent certain tranquilizers, analgesics, and antidepressants. Thus, smokers may need larger than normal doses of these drugs. When they stop smoking, dosage of these drugs may have to be changed.

  Smoking also can affect certain diagnostic tests, such as red and white blood cells counts and blood clotting time determinations.

- *What is the effect of mixing alcohol and drugs?* Chronic use of alcohol can cause changes in the liver that speeds up the metabolism of some drugs, such as anticonvulsants, anticoagulants, and diabetes drugs. They become less effective because they do not stay in the body long enough.

Prolonged alcohol abuse can also damage the liver so that it is less able to metabolize or process certain drugs. In that case, the drugs stay in the system too long. This is especially serious when the drugs are phenothiazines (antipsychotic drugs), which can cause liver damage.

Alcohol is a central nervous system drug (CNS) depressant. Alcohol taken along with another CNS depressant drug can affect performance skills, judgment, and alertness. If the mixture includes overdoses of barbiturates, diazepam (Valium) or propoxyphene (Darvon), the result can be fatal.

A person who has developed a tolerance to the sedative effects of alcohol may need larger doses of tranquilizers or sleeping pills to get the desired effect. This can lead to an overdose without the person being aware of it.

Similarly, alcoholics and patients with alcohol in their system need larger amounts of anesthetics to induce sleep. Once such a patient is "under," his sleep is deeper and lasts longer.

- *Will the drug affect the results of laboratory tests? Are any tests required with this drug—such as to check for liver or kidney function?* Drugs can affect the results of clinical laboratory tests. For example, excess use of laxatives can affect tests to determine calcium or bone metabolism. Penicillin can result in false readings of protein in the urine, a sign of kidney disease. Large doses of vitamin C can produce false results in a urinary glucose test for diabetes.

It is very important that you know the answers to these questions. Your personal well-being is involved. Make sure you do not find yourself in the position of not knowing what is really wrong with you and what the future might hold after being treated by a physician; what treatment he is using; what the alternatives might be; and what drugs he is prescribing and their purposes, actions, possible side effects, and potential danger. Being informed about the nature of your illness and the steps you should take to treat it will enable you to help yourself and your physician to alleviate it and eliminate needless worries and anxieties that might impede your recovery.

WHAT WOMEN SHOULD ASK THEIR DOCTORS ABOUT MEDICATION

Some medications that women commonly take can affect the way other drugs work. The following are some of the questions women should ask their physicians who are prescribing the medications for them:

- *If I am taking birth control pills, how will my newly prescribed drug be affected?* Birth control pills can counteract the effect of some drugs and increase the effect of others. In addition, some drugs may make birth control pills ineffective.
- *Would it be better to use a different form of birth control, instead of the pill,*

while taking this drug? The answer varies from person to person. Discuss it with your doctor.

- *If I am taking estrogen, will this affect my new medication?* Estrogen affects other drugs the same way birth control pills do. Certain drugs, especially other hormones, can cause estrogen to become more potent. Also, birth control pills and estrogen can influence the results of thyroid tests—making it look like you have a thyroid problem when you really don't.
- *Should I take this drug during my menstruation?* Aspirin and drugs that contain aspirin can increase bleeding during menstruation.
- *Will this drug cause an increase in premenstrual tension (PMT)?* Any drug that makes the body retain sodium or contains a lot of sodium can make PMT worse. And diuretics that make you lose excessive amounts of potassium can have the same effect.
- *Will this drug cause any distinct hormonal changes?* Certain tranquilizers can change the pituitary hormones, making a woman sluggish, tired, and cold, among other things.
- *Will this drug have any effect on my attempts to get pregnant—or will it affect my unborn baby?* Most drugs will affect your baby if you become pregnant while taking them. If you're trying to get pregnant, then you should talk to your doctor before he prescribes a drug.
- *What effect could this drug have on menopause?* Some drugs, such as nicotinic acid or any vasodilator, could make the symptoms of menopause even worse, causing more hot flashes, more headaches, and more irritability.
- *Will this drug cause unwanted hair growth on parts of my body?* Some drugs, such as certain male hormones, will cause hair to grow on women's faces.
- *Will this drug affect my sexual drive?* Certain hormones can cause an increase in sexual desire.

By asking the proper questions, you can do much to maximize the effectiveness of the medication you are being prescribed as well become alert to and educated about its possible side effects.

DRUG SAFETY

Whether you are purchasing prescription or over-the-counter drugs, there are certain measures you can take to make sure that the drugs you buy are safe to take and are taken safely. *Do not buy or take a product if:*

- The plastic is ripped.
- The plastic seal around the top of the bottle is stretched, torn, or missing.
- The inner seal is ripped or gone.
- The cotton plug looks unusual or is out of place.

- The tablets or capsules have unusual spots, cracks, or dents—or are of different sizes.
- The capsules have fingerprints, a dull look about them, or the printed letters don't line up.
- The tablets are moist rather than dry.

Never:

- Take drugs without reading and understanding the label. If you have vision problems, ask for large typing on labels. You might also want to request a duplicate, large-print label on a flat surface, such as a medication information sheet or a blank piece of paper. Don't skip doses and make sure you finish the course of the medication as prescribed, unless your doctor tells you otherwise. Consult with your doctor on this matter. Don't cut pills in half to make them last longer unless your physician allows you to do it. Ask your doctor first because not all drugs can be split.
- Take drugs in the dark. Put a light on and wear glasses, if necessary.
- Take drugs prescribed for someone else.
- Take drugs that have been sitting in your medicine chest for a long time. Check the expiration dates.
- Keep different drugs in similar containers, put drugs in an incorrectly marked container, or mix different drugs in the same pillbox. You could take too much of one medication, take too little of another, and forget which drug is for what. Remember, the original bottle is tinted or opaque to keep out light, which can degrade many medicines, and the storage instructions should be on the container and package insert.

Always:

- Keep track of the medicines you take, their dosage, when and how often you take them, and the name of the pharmacy. Use a memory aid such as a written checklist to help you, and keep it in a place that is handy to you. Write out a daily medication schedule or ask the pharmacist for a chart to fill in, or logs, weekly pillboxes (known as dosettes), special blister packs, or portable alarm systems such as on your cell phone or Palm Pilot to help you organize and remember to take the medications. Take the medications at a regularly scheduled time each day. Develop a routine that is easy to remember such as mealtimes, if the medications must be taken with food, or during a favorite television program or at bedtime. Post notes to yourself on the refrigerator or other places you regularly look at to remember your regimen until you establish this routine.
- Tell your physician about *all* the medicines and drugs you're taking, including vitamins, herbal products, eye drops, and over-the-counter medications. Reg-

ularly consult with your doctor to determine if you really need all the drugs you are taking.
- Leave drugs in their original containers with directions.
- Before taking each dose, read and follow the directions on the label to make sure you have the right drug. Pay attention to drug interactions. Ask the physician to write clearly the medication's purpose on any prescription. Always try to fill your prescription at the same pharmacy. If you should spend part of the year in another area, have your records transferred there from your home pharmacy. In this manner a complete record of the medications you are taking as well as those you have taken can be maintained and the pharmacist can assist you in regard to any questions you may have relating to your prescription regimen.
- Be careful when pouring liquid medications, so the instructions aren't wiped out by drippy syrup.
- Swallow tablets and capsules with a full glass of water while standing. Don't chew or break pills unless instructed to do so.
- Flush unused drugs down the toilet after the expiration date. While some authorities fear that a potential environmental hazard may result from this method, they suggest using trash to get rid of unused drugs by breaking up the capsules and crushing tablets, putting the remains back in the original container with its child-resistant cap, and then taping it up and double bagging it before tossing it away. Another method is to check if local household hazardous-waste collection programs—where you would get rid of old batteries and other materials—accept expired medicine. Or ask whether your local pharmacy might accept the return of such expired medicines for incineration.[5]
- Keep medicines away from your bedside. Make it necessary for yourself to get up to take them. Drugs and medicines on the nightstand are dangerous because an overdose may occur if the medication is accidentally repeated while sleepy.[6]

By following the previous suggestions, you will be able to obtain the most beneficial use from your prescriptions or other medicines. To learn more about prescription and over-the-counter drugs, as well as drug interactions, you can go to the Food and Drug Administration Web site at http://www.fda.gov. Click on "Information for Consumers" and then on "D" for a report on drug interactions. For additional information on drugs, you can go to the National Council on Patient Information and Education (NCPIE) at http://www.talkaboutrx.org and the AARP at http://www.aarp.org, clicking on "Health and Wellness" and then on "Prescription Drugs." And for information on nonprescription products, as already noted, you can go to http://www.bemedwise.org.

HOW TO REDUCE YOUR PRESCRIPTION DRUG BILL

"Melvin, I can't believe what I am paying for some of my prescription drugs today. I'm reaching a point where I sometimes feel, do I eat today or buy my medicine? I really feel helpless. I can't control their costs, but I need these drugs to stay well. It's funny we complain about the price we pay for medicine, but we don't complain about the same medicine if it cures us. Is there any answer to this dilemma? Perhaps, if I knew how to manage their costs, I could live with their prices and within my budget so I wouldn't have to consider whether I eat or buy my medication."

"Dick, there are steps you can take to control the costs of your medication."

Once you have received a prescription, there are several measures you and your physician can take to reduce your personal drug bill. *You can ask your physician whether:*

- He is aware of a generic drug product that will produce the same medical therapy for which the brand-name drug is being prescribed. What is the difference in price? If there is such a generic drug product available, find out whether your state permits its substitution and whether your physician will recommend such a change. If there is no generic available, ask your physician if there is an older, less expensive drug that can accomplish the same treatment therapy just as well.
- He can recommend pharmacies in your local area that offer quality drugs at lower costs. There can be huge price differences among drugstores, even among stores in the same neighborhood. If your physician cannot make a recommendation, telephone area pharmacies yourself to compare prices. If another pharmacy has a lower price, see if yours will match it. Also, take advantage of pharmacy discount programs. Ask the pharmacist if you might qualify for any pharmaceutical company discount program or government assistance program. Drugs tend to cost less in megadiscount stores than they do in drugstore chains and independent pharmacies. They also may cost less in pharmacies in cities than they do in the suburbs and rural areas.
- He has any prescription drug samples from the pharmaceutical companies. In this way, you do not have to purchase your initial supply. Also, you can test the medication for its effectiveness before you purchase a large supply and report your findings to your physician. He may wish to prescribe another medication that might be useful in alleviating your ailment. Thus, until you know how you respond to a new medication, fill your prescription with smaller quantities, then buy larger quantities to limit dispensing fees and other charges.

There are also other sources to help you learn about a drug's effectiveness. Evidence-based research is quickly emerging as an important tool to assess which medicines are most effective. Evidence-based research reviews are objective research that analyzes all clinical studies performed by universities, drug companies, and others on sets of drugs used to treat the same medical condition. Each review lays out the best evidence on how effective and safe each drug is. In addition to prices, the following Web sites provide patients with information on common ailments like high cholesterol, heartburn, or chronic pain so that patients can talk more knowledgeably with their physicians about the best drug for their condition at the right price. To learn how similar drugs for common conditions compare, based on Oregon's Drug Effectiveness Review project, go to:

- AARP's "Choosing the Right Prescription Drug" at http://www.aarp.org/ ResearchRx
- Consumer's Union's 'Best Buy Drugs" at http://www.crbestbuydrugs.org
- Oregon's project reports can be read in full at http://www.oregonrx.org

Oregon's Drug Effectiveness Review Project based at the Oregon Health and Sciences University in Portland is one of the leading centers in the country studying the effectiveness of medicine through evidence-based research. Experts state that evidence-based research is not perfect, so that when Oregon believes that there is not good evidence, the Oregon reports say so.

Finally, don't insist that your doctor prescribe a drug seen in an advertisement which may be heavily marketed and cost more than the alternatives, for little or no benefit. Instead, ask about it and encourage the doctor to make a sensible choice for you.

Once you have ascertained a drug's effectiveness in your treatment, you can sometimes save money by buying as large a quantity as will remain fresh at the rate you use it. If you have a chronic condition, ask you doctor if a ninety-day supply of the medication would be appropriate. Typically, the price of a prescription equals the price of the drug plus the pharmacist's dispensing fee. If you purchase your drugs in volume, as already noted, you may eliminate dispensing fees. However, remember that it is dangerous to keep unused drugs around the house or to use them after the expiration date. So make sure your doctor says buying in volume is permissible.

Also, because some medications cost about the same regardless of strength, ask your doctor, whenever possible, if he/she might prescribe the drugs you need in double strength or dosage, then cut each pill in half with a plastic pill cutter that you can buy at any pharmacy (you cannot do this with capsules or long-acting, time-release pills) to save money. The following characteristics make pills dangerous or hard to split:

- *Shell*: Capsules, extended release pills, and pills having a safety coating.
- *Size and shape*: Triangles, or other unusual shapes, spheres, and pills having a thick coating.
- *Strong dose response*: A small dose change—if you don't split evenly—has a big effect.
- *Patient ability*: Poor eyesight, trembling hands, cognitive problems.

Another way to reduce your drugs bills today is through prescription discount cards. Hundreds of these cards are on the market; none of them are regulated. Many are aimed at the uninsured or those whose health plan does not cover prescription drugs. Some manufacturers make it relatively easy to obtain a card, while others create a lot of obstacles such as having your physician rather than yourself submit a card or having you fill out lengthy financial forms. Once your application is approved, usually you will receive a three-month supply of medications at a time. When you use up your three-mouth supply, some companies automatically renew your medications, while others make you start all over again in terms of the application process. Periodically companies will change their eligibility requirements and other rules. Some cards target Medicare patients. Some cards charge an enrollment fee, most a monthly fee or an annual fee, and some charge both. Some offer free cards. Some have age or income restrictions. Some require only name, address, and credit card numbers. Not all cards provide prescription drug coverage. Not all pharmacies accept all cards. And the cards only rarely deliver the "up to 65 percent" or greater savings that some advertise. Many of the largest discounts are available only for certain medications at certain pharmacies in certain cities on certain days, and because prices change every day, patients rarely have the information they need to decide, up front, whether a card is worth the trouble—or in some instances, the monthly fee. But regardless of the card you choose, make sure you and your physician have the widest possible choice of medications. To do so, choose a card that has an "open formulary"—an unrestricted list of drugs. A reference to a "preferred drug list" in an advertisement or a brochure means fewer medication choices for you and your physician. The following is a snapshot of the various sources that patients may use in seeking discounts on prescriptions drugs.

Prescription Discount Cards

If you are over sixty-five years of age, request a senior citizen discount at your pharmacy. Many stores offer this benefit. NeedyMeds, Inc. at http://www.needymeds .com gives tips on how to get free or discounted medications directly from drug companies. Also, the Pharmaceutical Research and Manufacturers of America (PhRMA) has information on drug assistance programs. Telephone 1-800-762-4636, or write the PhRMA at 1100 15th St. NW, Washington, DC 20005, or visit it on the Web at http://www.phrma.org. In addition, many drug makers offer free supplies of their own products to Medicare enrollees without drug coverage. Income limits apply. For a free directory, call 1-800-762-4636 or go to http://www.helpingpatients .org. Also, nearly all pharmaceuticals companies will provide free medicine, regardless of age, to the most needy. You can log on to http://www.freemedicineprogram .com to find out if you qualify. For details of drug company cards for low-income seniors with no drug coverage, go to http://www.rxassist.org or telephone the following numbers: GlaxoSmithKline's Orange Card 1-888-672-6436; Eli Lilly's LillyAnswers 1-877-795-4559; Pfizer's UShare Medicare Prescription Drug Discount Card, 1-800-717-6005; Novartis's CareCard, 1-866-974-2273; or the Together

Rx Card 1-800-865-7211, or visit http://www.Together-Rx.com, which offers percentage discounts on a range of drugs. Most will accept Medicaid and will bill the state directly for your prescription; your pharmacist cannot charge you for any portion of this cost. Remember, there are many legitimate companies that charge a reasonable fee for helping people who need assistance with obtaining their medications through patient assistance programs. However, there are also a few organizations that make outrageous claims about free medicine and claim to be able to help any person obtain any drug. They not only charge very high fees but also do not provide the drugs or information. To learn more about such organizations, go to the Web site of the Federal Trade Commission at http://www.ftc.org and write "free medicines" in the Web site's search box. If you want to file a complaint with the FTC or learn more about these and other consumer issues, you can telephone the Federal Trade Commission agency at 1-877-382-4357 or TTY 1-866-653-4261.

In addition to the previous discount cards, by the spring of 2004 a new prescription drug card became available to senior citizens. It was part of the massive Medicare Prescription Drug, Improvement, and Modernization Act of 2003 (Public Law 108-173) that President Bush signed into law on December 8, 2003. The cards are scheduled to be phased out during 2006 after the start of a new prescription drug benefit in the Medicare program (January 1, 2006) and are issued by insurance companies, wholesale and retail pharmacies, and pharmacy benefit managers that now administer drug insurance programs for companies and the government. Critics state the cards would save seniors very little since the cards do not take into consideration inflation of drug prices, while the Bush administration claims the cards can reduce out-of-pocket expenses by 15 to 25 percent. Unlike discount cards now available, this program allows a Medicare recipient to sign up for only one card. Participants pay an amount that cannot exceed $30 a year to join. The cards are likely to offer different discounts for different drugs made by different pharmaceutical companies. Participants will have to select a card based on which card matches best with their prescription drugs. Pricing information will be posted and updated on the Medicare Web site (http://www.Medicare.gov) and also will be available from the Medicare help line (tel: 1-800-MEDICARE). A principal problem is that prices and the prescriptions covered by a card may change at any time, but the law says participants can choose a different card only during the annual enrollment period or under exceptional circumstances, such as long-distance moving. Medicare rules allow prescription drug card sponsors to change prices once a week without any warning to cardholders, thus making it difficult for Medicare beneficiaries to decide which cards offer the best prices for the medicines they take, so that a card that is best for a senior citizen one week may not the best card for that person the following week.

Prescription Assistance Programs

If you are eligible for Medicaid, present your card to the pharmacist. Most will accept Medicaid and will bill the state directly for your prescription; as already noted, your pharmacist cannot charge you for any portion of this cost. If you do not qualify for Medicaid, find out if your state has established a program to help low-income elderly and disabled patients with the costs of prescription drugs. Depending upon your state, you may have to pay a deductible before the coverage begins; you may have to pay a copayment or coinsurance, and there might be a low limit on benefits. Telephone your state health department or the local Area Agency on Aging (the telephone number is in your telephone book) or contact the Eldercare Locator at 1-800-677-1116 or go to http://www.benefitscheckup.org to find programs for which you may qualify. New Jersey and Pennsylvania's Pharmaceutical Assistance Contract for the Elderly (PACE) program subsidize all prescription drugs for seniors who meet income requirements. Others, in California, Vermont, and Florida, for example, require most pharmacies to sell drugs at slight discounts to poor seniors. Missouri offers tax credits. It is possible that your state has similar programs. Make sure you find out. The National Conference of State Legislatures' Web site, at http://www.ncsl.org offers information on state drug assistance programs for older people. Or call your state health department or agency on aging or go to http://www.benefitscheckup.org to find programs for which you may qualify.

The Partnership for Prescription Assistance Program is another source of aid that can help persons who are having difficulty paying for healthcare services including the costs of prescriptions drugs. This group brings together America's pharmaceutical companies, doctors, other healthcare providers, patient advocacy organizations, and community groups to help qualifying patients who do not have prescription coverage obtain the medicines they require through public or private programs that meet their needs. This collaboration includes, but is not limited to, the American Academy of Family Physicians, the American Cancer Society, Easter Seals, the United Way, the American Autoimmune Related Disease Association, the Lupus Foundation of America, the NAACP, the National Alliance for Hispanic Health, and the National Medical Association. As of 2006, The Partnership for Prescription Assistance offers a single point of access to more than 475 public and private patient assistance programs, including more than 150 programs offered by pharmaceutical companies. The mission of this organization is to increase awareness of public assistance programs and increase the enrollment of those who are eligible to be helped. To contact the Partnership for Prescription Assistance Program, you may telephone 1-888-477-2669 or visit its Web site at http://www. pparx.org.

Veterans and Military Benefits

If you are a veteran, telephone 1-877-222-8387 or go to http://www.va.gov. If you are a military retiree or dependent, including a widow or a divorced spouse, you become eligible for TRICARE Senior Pharmacy Program. Telephone 1-800-538-9552 or go to http://www.tricare.osd.mil. TRICARE beneficiaries can obtain their medicine through the national Mail-Order Pharmacy. You don't have to enroll in the program; a military identification card is all you need. Just send in your prescription and a Patient Profile Registration Form, which beneficiaries can receive by telephoning 1-800-903-4680. You can also visit your local drugstore, as long as it is part of the TRICARE network, though your costs will increase this way. If you have access to a military treatment facility pharmacy, you can obtain the medicine for free. Before using this program, make sure you update your address with the Defense Enrollment Eligibility Reporting System (DEERS). You can do so by telephoning 1-800-538-9552 or by visiting http://www.tricare.osd.mil/DEERS/default .cfm. If you do not provide your current address, you will not receive updated information on the program. For more information about TRICARE, you can telephone 1-877-363-6337 or go to http://www.tricare.osd.mil.

Discount Mail-Order Programs

There are many mail-order programs, including AARP's program, at 1-800-289-8849 or http://www.aarppharmacy.com, and Medco Health, at 1-877-733-6765 or http://www.yourxplan.com. Compare prices among several plans at http://www .destinationrx.com.

Two American nonprofit organizations help Americans of any age fill prescriptions from licensed Canadian pharmacies by mail order: the Minnesota Senior Federation, at 1-877-645-0261, extension 5024, or http://www.mnseniors.org, and the United Health Alliance, at 1-866-633-7482 or http://www.medicineassist.org. Americans also travel to Canada and Mexico to save money on medications. In Canada, pharmacies will only fill prescriptions written by Canadian doctors (though most pharmacies will help you get in touch with a Canadian physician to do so). But be sure to go to a licensed pharmacy and purchase the correct drug at the correct dosage. Also, remember that some prescriptions are available over-the-counter in other countries at substantial savings. Just make sure that your doctor does not object to your buying drugs abroad, and make sure you are buying the correct medication at the correct dosage. Although the federal government does not look positively upon this situation, US law permits travelers to import a three-month supply of medicine for personal use, as long as they have valid prescriptions from their doctors at home. Also find out if the Food and Drug Administration has approved the drug for its intended use in the United States. While many Americans may assume that new drugs inevitably work better than old drugs, such a belief is not necessarily true. In order to obtain ratings and profiles of mail-order and online pharmacies in the United States, Canada, or foreign countries, you should visit http://www.pharmacy checker.com. Here you can learn which domestic and foreign pharmacies have licenses and provide proper privacy, security, and reliable contact information. This independent site also lists the prices of prescription medicines so that you can compare prices and determine which are best for you.

Other Sources

Other sources of prescription drug information include the Robert Wood Johnson Foundation, which sponsors a Web site that gives information on national and state-based medication assistance programs: http://www.rxassist.org. Another source is the Consumers Union, publisher of *Consumers Reports*, which gives advice on making cost-effective prescription drug decisions at its Web site, http://www.crbest buydrugs.org. Rather than performing the evaluation of drugs themselves, the Consumers Union relies on the drug safety and effectiveness reviews done for twelve states by the Center for Evidenced Based Policy (http://www.ohsu.edu), which itself is part of the Oregon Health and Science University. For price information, the Web site uses national averages compiled by NDCHealth. Consumers are encouraged to download the information and discuss it with their doctors. The National Association of Boards of Pharmacy (NABP) offers a list of approved Internet pharmacy sites where you can fill prescriptions with confidence. Its site is located at http://www.nabp.net. Remember, there are many illegal Internet pharmacies overseas that are beyond the reach of US law enforcement, so you have no guarantee that their products are safe and effective. Some may come with no instructions or warnings. The pharmacies the National Association of Boards of Pharmacy sanctions are professional operations that adhere to all federal and state laws. They have licensed pharmacists on call; they protect patient confidentiality; and they follow industry standards for the safe storage and shipping of medicine. Some very good bargains are available at http://www.drugstore.com and http://www.familymeds.com. There are also Web sites for chain drugstores such as http://www.cvs.com, http://www. walgreen.com, and http://www.eckerd.com. A complete list of Web sites is available at http://www.napb.org/vipps. The acronym VIPPS stands for Verified Internet Pharmacy Practice Sites.

Also, for a small annual fee, the AARP offers its members a discount card that enables seniors to get reduced-cost drugs at thousands of pharmacies across the country. If you are enrolled in any of AARP's health insurance plans, you have free access to its Prescription Saving Service, which offers discounts on prescription drugs through the mail or at thousands of pharmacies throughout the country. If you don't have an AARP-sponsored insurance plan, you can pay a small annual fee and join an identical AARP program called Member Choice. Both programs offer additional benefits, including telephone consultation with pharmacists and drug utilization review to make sure none of your medicines interact dangerously with each other. For more information call the AARP toll-free at 1-800-456-2277 or visit it on the Web at http://www.aarp.org, or more specifically click on http://www.aarp pharmacy.com. Find out if the AARP has published any booklets on the prescription drug discount cards. Another group that requires a small fee is the Medicine Program, which offers detailed individualized assistance for people applying for free or discounted prescription drugs from major drug companies. For more information, write the Medicine Program at P.O. Box 515, Doniphan, MO 63935-0515, or call them at 1-573-996-7300, or visit it on the Web at http://www.themedicineprogram .com. Another informative site, available for a small annual fee, is http://www. rxaminer.com, which offers cost-cutting ideas for getting hundreds of commonly prescribed medications. Lastly, if your income is too large to qualify for a state or drug company–sponsored program and you are not a veteran, you might want to look into joining a private plan such as WellRx (click on http://www.wellrxcard .com), which charges an annual fee and offers discounts. But before joining any plan, examine your purchasing needs and plan membership fees to make sure you will save money, because while some private programs do offer generous savings on generic drugs they do not always do so in regard to brand name drugs.

Finally, as already mentioned and this cannot be emphasized enough, shop around for the best drug prices. Call five or six local pharmacies to compare prices when you are filling a prescription. Understand that just because a pharmacy gives you the best price on one drug, it won't necessarily offer the best prices on other drugs. Also, be aware that pharmacies providing such services as free or emergency delivery or twenty-four-hour service may charge slightly more.

SELECTING A PHARMACIST

Another way to get more for your money when purchasing drugs is to find a family pharmacist you like and stay with him. This allows your pharmacist to maintain family medication records to protect you against adverse drug reactions and to determine whether you are taking too many or the wrong combination of medicines. He can also advise you on all drug purchases—including the nonprescription drugs you purchase regularly for self-medication—and possibly help to reduce your spending on over-the-counter drugs you do not need. In addition to finding out whether your pharmacist maintains patient medication profiles, you should determine whether the pharmacist offers emergency prescription service, whether the pharmacy delivers and allows you to charge drug purchases, and whether the pharmacist is willing to answer your questions about drugs. While additional services may increase the cost of your medications, these diverse services will affect the quality of care you receive from the pharmacist. It is up to you to decide whether they are worth the extra expense.

Your pharmacist can serve as your patient counselor so that you can get the maximum therapeutic benefits from your medication. He can ensure that you understand the purpose, proper use, and expected outcomes from your drug therapy. Also be aware that as of January 1, 2006, a provision in the Medicare Prescription Drug, Improvement, and Modernization Act of 2003 mandates that pharmacists in hospitals or long-term healthcare pharmacies are to be paid when they consult with Medicare patients who take multiple drugs for chronic illness. As with your doctor, make sure that the pharmacist reviews the following pertinent aspects for each medication in your drug regimen, whether the medication is a prescription or over-the-counter:

- The medication's trademark name, generic name, common synonym, or other descriptive name(s).
- Its intended use and expected action. What to do if the expected action does not occur.
- The route, dosage form, dosage, and administration schedule (including duration of therapy).
- Directions for preparation.
- Directions for administration.
- Precautions to be observed during administration.
- Common adverse effects that may be encountered, including their avoidance and the action required if they occur.
- Techniques for self-monitoring of drug therapy.
- Proper storage.
- Potential drug-drug or drug-food interactions or contraindications.
- Issues related to radiologic and laboratory procedures (e.g., timing of doses and potential interference with interpreting results).
- Prescription refill information.
- Any other information peculiar to the specific patient or drug.[7]

When a pharmacist sells you a prescribed medication, a fee for his services arises from his dispensing the prescription, buying and stocking drugs, making deliveries to your home if this be the case, and maintaining your monthly charge accounts. This fee is added to the pharmacy's cost of the dispensed medication. (The fee system has generally replaced the older markup system, which, because it varied with drug prices, might have tempted a pharmacist to dispense a more costly product.) The fee varies, depending upon geographical location and other factors. However, you can ask your pharmacist and other pharmacists in your community what their dispensing fees are in order to compare the costs. How does the pharmacist's pricing policy fit your needs? If you have complaints about the dispensing fee practices of a pharmacist and drug prices or even about the prescribing practices of a physician, you should contact your state board of pharmacy and local medical society, respectively.

A pharmacist is a graduate of either a five- or a six-year college of pharmacy where he or she was trained in the science of preparing medicine. This academic training includes the basic sciences such as biology, chemistry, physics, and mathematics as well as pharmacology, physiology, anatomy, and biochemistry. Pharmacy students, like their physician counterparts, also work with patients in a medical setting as part of their professional training prior to seeking employment as full-fledged pharmacists. Years ago these professionals filled prescriptions by compounding different drugs in specific quantities; since World War II this time-consuming method has become outdated. Most medicines today are prepared by large manufacturing companies, and pharmacists no longer need to use their scientific skills to compound drugs. Thus, the professional role of the pharmacist has changed over the years.

Today, more and more pharmacists are emerging as health counselors who can be a source of valuable information for you and your family. Some pharmacists, for example, are routinely quizzing diabetic patients about symptoms that could signal a need for closer medical attention, while others are administering immunizations for pneumonia and influenza. Other considerations when choosing a pharmacist and the pharmacy include:

- Does the pharmacy provide screenings and monitoring for hypertension and other problems? Does it maintain patient profiles, medication information sheets, and medication reminder programs (including costs).
- Does it sell and fit patients for crutches and other devices?
- Are the hours and location convenient? What about its dispensing fee? Too high, low, or reasonable compared to other pharmacies?
- If you are as senior citizen, does the pharmacy offer discounts?
- Does it provide delivery services (an important consideration if you are elderly or have small children)? Are they free?
- Can you charge your purchases to an account or use a prescription drug plan or Medicaid?

Choosing a pharmacist and a pharmacy can be as important to your health as selecting a family doctor or dentist, so do not settle for one who is too busy to serve you. You may have to shop around until you find a pharmacist who keeps patient medication records and offers drug consultations—but when you do, visit him regularly in order to establish a personal and trusting relationship. Also, keep your doctor's and pharmacy's telephone numbers by the phone in case you need to reach them in an emergency.

Although there is no standard form, a medication record should contain the customer's name, age, weight, and height as well as information about drug allergies and sensitivities. It should also list all the prescription and nonprescription drugs regularly used by the patient. With all these facts readily available, the pharmacist can make a professional judgment when new drugs are prescribed or old prescriptions refilled. Patient medication records can even help the pharmacists advise you on seemingly casual nonprescription purchases such as aspirin as well as on the importance of taking prescribe drugs regularly. Records are kept confidential, but clients may ask to have their prescription records printed out to help make medical claims on their taxes. Your pharmacist may do this for you. Today, such information may be computerized. Computerized patient-profile systems designed to keep detailed records and monitor potential drug interactions are becoming commonplace. Such profiles can also state whether safety caps are needed, whether generic drugs can be substituted, and what insurance company should be billed.

If you have a problem opening childproof bottle caps, ask your pharmacist to substitute an easy-to-open cap for you. Most pharmacies carry both kinds of bottle caps and will gladly substitute for you, if you ask. Remember, your pharmacist is there to help you. Do not be afraid to ask as many questions as you must until you understand when and how to take your medication. After all, you are paying for the pharmacist's services and your health is involved.[8]

ONLINE PHARMACIES

If you decide to purchase you medications online at an Internet Web site, be very careful that the online pharmacy is not selling prescription drugs without proper medical protections. Unlike legitimate sites, these illegitimate sites—many operating in foreign countries—sell prescription drugs without a prescription or other physician involvement. In other words, they will dispense a medication without requiring you to mail in a prescription, or they may not contact your doctor to obtain a valid prescription orally. Some send medication based solely on an online questionnaire without you having a preexisting relationship with a physician and the benefit of an in-person physical examination. A legitimate Internet pharmacy requires a prescription from the patient's physician and checks the prescription with the doctor. Consumer-patients or their doctors can send in prescriptions by fax, mail, telephone, or e-mail. The prescription is mailed to the person's home or, in many instances, is available to be picked up at a local drugstore. It is very important that your doctor be involved with the Internet pharmacy. Your physician not only can make sure that the medicine is correct but also can reduce the possibility of the new prescription drug interacting adversely with medicine you are already taking. As other precautions against illegitimate pharmacy sites, consumers should avoid sites that fail to state the names and telephone numbers of physicians or pharmacists who can answer their questions or doesn't have a toll-free telephone number as well as a posted street address. Avoid a site that does not advertise the availability of pharmacists for medication consultation. You should also avoid sites that offer unrealistic claims or ask personal history questions that are intended to look like professional medical reviews but are not. You should also be suspicious of Internet sites that sell a limited number of medications or specialize or chiefly sell drugs for hair growth, weight loss, depression, and other conditions that many people find embarrassing, which illegitimate sites depend on to attract customers. Be a wise consumer-patient and discuss any drug purchases with your doctor. Make sure the drugs you are purchasing are not counterfeit medications. First, know the color, size, shape, and taste of your prescription drugs. Check any differences with your doctor. Second, check for altered or unsealed containers or changes in packaging or labels. The National Consumers League Web site has more information on this subject at http://www .nclnet.org. Finally, as already noted, to determine whether or not the Internet pharmacy is legitimate, seek such information on the Food and Drug Administration Web site at http://www.fda.gov, or try http://www.nabp.net, the Web site of the National Association of Boards of Pharmacies, which describes the organization's Verified Internet Pharmacy Practice Sites (VIPPS) and lists the online drugstores that carry its seal. Click on "VIPPS." Consumers can also write to the National Association of Boards of Pharmacies at 1600 Feehanville Drive, Mt. Prospect, IL 60056, or telephone 1-847-391-4406.

MEDICATION ERRORS

The purpose of drug therapy is the achievement of defined therapeutic outcomes that improve a patient's quality of life while minimizing patient risk. However, there are inherent risks, both known and unknown, associated with the therapeutic use of drugs (prescription and nonprescription) and drug administration devices. The incidents or hazards that result from such risks include adverse drug reactions and medication errors. The latter can adversely affect the patient's view of the healthcare system and increase healthcare costs. Errors occur from lack of knowledge, substandard performance and mental lapses, or defects or failures in systems. Medication errors include prescribing errors, dispensing errors, medication administration errors, and patient compliance errors. While many medication errors are probably undetected, some can result in serious patient morbidity (sickness) or mortality. Some of the common causes of medication errors include:

- ambiguous drug strength designated on labels or in packaging
- drug product nomenclature (look-alike or sound-alike names, use of lettered or numbered prefixes, and suffixes in drug names)
- equipment failure or malfunction
- illegible handwriting
- improper transcription, such as misplacing a decimal point or knowing the right dose but writing the wrong dosage
- inaccurate dosage calculation
- look-alike packaging
- inadequately trained personnel
- ignorance of drug interactions
- inappropriate abbreviations used in prescribing
- labeling errors
- excessive workload in organization
- lapses in individual performance
- medication unavailable[9]

It has been estimated that 1 percent of hospitalized patients suffer adverse events as the result of medical mismanagement and that drug-related complications are the most common kind of adverse event. For example, on February 15, 2006, the United States Pharmacopeia, a nonprofit organization that sets standards for drugs and pharmacy procedures, released a report that noted that communication breakdowns and improperly programmed IV pumps cause harmful medication errors in hospital intensive care units. Many of the prescribing errors were associated with such issues as writing orders that were incomplete or incorrect, illegible hand-writing, using abbreviations that were misinterpreted, and a lack of familiarity with some drug information. *Therefore, the following recommendations for preventing medication errors are suggested for physicians and other prescribers*:

- To determine appropriate drug therapy, prescribers should
    - ▼ stay abreast of the current state of medical knowledge;
    - ▼ consult with pharmacists and other physicians; and
    - ▼ participate in continuing professional education programs and other means.

    It is especially crucial to seek information when prescribing for conditions and diseases not typically experienced in the prescriber's practice.
- Prescribers should evaluate the patient's total status and review all existing drug therapy before prescribing new or additional medications to ascertain possible antagonistic or complementary drug interactions. To evaluate and optimize patient response to a prescribed therapy, appropriate monitoring of clinical signs and symptoms and relevant laboratory data is necessary.
- In hospitals, prescribers should be familiar with the medication-ordering system (e.g,. the formulary system, the list of medications for which the health plans pays), allowable delegation of authority, procedures to alert nurses and others to new drug orders that need to be processed, standard medication times, and approved abbreviations.
- Drug orders should be complete. They should include the following:
    - ▼ patient name
    - ▼ generic drug name
    - ▼ trademarked name (if a specific product is required)
    - ▼ route and site of administration
    - ▼ dosage form
    - ▼ dose strength
    - ▼ quantity
    - ▼ frequency of administration
    - ▼ prescriber's name

The desired therapeutic outcome for each drug should be expressed when the drug is prescribed. Prescribers should review all drug orders for accuracy and legibility immediately after they have prescribed them. As a patient, you also have a responsibility. Make sure when you are looking at the prescription and medicine bottle that your name is correct, the name of the medication is correct, the dosage is the same as the physician told you, and the instructions are understandable and clear. Doctors and pharmacists often communicate in Latin. The following Latin terms, their abbreviations, and their meanings should help you understand their dialogue and your prescription.

Latin	*Abbreviation*	*Meaning*
ante cibum	ac	before meals
bis in die	bid	twice a day
gutta	gt	drop
hora somni	hs	at bedtime
oculus dexter	od	right eye
oculus sinister	os	left eye
per os	po	by mouth
post cibum	pc	after meals
pro re nata	prn	as needed
quaque 3 hora	q3h	every three hours
quater in die	qid	four times a day
ter in die	tid	three times a day

- Care should be taken to ensure that the intent of medication orders is clear and unambiguous. Prescribers should
  - ▼ Write out instructions rather than using nonstandard or ambiguous abbreviations. For example, write "daily" rather than "qd," which could be misinterpreted as qid (which would cause a drug to be given four times a day instead of once) or as od (for right eye).
  - ▼ Not use vague instructions, such as "take as directed," because specific instructions can help differentiate among intended drugs.
  - ▼ Specify exact dosage strengths (such as milligrams) rather than dosage form units (such as one tablet or one vial). An exception would be combination drugs products, for which the number of dosage units should be specified.
  - ▼ Prescribe by standard nomenclature, using the drug's generic name (United States Adopted Name, USAN), official name, or trademarked name (if deemed medically necessary). Avoid the following:
    - ■ locally coined names (e.g., Dr. Doe's syrup)
    - ■ chemical names (e.g., 6-mercaptopurine [instead of mercaptopurine] could result in a sixfold overdose if misinterpreted)
    - ■ unestablished abbreviated names (e.g., "AZT" could stand for zidovudine, azathioprine, or aztreonam)
    - ■ acronyms
    - ■ apothecary or chemical names
  - ▼ A leading zero should always precede a decimal expression of less than one (e.g., 0.5 ml). Conversely, a terminal zero should never be used (e.g., 5.0 ml), since failure to see the decimal could result in a tenfold overdose. When possible, avoid the use of decimals (e.g., prescribe 500 mg instead of 0.5 g).
  - ▼ Spell out the word "units" (e.g., 10 units regular insulin), rather than writing "u," which could be misinterpreted as a zero.

- Written drug or prescription orders (including signatures) should be legible. Prescribers with poor handwriting should print or type medication or prescription orders if direct order-entry capabilities for computerized systems are unavailable. A handwriting order should be completely readable (not merely recognizable through familiarity). An illegible handwritten order should be regarded as a potential error. If it leads to an error of occurrence (i.e., the error actually reaches the patient), it should be regarded as a prescribing error.
- Verbal drug or prescription orders (i.e., orders that are orally communicated) should be reserved only for those situations in which it is impossible or impractical for the prescriber to write the order or enter it into the computer. The prescriber should dictate verbal orders slowly, clearly, and articulately to avoid confusion. Special caution is urged in the prescribing of drug dosages in the teens (e.g., a 15-meq dose of potassium chloride could be misheard as a 50-meq dose). The orders should be read back to the prescriber by the recipient (i.e., the nurse or pharmacist, according to organizational policies). When read back, the drug name should be spelled to the prescriber, and when directions are repeated, no abbreviations should be used (e.g., say "three times daily" rather than "tid"). A written copy of the verbal order should be placed in the patient's medical records, if in an institution, and later confirmed by the prescriber in accordance with applicable state regulations and hospital policies.
- When possible, drugs should be prescribed for administration by the oral route, rather than by injection.
- When possible, the prescriber should talk with the patient or caregiver to explain the medication prescribed and any special precautions or observations that might be indicated, including any allergic or hypersensitivity reactions that might occur.
- Prescribers should follow-up and periodically evaluate the need for continued drug therapy for individual patients.
- Instructions with respect to "hold" orders for medications should be clear.[10]

Patients also can assume an important role in preventing medication errors. Patients (or their authorized caregivers or designees) have the right to know about all aspects of their care, including drug therapy. When patient status allows, healthcare providers should encourage patients to take an active role in their drug use by questioning and learning about their treatment regimens. Generally, if patients are more knowledgeable, anxieties can be alleviated and errors in treatment may be prevented. *The following suggestions are offered to help patients whose health status allows, and their caregivers, make the best use of medications:*

- Patients should feel free to ask questions about any procedures and treatments received.
- Patients should learn the names of the drug products that are prescribed and

administered to them, as well as dosage strengths and schedules. It is suggested that patients keep a personal list of all drug therapy, including prescribed drugs, nonprescription drugs, home remedies, and medical records. Patient should also maintain lists of medications that they cannot take and the reasons why. This information should be shared with the healthcare provider. Patients should be assertive in communicating with healthcare providers when anything seems incorrect or different from the norm.

- After counseling from an authorized healthcare provider about the appropriateness of the medication, patients should take all the medications as directed.[11]

By working with healthcare providers, patients can do much to help prevent medication errors.

AVOIDING ADVERSE DRUG REACTIONS

One important area in which your pharmacist, through his patient medication records, and your physician can be of great assistance is helping you avoid adverse drug reactions if you are taking more than one medication at the same time. The results of some drug interactions are not important. Others, however, can mean the difference between successful and unsuccessful treatment if the medication does not work; can produce a false reading of a laboratory test; can cause unexpected and possible serious, even fatal, side effects; or can set off puzzling or misleading symptoms.

Although the Food and Drug Administration (FDA) requires that the manufacturer of a new drug prove its safety and effectiveness, the drug producer does not routinely carry out, and is not required by law to carry out, tests for safety and effectiveness that involve simultaneous use of several drugs. One reason is that the whole problem of drug interactions is relatively new and not totally understood; another is that it is an endlessly complicated business. However, as factual knowledge about potentially significant drug interactions emerges, the FDA requires that such information be reflected in the label that accompanies nonprescription (over-the-counter) medication and the labeling information available to pharmacists and physicians for prescription drugs. The FDA also publishes a widely distributed monthly collection of data about interactions and other important effects of drugs.[12]

Drugs interact in a number of ways. One drug may make another drug act faster or slower, more powerfully or less powerfully, than it normally would. One drug may change the effect another drug has on the body. A fairly common way in which one drug acts on another is by affecting the way it is absorbed, distributed, or broken down (metabolized) by the body. In addition to these latter effects, one drug can also either inhibit or hasten the excretion of another, and thus either exaggerate or reduce its effect.

When a number of drugs are being taken, consideration must be given to their cumulative impact. This so-called additive reaction is especially important if the drugs are similar in their general effect. Some drugs, when combined, produce reactions that go beyond what one might assume would result from adding the effect of one drug to another. This type of action, in which the effects from two drugs are not simply added to each other but are multiplied, is called *potentiation*. This reaction can greatly accelerate the helpful effect of a drug, on the one hand, but also can become one of the most dangerous forms of interaction. A number of deaths of otherwise healthy persons have been reported that resulted from potentiation—especially through mixing alcohol with sleeping aids, pain relievers, or tranquilizers.

Another important unwanted drug reaction occurs when a drug affects the body chemistry in a way that skews or confuses the results of the diagnostic tests. Ordinary nonprescription drugs can have this confusing effect and so can vitamins. For example, laboratory tests to determine a patient's calcium or bone metabolism can be affected by an excess use of laxatives. Vitamins A, D, and K, as well as such common over-the-counter drugs as aspirin, can produce false positive or negative readings in a great number of important tests used by physicians to diagnose illness. And large doses of vitamin C can produce false negative urinary glucose tests, which can hide a diabetes condition.[13]

Therefore, you must do everything within your ability to protect yourself against harmful drug interactions. Here are several suggestions. Although some have been mentioned previously, they cannot be emphasized enough.

- When your physician prescribes a drug for you, make sure he knows what other drugs you are taking—both prescription and nonprescription—as well as vitamins and herbal products. All of them. Remember that the words "drug" and "medicine" mean the same thing, and alcohol is a drug. Headache remedies, cold medicines, laxatives, and other nonprescription medicines are drugs. When your physician asks, "Are you taking any other medicines?" no drug is too unimportant to mention. Some authorities suggest writing a continuing inventory (including dosages and dates) in a notebook where relatives or friends can find it in an emergency.

- Go to *one* pharmacy for all your prescriptions. Ask your pharmacist to keep a complete record of all your prescription and nonprescription medications. Even if your pharmacist is rushed, ask the pharmacist to double-check interaction information for a new prescription.

- Do not start taking a second drug unless your physician knows about it. If you go into a hospital, be sure the staff carefully checks your hospital identification bracelet before you take any medications. It is also a good idea to tell your pharmacist when he fills a prescription what other drugs you are taking. He may wish to set up a personal record so that he can tell at a glance whether you might be exposed to a drug interaction.

- Do not take a drug prescribed for someone else because it is "good for a stomach pain" or whatever else is troubling you. The drug in that prescription may interact with something else you are taking, or it may not be suitable for you or your ailment.

- Read the label as well as any package inserts. Over-the-counter (OTC) drugs are required by the Food and Drug Administration to contain information about significant drug interactions. Most OTC medications are meant for short-term use; are generally cheaper, though not always, than prescription medicines; and eliminate the cost of seeing a doctor for a prescription. However, if the problem lingers on even with the use of the OTC medicine, that's the time your should go to your doctor.[14] More than three hundred thousand nonprescription medicines are presently sold in the United States, according to the nonprescription Drug Manufacturers Association. More than four hundred of these products use ingredients or dosages that were available only by prescription in the mid-1970s. The five most commonly purchased OTC medications include internal analgesics, (i.e., aspirin); cough and cold remedies to alleviate such ailments as congestion, sneezing, and running nose; antacids to ease stomach discomfort; laxatives to treat constipation; and skin medications to lessen itching, rashes, dryness, or acne. Other popular over-the-counter products include contact lens solutions, antiseptic mouthwashes, dandruff medicated shampoos, diet aids, and foot preparations.[15] Before taking any OTC medication, experts advise:
  - ▼ After reading the label, follow instructions carefully.
  - ▼ Consult your doctor if you notice undesirable side effects. Often, alternative drugs can be used.
  - ▼ Never use drugs to enhance personal performance or to hide pain. Pain is the body's signal that something is wrong; if you try to block it out, you're setting yourself up for serious injury.
  - ▼ Check caffeine content. If you take OTC drugs that have caffeine content in combination with foods that contain caffeine—such as coffee, chocolate, and colas—you could overload yourself with the stimulant.
  - ▼ Popular diet pills Accutrim and Dexatrim are stimulants. The main ingredient is actually a decongestant used for its appetite suppressant properties, then combined with caffeine. It is common for dieters to take more than the recommended doses, and they are asking for trouble.
  - ▼ Stimulants, such as caffeine and pseudoephedrine, elevate heart rate and are found in many nonprescription cold medicines, such as decongestants, and in other OTC remedies as extra ingredients. At high doses, OTC stimulants may result in undesirable effects like impaired concentration, insomnia, accelerated dehydration, and dangerously elevated blood pressure or heartbeat irregularities.
  - ▼ Antihistamines, which make people drowsy, also may cause problems for exercisers. While the label often tells you not to operate machinery, it is also a poor idea to go cycling or roller-skating for exercise after taking one.
  - ▼ Diuretics in preparations such as Pamprin or Midol cause the body to eliminate water. Exercisers taking these pills should drink plenty of

water, especially in warm weather since excessive water loss—dehydra-tion—can be a serious health risk.[16]

▼ Remember that drugs have three names: the chemical name, which usu-ally is not given on the label; the generic name, which is the official, established name for that drug; and the proprietary name or trademarked brand name for that drug. It is important to remember this because the warnings printed on labels give the generic name. Thus, a number of nonprescription medicines such as antacids warn against taking medi-cine with tetracycline, which is the generic name of an antibiotic. How-ever, Achromycin, Azotrex, Kesso-Tetra Syrup, Sumycin, Panmycin, Tetrastatin, and over a dozen others are proprietary or brand names for tetracycline. So, unless you know the generic name as well as the pro-prietary or brand name, you may be exposing yourself to a drug interac-tion. To avoid this, ask your physician or pharmacist to tell you the generic name of any prescription drugs you may be taking.

▼ It is also worth remembering that many drugs contain more than one ingredient. Empirin, a medicine widely used for relief of simple headaches and other discomforts, contains aspirin as well as phenacetin and caffeine.[17]

Finally, since knowledge about drug interactions is by no means complete and individuals differ in their reaction to drugs, you might experience a reaction to a mixture of drugs that is heretofore unknown, not only to your physician and your pharmacist, but to the medical professional generally. So if you are taking more than one drug and you become ill, be sure to report it to your physician and pharmacist. Drugs sometimes are prescribed so they will interact and produce a desired result. But be careful and be alert. Your physician and your pharmacist are there to help you. Use them.

FOOD AND DRUG INTERACTIONS

Drugs can not only interact with other drugs to produce adverse effects but also, according to the Food and Drug Administration, drugs interacting with the food you eat can produce negative results. The extent of interaction between foods and drugs depends upon the drug dosage and on the individual's age, size, and specific med-ical condition. In general, though, the presence of food in the stomach and intestines can influence a drug's effectiveness by slowing down or speeding up the time it takes the medicine to go through the gastrointestinal tract to the site in the body where it is needed. Food also contains natural and added chemicals that can react with cer-tain drugs in ways that make the drug virtually useless. Some reactions can be absolutely dangerous, triggering a medical crisis or, in rare instances, even death.[18]

A major way food affects drugs is by enhancing or impeding absorption of the drug into the bloodstream. According to the FDA, the following are examples of the problems caused by food and drug interaction:

- A classic example of food interfering with drug absorption is the one between dairy products and tetracycline compounds. The calcium in milk, cheese, and yogurt impairs the absorption of tetracycline (an antibiotic).
- Oral contraceptives are known to lower blood levels, folic acid, a member of the vitamin B family, and vitamin B$_6$. The depletion is usually not serious enough to cause symptoms. They also can decrease the absorption of vitamin C. Women who take birth control pills would be wise to include dark green leafy vegetables in their diet.
- Chronic use of antacids containing aluminum can cause phosphate depletion, leading to weakness, malaise, and loss of appetite.
- Taking some iron supplements with citrus juices or fruits containing ascorbic acid enhances the absorption of iron.
- In general, it is not wise to take drugs with soda pop, acid fruit, or vegetable juices unless you check with your physician first. These beverages can result in excess acidity that may cause some drugs to dissolve quickly in the stomach—instead of in the intestines, where they can be more readily absorbed into the bloodstream. Caffeine, found in coffee, tea, and many soft drinks, can stimulate the production of stomach acid, so it is best not take pills with a caffeinated liquid.
- Excessive consumption of foods high in vitamin K, such as liver and leafy green vegetables, could hinder the effectiveness of anticoagulants. Vitamin K promotes the clotting of the blood, working in direct opposition to these drugs, which are intended to prevent clotting.
- Some foods, such as soybeans, rutabagas, brussels sprouts, turnips, cabbage, and kale contain substances known as goitrogens that inhibit production of the thyroid hormone and thus can produce goiter. Scientists suggest caution in eating these foods when taking thyroid medications.
- A very hazardous food-drug interaction is one between monoamine oxidase (MAO) inhibitors, drugs often prescribed for depression and high blood pressure, and such foods as aged cheese, Chianti wine, and chicken livers. MAO inhibitors can react with a substance called tyramine in these foods and force the blood pressure to dangerous levels, sometimes causing severe headaches, brain hemorrhage, and, in extreme cases, death. To prevent a possible reaction, the FDA suggests that anyone taking MAO inhibitor drugs should avoid aged and fermented foods, including pickled herring; fermented sausages, such as salami and pepperoni; sharp or aged cheeses; yogurt and sour cream; beef and chicken livers; broad beans, such as fava beans; canned figs; bananas; avocados; soy sauce; active yeast preparations; beer; Chianti wine; sherry and other wines in large quantities. MAO inhibitors also are suspected of reacting adversely with cola beverages, coffee, chocolate, and raisins.

- Natural licorice is another substance whose continuous excessive use may raise your blood pressure or counteract the effect of medication for high blood pressure. Although most American manufacturers now use a synthetic flavoring, many imported products like candy and some medications still may use licorice from natural sources. If you have high blood pressure, carefully read the label to determine the product's ingredients.
- Alcohol, which is actually a drug itself, although not regulated as a drug under the Food, Drug, and Cosmetic Act, does not mix well with a wide variety of medications, such as antibiotics; anticoagulants; antidiabetic drugs, including insulin; antihistamines; high blood pressure drugs; MAO inhibitors; and sedatives. Alcohol combined with antihistamines, tranquilizers, or antidepressants causes excessive drowsiness that can be especially hazardous to someone driving a car, operating machinery, or performing some other task that requires mental alertness. A good rule of thumb is to avoid alcoholic beverages when taking any type of prescription or over-the-counter medication.
- Aspirin reduces pain, fever, and inflammation. Because aspirin can cause stomach irritation, avoid alcohol. To avoid stomach upset, take with food. Do not take with prune juice.
- Corticosteroids. Cortisone-like drugs are used to provide relief to inflamed areas of the body. Avoid alcohol because both alcohol and corticosteroids can cause stomach irritation. Also, avoid foods high in sodium (salt). Check labels on food packages for sodium. Take with food to prevent stomach upset.
- Vasodilators are used to relax veins and/or arteries to reduce the work of the heart. Use of sodium (salt) should be restricted for medication to be effective. Check labels on food packages for sodium.
- Antihypertensive medications relax blood vessels, increase the supply of blood and oxygen to the heart, and lessen its workload. They also regulate heartbeat. Use of sodium (salt) should be restricted for medication to be effective.
- Methenamine is used to treat urinary tract infections. Cranberries, plums, prunes, and their juices help the action of this drug. Avoid citrus fruits and citrus juices. Eat foods with protein, but avoid dairy products.
- Metronidazole (brand name is Flagyl) is an anti-infective that is used to treat intestinal and genital infections caused by bacteria and parasites. Do not take alcohol while using this drug because it may cause stomach pain, nausea, vomiting, headache, flushing or redness of the face.
- Penicillins are antibiotics used for treatment of a wide variety of infections. Amoxicillin and bacampicillin may be taken with food; however, absorption of other types of penicillins is reduced when taken with food.
- Sulfa drugs are anti-infectives that are used to treat stomach and urinary infections. Avoid alcohol, since the combination may cause nausea.
- Erythromycin is an antibiotic used to treat a wide variety of infections, including those of the throat, ears, and skin. Erythromycin varies in its reaction with food; consult your doctor or pharmacist for instructions.

- Ibuprofen and other anti-inflammatory agents. These reduce pain and reduce inflammation and fever. These drugs should be taken with food or milk because they can irritate the stomach. Avoid taking the medication with those foods or alcoholic beverages that tend to bother your stomach.
- Indomethacin is used to treat the painful symptoms of certain types of arthritis and gout by reducing inflammation, swelling, stiffness, joint pain, and fever. This drug should be taken with food because it can irritate the stomach. Avoid taking the medication with the kinds of foods or alcoholic beverages that tend to irritate your stomach.
- Piroxicam is used to treat pain, inflammation, redness, swelling, and stiffness caused by certain types of arthritis. This medication should be taken with a light snack because it can cause stomach irritation. Avoid alcohol because it can add to the possibility of stomach upset.
- Codeine is narcotic that is contained in many cough and pain relief medicines. Codeine suppresses coughs and relieves pain, and is often combined with aspirin and acetaminophen in medications.
- Narcotics are used to relieve pain. Do not drink alcohol because it increases the sedative effect of the medications. Take these medications with food because they can upset your stomach.[19]

Just as some foods can affect the way drugs perform in the body, so *drugs can affect the manner in which the body uses food*. Drugs may act in various ways to impair proper nutrition—by hastening excretion of certain nutrients, by hindering absorption of nutrients, or by interfering with the body's ability to convert nutrients into usable forms. Nutrient depletion of the body takes place gradually, but for those taking drugs over a long period of time, these interactions can lead to deficiencies of certain vitamins and minerals, especially in children, the elderly, those with poor diets, and the chronically ill. The following represent a few examples of this food-drug interaction:

- Anticonvulsant drugs used to control epilepsy can lead to deficiencies of vitamin D and folic acid because they increase the turnover rate of these vitamins in the body.
- Mineral oil, an old-fashioned laxative used widely by elderly people and in nursing homes, can hinder absorption of vitamin D. It is reported that as little as 20 milliliters (4 teaspoons) of mineral oil twice daily can interfere with the absorption of vitamin D, vitamin K, and carotene, a substance the body converts to vitamin A.
- Drugs readily available without prescription, such as antacids to treat gastric upset, also can lead to nutritional problems. Chronic use of antacids without a doctor's supervision can cause phosphate depletion, a condition that in its milder form produces muscle weakness and in more severe form leads to vitamin D deficiency. Antacids, even those containing calcium and taken as

calcium supplements may cause constipation, already a problem for many older people because of reduced intestinal function.[20]

- Long-term use of diuretics, or "water pills," to treat such conditions as congestive heart failure, can lead to serious potassium depletion. If the potassium loss is not corrected in heart patients taking digitalis, the heart may become more sensitive to the effects of the drug. People taking diuretics regularly are advised to eat foods that are good sources of potassium. These include tomatoes and tomato juice, oranges and orange juice, dried apricots, cantaloupes, figs, raisins, bananas, prunes, potatoes, sweet potatoes, and winter squash.[21]

Modifying your diet to include more foods that are rich in vitamins and minerals which may be depleted by certain drugs generally is preferable to taking vitamin or mineral supplements. Fortunately, the diets of most Americans are sufficiently well balanced that the threat of drug-related nutritional deficiencies can easily be cured. However, *as a preventive measure there are certain steps that consumers can take to prevent adverse drug-food interactions.* Although some have been mentioned previously, they are important enough to be repeated:

- Read the labels on over-the-counter drugs and the package inserts included with prescription drugs to see whether they contain any information in regard to food-drug interactions with that particular medication.
- Follow your doctor's orders about when to take drugs and what foods or beverages to avoid while taking medications. If he does not mention any when he prescribes a medication for you, ask your physician if there are any foods or drugs to avoid when taking your medication.
- While taking drugs, be sure to tell you doctor about any unusual symptoms that follow eating particular foods.
- Maintain a well-balanced diet, including a wide variety of foods. Use of a needed drug, even on a long-term basis, is less likely to cause depletion of vitamins and minerals if your overall nutritional status is good.[22]

Drug labeling and informed professionals can be helpful to you, but your physician and pharmacist cannot monitor your eating habits. Remember that warnings about food-drug interactions are only as good as your willingness to pay attention to them.

UNDERSTANDING ANTIBIOTIC DRUGS

As already noted, one classification of drugs affected by food-drug interactions is the antibiotics. If any class of drugs deserves the title "wonder drug," antibiotics might be the most likely candidate. Their discovery has been called the greatest single advance in the history of medicine, and they are among the most frequently prescribed medications in this country. Before their advent, diseases and illnesses such as bacterial pneumonia, typhoid fever, "strep" throat, whooping cough, tuberculosis, meningitis, and various infections of the genitourinary tract, for example, took a terrible toll in terms of lives lost or lives damaged by the side effects of these diseases. Today, as a result of antibiotics, deaths from these and other severe infections are rare.

According to the Food and Drug Administration, an antibiotic drug is "any drug . . . containing a quantity of any chemical substance which is produced by a microorganism and which has the capacity to inhibit or destroy microorganisms in dilute solutions." [23] The word *antibiotic* is derived from the Latin *antibiosis*, which means "against life." While antibiotics have been very effective in treating and preventing human illnesses, they also have had wide applications in veterinary medicine and in agriculture. Today, there are many antibiotics on the market that come in various dosage forms, including tablets, liquids, and injectables.

The Food and Drug Administration monitors antibiotics more closely than any other class of drugs, except insulin. Every batch of every antibiotic made for human use, and some intended for veterinary use, must be certified by the agency before it goes to the marketplace. Insulin also must be batch certified before it is sold. Exactly which tests are performed depend upon the kind of antibiotic. Bulk antibiotics receive the most extensive testing for potency, purity, and other stability factors. Tablets or capsules may be tested only for potency and moisture content, while a solution or suspension for injection may be tested for potency acidity, pyrogens (fever-producing substances), toxicity, and sterility. Some products require special tests. Ointments for the eye, for example, are checked for the presence of metal fragments. In addition to the batch testing performed by the FDA, the manufacturers of the antibiotics must perform the same analyses before submitting the batch samples to the government agency. According to the government's Code of Federal Regulations, a batch is defined as "a specific quantity of drug or other material that is intended to have uniform characteristics and quality, within specified limits, and is produced according to a single manufacturing order during the same cycle of manufacturing."

The Food and Drug Administration's certification of a sample of antibiotics involves the following procedures. When a drug manufacturer submits an application to the Food and Drug Administration to market a new antibiotic, it must submit proof of the drug's safety and efficacy. If the FDA's review of the drug application sustains the manufacturer's claims, the FDA develops a set of specifications called monographs, which is published in the *Federal Register* and enters the Code of Federal Regulations. A sample of each antibiotic batch that the drug manufacturer produces is then tested against these specifications, and if the sample meets these specifications, the Food and Drug Administration certifies this fact. This procedure is called batch certification. However, if the Food and Drug Administration observes that the drug manufacturer is not following the FDA's Good Manufacturing Practice regulations, the FDA will not certify such a batch even though it meets the government's specifications. In the case of insulin, the United States Pharmacopeia, a private organization, has developed over the years, with authority from Congress, a set of specifications against which a sample batch of insulin is tested.

Despite the impressive record of antibiotics in alleviating illness, they still can be misused as well as cause adverse reactions in some patients. For example, some antibiotics may cause allergic reactions ranging from mild rash to death. Penicillin is the worst offender in this regard, producing the highest incidence of severe and fatal reactions. Tetracyclines can cause staining of children's teeth if they are exposed to these drugs before they reach eight years of age. A child can be affected before birth if the expectant mother takes any of the tetracyclines. One other side effect associated with tetracyclines is that they make the user especially sensitive to sunlight. Another antibiotic, chloramphenicol, produces an unusual reaction in some people, causing a deterioration of the blood-making marrow in the bones. Information prepared for doctors and other health professionals now includes warnings in boldface type to alert them to use this drug only for serious infections. Also, the antibiotic oral clindamycin carries with it the risk of precipitating severe colitis. As a final example, another adverse effect that sometimes appears with the use of antibiotics is the development of "super infections." These occur because the antibiotic kills some, but not all, bacteria. Normally, the body contains varieties of bacteria that hold each other in check. No one type can multiply to the point where it causes harm. But if one group of bacteria is eliminated by antibiotic treatment, the surviving groups have less competition for the resources they need to survive. They can then multiply explosively and produce a secondary infection. This is especially serious if the bacteria causing the secondary infection have developed resistance to antibiotics. Bacteria, normally sensitive to certain antibiotics, can through repeated exposure or misuses of the drugs build up a resistance to the effects of the antibiotics and transmit such resistance to other bacteria of the same or different types. Bacteria can also develop resistance to more than one antibiotic, and this multiresistance also can be passed on. Certain substances, such as heavy metals or sulfas, can cause transmission of multiple antibiotic resistance; as a result, the antibiotics will not be able to fight the infections caused by those bacteria that are now resistant to them.[24] Thus, great caution must be exercised when you are using antibiotics. *Toward this end, the Food and Drug Administration has the following advice for patients taking antibiotics:*

- Most antibiotics should be taken on an empty stomach, one-half to one hour before meals or two hours after meals. Most pharmacists put stickers on the bottle about these things. As already noted, food in the stomach interferes with the absorption of the drug. Do not take tetracyclines with dairy products or with antacids containing aluminum, calcium, or magnesium.
- Take all the antibiotics prescribed, exactly as prescribed, and around the clock. Do not miss a dose, since the effectiveness of the drug depends upon keeping the proper amount of it in your system Do not stop after a few days just because you feel better. If you stop too soon, not all the disease-causing bacteria will be destroyed and reinfection can occur.
- Follow directions for storage very carefully. Some antibiotics need to be refrigerated.

- Keep liquids tightly closed. Shake well before using.
- Do not keep antibiotics beyond their expiration date. This is especially true for tetracyclines because they can cause adverse reactions when they are outdated.
- As already mentioned, do not give anyone else any antibiotic especially prescribed for you. Infections caused by different bacteria may have similar symptoms, but the different bacteria may not be sensitive to the same antibiotic. Thus, your antibiotic will not do the other person any good and may do harm.
- Do not ask for or expect any antibiotic to treat the common cold or simple upper respiratory infections. Antibiotics are not effective against illness caused by viruses.[25]

By understanding the nature of antibiotics and knowing how to use the medicine wisely, you can do much to alleviate the illness for which it is being prescribed. If you have any questions concerning the purpose, possible side effects, method of administration, or other matters pertaining to the prescribed antibiotic, be sure to ask your physician or your pharmacist.

PRESCRIBING FOR THE ELDERLY

Between the years 2010 and 2030, experts project that one in five Americans will be sixty-five years or older. The number of sixty-five- to eighty-four-year-olds will rise to 57 million, an increase of 73 percent, while the number of Americans over eighty-five years of age is expected to almost double by the year 2010. As the elderly population increases, so may patient compliance, adverse reactions, and inappropriate prescribing problems that are often seen in this age group. A Harvard Medical School study published in July 1994 noted that more than 1.35 million Americans over the age of sixty-five received more than one of the inappropriate medications in the study. Researchers estimated that more than six million people over the age of sixty-five who are not institutionalized may be exposed to hazardous prescription drugs each year. In addition to inappropriate medications, a bigger problem may be that elderly patients are prescribed the right drug but in the wrong dose and for too long a time or prescribed something that might interact dangerously with other medications, including over-the-counter drugs.[26] One of the largest categories of drugs on the Harvard Medical School study list of twenty inappropriate medications was sedatives and sleeping pills (including Valium and Librium)—medications whose long duration keeps many seniors sleepy all day and prone to confusion, falls, and hip fractures. Rather than relying on sleeping pills, older people should reduce coffee and tea consumption, increase daily exercise, and eliminate daytime naps if they have trouble sleeping at night. More important, they need to be willing to accommodate to a new sleeping pattern and realize that as people age they often require fewer hours of sleep and not as deep a sleep as in their younger years. The next largest group of drugs,

Darvon and Darvocet, were prescribed for 1.3 million elderly patients. The study characterized these medications as "addictive narcotics" that are no more effective than aspirin for pain but can cause respiratory failure at low doses when combined with alcohol and also can cause seizures and heart problems. In addition, according to the study, antidepressants such as Elavil, Limbitrol, Triavil, Etrafon, and Endep can cause difficulty in urinating, dizziness, and drowsiness that may cause falls and worsen glaucoma. Diabinese, a pill to lower blood sugar in diabetics, can cause dangerous fluid retention. Indocin, a pain reliever and anti-inflammatory drug, can cause confusion, headaches, and leave the patient with a high risk of bleeding from the stomach, according to the study. Persantine, a blood thinner that is useless except for patients with artificial heart valves, according to the Harvard study, and dispensed to about eighteen million seniors, was another commonly prescribed drug on the inappropriate list. It's not just doctors who can sometimes overlook potential problems from combining medications. Many patients demand medications to treat symptoms when a nondrug therapy might work better. So anytime a medicine is prescribed, ask if it is necessary, safe, and has side effects.[27]

In a 1988 study of the elderly population, 40 to 45 percent of older patients did not take their prescribed medication properly. In addition, studies have found that problems caused by noncompliance may result in costs of up to $20 billion per year. The most prevalent chronic conditions in Americans aged sixty-five and over include arthritis, hypertension, heart disease, hearing loss, influenza, orthopedic impairment, cataracts, chronic sinusitis, depression, cancer, diabetes, visual impairment, and urinary incontinence.[28]

At the present time, sixty-four million people over fifty years of age use one-half of all the medical care administered annually. As patients pass the age of fifty, the prescription drugs they have routinely taken can result in adverse reactions. The fact that the ability to metabolize some drugs decreases with age is well documented. Decreasing organ function, muscle mass, renal function, and even cardiac output all impact upon the elderly's ability to metabolize these agents. The increased number of medications used by the elderly, as well as the fact that they are more sensitive to certain drug classes than younger patients (i.e., anticoagulants and psychoactive drugs), makes prescribing for the elderly a wholly different scenario. The *following prescribing principles have been suggested by Partners for Health Aging, a program developed by a division of Merck & Co., Inc., to increase health providers' and pharmacists' understanding of the effects of prescription drugs in elderly patients.*

- Prescribe only when a symptom or disease is serious enough to warrant treatment.
- Prescribe only when therapy is likely to be effective.
- Have a set goal for each drug. If it is not effective in reaching that goal, adjust dosage, stop, or change therapy.
- Avoid medications that pose especially high risk to older persons. These include anticholinergics, long-acting benzodiazepines, and narcotics.

- Chart medication use and active diagnoses and screen for both drug-drug and drug-disease interactions.
- When necessary, simplify a medication schedule to improve compliance.
- Consider the preventive health aspects of medications.
- Be suspicious that a change in function or cognition, or new symptom may be caused by a medication.
- Adjust doses and frequencies of administration for age-related changes in distribution, and diminished hepatic and renal clearance.[29]

One of the problems physicians encounter in prescribing drugs is patient addiction to the medication. Physicians who prescribe potentially addicting drugs in any patient population should be aware that problems can and do develop and that the elderly are the most sensitive to medication effects. Reevaluation of pharmacologic agents for effectiveness and potential problems should be done at regular intervals. Open-ended prescriptions should not be provided for potentially addictive drugs. The following have been suggested as some considerations in the rational use of potentially addictive prescription drugs in the elderly population:

- Does the diagnosis, distress, and disability warrant the drug use?
- Have appropriate nonpharmacologic therapies been used when indicated?
- Have pharmacologic agents with less potential for long-term problems and dependence been used if appropriate (for example, buspirone hydrochloride for anxiety or nonopioid analgesics for pain)?
- Is the drug yielding an acceptable therapeutic response with the use of appropriate doses (often lower in elderly than in younger patients), and if not, have the diagnosis and treatment been reconsidered?
- Has the patient had other drug or alcohol dependence or abuse problems in the past (a major relative contraindication to use of addictive drugs)?
- Do any findings suggest addiction to the prescribed drug (for example, hoarding of drugs, uncontrolled dose escalation, or obtaining drugs from multiple physicians)?
- Are other drug impairments (such as memory or psychomotor difficulties) apparent?
- Can a family member or significant other confirm the effectiveness of the drug as well as the absence of impairment or addiction?
- Would tapering the dose of the drug (after an appropriate trial) help determine whether problems are related to the drug or whether further treatment is needed?

In a poorly functioning elderly patient who is taking potentially addicting medication, the managing physician may need to taper the dose and then discontinue the therapy to clarify the role of the medication in the problem. The withdrawal may be difficult; after discontinuation, several weeks may be needed to assess whether the drug was causing all or part of the difficulty, because of prolonged symptoms related to the withdrawal. Patients with potential addiction to prescription drugs should be referred early to appropriate psychiatric, addiction, and pain management services as needed. The many-sided nature of prescription drug dependence in the elderly often necessitates a team approach or referral to a center that can coordinate the various aspects of evaluation and treatment. The potential for prescription drug dependence among the elderly requires the physician to monitor the use of such agents in this population.[30]

GETTING THE BEST RESULTS FROM YOUR PRESCRIPTION

In addition to heeding warnings about adverse drug and food interactions and using the knowledge gleaned from your pharmacist and your physician in regard to drug quality, there are other ways in which you as a consumer can get the most effective use from your medication. The Food and Drug Administration has the following suggestions, some of which require repetition:

- Make sure you understand all the directions printed on the drug container. If vision is a problem, ask the pharmacist to use large type.
- Keep a daily or weekly record of all medications you are taking. The chart should show the name of the drug, the time it should be taken, and the number of pills to take. Or you can begin each day by placing your daily dosage of medicine in a small cup. Thus, if you forget whether you've taken some medication that day, you can refer back to the chart or the cup and avoid a possibly dangerous overdose. *Before using any container system,* check with your pharmacist or your doctor about whether your medicines will deteriorate if left out in the open for a few hours. Some drugs like nitroglycerine lose their strength if exposed to the open air; others must be kept refrigerated. If you have children in your home, you should be wary of using any container system since it requires leaving medicines out in the open.
- If you become sick and your symptoms appear to be the same as in a previous illness, consult your physician before taking any medication. Although you might think you have the same illness as before, you could be in trouble if you guess wrong and take leftover medication prescribed for that earlier treatment.
- Always keep medicines in locked cabinets or out of reach of children. Many drugs come in safety packaging that is hard for children to open: if you have children in the home, be sure you ask for it. If you have trouble opening the container, ask your pharmacist to show you how. If it is too difficult to open the "childproof" closures and there are no children at home, ask if he can provide a conventional cap. Make sure you reseal your medicine bottles tightly after each opening to cut down on the leakage of air into the bottle. Air interacts with medications and can change them chemically, reducing their effectiveness. In addition, screw-on caps are better than snap-on lids or plastic

blister packs for reducing the leakage of air into medicine bottles. Also, when you give your children medicine, never refer to it as "candy" or something else they like. Similarly, never take medicine in front of your child. They may try to get more of it when they are alone. It only takes a moment for a child to swallow an overdose.

Never give your child adult doses of medication. In view of your child's age and weight, ask your doctor about the correct doses for your child, because while pediatric doses are almost always lower than adult medication, they are not necessarily lower by half.

When giving a child medication by mouth, use an oral syringe, not a hypodermic one. Hypodermic syringes have small, clear caps that, if not removed, can cause a child to choke. Oral syringes have colored caps for easier viewing.

Monitor the amount of medicine older children are taking to get rid of headaches. Excessive use of some over-the-counter pain relievers can result in gastrointestinal bleeding, while others can cause organ failure. If not sure, read the medication label or consult with your pharmacist on the proper use of the medication.

If a child has flu symptoms, avoid substituting aspirin for acetaminophen because it could result in Reye's syndrome, a serious but rare illness.

Never give concentrated infants' drops to children who are older than three years of age. Use children's liquids or chewable tablets.

- Don't assume that your bathroom medicine chest is the right place to keep your drugs. The moisture from the bathtub and shower may cause them to deteriorate. Also, avoid storing drugs in a kitchen closet or drawer, since the kitchen is too warm. Ask your pharmacist how specific medicines should be stored. Don't keep old or expired medicines in your medicine chest.
- Take your medicine according to the schedule printed on its label. If you miss a dose, don't catch up by doubling the next one without consulting your doctor or pharmacist. The timing of your doses can have an important effect on the success of the treatment. Ask your doctor what you should do if you forget to take a dose.
- Don't stop taking your medication just because you're feeling better. You may prevent the drug from doing its work completely, which may lead to a flare-up of the original problem.
- Don't take more—or less—than the prescribed amount of any drug.
- Never take medicine without checking the label to make sure you are taking the correct one. Also, check drug labels for specific instructions or warnings, such as "do not take on an empty stomach" or "do not take with milk." Do not take "look-alikes" and do not take medicine at night without turning on the light.
- If you have trouble swallowing a drug in tablet form and it doesn't come as a liquid, don't automatically crush it and take it with water. While this may be all right sometimes (ask your pharmacist), often tablets are in a wax bonding

agent that allows the active ingredients to leach out slowly. Other tablets have a special coating so they won't dissolve until they reach the intestine.

- Drink a full glass of water when swallowing medication. It helps dissolve the drug and send it into your bloodstream. There can be danger in taking medication without water. Also, ideally some drugs should be taken on an empty stomach to speed absorption, while others are better absorbed with a meal. Check with a doctor if you are not sure how your drug should be taken.

- Don't expect a medicine to make you feel better instantly. If a drug is not doing what it is supposed to do for you, check with your doctor. You may need a different dosage or a different drug.

- If you have an unexpected symptom—rash, nausea, dizziness, headache, drowsiness or more symptoms such as prolonged vomiting, bleeding, marked weakness, or impaired vision or hearing—these are warning signals that the drug is causing problems. When a reaction is unexpected or severe, a doctor should be consulted.

- If you are taking several different drugs and have difficulty remembering when and how to take them, your pharmacist may be able to provide you with a handy checklist.

- A prescription medicine is prescribed for you only. Never let anyone else take it, even if their symptoms seem to be the same as yours. The other person may be suffering from an entirely different problem—and certainly has a different medical history—and taking your medicine could be very dangerous.

- Do not transfer medicines from the containers in which they were dispensed. These containers are designed to keep the drug properly protected. Multipurpose pillboxes or other containers may not be suitable. Also, keep medicine away from household products. Many of the containers look alike.

- Do not keep prescription drugs you no longer need. If you have medicines left over, destroy them, especially after their expiration date—after which the medication is no longer sure to be fully effective, or may be harmful. When purchasing an over-the-counter drug, always select the package with the most distant expiration date.

- When physicians write the names of drugs on prescription slips, a misreading by the pharmacist or a slight misspelling by the physician can be dangerous. To avoid these possible mistakes and to receive the right drug from the pharmacist, tell the pharmacist the disease for which the drug is being prescribed.

- Do not use a medicine that seems off-color or stale after you purchase it. Return it to the pharmacy. If you believe a medicine has gone bad or is otherwise harmful before its expiration date, do not just throw it out—report it to either the headquarters of the Food and Drug Administration, 5600 Fischers Lane, Rockville, MD 20857, or its office in your area, which can be found by looking in telephone book under US Government, Department of Health and Human Services, Food and Drug Administration. Promptly report the problem, giving your name, address, and telephone number; state clearly what appears to be wrong; list any code numbers that appear on the container; give the name and address of the store where the article was bought and the date of purchase; save whatever remains of the product for possible examination by the Food and Drug Administration; and hold any unopened container of the product bought at the same time. This advice also applies to nonprescription over-the-counter drugs as well. Finally, if you are in possession of contaminated, mislabeled, or suspect products made and/or sold exclusively within a state, you should also contact the local or state health department or similar law enforcement agency listed in the telephone book.

- Unlike over-the-counter medicine, prescription drugs generally are not required to include printed information directed to the patient. But for some prescription drugs such as oral contraceptives and estrogens, the Food and Drug Administration requires that information on the use of the product be given to the consumer in the form of a leaflet or brochure that must accompany the product when the prescription is filled. Such "patient package inserts" are provided so the consumer can be fully informed about the benefits and possible hazards involved in the use of the drug and can make an informed decision about whether to use it and what to watch out for while taking it. If there is a patient package insert with a drug that has been prescribed for you, be sure to read it carefully. If after reading the patient package insert you have additional questions, consult your physician or your pharmacist.[31]

- Try to fill all your prescriptions at the same pharmacy. Many pharmacies now keep computerized records of what drugs their customers are taking. They are the first line of defense against dangerous interaction.

- Be sure that someone close to you knows exactly what medications you are taking. Your family or friends should have the name of someone to call if your behavior or condition changes. Toxic reactions can be halted, even reversed, if recognized in time.

- Take the medicine exactly the way the physician instructs. If you do not understand, ask your pharmacist to go over it with you. If this interferes with your lifestyle or the medicine makes you feel sick, or if you don't think it is helping or think you are taking too many drugs already and don't want to take this one, tell your doctor at once.[32]

- Always look at your prescription before you leave your doctor's office. If you cannot read it, ask your doctor to print the information above the writing.

  ▼ The *first word* is always the name of the drug.

  ▼ *Next is the dosage form* (pills, capsules, or other kind of formulation) and the strength of the drug, such as 250 mg (milligrams).

  ▼ *Next is the quantity* the pharmacist will dispense (such as 15 capsules or 50 pills) followed by the directions for their use.

  ▼ *In writing out the name of the prescribed drug* your physician will use either the manufacturer's trade name or the generic (common name). He may also use a lot of *abbreviations on the prescription*. For example, in regard to dosage forms, he may write "cap" for capsules and "tab" for tablets while liquids are denoted as "el" for elixir, "sy" for syrup, or "sol" for solution.

▼ *In terms of directions*, if the drug is to be taken three times a day for seven days, the physician may write "#21" or "21." Refill information may also be indicated in an abbreviated form as "Refill 2x," meaning the patient can obtain the same amount of the drug two more times without obtaining a new prescription. Or you may observe on the prescription blank printed letters, followed by numbers, followed by printed letters such as REP 0-1-2-3 PRN. These also indicate the number of times your prescription can be refilled. Thus, if the number "zero" is circled, it means your prescription cannot be refilled; but if the numbers 1, 2, or 3 are circled, it means that your prescription can be refilled that many times before you must obtain a new prescription from your physician.

▼ Finally, *the abbreviation "Sig"* on the prescription blank is followed by the instructions the physician is telling the pharmacist to put on the medication label so that the patient will know how to use the medication.[33]

Also, the guidelines listed herein are relevant whether you are taking the medications either at home or abroad. But if you are traveling abroad, there are just a few more guidelines of which you should be aware. Don't place your medications in checked luggage—keep them with you. Bring along more than enough for your trip as a backup to your original supply. Before you leave, review your dosage schedule with your doctor or your pharmacist and ask about any other relevant health matters in regard to the areas to which you are traveling, such as how the change in time zones may affect your taking the medication. Keep a list of all the medications and dietary supplements that you are taking with you in the event that something is misplaced or lost and must be replaced abroad.

Remember, the medicine with which your physician is treating your illness can produce the most beneficial results or the most adverse reactions, depending upon how you use rather than abuse the drug. Do not take more medication than your physician prescribes. Should you forget to take medication, do not take twice the dosage the next day in an attempt to catch up. Any medication, whether prescribed or purchased over-the-counter, can either help you or harm you. That decision is yours. But your pharmacist and your physician can provide you with all the necessary information that will allow you to make the most effective use of the drug. Seek and use their advice—and benefit from their skills and knowledge.

NOTES

1. "FDA Chief Says Generic, Brand Rx's Nearly Equal," *AMA News*, November 21, 1977, p. 3.

2. Kathleen Day, 'Maryland Terminates Contract with Drug Prescription Firm: Medco Lacks Pharmacy Network to Fulfill Terms of Deal, State Says," *Washington Post*, December 28, 1995, p. D9.

3. Annabel Hecht, "Generic Drugs: How Good Are They," *FDA Consumer* 12, no. 1 (February 1978).

4. US Department of Health, Education, and Welfare, *We Want You to Know about Prescription Drugs* (Washington, DC: Food and Drug Administration, 1978).

5. *Inside Health* (Washington, DC: Washington Internal Medicine Group, Fall 1986), p. 2; Lauren Neergaard, "New Advice on How to Dump Old Medicines," *Washington Senior Beacon*, November 2003, p. 4.

6. Raymond Schuessler, "Is There More to Taking Medicine Than You Realize?" *Your Life and Health*, March 1983, p. 19; Peggy Eastman, "Rx: Misuses a New Peril," *AARP Bulletin* 43, no. 7 (July–August 2002): 12–13.

7. "ASHP Guidelines on the Pharmacist-Conducted Patient Counseling," *American Journal of Hospital Pharmacology* 50, no. 3 (March 1993): 505–506.

8. Florence and Gerald Schumacher, "Rx for Choosing a Pharmacist," *Family Health/Today's Health* 9, no. 6 (June 1977): 48–49.

9. "ASHP Guidelines on Preventing Medication Errors in Hospitals," *American Journal of Hospital Pharmacology* 50, no. 2 (February 1993): 305–307.

10. Ibid., pp. 309–10; Steven Slon, "How to Be Drug Smart," *AARP Consumer Guide*, p. 8 (undated); and "Communication Breakdowns and Improperly Programmed IV Pumps Cause Harmful Medication Errors in Hospital Intensive Care Units," Pharmacopeia news release, February 15, 2006, p. 1.

11. "ASHP Guidelines on Preventing Medication Errors in Hospitals," pp. 311–12.

12. Timothy J. Larkin, "Mixing Medicines? Have a Care!" *FDA Consumer* 10, no. 2 (March 1976).

13. Ibid.

14. Dan Sperling, "Prescriptions Go Over-the-Counter," *USA Today*, May 22, 1984, p. 5D.

15. "Over-the-Counter Drugs," *Washington Post/Health*, October 15, 1991, p. 5.

16. Carol Krucoff, "Exercise Caution: Over-the-Counter Drugs Can Affect the Body's Response to Activity," *Washington Post/Health*, June 16, 1992, p. 20.

17. Larkin, "Mixing Medicines? Have a Care!"

18. Phyllis Lehmann, "Food and Drug Interactions," *FDA Consumer* 12, no. 2 (March 1978).

19. *Food and Drug Interactions* (Washington, DC: Food and Drug Interactions, American Pharmaceutical Association, Food and Drug Administration, Food Marketing Institute and National Consumer League, undated).

20. Sandy Rovner, "Drugs and Nutrition," *Washington Post/Health*, January 29, 1986, p. 9.

21. Lehmann, "Food and Drug Interactions."

22. Ibid.

23. Annabel Hecht, "Antibiotics—Oft Gone Astray," *FDA Consumer* 14, no. 6 (July–August 1980): 24.

24. Ibid., p. 25.

25. Ibid., pp. 25–26.

26. Mary Beth Franklin, "Mixing Medicines: Drug Interactions Can Cause Confusion, Drowsiness, Falls," *Washington Post/Health*, October 25, 1994, p. 12.

27. Ibid., pp. 12–13.

28. Elizabeth C. Meszaros, "The Onslaught of the Elderly: MCOs Prepare for America's Fastest Growing Demographic with Special Drug Programs," *Managed Care* (July 1995): S13, S14, S16.

29. Ibid., p. 15.

30. Stephen M. Juergens, "Prescription Drug Dependence among Elderly Persons," *Mayo Clinic Proceedings* 69, no. 12 (1994): 1216–18.

31. US Department of Health, Education, and Welfare, *We Want You to Know about Prescription Drugs*; Dianne Hales, "Take Your Meds—the Right Way," *Parade*, February 13, 2005, p. 15.

32. Sandy Rovner, "Healthtalk: Drugs and the Elderly," *Washington Post*, January 22, 1982, p. C5.

33. Annabel Hecht, "On Reading Prescriptions," *FDA Consumer* 10 no. 10 (December 1976–January 1977): 17–18.

DIRECTORY OF INFORMATIONAL WEB SITES BY CHAPTER

TOPIC/AGENCY	WEB SITE

Chapter One: Physician Care

American Academy of Family Physicians	http://www.familydoctor.com
American Academy of Home Care Physician	http://www.aahcp.org
American Academy of Pediatrics	http://www.aap.org
American Association of Geriatric Psychiatrists	http://www.aagponline.org
American Geriatrics Society	http://www.americangeriatrics.org
American Self-Help Clearinghouse (offers referrals to self-help clearinghouses nationally, maintains database of national and international self-help headquarters, offers assistance to persons interested in starting new groups, and publishes directory of national support groups)	http://www.mentalhelp.net/selfhelp and http://selfhelpgroups.org
Board certification in various medical specialties American Medical Association American Board of Medical Specialties	http://www.ama-assn.org http://www.abms.org
College of American Pathologists (accredited medical testing laboratories)	http://www.cap.org

Complaints or disciplinary actions taken against physicians	http://www.docboard.org and http://www.healthcarechoices.org http://www.massmedboard.org (state of Massachusetts),
Pay-for-use sites with similar information	http://www.checkbook.org, and http://www.Docinfo.org
Directory of Medicare Participating Physicians	http://www.medicare.gov
Federal government gateways to information on health issues, health care programs, and organizations	http://www.HealthierUS.gov
Federation of State Medical Boards (physician licensure)	http://www.fsmb.org
Greater Midwest Region of the National Network Libraries of Medicine (supported links to health Web sites by medical topics, professions, and scientific fields)	http://www.healthweb.org
Harvard Medical School (information and practical advice on staying healthy)	http://www.intelihealth.com
Health resources for consumers, physicians, nurses, and educators	http://www.WebMD.com
History and Training of a Physician	http://www.healthgrades.com
Information about men's health, women's health, and treatments for different medical conditions	http://www.thehealthpages.com http://www.medicinenet.com
Information for senior citizens' medical conditions	http://www.nihseniorhealth.gov
Joint Commission on Accreditation of Healthcare Organizations (accredited medical testing laboratories)	http://www.jcaho.org
Mayo Clinic (family medical history)	http://www.mayoclinic.com
Medical Library Associations (Web sites suggested by librarians)	http://www.mlanet.org

MedlinePlus (information about medical illness operated by the US National Library of Medicine and the National Institutes of Health) http://www.medlineplus.gov

Mental Health Directory (links to mental health professionals in community) http://www.mentalhealth.net

National Association of Home Care & Hospice (homecare physicians and other homecare information) http://www.nahc.org

National Breast Cancer Foundation (free or low-cost mammograms for low-income women in inner cities) http://www.nationalbreastcancer.org

National Cancer Institute http://www.cancer.gov
and http://www.cancer.gov/cancertopics/screening

National Center for Complementary and Alternative Medicine (herbs, acupuncture, and other treatments) http://www.nccam.nih.gov

National Guideline Clearinghouse (medical treatment guidelines) http://www.guideline.gov

National Health Service Information Center (links to more than 1,500 health-related organizations on illness, treatment, and other information) http://www.healthfinder.gov

National Institutes of Health (links to all major NIH Institutes) http://www.nih.gov

National Institutes of Health (health information) http://www.health.nih.gov

National Institutes of Mental Health (broad range of mental health topics) http://www.mentalhealth.gov

National Library of Medicine (clinical trials) http://www.clinicaltrials.gov

National Self-Help Clearinghouse http://www.selfhelpweb.org

New York Online Access to Health (medical conditions and health issues listed alphabetically) http://www.noah.health.org

Physician-Patients Communications Network	http://www.medem.com
Prevent Blindness America	http://www.preventblindness.org
Stanford University's Medical Center's Health Library (information on illness or treatment)	http://healthlibrary.stanford.edu
US Administration on Aging (Eldercare Locator)	http://www.eldercare.gov
US Agency for Healthcare Research and Quality (click on "Interactive Preventive Services Selector" for federal guidelines on illness)	http://www.ahrq.gov/clinic
US Centers for Disease Control & Prevention (CDC)	http://www.cdc.gov
Violation of Medical Privacy Records (filing complaint to the Office of Civil Rights, US Department of Health and Human Services)	http://www.hhs.gov/ocr/hipaa
Violation of Medical Privacy Records (obtaining a model complaint from Georgetown University's Health Privacy Project, Washington, DC)	http://www.healthprivacy.org

Chapter Two: Dental Care

American Academy of Pediatric Dentistry	http://www.aapd.org
American Dental Association	http://www.ada.org
Dental care and dental health insurance	http://www.medlineplus.gov

Chapter Three: Traditional Private Health Insurance

America's Health Insurance Plans (Guide to Health Insurance)	http://www.ahip.org
Coalition against Insurance Fraud	http://www.insurancefraud.org
Community health centers (primary care)	http://www.bphc.hrsa.gov

Free community clinics and healthcare
coverage for medically underserved and
uninsured in the United States

http://www.uniteforsight.org/
freeclinics.php
http://www.nlm.nih.gov/MedlinePlus

in foreign countries

http://dir.yahoo.com/Health/Medicine/
(a directory of international medical
care organizations)
Organizations/International_Relief_and_
Development
(International Red Cross and
Red Crescent)
http://www.ifrc.org/address/directory.asp

Georgetown University Health Policy Institute
(consumer guides by state for buying and
keeping health insurance)

http://www.healthinsuranceinfo.net

Guide for handling and disputing a rejected
medical claim with a health insurance provider

http://www.medicarerights.org
and http://kff.org/consumerguide

Health insurance coverage information
for uninsured Americans

http://www.healthinsurance.org
http://www.covertheuninsured.org

Health insurance price quotes and
other information

http://www.insure.com
http://www.medhealthinsurance.com

Health Savings Accounts

http://www.Treas.gov

National Association of Insurance Commissioners http://www.naic.org

Public and private benefit programs,
including health insurance, by state
for older adults (55 years and older)

http://www.BenefitsCheckUp.org

State children's health insurance programs

http://www.insurekidsnow.gov/states.htm

US Agency for Healthcare Research and Quality
(basic health insurance information as well as
other consumer health, clinical, specific
populations, quality, and patient safety information)

http://www.ahcpr.gov

Chapter Four: Managed Care

America's Health Insurance Plans (managed care) http://www.ahip.org

Health Administrative Responsibility Project   http://www.harp.org

Health Maintenance Organization (handling
disputes with employer and private health plans
—Consumers Union)
http://www.consumersunion.org/
health/hmo-review

Health Maintenance Organization—handling
disputes with employer and private health
plans (Kaiser Family Foundation)
http://www.kff.org/consumerguide

Medicare's Health Maintenance Organizations
http://www.Medicare.gov

National Business Group on Health
http://www.wbgh.org

National Committee for Quality Assurance
http://www.ncqa.org

Service and quality of health maintenance
organizations and point-of-service plans
http://www.usnews.com

Chapter Five: Medicaid and Medicare

Center for Medicare Advocacy
(Medicare prescription drug benefit)
http://www.medicareadvocacy.org

Centers for Medicare and Medicaid Services
(Medicare prescription drug benefit)
http://www.Medicare.gov

Medicaid program information
http://www.cms.hhs.gov/Medicaid

Medicare program information
http://www.Medicare.gov

Medicare Prescription Drug Benefit and
Outreach Education Project
http://www.medicarerxoutreach.org

Medicare Prescription Drug Benefit Program
(ratings, forum questions, reviews, and
information by state)
http://www.MedicareDrugPlans.com

Medicare Prescription Drug Benefit Program
Assistance for Low-Income Recipients
http://www.BenefitsCheckUp.org/rx

Medicare Rights Center (Medicare prescription
drug and other benefit information)
http://www.medicarerights.org

Medicare Rx Education Network (Medicare
prescription drug benefit)
http://www.medicarerxeducation.org

Medicare Today (Medicare prescription drug benefit program and other information)   http://www.medicaretoday.org

National Academy of Elder Law Attorneys (care of the elderly)   http://www.naela.org

Prescription drug discount cards   http://www.medicare.gov

Prescription drug discount cards, mail-order discount pharmacies in the United States and Canada, prescription drug price comparison Web sites, national and state prescription drug assistance programs   http://www.medicarerights.org/rxframeset.html

Quality and effectiveness of prescription drugs (useful for Medicare Part D drug plan and other drug information)   http://www.crbestbuydrugs.org

Rating pharmacies and drug prices   http://www.pharmacychecker.com

State health insurance assistance program (counseling assistance on Medicare Part D drug plan and assistance to persons with Medicare and their families)   http://www.shiptalk.org

Social Security (Medicare prescription drug benefit)   http://www.socialsecurity.gov/organizations/medicareoutreach2

State Quality Improvement Organizations (formerly named Peer Review Organizations)   http://www.cms.hhs.gov/qio

US Administration on Aging Eldercare Locator (information on Medicare prescription drug program and assistance in your community)   http://www.eldercare.gov

Chapter Six: Surgery and Second Opinion Surgical Programs

Accreditation Association for Ambulatory Health Care   http://www.aaahc.org

American Association for Accreditation of Ambulatory Surgical Facilities, Inc.   http://www.aaaasf.org

American College of Surgeons   http://www.facs.org

Best Treatment Guide British Medical Journal/   http://www.besttreatments.co.uk
British National Health Service
in the United States   http://www.MyUHC.com
                                                (member United Health Group)
                                                or http://www.ConsumerReportsHealth
                                                .org (subscription)

Federated Ambulatory Surgical Association   http://www.fasa.org

Joint Commission on Accreditation of   http://www.jcaho.org
Healthcare Organizations

National Guideline Clearinghouse   http://www.guideline.gov

Physicians profiles, New York State   http://www.nydoctorprofile.com

Chapter Seven: Hospital Care

America's Best Hospitals ranking   http://www.usnews.com
(*U.S. News & World Report*)

Billing procedure codes   http://www.cdc.gov/nchs/icd9.htm

Equifax (credit rating)   http://www.equifax.com

Experian (credit rating)   http://www.experian.com

Guide to Hospitals (*Consumer's Checkbook*)   http://www.checkbook.org

Health Care Choices (report card)   http://www.healthcarechoices.org

Hospital Compare (Medicare)   http://www.hospitalcompare.hhs.gov

Hospital Profile Consumer Guide   http://www.hospitalprofiles.org

Hospital report cards   http://www.healthgrades.com

Hospitals with computerized drug ordering   http://www.leapfroggroup.org
systems, hospital quality ratings, and safety,
quality, and affordability in healthcare

Medicare benefits   http://www.Medicare.gov

National Association of Attorneys General   http://www.naag.org

Quality Check (Joint Commission on Accreditation of Healthcare Organizations)	http://www.jcaho.com

State Hospital Information

California	http://www.oshpd.state.ca.us
Maryland	http://hospitalguide.mhcc.state.md.us
New Jersey	http://www.state.nj.us/health
New York	http://hospitals.nyhealth.gov http://www.health.state.ny.us/nysdoh/healthinfo/index.htm
Pennsylvania	http://www.phc4.org
Texas	http://www.dshs.state.tx.us
Virginia	http://www.vhi.org
Wisconsin (southcentral)	http://www.qualitycounts.org
TransUnion (credit rating)	http://www.transunion.com

Chapter Eight: Nursing Home Care

AARP (Legal Services Network)	http://www.aarp.org/lsn
A.M. Best (insurance companies)	http://www.AMBest.com
American Association of Homes and Services for the Aging	http://www.aahsa.org
American College of Health Care Administrators	http://www.achca.org
American Health Care Association	http://www.ahca.org
Fitch Ratings (insurance companies)	http://www.fitchratings.com
Long-term care insurance (federal government employees and retirees)	http://www.ltcfeds.com
Long-term care ombudsman program (state or local government) and other aging issues	http://www.aoa.dhhs.gov
Medicare's Nursing Home Compare	http://www.medicare.gov/nhcompare/home.asp
Moody's Investor Services (insurance companies)	http://www.moodys.com
National Academy of Elder Law Attorneys	http://www.naela.org

National Citizens' Coalition for Nursing Home Reform — http://www.nursinghomeaction.com

Nursing Home Patient Advocacy Organizations by State (citizen groups not affiliated with nursing home industry or federal and state governments) — http://www.nhadvocates.org

SafetyForum (click on "Nursing Home Abuse Action Group") — http://www.safetyforum.com

Standard & Poor's Insurance Rating Services (insurance companies) — http://www.standardandpoors.com

Weiss Ratings (insurance companies) — http://www.weissratings.com

Chapter Nine: Homecare and Hospice Care

American Association of Daily Money Managers — http://www.aadmm.com

American Association of Homes and Services for the Aging (assisted living information) — http://www.aahsa.org

American Association of Retired Persons (AARP) — http://www.aarp.org

Assisted Living Federation of America — http://www.alfa.org

Consumer Consortium on Assisted Living — http://www.ccal.org

Eldercare Locator (US Administration on Aging) — http://www.eldercare.gov

Home Health Compare (Medicare) — http://www.Medicare.gov

Long Term Care Community Coalition (former Nursing Home Community Coalition) — http://www.ltccc.org and http://www.nursinghome411.org

National Adult Day Services Association, Inc. — http://www.nadsa.org.

National Association of Professional Geriatric Care Manager — http://www.caremanager.org

National Center for Assisted Living — http://www.ncal.org

National Hospice and Palliative Care Organization — http://www.nhpco.org

Program of All-Inclusive Care for the Elderly (PACE)

http://www.cms.hhs.gov/pace

Social Health Maintenance Organizations (SHMO)

http://www.Medicare.gov/nursing/alternatives/shmo.asp

US Administration on Aging

http://www.aoa.dhhs.gov

Chapter Ten: Prescription Drugs

AARP (information on drug safety, effectiveness, and cost)

http://www.aarp.org/Researchrx and http://www.aarp.org/health/comparedrugs

Canadian Mail-Order and Other Countries
Minnesota Senior Federation
United Health Alliance

http://www.mnseniors.org
http://www.medicineassist.org

Comparison of prescription drug prices at pharmacies in New York State (Office of NY State Attorney General)

http://www.nyagrx.org

Consumer's Union (Best Buy Drugs)

http://www.crbestbuydrugs.org

Counterfeit Medicines National Consumers League

http://www.nclnet.org

Discount Mail Order Programs
AARP
Comparison of several plans
Medco Health

http://www.aarppharmacy.com
http://www.destinationrx.com
http://www.yourxplan.com

Drug Safety and Effective Reviews–Center for Evidence Based Policy-Oregon Health and Science University

http://www.ohsu.edu

Federal Trade Commission (false free medicine claims)

http://www.ftc.gov

Food and Drug Administration

http://www.fda.gov

Internet Pharmacies
CVS Pharmacy
Eckerd Pharmacy
Walgreen Pharmacy

http://www.cvs.com
http://www.eckerd.com
http://www.walgreen.com

National Association of Boards of Pharmacies (list of Web sites)

http://www.nabp.net/vipps

Quality pharmacies

http://www.drugstore.com
http://www.familymeds.com

Medicare drug coverage

http://www.Medicare.gov

Medication information for senior citizens

http://www.nihseniorhealth.gov

National Council on Patient Information
and Education (safe and appropriate
use of medicines)

http://www.talkaboutrx.org

Nonprescription medications and other drugs

http://www.bemedwise.org

Oregon's Drug Effectiveness Review Project

http://www.oregonrx.org

Online and mail-order pharmacies
(ratings, profiles and prescription drug price
comparisons in the United States, Canada,
and other foreign countries)

http://www.pharmacychecker.com

Partnership for Prescription Assistance
Programs (links to public and private programs
for low-cost or free prescriptions for those
without any prescription drug coverage)

http://www.pparx.org

Senior Citizen Prescription Drug Assistance Programs
Discount cards for low-income seniors
http://www.rxassist.org
Free and discounted drugs from drug companies
http://www.needymeds.com
Free and discounted drugs from drug companies
http://www.themedicineprogram.com
Free medicine from drug companies
http://www.freemedicineprogram.com
Percentage discounts on prescription drugs
http://www.Together-Rx.com
Pharmaceutical assistance program eligibility
http://www.helpingpatients.org
Pharmaceutical Research and Manufacturers
of America—drug assistance programs

http://www.phrma.org

Prescription discount card pricing (Medicare)

http://www.Medicare.gov

State Prescription Drug Assistance Programs
Finding state programs
http://www.BenefitsCheckUp.org
National Conference of State Legislatures
http://www.ncsl.org
Safe Use of Medicine
http://www.aarp.org/wiseuse

Reducing Prescription Drug Costs

http://www.rxaminer.com

Volunteers in Health Care (directory of patient assistance programs and free and low-cost medicines)

http://www.rxassist.org

WellRx (US and Canadian mail order prescription drug services)

http://www.wellrxcard.com and http://www.prescriptionpoint.com

Veteran and Military Benefits
TRICARE Senior Pharmacy Program
US Department of Defense Eligibility Enrollment System (DEERS)

http://www.tricare.osd.mil
http://www.tricare.osd.mil/ DEERS/default.cfm

US Department of Veterans Affairs (Veterans Administration)

http://www.va.gov

DIRECTORY OF HEALTH-RELATED ORGANIZATIONS

In order to find out more about the various groups that constitute our healthcare system, you should visit their Web sites, telephone, or write to their executive directors or the public affairs offices. They can inform you about the group as a whole and supply the names and addresses of their affiliated state associations, where appropriate, whom you also may wish to contact.

CONSUMER GROUPS

Consumer Federation of America
1620 I St. NW
Suite 200
Washington, DC 20036
http://www.consumerfed.org
Tel: 1-(202)-387-6121

FamiliesUSA
1201 New York Ave. NW
Suite 1100
Washington, DC 20005
http://www.familiesusa.org
Tel: 1-(202)-628-3030

National Consumers League
1701 K St. NW
Suite 1200
Washington, DC 20006

http://www.nclnet.org
Tel: 1-(202)-835-3323

Public Citizen Health Research Group
(A Ralph Nader–affiliated organization)
1600 20th St. NW
Washington, DC 20009
http://www.citizen.org
Tel: 1-(202)-588-1000

DENTISTRY

Academy of General Dentistry
211 East Chicago Ave.
Suite 900
Chicago, IL 60611
http://www.agd.org
Tel: 1-(888)-243-3368

American Academy of Pediatric
  Dentistry
211 East Chicago Ave.
Suite 700
Chicago, IL 60611
http://www.aapd.org
Tel: 1-(312)-337-2169

American Dental Association
211 East Chicago Ave.
Chicago, IL 60611
http://www.ada.org
Tel: 1-(312)-440-2500

THE ELDERLY

Alliance for Retired Americans
815 16th St. NW
Fourth Floor
Washington, DC 20006
http://www.retiredAmericans.org
Tel: 1-(202)-637-5399

American Association of Retired Persons
601 E St. NW
Washington, DC 20049
http://www.aarp.org
Tel: 1-(888)-687-2277

American Geriatrics Society
Empire State Building
350 Fifth Ave.
Suite 801
New York, NY 10018
http://www.americangeriatrics.org
Tel: 1-(212)-308-1414

American Society on Aging
833 Market St.
Suite 511
San Francisco, CA 94103

http://www.asaging.org
Tel: 1-(415)-974-9600

Gray Panthers
1612 K St. NW
Suite 300
Washington, DC 20006
http://www.graypanthers.org
Tel: 1-(800)-280-5362
Tel: 1-(202)-737-6637

National Asian Pacific Center on Aging
Melbourne Tower
Suite 914
1511 3rd Ave.
Seattle, WA 98101
http://www.napca.org
Tel: 1-(800)-336-2722
Tel: 1-(206)-624-1221

National Association of Area Agencies
  on Aging
1730 Rhode Island Ave. NW
Suite 1200
Washington, DC 20036
http://www.n4a.org
Tel: 1-(202)-872-0888

National Association of Professional
  Geriatric Care Managers
1604 North Country Club Rd.
Tucson, AZ 85716
http://www.caremanager.org
Tel: 1-(520)-881-8008

National Association of State Units on
  Aging
1201 15th St. NW
Suite 350
Washington, DC 20005
http://www.nasua.org
Tel: 1-(202)-898-2578

National Caucus and Center on Black
  Aged, Inc.
1220 L St. NW
Suite 1200
Washington, DC 20005
http://www.ncba-aged.org
Tel: 1-(202)-637-8400

National Council on the Aging
300 D St. SW
Suite 801
Washington, DC 20024
http://www.ncoa.org
Tel: 1-(202)-479-1200

National Hispanic Council on Aging
1341 Connecticut Ave. NW
Suite 402
Washington, DC 20036
http://www.nhcoa.org
Tel: 1-(202)-429-0787

National Indian Council on Aging
10501 Montgomery Blvd. NE
Suite 210
Albuquerque, NM 87111
http://www.nicoa.org
Tel: 1-(505)-292-2001

National Women's Health Network
514 10th St. NW
Suite 400
Washington, DC 20004
http://www.nwhn.org
Tel: 1-(202)-628-7814

Older Women's League
3300 North Fairfax Dr.
Suite 218
Arlington, VA 22201
http://www.owl-national.org
Tel: 1-(703)-812-7990

United Seniors Health Council Program
National Council on the Aging
300 D St. SW
Suite 801
Washington, DC 20024
http://www.ncoa.org
Tel: 1-(202)-479-1200

HEALTH INSURANCE

America's Health Insurance Plans
601 Pennsylvania Ave. NW
South Building, Suite 500
Washington, DC 20004
http://www.ahip.net
Tel: 1-(202)-778-3200

Blue Cross–Blue Shield Association
225 North Michigan Ave.
Chicago, IL 60601
http://www.bluecross.com
Tel: 1-(312)-540-0460

Delta Dental Plans Association
1515 West 22nd St.
Suite 1200
Oak Brook, IL 60523
http://www.deltadental.com
Tel: 1-(630)-574-6001

National Association of Insurance
  Commissioners
2301 McGee St.
Suite 800
Kansas City, MO 64108
http://www.naic.org
Tel: 1-(816)-842-3600

HEALTH MAINTENANCE ORGANIZATIONS

America's Health Insurance Plans
601 Pennsylvania Ave. NW
South Building, Suite 500
Washington, DC 20004
http://www.ahip.net
Tel: 1-(202)-778-3200

National Committee for Quality Assurance
2000 L St. NW
Washington, DC 20036
http://www.ncqa.org
Tel: 1-(202)-955-3500

HOME HEALTHCARE

Assisted Living Federation of America
1650 King St.
Suite 602
Alexandria, VA 22314
http://www.alfa.org
Tel: 1-(703)-894-1805

Consumer Consortium on Assisted
  Living
2342 Oak St.
Falls Church, VA 22046
http://www.ccal.org
Tel: 1-(703)-533-8121

National Association for Home Care &
  Hospice
228 7th St. SE
Washington, DC 20003
http://www.nahc.org
Tel: 1-(202)-547-7424

HOSPICE CARE

Children's Hospice International
901 North Pitt St.
Suite 230
Alexandria, VA 22314
http://www.chionline.org
Tel: 1-(703)-684-0330

National Hospice and Palliative Care
  Organization
1700 Diagonal St.
Suite 625
Alexandria, VA 22314
http://www.nhpco.org
Tel: 1-(800)-658-8898
Tel: 1-(703)-837-1500

HOSPITALS

American Hospital Association
One North Franklin St.
Chicago, IL 60606
http://www.aha.org
Tel: 1-(312)-422-3000

Catholic Health Association of the
  United States
4455 Woodson Rd.
St. Louis, MO 63134
http://www.chausa.org
Tel: 1-(314)-427-2500

Federation of American Hospitals
  (proprietary hospitals)
801 Pennsylvania Ave. NW
Suite 245
Washington, DC 20004
http://www.americashospitals.com
Tel: 1-(202)-624-1500

Joint Committee on Accreditation of
Healthcare Organizations
One Renaissance Blvd.
Oak Brook Terrace, IL 60181
http://www.jcaho.org
Tel: 1-(630)-792-5000

National Association of Children's Hospitals and Related Institutions, Inc.
401 Wythe St.
Alexandria, VA 22314
http://www.childrenshospitals.net
Tel: 1-(703)-684-1355

National Association of Public Hospitals and Health Systems
1301 Pennsylvania Ave. NW
Suite 950
Washington, DC 20004
http://www.naph.org
Tel: 1-(202)-585-0100

VHA, Inc.
PO Box 140909 (mailing address)
Irving, TX 75014
220 E. Las Colinas Blvd. (location)
Irving, TX 75039
http://www.vha.com
Tel: 1-(972)-830-0000

MEDICINE

American Academy of Family Physicians
11400 Tomahawk Creek Pkwy.
Leawood, KS 60211
http://www.familydoctor.org
Tel: 1-(800)-274-2237

American Board of Medical Specialties
1007 Church St.
Suite 404

Evanston, IL 60201
http://www.abms.org
Tel: 1-(847)-491-9091

American Medical Association
515 North State St.
Chicago, IL 60610
http://www.ama-assn.org
Tel: 1-(800)-621-8335

American Medical Group Association
1422 Duke St.
Alexandria, VA 22314
http://www.amga.org
Tel: 1-(703)-838-0033

American Osteopathic Association
142 East Ontario St.
Chicago, IL 60611
http://www.osteopathic.org
Tel: 1-(800)-621-1773

Medical Group Management Association
104 Inverness Terrace East
Englewood, CO 80112
http://www.mgma.com
Tel: 1-(877)-275-6462
Tel: 1-(303)-799-1111

National Medical Association
1012 10th St. NW
Washington, DC 20001
http://www.nmanet.org
Tel: 1-(202)-347-1895

NURSING HOMES

American Association of Homes and
Services for the Aging
2519 Connecticut Ave. NW
Washington, DC 20008

http://www.aahsa.org
Tel: 1-(202)-783-2242

American College of Health Care
Administrators
300 North Lee St.
Suite 301
Alexandria, VA 22314
http://www.achca.org
Tel: 1-(703)-739-7900

American Health Care Association
1201 L St. NW
Washington, DC 20005
http://www.ahca.org
Tel: 1-(202)-842-4444

Long Term Care Community Coalition
242 West 30th St.
Suite 306
New York, NY 10001
http://www.ltccc.org
http://www.assisted-living411.org
http://www.nursinghome411.org
Tel: 1-(212)-385-0355

National Center for Assisted Living
(Affiliated with the American Health
Care Association)
1201 L St. NW
Washington, DC 20005
http://www.ncal.org
Tel: 1-(202)-842-4444

National Citizen's Coalition for
Nursing Home Reform
1828 L St. NW
Suite 801
Washington, DC 20036
http://www.nursinghomeaction.org
Tel: 1-(202)-332-2276

NURSES

American Nurses Association
8515 Georgia Ave.
Suite 400
Silver Spring, MD 20910
http://www.ana.org
Tel: 1-(301)-628-5000

National League for Nursing
61 Broadway Ave.
New York, NY 10006
http://www.nln.org
Tel: 1-(800)-669-1656
Tel: 1-(212)-363-5555

OCCUPATIONAL THERAPY

American Occupational Therapy Association, Inc.
4720 Montgomery Lane
PO Box 31220
Bethesda, MD 20824
http://www.aota.org
Tel: 1-(301)-652-2682

OPTOMETRY

American Optometric Association
243 N. Lindbergh Blvd.
First Floor
St. Louis, MO 63141
http://www.aoa.org
Tel: 1-(800)-365-2219

PHARMACY

American Pharmacists Association
2215 Constitution Ave. NW
Washington, DC 20037

http://www.aphanet.org
Tel: 1-(202)-628-4410

American Society of Health System
  Pharmacists
7272 Wisconsin Ave.
Bethesda, MD 20814
http://www.ashp.com
Tel: 1-(301)-657-3000

PHYSICAL THERAPY

American Physical Therapy Association
1111 North Fairfax St.
Alexandria, VA 22314
http://www.apta.org
Tel: 1-(800)-999-2782
Tel: 1-(703)-684-2782

PODIATRY

American Podiatric Medical Association
9312 Old Georgetown Rd.
Bethesda, MD 20814
http://www.apma.org
Tel: 1-(301)-571-9200

SURGERY

Accreditation Association for Ambulatory Health Care
3201 Old Glenview Rd.
Suite 300
Wilmette, IL 60091
http://www.aaahc.org
Tel: 1-(847)-853-6060

American Association for Accreditation
  of Ambulatory Surgery Facilities, Inc.

5101 Washington St.
Suite 2F
Gurnee, IL 60031
http://www.aaaasf.org
Tel: 1-(888)-545-5222

Federated Ambulatory Surgical Association
700 North Fairfax St.
Alexandria, VA 22314
http://www.fasa.org
Tel: 1-(703)-836-8808

OTHER ORGANIZATIONS

American Association of Blood Banks
8101 Glenbrook Rd.
Bethesda, MD 20814.
http://www.aabb.org
Tel: 1-(301)-907-6977

American Orthotics and Prosthetics
  Association
330 John Carlyle St.
Suite 200
Alexandria, VA 22314
http://www.opoffice.org
Tel: 1-(571)-431-0876

American Public Health Association
800 I (Eye) St. NW
Washington, DC 20001
http://www.apha.org
Tel: 1-(202)-777-2742

American Public Human Services
  Association
810 First St. NE
Suite 500
Washington, DC 20002
http://www.aphsa.org
Tel: 1-(202)-682-0100

National Adult Day Services Association, Inc.
2519 Connecticut Ave. NW
Washington, DC 20008
http://www.nadsa.org
Tel: 1-(800)-558-5301

National Association of Community
Health Centers, Inc.
7200 Wisconsin Ave.
Suite 210
Bethesda, MD 20814
http://www.nachc.org
Tel: 1-(301)-347-0400

National Business Group on Health
50 F St. NW
Washington, DC 20001
http://www.wbgh.org
Tel: 1-(202)-628-9320

National Council for Community
Behavioral Health Care
12300 Twinbrook Pkwy.
Rockville, MD 20852
http://www.nccbh.org
Tel: 1-(301)-984-6200

National Council on Patient Information and Education
(information about medicines)
4915 Saint Elmo Ave.
Bethesda, MD 20814
http://www.talkaboutrx.org
Tel: 1-(301)-656-8565

National Health Council
1730 M St. NW
Washington, DC 20036
http://www.nhcouncil.org
Tel: 1-(202)-785-3910

National Rural Health Association
521 East 63rd St.
Kansas City, MO 64110
http://www.nrharural.org
Tel: 1-(816)-756-3140

US Chamber of Commerce
1615 H St. NW
Washington, DC 20062
http://www.uschamber.com
Tel: 1-(202)-659-6000

US Pharmacopeia
(Official standard-setting authority for
prescription and over-the-counter
drugs, dietary supplements, and other
healthcare products sold and manufactured in the United States)
12601 Twinbrook Pkwy.
Rockville, MD 20852
http://www.usp.org
Tel: 1-(800)-227-8772
Tel: 1-(301)-881-0666

United Way of America
701 North Fairfax St.
Alexandria, VA 22314
http://www.unitedway.org
Tel: 1-(703)-836-7100

SELECTED DISEASES

Alzheimer's Association, Inc.
225 North Michigan Ave.
Seventeenth Floor
Chicago, Il 60611
http://www.alz.org
Tel: 1-(800)-272-3900
Tel: 1-(312)-335-8700

American Cancer Society
1599 Clifton Rd. NE

Atlanta, GA 30329
http://www.cancer.org
Tel: 1-(800)-227-2345

American Diabetes Association
1701 North Beauregard St.
Alexandria, VA 22311
http://www.diabetes.org
Tel: 1-(800)-342-2383

American Foundation for the Blind
11 Penn Plaza
New York, NY 10001
http://www.afb.org
Tel: 1-(212)-502-7600

American Heart Association
7272 Greenville Ave.
Dallas, TX 75231
http://www.amhrt.org
Tel: 1-(800)-242-8721

American Lung Association
61 Broadway Ave.
Sixth Floor
New York, NY 10006
http://www.lungusa.org
Tel: 1-(212)-315-8700

American Psychiatric Association
1000 Wilson Blvd.
Suite 1825
Arlington, VA 22209
http://www.psych.org
Tel: 1-(703)-907-7300

American Speech—Language—
 Hearing Association
10801 Rockville Pike
Rockville, MD 20852
http://www.asha.org
Tel: 1-(800)-498-2071
Tel: 1-(301)-897-5700 (TTY)

Arthritis Foundation
PO Box 7669
Atlanta, GA 30357
http://www.arthritis.org
Tel: 1-(800)-568-4045
Tel: 1-(404)-872-7100
Tel: 1-(404)-965-7888

Asthma and Allergy Foundation of
 America
1233 20th St. NW
Washington, DC 20036
http://www.aafa.org
Tel: 1-(202)-466-7643

Crohn's and Colitis Foundation of
 America
386 Park Ave. S.
Seventeenth Floor
New York, NY 10016
http://www.ccfa.org
Tel: 1-(800)-932-2423

Cystic Fibrosis Foundation
6917 Arlington Rd.
Bethesda, MD 20814
http://www.cff.org
Tel: 1-(800)-344-4823
Tel: 1-(301)-951-4422

Easter Seals
230 West Monroe St.
Chicago, IL 60606
http://www.easter-seals.org
Tel: 1-(800)-221-6827
Tel: 1-(312)-726-6200

Epilepsy Foundation of America
4351 Garden City Dr.
Landover, MD 20785
http://www.efa.org
Tel: 1-(301)-459-3700

Eye-Bank Association of America, Inc.
1015 18th St. NW
Suite 1010
Washington, DC 20036
http://www.restoresight.org
Tel: 1-(202)-775-4999

Huntington's Disease Society of
   America
505 Eighth Ave.
Suite 902
New York, NY 10018
http://www.hdsa.org
Tel: 1-(212)-242-1968
Tel: 1-(800)-345-4372

March of Dimes
1275 Mamaroneck Ave.
White Plains, NY 10605
http://www.modimes.org
Tel: 1-(914)-428-7100

Muscular Dystrophy Association-USA
National Headquarters
Tucson, AZ 85718
http://www.mdausa.org
Tel: 1-(800)-344-4863

National Alliance for Hispanic Health
1501 16th St. NW
Washington, DC 20006
http://www.hispanichealth.org
Tel: 1-(202)-387-5000

National Council on Alcoholism and
   Drug Dependence
22 Cortlandt St.
Suite 801
New York, NY 10007
http://www.ncadd.org
Tel: 1-(212)-269-7797

National Deaf Education Network &
   Clearinghouse
Laurent Clerc National Deaf Education
   Center
Gallaudet University
800 Florida Ave. NE
Washington, DC 20002
http://clerccenter.gallaudet.edu/InfoToGo
Tel: 1-(202)-651-5051
Tel: 1-(202)-651-6052 (TTY)

National Kidney Foundation
30 East 33rd St.
New York, NY 10016
http://www.kidney.org
Tel: 1-(800)-622-9010

National Mental Health Association
2001 N. Beauregard St.
Twelfth Floor
Alexandria, VA 22311
http://www.nmha.org
Tel: 1-(703)-684-7722

National Multiple Sclerosis Society
733 3rd Ave.
New York, NY 10017
http://www.nmss.org
Tel: 1-(800)-344-4867

National Rehabilitation Association
633 South Washington St.
Alexandria, VA 22314
http://www.nationalrehab.org
Tel: 1-(703)-836-0850

Self-Help for Hard of Hearing People,
   Inc.
7910 Woodmont Ave.
Bethesda, MD 20814
http://www.shhh.org
Tel: 1-(301)-657-2248
Tel: 1-(301)-657-2249 (TTY)

United Cerebral Palsy Association, Inc.
1660 L St. NW
Suite 700
Washington, DC 20036
http://www.ucpa.org
Tel: 1-(800)-872-5827
Tel: 1-(202)-973-7197

FEDERAL GOVERNMENT: CONSUMER HEALTH INFORMATION CENTERS

Alzheimer's Disease Education and
  Referral Center
PO Box 8250
Silver Spring, MD 20907
http://www.alzheimers.org
Tel: 1-(800)-438-4380
Tel: 1-(301)-495-3311

Clearinghouse for Occupational Safety
  and Health Information
4676 Columbia Pkwy.
Cincinnati, OH 45226
http://www.cdc.gov/niosh
Tel: 1-(800)-356-4674
Tel: 1-(513)-533-8328

Clearinghouse on Disability Information
550 12th St. SW
Room 5153
Washington, DC 20202
http://www.ed.gov
Tel: 1-(202)-245-7307

Communicable Disease Center (CDC)
National HIV/AIDS Clearinghouse
  (also covers sexually transmitted diseases and tuberculosis)
PO Box 6003
Rockville, MD 20849

http://www.cdcnpin.org
Tel: 1-(800)-458-5231
Tel: 1-(301)-562-1098

Food and Drug Administration
Office of Consumer Communications
5600 Fischers Lane
Rockville, MD 20857
http://www.fda.gov/cder
Tel: 1-(301)-827-4573
Tel: 1-(888)-463-6332

Food and Nutrition Information Center
National Agricultural Library Building
US Department of Agriculture
10301 Baltimore Ave.
Beltsville, MD 20705
http://www.nal.usda.gov/fnic
Tel: 1-(301)-504-5719

Genetic & Rare Diseases Information
  Center
PO Box 8126
Gaithersburg, MD 20898
http://rarediseases.info.nih.gov
http://www.genome.gov (National
  Human Genome Institute)
http://www.rarediseases.org (National
  Organization for Rare Diseases)
Tel: 1-(888)-205-2311

National Arthritis and Musculoskeletal
  and Skin Diseases Information
  Clearinghouse
1 AMS Circle
Bethesda, MD 20892
http://www.niams.nih.gov
Tel: 1-(301)-495-4484

National Cancer Institute
Office of Cancer Communications
31 Center Dr. MSC 2580
Building 31, Room 10A07

Bethesda, MD 20892
http://www.cancer.gov
Tel: 1-(800)-422-6237

National Center for Chronic Disease
Prevention and Health Promotion
Technical Information and Editorial
Services Branch
Centers for Disease Control and
Prevention
4770 Buford Hwy. MS K13
Atlanta, GA 30341
http://www.cdc.gov
Tel: 1-(770)-488-5080

National Center for Complementary
and Alternative Medicine Information
Clearinghouse
PO Box 7923
Gaithersburg, MD 20898-7927
http://www.nccam.nih.gov
Tel: 1-(888)-644-6226

National Clearinghouse for Alcohol and
Drug Information
PO Box 2345
Rockville, MD 20847-2345
http://www.health.org
Tel: 1-(800)-729-6686
Tel: 1-(301)-468-2600

National Clearinghouse on Child Abuse
and Neglect Information
1250 Maryland Ave. SW
Washington, DC 20447
http://nccanch.acf.hhs.gov
Tel: 1-(800)-394-3366
Tel: 1-(703)-385-7565

National Clearinghouse on Primary
Care Information
c/o Circle Solutions
2070 Chain Bridge Rd.
Suite 450

Vienna, VA 22182
http://bphc.hrsa.gov
Tel: 1-(888)-275-4772
Tel: 1-(703)-821-8955

National Diabetes Information
Clearinghouse
1 Information Way
Bethesda, MD 20892
http://www.diabetes.niddk.nih.gov
Tel: 1-(301)-654-3327

National Digestive Diseases Education
and Information Clearinghouse
2 Information Way
Bethesda, MD 20892
http://www.digestive.niddk.nih.gov
Tel: 1-(301)-654-3810

National Health Information Center
(locates health information for
public)
PO Box 1133
Washington, DC 20013
http://www.health.gov/nhic
http://www.healthfinder.gov
Tel: 1-(800)-336-4797
Tel: 1-(301)-565-4167

National Heart, Lung, and Blood
Institute Information Center
PO Box 30105
Bethesda, MD 20824-0105
http://www.nhlbi.nih.gov
Tel: 1-(301)-592-8573

National High Blood Pressure
Education Program
NHLBI Health Information Center
PO Box 30105
Bethesda, MD 20824-0105
http://www.nhlbi.nih.gov/hbp/index.html
Tel: 1-(301)-592-8573

National Information Clearinghouse on
Children Who Are Deaf-Blind
345 North Monmouth Ave.
Monmouth, OR 97361
http://www.dblink.org
Tel: 1-(800)-438-9376
Tel: 1-(800)-854-7013 (TTY)

National Injury Information
Clearinghouse
US Consumer Product Safety
Commission
4330 East West Hwy.
Bethesda, MD 20814
http://www.cpsc.gov
Tel: 1-(800)-638-2772
Tel: 1-(800)-638-8270 (TTY)

National Institute of Allergy and
Infectious Diseases
Office of Communications
31 Center Dr. MSC 2520
Bethesda, MD 20892
http://www.niaid.nih.gov
Tel: 1-(301)-496-5717

National Institute of Mental Health
Information Resources and Inquiries
Branch
6001 Executive Blvd. MSC 9663
Bethesda, MD 20892-9663
http://www.nimh.nih.gov
Tel: 1-(866)-615-6464
Tel: 1-(301)-443-4513

National Institute on Aging Information
Center
PO Box 8057
Gaithersburg, MD 20898
http://www.nia.nih.gov
Tel: 1-(800)-222-2225

National Institute on Deafness and
Other Communication Disorders
Information Clearinghouse
1 Communication Ave.
Bethesda, MD 20892
http://www.nidcd.nih.gov
Tel: 1-(800)-241-1044

National Kidney and Urologic Diseases
Information Clearinghouse
3 Information Way
Bethesda, MD 20892-3580
http://www.kidney.niddk.nih.gov
Tel: 1-(800)-891-5390
Tel: 1-(301)-654-4415

National Maternal and Child Health
Clearinghouse
c/o Circle Solutions
2070 Chain Bridge Rd.
Suite 450
Vienna, VA 22182
http://www.ask.hrsa.gov
Tel: 1-(888)-275-4772
Tel: 1-(703)-356-1964

National Oral Health Information
Clearinghouse
1 NOHIC Way
Bethesda, MD 20892
http://www.nidcr.nih.gov
Tel: 1-(301)-402-7364

National Osteoporosis and Related
Bone Diseases National Resource
Center
1232 22nd St. NW
Washington, DC 20037
http://www.niams.nih.gov/bone
Tel: 1-(800)-624-2663
Tel: 1-(202)-223-0344

National Rehabilitation Information
    Center
4200 Forbes Blvd.
Suite 202
Lanham, MD 20706
http://www.naric.com
Tel: 1-(800)-346-2742

National Resource Center for Home-
    lessness and Mental Illness
7500 Old Georgetown Rd.
Bethesda, MD 20814
http://www.nrchmi.samhsa.gov
Tel: 1-(800)-444-7415

National Second Surgical Opinion
    Program
US Department of Health and Human
    Services
330 Independence Ave. SW
Washington, DC 20201
http://www.medicare.gov
Tel: 1-(800)-633-4227
Tel: 1-(877)-486-2048

National Sudden Infant Death
    Syndrome Resource Center
c/o Circle Solutions
2070 Chain Bridge Rd.
Suite 450
Vienna, VA 22182
http://www.sidscenter.org
Tel: 1-(866)-866-7437
Tel: 1-(703)-821-8955

National Women's Health Information
    Center
8270 Willow Oaks Corporate Dr.
Fairfax, VA 22031
http://www.womenshealth.gov
Tel: 1-(800)-994-9662

Office on Smoking and Health
Centers of Disease Control and
    Prevention
National Center for Chronic Disease
    Prevention and Health Promotion
Mailstop K-50
4770 Buford Hwy. NE
Atlanta, GA 30341
http://www.cdc.gov/tobacco
Tel: 1-(770)-488-5705, option 3

President's Council on Physical Fitness
    and Sports
Dept. W
200 Independence Ave. SW
Room 738-H
Washington, DC 20201
http://www.fitness.gov
Tel: 1-(202)-690-9000

US Federal Citizen Information Center
    (FCIC)
    (publishes free *Consumer Informa-
    tion Catalog*)
PO Box 100
Pueblo, CO 81002
http://www.pueblo.gsa.gov
Tel: 1-(888)-878-3256

GLOSSARY

access. An individual's or a group's ability to obtain medical care.

accident. An event or occurrence that could not be anticipated in advance and did not happen on purpose.

accidental bodily injury. Injury to the body as a result of an accident.

accidental death and dismemberment insurance. Insurance that provides payment to an insured in the event of death or specific bodily injury resulting from an accident.

accidental means. The unexpected and unforeseen cause of an accident. The "means" that caused the mishap must be accidental in order to claim benefits under the policy.

accident insurance. A form of health insurance that insures against financial loss resulting from an accident.

accreditation. A process where a program of study or an institution is recognized by an outside group as meeting certain predetermined standards. Accreditation is often performed by organizations created for the purpose of assuring the public of the quality of the accredited institution or program. Accreditation may either be permanent or given for a specified period of time.

accumulation period. A specified period of time, such as ninety days, during which the insured person must incur eligible medical expenses at least equal to the deductible amount in order to establish a benefit period under a major medical expense or comprehensive medical expense policy.

acquisition cost. The immediate cost of issuing a new insurance policy, including the cost of clerical work, the agent's commission, and medical inspection fees.

actual charge. The amount a physician or other practitioner actually bills a patient for a particular medical service or procedure. The amount may differ from the customary, prevailing, and/or reasonable charges under public or private insurance programs.

actuary. A technical expert trained in the insurance field who is responsible for calculating premium rates, reserves, and dividends, as well as conducting various other statistical studies.

acute care. Medical treatment that is provided to persons whose illnesses or health problems are of a short-term or episodic nature. Acute care facilities are those institutions that treat persons with short-term health problems.

acute disease. A disease that is distinguished by a single episode of a relatively short duration from which the patient returns to his/her normal or previous state and level of activity.

adjustable premium. A premium that an insurance company may modify under certain special conditions in accordance with a policy provision.

administrative service only (ASO) plan. An arrangement under which an insurance carrier or an independent organization will, for a fee, handle the claims and benefits paperwork for a self-insured group and insure against a certain level of large unpredictable claims.

adverse selection. The tendency of persons with poorer-than-average health expectations to apply for or continue insurance to a greater extent than do persons with average or better health expectations.

age limits. Stipulated minimum and maximum ages below and above which an insurance company will not accept applications or may not renew policies.

agent. An insurance company representative licensed by the state who solicits, negotiates, or effects contracts of insurance and services the policyholder for the insurer.

aggregate indemnity. The maximum dollar amount that may be collected for any disability or period of disability under an insurance policy.

allocated benefits. Benefits for which the maximum amount payable for specific services is itemized in the contract.

allowable costs. Items or elements of an institution's costs that are reimbursable under a payment formula.

alternate delivery system. Systems of delivering healthcare that are less expensive than inpatient, acute care hospitals. Examples of such systems are skilled and intermediary nursing facilities, hospice care, and homecare services.

ambulatory care. All kinds of health services that are provided on an outpatient basis, in contrast to services provided in the home or to persons who are inpatients and receive services that require an overnight stay in an institution such as a hospital.

amendment. A document that alters the provisions of an insurance contract that both the insurer and the policyholder have signed.

ancillary services. Supplemental services, including laboratory, radiology, physical therapy, and inhalation therapy, that are provided in conjunction with medical or hospital care.

application. A signed statement of facts requested by an insurance company on the basis of which the company decides whether or not to issue a policy. This, then, becomes part of the health insurance contract if the policy is issued.

assigned benefits. Signing a paper allowing your insurance company to make payments for your medical treatment directly to your hospital or your physician. Otherwise, the money will be paid to you when you turn in your bills and claim forms to the company.

assignment. A process in which a Medicare beneficiary agrees to have Medicare's share of the cost of a service paid directly or assigned to a doctor or other provider, and the provider agrees to accept the Medicare-approved charge as payment in full.

association group. A group formed from members of a trade or professional association for group insurance under one master health insurance contract.

behavioral healthcare. The delivery of mental health services and other services to treat chemical dependency (substance abuse).

beneficiary. A person or persons designated by the policyholder to receive a specified cash payment upon the policyholder's death. Also, a person who is eligible to receive or is receiving benefits from an insurance policy or health maintenance organization. This usually includes both people who themselves have contracted for benefits and their eligible dependents.

benefit. An amount an insurance company pays to a claimant, assignee, or beneficiary when the insured experiences a loss.

benefit period. The period of time for which payments for benefits that an insurance policy covers are available.

binding receipt. A receipt given for a premium payment accompanying the application for insurance. If the policy is approved, this binds the company to make the policy effective from the date of the receipt.

blanket contract. A contract of health insurance affording benefits, such as accidental death and dismemberment, for all of a class of persons not individually identified. It is used for such groups as athletic teams, campers, and as a travel policy for employees.

blanket medical expense. A provision that entitles the insured person to collect up to a maximum established in the policy for all hospital and medical expenses incurred, without any limitations on individual types of medical expenses.

Blue Cross. An independent, nonprofit membership corporation providing protection against the costs of healthcare.

Blue Shield. An independent, nonprofit membership corporation providing protection against the cost of surgery and other items of medical care.

board certified. A designation a medical specialist receives upon completing a required course of training and experience (residency) and passing a test in his or/her specialty. Persons who have met all the requirements except examination are called "board eligible."

broker. An insurance solicitor, licensed by the state, who places business with a variety of insurance companies and who represents the buyers of insurance rather than the companies even though he is paid commissions by the companies.

business insurance. A policy that primarily provides coverage of benefits to a business as contrasted to an individual. It is issued to indemnify a business for the loss of services of a key employee or a partner who becomes disabled.

capital sum. The maximum amount payable in one sum in the event of accidental dismemberment. When a contract provides benefits for various kinds of dismemberment, each benefit is an amount equal to, or a fraction of, the capital sum. Dismemberment may include loss of eyesight or a limb.

capitation. A method of paying for health services in which a physician or a hospital is paid a fixed, per capita amount for each person served in a particular plan without regard to the actual number or nature of the services provided to each person.

carrier. A private organization, usually an insurance company, that finances healthcare. Also pays Medicare Part B bills; Fiscal Intermediary pays Part A bills.

case management. An approach designed to provide effective treatment to meet the specific needs of people with serious medical problems. Benefits not traditionally covered (for example, medical equipment) may be provided to promote cost effectiveness.

categorically needy. Persons who are both economically needy and members of certain categories or groups, such as the aged, the blind, or the disabled, eligible to receive public assistance.

certificate of insurance. A document delivered to the insured person that summarizes the benefits and principal provisions of the group plan.

certification. The process by which a governmental or nongovernmental agency or association assesses and recognizes an individual, institution, or educational program as meeting predetermined standards. Such recognition is called "certification." It is essentially similar to accreditation, except that certification is usually applied to individuals and accreditation is applied to institutions. Certification programs are generally nongovernmental and, unlike licensure programs, do not prevent the uncertified from practicing.

Children's Health Insurance Program (CHIP). Established by the Balanced Budget Act of 1997, this program was designed for families who earn too much money to qualify for Medicaid but cannot afford to buy health insurance for their children. The insurance is designed to be available to children in working families, including families with a variety of immigration statuses. For little or no cost, the insurance pays for doctor visits, prescription medicines, hospitalizations, and other benefits. States can use CHIP funds to expand Medicaid eligibility to children who did not previously qualify for the program, establish a separate children's health insurance program, or combine both the Medicaid and the separate program options.

claim. A demand to the insurer by the insured person for the payment of benefits under a policy.

clinical practice guideline. A utilization and quality management mechanism whose purpose is to help providers decide about the most appropriate course of treatment for a specific clinical case.

closed-panel HMO. An HMO in which physicians are either on salary as employees or are a part of a group of physicians that contracts with the HMO.

coding errors. Errors of documentation in which medical treatments are not correctly coded or the codes that are used to describe the procedures are different from those used to note the diagnosis.

coinsurance. A policy provision frequently found in major medical insurance by which both the insured person and the insurer share, in a specified ratio, the covered losses of the policy.

community rating. A method of establishing health insurance premiums using the average cost of actual or anticipated health services for all subscribers within a specific geographic locality. The premium does not differ for different groups or subgroups of subscribers on the basis of their specific claims experience.

competitive medical plan (CMP). A state-licensed entity, other than a federally qualified health maintenance organization, that signs a Medicare risk contract and agrees to assume financial risk for providing care to Medicare beneficiaries on a prospective, prepaid basis.

comprehensive major medical insurance. A policy designed to give the protection offered by both a basic and a major medical health insurance policy. It is characterized by a low deductible amount, a coinsurance feature, and high maximum benefits, up to $250,000 or more.

concurrent review. Review of the medical necessity of hospital or other health facility admissions upon or within a short period of time following an admission and the periodic review of services provided during the course of treatment.

conditionally renewable policy. Policies with this provision are no longer sold, but older policies may still be in force. When a policy is conditionally renewable, an insurance company agrees to continue insurance for an individual policyholder as long as it continues to insure everyone in the same state holding the same kind of policy. This is not a guarantee of continued coverage, and policyholders have better protection with a policy that is guaranteed renewable.

confining sickness. An illness that confines an insured person to his or her home or to a hospital.

consideration. One of the elements of a binding contract. Consideration is acceptance by the insurance company of the payment of the premium and the statements made by the prospective policyholder in the application.

Consolidated Omnibus Budget Reconciliation Act of 1986 (COBRA—Public Law 92-272). A federal law that requires employers to offer continued health insurance coverage to certain employees and their beneficiaries whose group health insurance coverage has ended. The law applies to employers with twenty or more eligible employees. Typically, it makes continued coverage available up to eighteen or thirty-six months. COBRA enrollees may be required to pay 100 percent of the premium, plus an additional 2 percent.

contributory plan. A group plan under which both the policyholder and the insurer share the plan's costs.

conventional health plan. A plan that provides all the benefits and issues certificates containing the insurance company's guarantees.

conversion privilege. The right given to an insured person to convert to individual insurance without evidence of medical insurability, usually upon termination of coverage under a group contract.

coordinated care plans. (CCPs). The Medicare Advantage option (Part C) that includes HMOs (with or without a point-of-service provision), preferred-provider organizations (PPOs), and a provider-sponsored organization (PSO).

coordination of benefits (COB). A method of integrating benefits payable under more than one group health insurance plan so that the insured person's benefits from all sources do not exceed 100 percent of the allowable medical expenses. That is, they are procedures and provision insurers use to avoid duplicate payment for losses under more than one insurance policy.

copayment. Another way of sharing medical costs. You pay a flat fee every time you receive a medical service (for example, $15 for every visit to the doctor). The insurance company pays the rest.

cost containment. An effort to reduce inefficiencies in the use, allocation, and delivery of healthcare services. Inappropriate use of health services, delivering services in more costly settings when less expensive settings are available, and not reducing health service costs by failing to use a different combination of resources leads to such inefficiencies.

cost sharing. Provisions of a health insurance policy that requires the insured or otherwise covered individual to pay some portion of the covered medical expenses such as copayments or coinsurance.

covered expenses. Most insurance plans, whether they are fee-for-service, HMOs, or PPOs, do not pay for all services. Some may not pay for prescription drugs. Others may not pay for mental healthcare. Covered services are those medical procedures the insurer agrees to pay for and are listed in the policy.

credentialing. The process of obtaining, reviewing, and making sure of a provider's credentials, including his training, licenses, and certifications, in order to determine whether the provider meets an organization's established criteria for being part of its network.

creditable prescription drug coverage. Drug coverage offered by other prescription drug plans that is as good as the standard prescription drug plan under Part D of the Medicare program—that is, prescription drug coverage such as from an employer or a union that pays out, on average, as much as or more than Medicare's standard prescription drug coverage.

custodial care. Assistance with bathing, dressing, eating, taking medicine, and similar personal needs. Custodial care can be provided by people without medical skills or training.

customary charge. One of the factors determining a physician's payment for a service under Medicare. It is calculated as the physician's median charge for that service over a prior twelve-month period.

customary, prevailing, and reasonable. A method of paying physicians under Medicare. Payment for a service is limited to the lowest of the physician's billed charge for a service, the physician's customary charge for services, or the prevailing charge for that service in the community. This is similar to the usual, customary, and reasonable system used by private insurers.

deductible. The amount of covered expenses that must be incurred by the insured person before benefits become payable by the insurer.

dental health maintenance organization (DHMO). An organization that delivers dental services to its members who have prepaid for these services through a network of providers.

dental point-of-service plan (Dental POS). A dental service plan that permits a member to use a dental health maintenance organization network or to seek care from a dentist not in the network, paying higher out-of-pocket costs to dentists who are not in the network.

dental preferred-provider organization (Dental PPO). An organization that provides dental care to its members through a network of dentists who charge discounted fees to plan members.

diagnosis-related groups (DRG). A system of classification for inpatient hospital services based on principal diagnosis, secondary diagnosis, surgical procedures, age, gender, and presence of complications. This system of DRG classification is used as a financing mechanism to reimburse hospitals and selected other providers for services rendered, typically based on the average cost of all patients within the DRG.

diagnostic and treatment codes. Codes that briefly and specifically describe each diagnosis and treatment that are also identified by a number.

disability. A condition that renders a person incapable of performing one or more duties of his or her regular occupation.

disability income insurance. A form of health insurance that provides periodic payments to replace income when the insured person is unable to work as a result of illness, injury, or disease.

discharge planning. Under managed care, this is the process of facilitating the transfer of a patient to a more cost-effective care facility after it is deemed that the patient no longer needs to remain in the hospital.

disease management. A system that coordinates preventive, diagnostic, and therapeutic efforts and whose purpose is to deliver cost-efficient, quality healthcare for a patient group that is at risk for a specific chronic illness or medical condition.

dismemberment. The loss of a limb or eyesight.

dispensing fee. A fee a pharmacist charges for filling a prescription.

double indemnity. A policy provision usually associated with death, which doubles the payment of designated benefits when certain kinds of accidents occur.

"doughnut hole." The financial coverage gap in the Part D Medicare prescription drug program where the beneficiary pays 100 percent of his/her drug costs.

dread disease insurance. Insurance providing an unallocated benefit, subject to a maximum amount, for expenses incurred in connection with the treatment of specified diseases, such as cancer, poliomyelitis, encephalitis, and spinal meningitis.

drug utilization review. A program that analyzes whether drugs are being used safely, effectively, and appropriately.

"dual choice" provisions. Stipulations in the HMO Act of 1973 which require that employers that cover their workforce of more than twenty-five employees with health insurance must offer their employees a choice of managed care or traditional health insurance.

duplication of coverage. When two or more policies provide protection for the same potential loss.

durable medical equipment. Prescribed medical equipment such as a wheelchair that can be used for an extended period of time.

Early and Periodic Screening, Diagnosis, and Treatment Program (EPSDT). A program required by law as part of the Medicaid program. The law requires that all states have in effect a program for eligible children under age twenty-one to determine their physical or mental defects and to provide such healthcare treatments and other measures to correct or make better defects and to discover chronic conditions. The state programs also have active outreach components to inform eligible persons of the benefits available to them, to provide screening, and, if necessary, to assist in obtaining appropriate treatment.

earned premium. That portion of a policy's premium payment for which the protection of the policy has already been given. For example, an insurance company is considered to have earned 75 percent of an annual premium after a period of nine months of the annual term has elapsed.

effective date. The date when insurance coverage starts.

elective benefit. A benefit payable in lieu of another; that is, a lump sum benefit may be allowed for specified fractures or dislocations in lieu of a weekly or monthly indemnity.

eligibility date. Date when a member of an insured group applies for coverage.

eligibility period. Time after the eligibility period (usually thirty-one days) during which a member of a group may apply for insurance coverage without providing evidence about whether the person is insurable or not.

eligible employees. Employees who meet the eligibility requirements for insurance coverage as stated in the group policy.

elimination period. A term used in disability income policies meaning a specified length of time at the beginning of disability during which no benefits will be payable.

Employee Retirement Income Security Act of 1974 (ERISA—Public Law 93-406). A law that mandates the disclosure of grievance and appeal requirements, and fiduciary standards for group life and health plans. It is sponsored by private (but not public) employers.

endorsement. See *rider*.

ethical drug. A drug that is advertised only to physicians and other prescribing health professionals.

evidence of insurability. Any statement or proof of a person's physical condition and/or other factual information affecting his or her acceptance for insurance.

exclusions. Specific hazards or conditions listed in the insurance policy for which the policy will not provide benefit payments.

exclusive-provider organization (EPO). An organization that provides coverage for services only from network providers.

experience. The percentage or ratio of claims to premiums for a specific period of time. Also, the actual cost of delivering healthcare services to a group during a period of coverage.

experience rating. A variation of premium rate, computed on the basis of past losses and expenses incurred by the insurance company in the settlement of claims and other expenses involving a particular group of risks.

experience refund. A provision in most group policies for the return of a portion of the premium to the policyholder because of lower than anticipated claims.

explanation of benefits. The coverage statement sent to covered persons listing services rendered, amounts billed, and payments made.

Extra Help. A special program under the Medicare Part D prescription drug program that offers low costs and continuous coverage to people with limited incomes who qualify. If approved, recipients are helped with their drug plan's monthly premium, yearly deductible, and prescription drug copayments. The US territories of Puerto Rico, the Virgin Islands, Guam, American Samoa, and the Northern Mariana Islands have their own rules for providing extra help to their residents.

family expense policy. An insurance policy that insures both the policyholder and his or her immediate dependents (usually spouse and children).

fee-for-service (FFS) payment system. A benefit payment system in which the insurance organization reimburses the group insurance member or pays the provider of the service(s) directly for each covered medical service after the plan member has incurred the medical expense.

first-dollar coverage. A hospital or surgical policy with no deductible amount—that is, coverage for the insured begins with the first dollar of expense incurred for the covered benefits.

formulary. A list of prescription drugs that a health plan covers subject to conditions and limits.

franchise insurance. A form of insurance in which individual policies are issued to the employees of a common employer or to the members of an association under an arrangement by which the employer or the association agrees to collect the premiums and remit them to the insurer.

fraternal insurance. A cooperative type of insurance provided by social organizations for their members.

gatekeeper. The primary care practitioner in a managed care organization who decides whether the patient has to see a specialist or requires other nonroutine services.

generic substitution. The substitution and dispensing of a generic drug for a brand-name drug because the generic is said to be therapeutically equivalent to its brand-name counterpart, with or without the physician's approval, depending upon state law.

grace period. A specified period after a premium payment is due in which the policyholder may make such payment and during which the protection of the policy continues.

group contract. A contract of insurance made with an employer or other entity that covers a group of persons identified as individuals by reference to their relationship to the entity.

group practice. A formal association of three or more physicians or other health professionals who provide health services, pool their practice's income, and redistribute it according to a prearranged plan.

guaranteed-renewable contract. A contract that the insured person has the right to continue in force by the timely payment of premiums for a substantial period of time, during which period the insurer has no right to make unilaterally any change in any provision of the contract, while the contract is in force, other than a change in the premium rate for classes of policyholders.

Health Care Quality Improvement Program (HCQIP). A program established by the Balanced Budget Act of 1997 that seeks to improve the quality of care that Medicare beneficiaries receive by requiring peer review organizations to make periodic quality reviews of Medicare coordinated care plans.

health insurance. A generic term applying to all types of insurance indemnifying or reimbursing costs of hospital and medical care or lost income arising from an illness or an injury. It is sometimes called accident and health insurance, accident or sickness insurance, or disability insurance.

Health Insurance Portability and Accountability Act of 1996 (HIPAA—Public Law 104-191). A federal law intended to improve the availability and continuity of health insurance coverage that, among other things, places limits on exclusions for preexisting medical conditions; allows certain individuals to enroll for available group health coverage when they lose other health insurance coverage or have a new dependent; prohibits discrimination in group enrollment based on health status; guarantees the availability of health insurance to small employers and the renewability of health insurance coverage in small and large group markets; and requires the availability of nongroup coverage for certain individuals whose group coverage is terminated.

health maintenance organization (HMO). An organization that provides a wide range of comprehensive healthcare services for a specified group at a fixed periodic payment. The HMO can be sponsored by the government, medical schools, hospitals, employers, labor unions, consumer groups, insurance companies, and hospital-medical plans.

Health Opportunity Account (HOA). This provision was established when the Deficit Reduction Act of 2005 became law (Public Law 109-171) on February 8, 2006. Similar to the Health Savings Account, Medicaid recipients can establish and use these accounts. State Medicaid programs contribute specified funds for adults and children to these accounts, with federal matching funds, so that a Medicaid recipient can pay for his or her medical expenses until he or she meets a deductible, after which Medicaid pays for the beneficiary's medical care with appropriate program copayments and other cost-sharing arrangements. This is a five-year demonstration project, in up to ten states, after which the secretary of the US Department of Health and Human Services can extend HOAs to all states and Medicaid beneficiaries if the secretary considers this project a success.

Health Plan Employer Data and Information Set (HEDIS). A core set of performance measures managed by the National Committee for Quality Assurance to assist employers and other health purchasers in evaluating health plan performance. It is also used by the federal agency Centers for Medicare and Medicaid Services to monitor the quality of care given by managed care organizations.

health savings account (HSA). Provision established by the enactment of the Medicare Prescription Drug, Improvement, and Modernization Act of 2003 (Public Law 108-173). HSA is a tax-sheltered savings account similar to an IRA, but earmarked for medical bills. Deposits are 100 percent tax deductible whether self-employed or not and can be easily withdrawn by check or debit card to pay routine medical bills with tax-free dollars. Larger medical expenses are covered by a low-cost, high-deductible health insurance policy. What is not spent from the account each year remains in the account and continues to increase in interest on a tax-favored basis to supplement retirement, just like an IRA. When combined with a low-cost, high-deductible health insurance policy (required), the health saving account is meant to replace a traditional high-cost health insurance policy (with its low copayments and many restrictions on medical choices). A health savings account allows the patient to have the freedom of choice to choose his or her own physician, as in a PPO, without extensive restrictions imposed by HMO-type plans.

Hill-Burton. A program named after the congressional sponsors of the Hospital Survey and Construction Act of 1946 (Public Law 79-725). The program provides federal support for modernizing hospitals and other health facilities in return for which hospitals have to provide a certain amount of free care each year.

home healthcare. A wide range of services provided at home, including part-time skilled nursing care, speech therapy, physical or occupational therapy, home health aides, and homemakers.

hospital benefits. Benefits provided under a policy for hospital charges incurred by an insured person because of an illness or an injury.

hospital indemnity. A form of health insurance that provides a stipulated daily, weekly, or monthly indemnity during hospital confinement. The indemnity is payable on an unallocated basis without regard to the actual expense of hospital confinement.

hospital-medical insurance. A term used to indicate protection that provides benefits toward the cost of any or all of the numerous healthcare services normally covered under various health insurance plans.

incontestable clause. An optional clause which may be used in noncancellable or guaranteed-renewable health insurance contracts providing that the insurer may not contest the validity of the contract after it has been in force for two (sometimes three) years.

indemnity benefits. A predetermined amount paid in the event of a covered loss.

Independent Practice Association (IPA) model health maintenance organization. A healthcare model that contracts with an entity, which in turn contracts with physicians, to provide healthcare services in return for a negotiated fee. Physicians remain in their existing individual or group practices, seeing both IPA enrollees and private-pay patients and are compensated on a per capita, fee schedule, or a fee-for-service basis.

individual insurance. Policies that provide protection to the policyholder and/or his or her family (as distinct from group and blanket insurance). Sometimes called personal insurance.

initial coverage. The amount a drug plan pays under the Medicare Part D prescription drug program prior to the beneficiary reaching the program's coverage gap ("doughnut hole").

injury independent of all other means. An injury resulting from an accident, provided that the accident was not caused by an illness.

inside limits. An insurance policy that will pay only a fixed amount for your hospital room, no matter what the actual rate, or will cover your surgical expenses only to a fixed limit, no matter the actual cost. In other words, if your policy has an inside limit of $500 per hospital day and you are in a $900-per-day hospital room, you will have to pay the difference.

insurance. Protection by written contract against the financial hazards (in whole or in part) of the happenings of specified chance events.

insurance company. Any corporation primarily engaged in the business of furnishing protection to the public.

insuring clause. The clause that sets forth the type of loss being covered by the policy and the parties to the insurance contract.

integration. When two or more benefit plans are brought together to avoid the duplication of payments.

intermediate care facility. A facility providing a level of care that is less than the degree of care and treatment that a hospital or a skilled nursing facility is designed to provide but greater than the level of room and board.

Joint Commission on Accreditation of Healthcare Organizations (JCAHO). An independent, private, not-for-profit organization that evaluates, sets standards for, and accredits hospitals, health plans, and other health organizations providing homecare, mental healthcare, ambulatory care, and long-term care services.

key person insurance. A policy that is tailored to protect a business against the loss of income that is due to the death or disability of an employee who occupies a significant position within the organization.

lapse. Termination of a policy upon the policyholder's failure to pay the premium within the time period required.

late penalty. The extra amount a person is charged in premiums if he or she does not enroll for the Medicare drug coverage when first becoming eligible, unless the person has creditable coverage under another drug plan.

legal reserve. The minimum reserve, as calculated under the state insurance code, that a company must maintain to meet future claims and obligations.

length of stay. The number of days, beginning from the day of admission to the day of discharge, that a patient is confined to a hospital or other facility for each episodic stay.

level premium. A premium that remains unchanged throughout the life of a policy.

lifetime disability benefit. A payment to help replace income lost by an insured person as long as he or she is totally disabled, even for a lifetime.

long-term care. A continuum of medical and social services designed to support the needs of people living with chronic health problems that affect their ability to perform everyday activities. Long-term care services include traditional medical services, social services, and housing. While the principal goal of long-term care is to restore an individual to a former level of functioning, long-term care also seeks to prevent deterioration and promote social adjustment to stages of decline. Medical services may be provided on an inpatient basis (rehabilitation, nursing home, mental hospital), an outpatient basis, or at home.

long-term disability income insurance. A provision to pay benefits to a covered disabled person as long as he or she remains disabled, usually exceeding two years.

loss-of-income benefits. Payments made to an insured person to help replace income lost through inability to work because of an insured disability.

mail-order pharmacy programs. Programs that deliver by mail medications that its members order at reduced cost.

major medical expense insurance. Health insurance to finance the expense of major illnesses or injuries. Characterized by large benefit maximums, ranging from up to $250,000 or no limit, the insurance, above an initial deductible, reimburses the major part of all charges for hospitals, doctors, private nurses, medical appliances, prescribed out-of-hospital treatments, drugs, and medicines. The insured person as coinsurer pays the remainder.

managed behavioral health organizations. An organization that uses managed care techniques in delivering behavioral health services.

managed care. Ways to manage cost, use, and quality of the healthcare system. All HMOs and PPOs, and many fee-for-service plans, have managed care. Organizations that use these techniques are called managed care organizations.

maximum allowable cost (MAC) list. Specified multisource prescription drugs that will be covered at the cost of a generic drug as established by a health plan. The plan periodically reviews and modifies this list and distributes it to participating pharmacies. The MAC list may require that the covered person pay the cost difference for a brand-name product.

maximum benefit amount. The limit your policy will pay.

maximum out-of-pocket expense. The money you will be required to pay a year for deductibles and coinsurance. It is a stated dollar amount set by the insurance company in addition to regular premiums.

Medicaid. State programs of public assistance to persons regardless of age whose income and resources are insufficient to pay for healthcare. Title XIX of the federal Social Security Act provides matching federal funds for financing state Medicaid programs, effective January 1, 1996.

medical error. A mistake that happens when a planned treatment or procedure is not delivered correctly or when the wrong treatment or procedure is carried out.

medically necessary. Services or supplies that are needed for the diagnosis or treatment of a patient's medical condition, are provided for the diagnosis and treatment of the patient's medical condition, meet the standards of good medical practice in the patient's local area, and are not mainly for the convenience of the patient or the doctor.

medically needy individuals. Persons who have enough income and resources to pay for their basic living expenses (and so do not need welfare) but not enough to pay for their medical care.

medical savings account (MSA). An account in which individuals can accumulate contributions to pay for medical care or insurance. Some states give tax-preferred status to MSA contributions, but such contributions are subject to federal income taxes.

Medicare. The hospital insurance system and the supplementary medical insurance for the aged created by the 1965 amendments to the Social Security Act and operated under the provisions of the act.

Medicare Advantage. Part C of Medicare and originally called Medicare+Choice, as created by the Balanced Budget Act of 1997. It permits contracts between the Centers for Medicare and Medicaid Services (formerly called the Health Care Financing Administration) and various kinds of managed care and fee-for-service organizations, including health maintenance organizations, preferred-provider plans, point-of-service plans, and private-fee-for-service plans that are also known as Medicare health plans.

Medicare-approved amount. In Part A and Part B of Medicare, this is the amount a doctor or a supplier can be paid, including what Medicare pays and the deductible, copayment, or coinsurance that the patient pays.

Medicare cost plan. This is a kind of HMO. If the patient receives services outside the plan's network without a referral, the person's Medicare-covered services will be paid for under the original Medicare plan (Part A and Part B), except the patient's plan pays for emergency services or urgently needed service outside the service area.

Medicare institution. A facility that meets Medicare's definition of a long-term care facility, such as a nursing home or a skilled nursing facility. This designation does not include assisted or adult living facilities, or residential homes.

Medicare Part D. The official name of the Medicare prescription drug program.

Medicare penalty. Under Medicare it is an amount added to an individual's monthly premium for Medicare Part B, or for a Medicare drug plan (Part D), if the person does not join when he or she is first able to do so. The individual pays this higher amount as long as that person has Medicare. There are some exceptions.

Medicare Prescription Drug, Improvement, and Modernization Act of 2003 (Public Law 108-173). This act created a prescription drug benefit under a new Part D of the Medicare program as well as transfered into Part D those elderly who qualify for prescription drug coverage under Medicaid. It also increased financial support for insurers to offer competition to the program, mandated a six-city trial of a partly privatized Medicare system by 2010, gave an extra $25 billion to rural hospitals, required higher fees from wealthier seniors, and added a pretax health savings account for working people.

Medicare Savings Programs. State programs for people with limited income and resources that pay Medicare premiums and, in some cases, may also pay for Medicare deductibles and coinsurance.

Medsupp (also called Medigap). Medicare supplemental insurance, or Medsupp, is private insurance that supplements or fills in many of the gaps in Medicare coverage. While Medsupp policies typically cover Medicare's deductibles and coinsurance amounts, they do not provide benefits for long-term care. This insurance is regulated by states, and insurers may only offer ten predetermined benefit plans, referred to as "A through J." The insurance is also called Medicare wrap.

Mental Health Parity Act of 1996 (MHPA—Public Law 104-204). A federal act that prohibits group plans that offer mental health benefits from applying more restrictive coverage for mental illness than for physical illness.

miscellaneous expenses. Expenses in connection with hospital insurance; hospital charges other than room and board, such as x-rays, drugs, laboratory fees; and other ancillary charges.

morbidity. A term used for sickness. A morbidity table shows the average number of illnesses befalling a large group of persons. It indicates the incidence of sickness and accident the way a mortality table shows the incidence of death.

National Practitioner Data Bank (NPDB). A database maintained by the federal government that contains information on physicians and other practitioners against whom medical malpractice claims have been settled and other disciplinary actions taken.

network. An affiliation of providers through formal and informal contracts and agreements. Networks may contract externally to obtain administrative and financial services. Also, a group of providers like physicians or hospitals that a managed care organization has contracted with to deliver medical services to its members.

Newborns' and Mothers' Health Protection Act of 1996 (NMHPA). A federal law which mandates that coverage for hospital stays for childbirth cannot be less than forty-eight hours for normal deliveries and ninety-six hours for births by cesarean section.

noncancellable or noncancellable and guaranteed renewable policy. An insurance policy that the insured person has the right to continue in force to a specified age, such as to age sixty-five, by the timely payment of premiums. During the specified period, the insurer has no right to unilaterally make any change in any provision of the policy while it is in force.

nonconfining sickness. An illness that prevents the insured person from working but which does not confine him to a hospital or to his home.

noncontributory plan. A group insurance plan in which the employer does not require that employees contribute to the cost of the plan.

nondisabling injury. An injury that may require medical care but does not result in loss of working time or income.

nonoccupational policy. A contract that insures a person against off-the-job accident or sickness. It does not cover disability resulting from injury or sickness covered by Workers' Compensation. Group accident and sickness policies are frequently nonoccupational.

nonprofit insurers. Persons organized under special state laws to provide hospital, medical, or dental insurance on a nonprofit basis. The laws exempt them from certain types of taxes.

notice of claim. A written notice you must give the insurance company when you have filed for medical expenses. It must be submitted within twenty days after the occurrence or start of such a loss or as soon thereafter as is reasonably possible.

open enrollment. A requirement under which a health plan must accept all who apply during a specific period each year.

open-panel HMO. An HMO in which a physician who meets the HMO's standards may sign up with the HMO as a provider of services. The physicians generally provide services out of their own offices and treat other patients in addition to HMO members.

optionally renewable contract. A contract of health insurance in which the insurer reserves the right to terminate the coverage at any anniversary or, in some cases, at any premium due date, but the insurer does not have the right to terminate coverage between such dates.

outline coverage. A description of policy benefits, exclusions, and provisions that makes it easier to understand a particular policy and compare it with others.

outpatient. A patient who receives ambulatory care at a hospital or other facility without being admitted to the facility.

overhead insurance. A type of short-term disability income contract that reimburses the insured person for specified, fixed, monthly expenses, normal and customary, in the operation and conduct of his business or office.

over-the-counter drug. A drug product that does not require a prescription under federal or state law.

Part D catastrophic coverage. A provision under which the Medicare prescription drug program covers almost all of a beneficiary's drug costs after the beneficiary has spent $3,600 out of pocket annually.

partial disability. An illness or an injury that prevents an insured person from performing one or more of the functions of his regular job.

participating physician. A physician who accepts assignment on all Medicare claims for one year.

peer review. The analysis of a clinician's care by a group of that clinician's professional colleagues.

peer review committees. Groups of physicians or other medical providers who advise insurers, patients, and physicians in disputes regarding what is a "reasonable and customary fee" for services rendered by medical providers other than those on the committee.

period of confinement. The time during which you receive care for a covered illness. The period ends when you have been discharged from care for a specified period of time, usually six months.

pharmacy benefit manager. A drug management company that administers drug plans and organizes the purchase, dispensing, and reimbursement of medicines for health insurers or other large purchasers of healthcare such as employers and unions.

physician's expense coverage. Coverage that provides benefits toward the cost of such services as doctor's fees for nonsurgical care in the hospital, at home, or in a physician's office and x-rays or laboratory tests performed outside of the hospital. Also called regular medical expense insurance.

point-of-service plan (POS). A health plan allowing the covered person to choose to receive a service from a participating or a nonparticipating provider, with different benefit levels associated with the use of participating providers. It is an HMO option that allows the beneficiary to use doctors and hospitals outside the plan for an additional cost.

policy. A legal document or contract that an insurance company issues to the insured person that states all the terms and conditions of the insurance.

policy term. That period for which an insurance policy provides coverage.

portability. A requirement that health plans guarantee continuous coverage without waiting periods for persons transferring to other plans.

preadmission. Having a patient undergo laboratory and other prescribing tests and examinations prior to being admitted to a medical facility as an inpatient.

preadmission certification. A process in which admission to a health institution is reviewed in advance to determine whether it is necessary and appropriate and to authorize a length of stay consistent with standards for evaluation.

precertification. A utilization management program whereby the provider of health services or the person who is insured contacts the insurer prior to being hospitalized or receiving surgery so that the insurer can decide whether or not it will pay for such services as well as recommend other courses of action.

preexisting condition. A physical and/or mental condition of an insured person that existed prior to the issuance of his policy. Many insurance plans will not cover preexisting conditions. Some will cover them only after a waiting period.

preferred-provider arrangement (PSA). As defined in state law, an arrangement between a healthcare insurer and a healthcare provider or a group of providers who agree to provide services to persons covered under the contract. It includes preferred-provider organizations (PPOs) and exclusive-provider organizations (EPOs).

preferred-provider organization (PPO). A combination of traditional fee-for-service and an HMO. When a patient uses the doctors and hospitals that are part of the PPO—these providers are called "preferred" and at other times "network" providers—the patient can have a larger part of his or her medical bills covered. Patients can use other doctors (out-of-network providers), but at higher cost.

premium. The periodic payment required to keep a policy in force.

prepaid group practice plan. A plan under which specified health services are rendered by participating physicians to an enrolled group of persons, with fixed periodic payment in advance made by or on behalf of each person or family. If a health insurance carrier is involved, it contracts to pay in advance for the full range of health services to which the insured is entitled under the terms of the health insurance contract. Such a plan is one form of a health maintenance organization (HMO).

primary care. General medical care that a patient receives directly without referral from another physician. It focuses on preventive care and the treatment of routine injuries and illnesses. It is basic or general care that emphasizes the point when the patient first seeks assistance from the medical system.

primary care physician. Usually your first contact for healthcare. This is often a family/general practice physician, an internist, or a pediatrician, but some women use their gynecologist. A primary care doctor monitors your health, diagnoses and treats minor health problems, and refers you to specialists if another level of care is needed.

principal sum. The amount payable in one sum in the event of accidental death and, in some cases, accidental dismemberment.

private fee-for-service plan (PFFS). A type of Medicare Advantage Plan (Part C) in which the patient can go to any Medicare-approved physician or hospital that accepts the plan's payment. The insurance company, rather than the Medicare program, decides how much it will pay and what the beneficiary pays for the services he or she receives. The beneficiary pays more for Medicare-covered benefits. The beneficiary may have extra benefits the original Medicare program does not cover. The original Medicare program has two parts: Part A (hospital insurance) and Part B (medical insurance).

probationary period. A specified number of days after the date of the issuance of an insurance policy during which coverage is not afforded for sickness. The purpose of the period is to eliminate coverage for sickness actually contracted before the policy went into effect.

Programs of All-Inclusive Care for the Elderly (PACE). PACE combines medical, social, and long-term care services for frail people. Some PACE programs may also provide Medicare prescription drug coverage. PACE is available only in states that have chosen to offer it under Medicaid.

proration. The adjustment of benefits paid because of a mistake in the amount of the premiums paid or the existence of other insurance covering the same accident or disability.

prospective payment. Any method of paying hospitals or other health programs in which amounts or rates of payment are established in advance for a definite period (usually a year). Institutions are paid these amounts regardless of the costs they incur.

provider. Any person (doctor, nurse, dentist) or institution (hospital or clinic) that provides medical care.

Provider-Sponsored Organization (PSO). A healthcare organization that a healthcare provider or a group of affiliated healthcare providers establish, organize, or operate to arrange for the delivery, financing, and administration of healthcare; that meets the requirements established by the Balanced Budget Act of 1997; and that has the authority to contract with Medicare.

qualified impairment insurance. A form of substandard or special class insurance that restricts benefits for the insured person's particular condition.

quality improvement organizations (QIO). Formerly named peer review organizations, QIOs in each state make determinations about hospital care and ambulatory surgical care. Paid and selected by the federal government, QIOs decide whether care provided to Medicare patients is medically necessary, is provided in the most appropriate setting, and is of good quality.

reasonable and customary charges. Healthcare fees consistent with average rates or charges for identical or similar services in a specified geographic area.

recredentialing. Reexamination by a delivery system such as a managed care plan of the qualifications of a provider and verification that provider still meets the standards for participating in the organization's network.

recurring clause. A provision in some health insurance policies that specifies a period of time during which the recurrence of a condition is considered a continuation of a prior period of disability or hospital confinement.

referral. Written permission from a primary care physician for the patient to see a specialist or get certain services. In many HMOs, the patient needs to obtain a referral before he or she can receive care from anyone except his or her primary care doctor. If the patient does not obtain a written referral first, the plan may not pay for his or her care.

regular medical expense insurance. See *physician's expense insurance.*

reimbursement. The process by which providers are paid for their services. Generally, providers are reimbursed by third parties who insure and represent patients.

reinstatement. The resumption of coverage under a policy that has lapsed.

renewal. Continuance of coverage under a policy beyond its original term by the acceptance of a premium payment for a new policy.

reserve. A sum set aside by an insurance company to assure the fulfillment of commitments for future claims.

rider. A legal document that modifies the protection of a policy, either expanding or decreasing its benefits or adding or excluding certain conditions from the policy's coverage.

risk. Any chance of loss.

risk (impaired or substandard). An insurance applicant whose physical condition does not meet the physical standards for normal health.

risk accident. An event or an occurrence that is unforeseen and unintended.

Section 1115 waivers. Waivers that states can obtain from the federal government that permit the states to establish demonstration projects such as in the area of managed care.

Section 1915(b) waivers. Waivers that states can receive from the federal government that permit the states to restrict a Medicaid recipient's choice of providers by using a primary care case manager or other arrangement.

self-insurance. A program in which an employer pays entirely for the insurance coverage of his employees rather buying insurance coverage from a commercial insurer. The ERISA Act of 1974 encouraged this avenue of self-insurance in private business.

senior citizen policies. Contracts insuring persons sixty-five years of age or over. In most cases these policies supplement the coverage afforded by the government under the Medicare program.

service benefit. An insurance benefit that fully pays the specific hospital or medical care services rendered.

short-term disability income insurance. A provision to pay benefits to a covered disabled person as long as he or she remains disabled, usually up to two years.

skilled nursing care. Daily nursing and rehabilitative care that can be performed only by, or under the supervision of, skilled medical personnel.

Social Security freeze. A long-term disability provision which guarantees that Social Security benefits will not be altered regardless of changes in the Social Security law.

special class insurance. Insurance for applicants of health insurance who cannot qualify for a standard policy by reason of impaired health.

special needs plan. A special kind of plan that provides more focused healthcare for specific groups of people, such as those who have both Medicare and Medicaid or those who reside in a nursing home.

special risk insurance. Coverage for risks or hazards of a special or unusual nature.

standard Medicare drug coverage. What the beneficiary pays in addition to what his or her plan pays for drugs.

state health insurance assistance plan. A state program that receives money from the federal government to give free local health insurance counseling to people with Medicare.

state insurance department. An administrative state agency that implements its jurisdiction's insurance laws and oversees (within the scope of these laws) the activities of insurers operating within the state.

stop-loss provision. A stipulation that some major medical policies with 80 percent–20 percent coinsurance will pay 100 percent of eligible expenses once your out-of-pocket outlay reaches a specified amount.

substandard health insurance. An individual policy issued to a person who cannot meet the normal health requirements of a standard health insurance policy. Protection is given in consideration of an increase in premium, through a waiver of medical condition, or under a special qualified impairment policy.

substandard risk. Persons who cannot qualify for the health requirements of a standard health insurance policy.

Supplemental Security Income (SSI) benefits. A monthly benefit paid by the Social Security Administration to people with limited income and resources who are disabled, blind, or age sixty-five or older. SSI benefits provide cash to meet basic needs for food, clothing, and shelter. SSI benefits are not the same as Social Security benefits, but the application for such benefits must be filed with the Social Security Administration.

surgical expense insurance. Health insurance policies that provide benefits toward the physician's or the surgeon's operating fees. Benefits usually consist of scheduled amounts for each surgical procedure.

surgical schedule. A list of cash allowances attached to an insurance policy that are payable for various types of surgery, with the maximum amounts based upon the severity of the operation.

surgicenter. A facility which serves outpatients requiring surgical treatment that exceeds the capability of the physician's office but not requiring hospitalization as an inpatient. Also known as ambulatory surgery, day surgery, and in-and-out surgery.

TDD. A term standing for a "Telecommunications Device for the Deaf." TTY is sometimes referred to as a mechanical teleprinter, and TDD is a modern electronic gadget that performs the same functions in a fraction of the size and weight.

telemedicine. Professional services given to a patient through an interactive telecommunication system by a practitioner at a distant site.

tertiary care. Services provided by highly specialized providers such as neurosurgeons that frequently require highly sophisticated equipment and support facilities as in an intensive care unit.

third-party administrator. An outside person or company (not a party to a contract) that maintains all records of individuals covered under an insurance plan and may pay claims as well.

third-party payer. Any payer for healthcare services other than the patient. This can be an insurance company, an HMO, a PPO, or the federal government.

time limit. The period of time during which a notice of claim or proof of a loss must be filed.

total disability. An illness or an injury that prevents an insured person from continuously performing every duty pertaining to his or her occupation or from engaging in any other type of work for remuneration. (This wording varies among insurance companies.)

travel accident policy. A limited contract covering only accidents while an insured person is travelling, usually on a commercial carrier.

TRICARE. Formerly called the Civilian Health and Medical Program of the Uniformed Armed Services or CHAMPUS, TRICARE is a US Department of Defense health program for active duty and retired uniform services members and their families.

TTY. A teletypwriter (TTY) is a communication device used by persons who are deaf, hard of hearing, or have a severe speech impairment. A TTY consists of a keyboard, a display screen, and a modem. Messages travel over regular telephone lines. People who don't have a TTY can communicate with a TTY user through a message relay center (MRC). An MRC has TTY operators available to send and interpret TTY messages.

unallocated benefit. A policy provision providing reimbursement up to a maximum amount for the costs of all extra miscellaneous hospital services but not specifying how much will be paid for each type of service.

unbundling. A coding device that involves dividing a procedure into payments for each part of the procedure rather than using a single code for the entire cost of the procedure itself.

underwriting. The process by which an insurer decides whether or not and on what basis it will accept an application for insurance.

unearned income. That portion of a premium the insurer has already received for which the protection of the policy has not yet been given.

uninsurables. High-risk persons who lack health insurance coverage through private insurance and who are not within the parameters of risk of standard health underwriting practices.

upcoding. Noting a code for a procedure or treatment whereby the provider can receive a higher reimbursement because it is more complex than the actual procedure or treatment for which the provider is paid less.

usual, customary, and reasonable fee. The amount that providers like physicians within a particular geographic region charge for a particular medical service. Traditional health insurance uses these fees as a basis for reimbursing providers like physicians and dentists.

utilization review. The evaluation of the medical necessity, effectiveness, and/or appropriateness of healthcare services and treatment plans.

waiting period. The duration of time between the beginning of an insured person's disability and the start of the policy's benefits. Also, a period of time an individual must wait either to become eligible for health insurance coverage or to become eligible for a given benefit after overall coverage has begun.

waiver. An agreement attached to a policy that exempts from coverage certain disabilities or injuries that are normally covered by the policy.

waiver of premium. A provision included in some policies that exempts the insured person from paying premiums while he is disabled during the life of the contract.

Workers' Compensation. Liability insurance that mandates certain employers to pay benefits and provide medical care to employees who suffer injuries on the job and to pay benefits to dependents of employees who were killed by occupational accidents.

written premiums. The entire amount of premiums due in a year for all policies issued by an insurance company.

Sources: Health Insurance Institute, *Source Book of Health Insurance Data, 1978–79* and *What You Should Know about Health Insurance*, Washington, DC, 1979, reprinted with permission of the Health Insurance Institute; US Department of Health and Human Services, *Checkup on Health Insurance Choices* (Washington, DC: Agency for Health Care Policy and Research, December 1992), pp. 19–20; *The Consumer Guide to Health Insurance*, (Washington, DC: Health Insurance Association of America, June 1992), pp. 22–25; US House of Representatives, *A Discursion Directory of Health Care* (Washington, DC: Subcommittee on Health and Environment of the Committee of Interstate and Foreign Commerce, February 1976); and US Department of Health and Human Services, *Medicare & You*, 2006 (Washington, DC: Centers for Medicare and Medicaid Services, 2006), pp. 30–61, 87–90.

INDEX

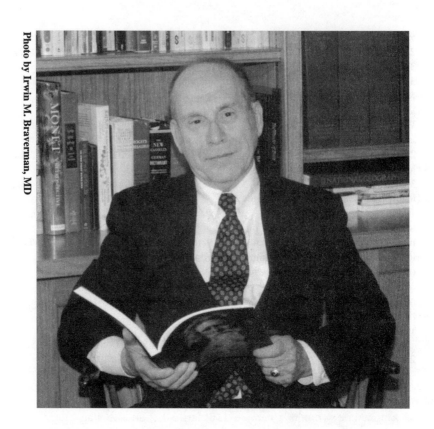

ABOUT THE AUTHOR

Jordan Braverman's career has spanned academia, the media, and public affairs. He has served as Director of Legislative and Health Policy Analysis at Georgetown University's Health Policy Center, along with similar health policy positions at the Pharmaceutical Manufacturers Association, the American Pharmaceutical Association, the Blue Cross Association, and the US Department of Health, Education, and Welfare.

Formerly managing editor of *Topics in Health Care Financing*, his newspaper columns were submitted in nomination for the Pulitzer Prize in journalism in 1994 and, along with his books and other writings, have been published or cited in such publications as the *Baltimore Sun, US News & World Report, Conference Board Magazine*, the *Washington Star*, the *Congressional Record*; spoken of on the floor of the US House of Representatives; and used by Walter P. Reuther, president of the United Automobile Workers Union, E. G. Marshall (film and stage actor), Congressman David Pryor (later US senator and governor of the state of Arkansas), and others in their own activities. He also appears on radio and television.

Jordan is a graduate of Harvard College. He received an MPH degree from Yale University School of Medicine (medical care administration) and a MSFS degree from Georgetown University's Graduate School of Foreign Service (international relations) and held the William Stoughton Scholarship at Harvard University's Graduate School of Design (urban planning/architecture).

His health books include *Crisis in Health Care* (nominated for the Kulp Book Award as one of the outstanding healthcare books published in 1978); *Nursing Home Standards: A Tragic Dilemma in American Health*; *Pharmaceutical Payment Plans: An Overview*; *Health Maintenance Organizations: New Choices for Receiving and Paying for Medical Care*; *State Health Insurance Plans: Is Anyone Listening* (as editor); *The Education of the Osteopathic Physician*; *The Consumer's Book of Health: How to Stretch Your Health Care Dollar*; and other publications. His books and other writings have been included in university curricula in the United States and abroad and used by private industry, the US Congress, federal and state governments, governor's councils, and health and nonhealth groups to improve, enact, or change governmental laws and regulations such as those relating to the quality of nursing home care or state laws to enable consumers to save money by allowing health providers to substitute and dispense therapeutically equivalent and effective lower-cost generic drugs for more expensive brand-name prescription drugs.

In addition, his history book, *To Hasten the Homecoming: How Americans Fought World War II through the Communication Media*, lauded by film and stage actress Nanette Fabray and dramatist Norman Corwin, was submitted in nomination for the Pulitzer Prize in Letters 1996, included in university curricula in the United States and abroad, and included in a Smithsonian Institution historical exhibit; his poem titled "Taps" has been placed into the historical archives of the Arlington National Cemetery; and his photography and other poetry, also commercially recorded and both winners of editor awards, have been published under such anthology titles as *The International Who's Who in Poetry* and *Best Photos of 2005*.

Jordan Braverman's biography has been published in Marquis' *Who's Who in America*, Marquis' *Who's Who in the World*, Marquis' *Who's Who in the East* (of the United States), the International Biographical Centre's (Cambridge, England) *Dictionary of International Biography*, *Outstanding People of the 21st Century*, *One Thousand Outstanding Intellectuals of the 21st Century*—and its companion title *One Thousand Outstanding Scholars of the 21st Century*—as well as in other biographical references both in the United States and abroad. Mr. Braverman lives in Washington, DC.

After many years in healthcare, thinking, writing, and working within it, my thoughts about the subject were (and still are) crystallized in the verse that I composed in 1978 for my book *Crisis in Health Care*, "The Most Precious Gift," which I chose as the epigraph to place in the front of this book. For, as my verse conceptualizes, health is a gift of unmeasurable value not only on an individual level but also on the collective level of an entire nation. As noted in the Apocrypha, Ecclesiasticus 30:15, "health and good estate of the body are above all gold," for according to nineteenth-century British prime minister and novelist Benjamin Disraeli, "the health of the people is really the foundation upon which all their happiness and all their powers as a state depend."